# Clinical Hematology and Fundamentals of Hemostasis

**D. HARMENING PITTIGLIO, Ph.D., M.T. (ASCP)**

Editor-in-Chief
Associate Professor
University of Maryland School of Medicine
Program in Medical Technology and Department of Pathology
Baltimore, Maryland
Clinical Assistant Professor
Georgetown University School of Medicine
Washington, D.C.

RONALD A. SACHER, M.D., F.R.C.P. (C)

Consulting Editor
Associate Professor of Medicine and Pathology
Georgetown University School of Medicine
Washington, D.C.

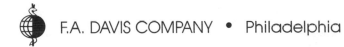
F.A. DAVIS COMPANY • Philadelphia

NOTE: As new scientific information becomes available through basic and clinical research, recommended treatments and drug therapies undergo changes. The author(s) and publisher have done everything possible to make this book accurate, up-to-date, and in accord with accepted standards at the time of publication. However, the reader is advised always to check product information (package inserts) for changes and new information regarding dose and contraindications before administering any drug. Caution is especially urged when using new or infrequently ordered drugs.

**Library of Congress Cataloging-in-Publication Data**

Clinical hematology and fundamentals of hemostasis.

Includes bibliographies and index.
1. Hematology.   2. Blood—Diseases.   3. Hemostasis.
I. Pittiglio, D. Harmening (Denise Harmening)
[DNLM: 1. Hematologic Diseases.   2. Hemostasis.
WH 100 C6413]
RB145.C536   1987         616.1′5         86-32897
ISBN 0-8036-6952-6

To all students, full-time, part-time, past, present, and future, who have touched and will continue to touch the lives of so many educators . . .

It is to you this book is dedicated in the hope of inspiring an unquenchable thirst for knowledge and love of mankind.

# Preface

This text is designed as a thorough and concise guide to clinical hematology and fundamentals of hemostasis. A practical and applied approach to the subject matter, with illustrative case histories, has been incorporated in an attempt to provide the reader with a working knowledge of contemporary hematology and coagulation. Two hundred and forty-five color plates demonstrating peripheral smears, bone marrow aspirates, gross morphology, and clinical manifestations enhance the text, providing a foundation for the interpretation and practice of clinical medicine. The teaching of normal and abnormal morphology is particularly emphasized, and characteristic laboratory profiles are presented for each major pathologic condition.

The first three chapters serve as an introduction to clinical hematology by focusing on normal hematopoiesis, red cell metabolism, and the pathogenesis of anemia. Beautiful illustrations depicting erythrocytic, myelocytic, lymphocytic, monocytic, plasmocytic, and megakaryocytic cell lines of maturation have been donated by Ann Bell from the University of Tennessee. These illustrations facilitate the application of the basic principles of cellular differentiation and maturation. The next 12 chapters are devoted to the subject of anemias, presenting the disease processes that lead to abnormal red cell morphology. A discussion of normal white cell physiology introduces the next section of text, which defines qualitative and quantitative white blood cell disorders and other hematologic diseases leading to abnormal white cell morphology. Bone marrow examination and interpretation concludes and summarizes the presentation of the pathologic processes of the various hematologic disorders.

The last group of chapters provides an overview of hemostasis including platelet structure and function, vascular and platelet disorders, defects of plasma clotting factors, von Willebrand's disease, and disseminated intravascular coagulation (DIC). Laboratory diagnosis and treatment of these hemorrhagic processes are presented in the text, and reinforced by illustrative case histories and color plates. Finally, a chapter on evaluation of red cell morphology and one on laboratory methods complete the scope of the book by serving as a quick guide to procedures routinely performed in the clinical hematology and hemostasis laboratories.

Several features of this textbook offer great appeal to students and educators. There are comprehensive outlines preceding each chapter, as well as an extensive glossary that provides easy access for defining hematologic terms. Case histories throughout the text serve to exemplify actual clinical situations, further illustrating important pathologic conditions. A table of normal values, found on the inside covers of this book, should prove to be an incredible time saver in the interpretation of patient laboratory data.

This book is a culmination of the tremendous efforts of a number of dedicated professionals who participated in this project by donating their time and expertise, because they cared about our common goal of improving patient care by providing a high-quality practical and usable textbook. In conclusion, this book has been designed to generate an "unquenchable thirst for knowledge" in all medical technologists, hematologists, and practitioners whose education, knowledge, and skills provide the public with excellent health care.

D. Harmening Pittiglio, Ph.D., M.T.(ASCP)

# Contributors

ANN BELL, M.S., S.H.(ASCP), C.L.SP.H.(NCA), Assistant Professor of Medicine, Professor of Clinical Laboratory Sciences, University of Tennessee, Memphis; Center for the Health Sciences, Division of Hematology/Oncology, Memphis, TN

MICHELE LYNNE BEST, B.S., M.T.(ASCP), Program Director, Medical Technology, Washington Hospital Center, Washington, DC

BETTY E. CIESLA, B.S., M.T.(ASCP), S.H.(ASCP), Instructor, University of Maryland, Program in Medical Technology, Baltimore, MD

THOMAS J. FORLENZA, M.D., Assistant Professor in Clinical Medicine, Downstate Medical Center, State University of New York, Attending, Hematology-Oncology, Woodhull Medical and Mental Health Center, Brooklyn, NY

ARMAND B. GLASSMAN, M.D., Professor and Chairman, Department of Laboratory Medicine; Acting Chairman, Department of Immunology and Microbiology; Assistant Dean, School of Applied Laboratory Sciences; Medical University of South Carolina, Charleston, SC

RALPH L.B. GREEN, B.APP.SCI.(MLS), F.A.I.M.L.S., Lecturer in Immunohematology, Department of Applied Biology, Royal Melbourne Institute of Technology, Melbourne, Australia

KATHRYN GRENIER-HUGHES, M.T.(ASCP), C.L.S.(NCA), Medical Technologist, University of Utah School of Medicine, Department of Pathology, Hematopathology Section, Salt Lake City, UT

SANDRA GWALTNEY-KRAUSE, M.A., M.T.(ASCP), Formerly Instructor, University of Maryland School of Medicine, Program in Medical Technology, Baltimore, MD

CHANTAL RICAUD HARRISON, M.D., Assistant Professor, Department of Pathology, University of Texas Health Science Center at San Antonio, San Antonio, TX

ERROL A. HOLLAND, M.B., B.CH., F.C.P.(SA), Division of Haematology, Georgetown University Medical Center; Washington, DC; Baragwanath Hospital and University of the Witwatersrand, Johannesburg, South Africa

ROBERT J. JACOBSON, M.D., F.A.C.P., Associate Professor of Medicine and Pathology, Chief, Division of Hematology, Georgetown University Hospital, Washington, DC

RICHARD P. JUNGHANS, Ph.D., M.D., Fellow in Hematology, Georgetown University Medical Center; Division of Cancer Treatment, National Cancer Institute, Bethesda, MD

JOETTE KIZER, M.L.T.(ASCP), Supervisor, Hemostasis Laboratory, Medical University of South Carolina, Charleston, SC

JOHN LAZARCHICK, M.D., Associate Professor of Clinical Pathology; Director, Hematology Division, Medical University of South Carolina, Charleston, SC

HARVEY LUKSENBURG, M.D., Chief, Section of Hematology, Georgetown Medical Service, District of Columbia General Hospital; Assistant Professor of Medicine, Georgetown University School of Medicine, Washington, DC

JOE MARTY, M.S., M.T.(ASCP), Technical Director, Hematopathology Laboratory, Department of Pathology, University of Utah School of Medicine, Salt Lake City, UT

JEANNINE R. MELOON, M.S., M.T.(ASCP), Program Director, Assistant Professor, and Chairperson, Department of Medical Technology, West Liberty State College, West Liberty, WV

MILKA MUKHOLVA MONTIEL, M.D., Professor of Pathology, Director of Clinical Laboratories and Hematology, University of Texas Health Science Center at San Antonio, San Antonio, TX

MARY LORING PERKINS, M.T.(ASCP), S.H., C.L.S.(NCA), Assistant Instructor, Department of Pathology, University of Utah, Salt Lake City, UT

D. HARMENING PITTIGLIO, Ph.D., M.T.(ASCP), Associate Professor, University of Maryland School of Medicine, Program in Medical Technology and Department of Pathology, Baltimore, MD; Clinical Assistant Professor, Georgetown University School of Medicine, Washington, DC

GAIL ROCK, M.D., Ph.D., Medical Director, Ottawa Centre, Canadian Red Cross; Associate Professor, Department of Medicine; Adjunct Professor, Department of Biochemistry, University of Ottawa, Ottawa, Ontario, Canada

NEAL ROTHSCHILD, M.D., Division of Hematology, Georgetown University Medical Center, Washington, DC

RONALD A. SACHER, M.D., F.R.C.P.(C), Associate Professor of Medicine and Pathology, Georgetown University Medical Center, Washington, DC

ROBERT M. SILGALS, M.D., Fellow, Division of Hematology, Georgetown University Medical Center, Washington, DC

ARTHUR J. SILVERGLEID, M.D., Medical and Executive Director, Blood Bank of San Bernardino and Riverside Counties, San Bernardino, CA; Associate Clinical Professor of Medicine, University of California (Los Angeles) School of Medicine, Los Angeles, CA

CATHERINE M. SPIER, M.D., Assistant Professor of Pathology, University of Arizona College of Medicine, Tucson, AZ

RONALD G. STRAUSS, M.D., Professor of Pathology and Pediatrics, University of Iowa College of Medicine; Medical Director, Elmer L. DeGowin Memorial Blood Center, University of Iowa Hospitals and Clinics, Iowa City, IA

JANIS WYRICK-GLATZEL, M.S., M.T.(ASCP), Instructor, University of Maryland School of Medicine, Program in Medical Technology, Baltimore, MD

S. ZAIL, M.B., B.Ch., M.D., FRCPath (Lond), Department of Haematology, School of Pathology of the South African Institute for Medical Research and the University of the Witwatersrand, Johannesburg, South Africa

HALLYE ZERINGER, M.T.(ASCP), S.H., Department of Hematology, Southern Baptist Hospital, New Orleans, LA

# Contents

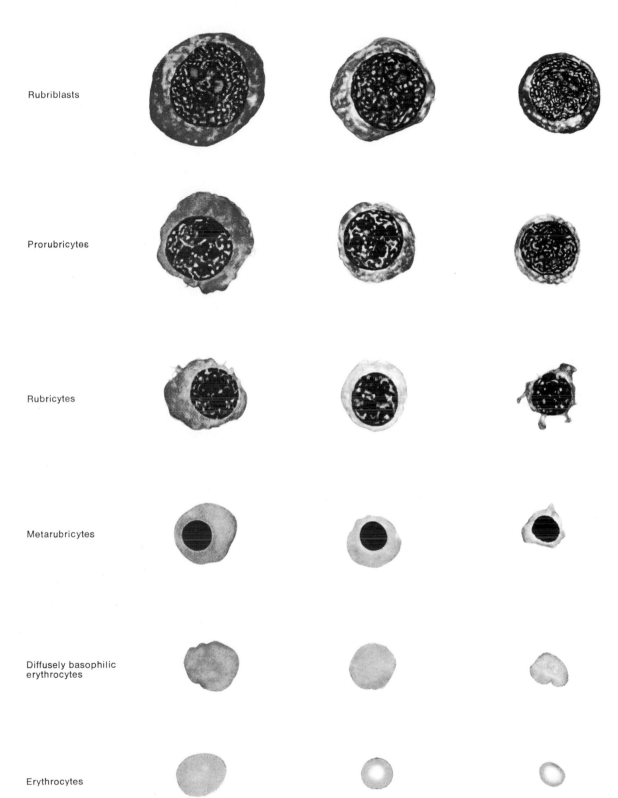

Figure 1. Erythrocytic system. (From Diggs, LW, Sturm, D, and Bell, A: Morphology of Human Blood Cells. Abbott Laboratories, Abbott Park, IL, 1985, with permission.)

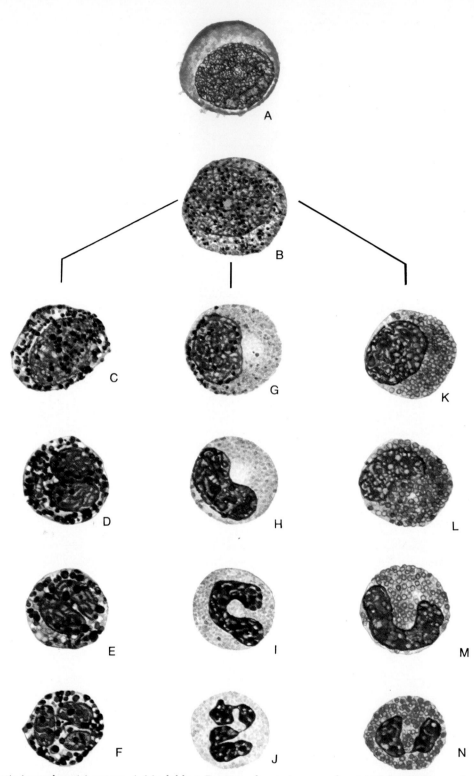

**Figure 2.** Myelocytic (granulocytic) system. *A*, Myeloblast; *B*, promyelocyte (progranulocyte); *C*, basophilic myelocyte; *D*, basophilic metamyelocyte; *E*, basophilic band; *F*, basophilic segmented; *G*, neutrophilic myelocyte; *H*, neutrophilic metamyelocyte; *I*, neutrophilic band; *J*, neutrophilic segmented; *K*, eosinophilic myelocyte; *L*, eosinophilic metamyelocyte; *M*, eosinophilic band; *N*, eosinophilic segmented. (From Diggs, LW, Sturm, D, and Bell, A: Morphology of Human Blood Cells. Abbott Laboratories, Abbott Park, IL, 1985, with permission.)

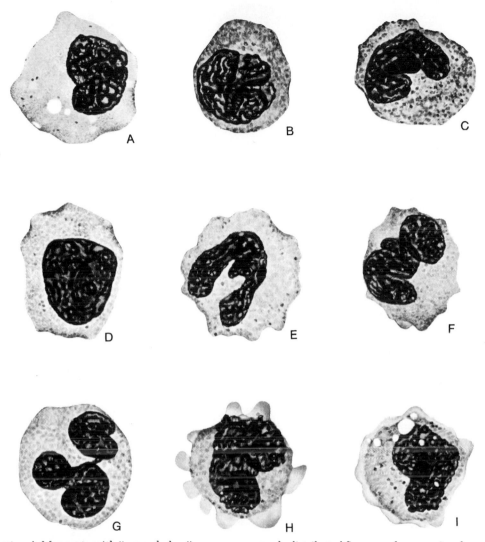

**Figure 3.** Monocytes. *A*, Monocyte with "ground-glass" appearance, evenly distributed fine granules, occasional azurophilic granules, and vacuoles in cytoplasm; *B*, monocyte with opaque cytoplasm and granules and with lobulation of nucleus and linear chromatin; *C*, monocyte with prominent granules and deeply indented nucleus; *D*, monocyte without nuclear indentations; *E*, monocyte with gray-blue color, band type of nucleus, linear chromatin, blunt pseudopods, and granules; *F*, monocyte with gray-blue color, irregular shape, and multilobulated nucleus; *G*, monocyte with segmented nucleus; *H*, monocyte with multiple blunt nongranular pseudopods, nuclear indentations, and folds; *I*, monocyte with vacuoles and with nongranular ectoplasm and granular endoplasm. (From Diggs, LW, Sturm, D, and Bell, A: Morphology of Human Blood Cells. Abbott Laboratories, Abbott Park, IL, 1985, with permission.)

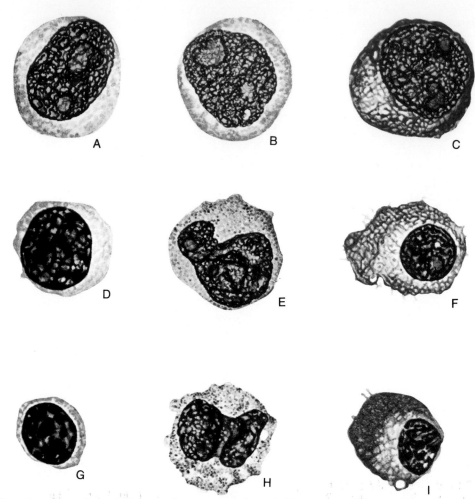

**Figure 4.** Lymphocytic, monocytic, and plasmocytic systems. *A*, Lymphoblast; *B*, monoblast; *C*, plasmoblast; *D*, prolymphocyte; *E*, promonocyte; *F*, proplasmocyte; *G*, lymphocyte with clumped chromatin; *H*, monocyte; *I*, plasmocyte. (From Diggs, LW, Sturm, D, and Bell, A: Morphology of Human Blood Cells. Abbott Laboratories, Abbott Park, IL, 1985, with permission.)

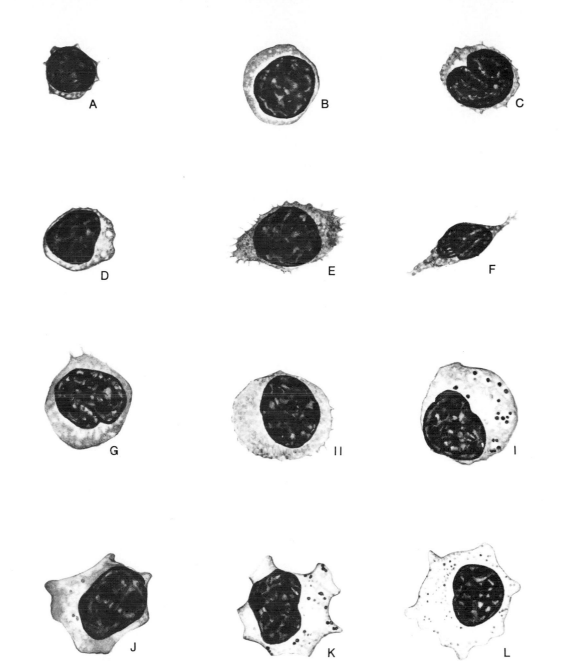

**Figure 5.** Lymphocytes. *A*, Small mature lymphocyte; *B*, lymphocyte of intermediate size; *C*, lymphocyte with indented nucleus; *D*, lymphocyte of intermediate size; *E*, lymphocyte with pointed cytoplasmic projections (frayed cytoplasm); typical nucleus; *F*, spindle-shaped and pointed cytoplasmic projections; *G*, large lymphocyte with indented nucleus and pointed cytoplasmic projections; *H*, large lymphocyte; *I*, large lymphocyte with purplish-red (azurophilic) granules; *J*, large lymphocyte with irregular cytoplasmic contours; *K*, large lymphocyte with purplish-red (azurophilic) granules and with indentations caused by pressure of erythrocytes; *L*, large lymphocyte with purplish-red (azurophilic) granules. (From Diggs, LW, Sturm, D, and Bell, A: Morphology of Human Blood Cells. Abbott Laboratories, Abbott Park, IL, 1985, with permission.)

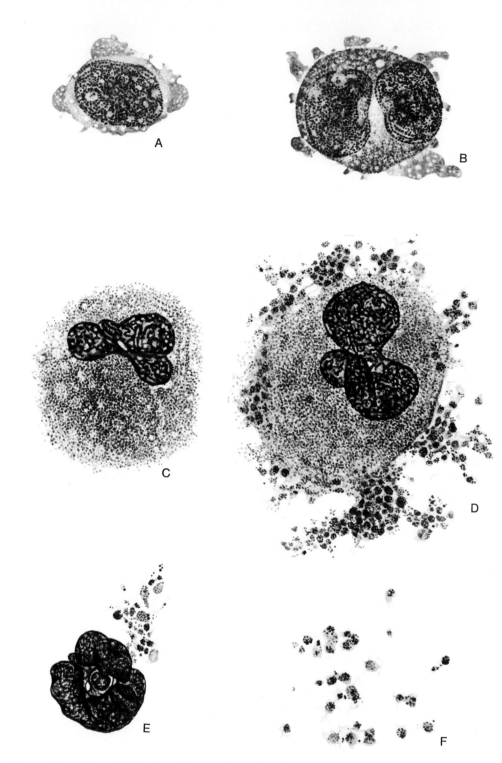

**Figure 6.** Megakaryocytic system. *A,* Megakaryoblast with single oval nucleus, nucleoli, and bluish foamy marginal cytoplasmic structures; *B,* promegakaryocyte with two nuclei, granular blue cytoplasm, and marginal bubbly cytoplasmic structures; *C,* megakaryocyte with granular cytoplasm and without discrete thrombocytes (platelets); *D,* metamegakaryocyte with multiple nuclei and with thrombocytes (platelets); *E,* metamegakaryocyte nucleus with attached thrombocytes; *F,* thrombocytes (platelets). (From Diggs, LW, Sturm, D, and Bell, A: Morphology of Human Blood Cells. Abbott Laboratories, Abbott Park, IL, 1985, with permission.)

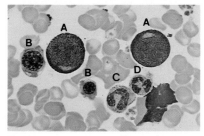

Fig. 7

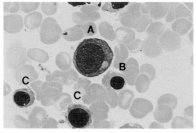

Fig. 8

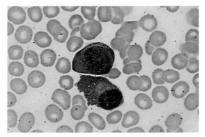

Fig. 9

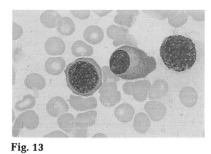

Fig. 10

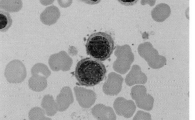

Fig. 11

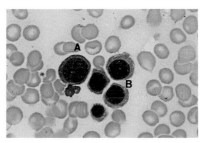

Fig. 12

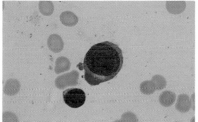

Fig. 13

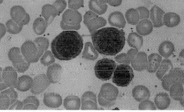

Fig. 14

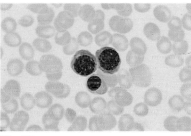

Fig. 15

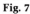
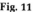

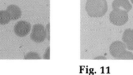

**Figure 7.** Two rubriblasts (*A*; note the perinuclear halo), two rubricytes (*B*), N. band (*C*), N. segmented (*D*).

**Figure 8.** Rubriblast (*A*), metarubricyte (*B*), two rubricytes (*C*).

**Figure 9.** Rubriblast (*center*), plasmocyte (*lower center*).

**Figure 10.** Rubriblast (*center*), lymphocyte (*lower center*).

**Figure 11.** Prorubricytes.

**Figure 12.** Prorubricyte (*A*), three rubricytes (*B*).

**Figure 13.** Prorubricyte (*left*), plasmocyte (*center*).

**Figure 14.** Prorubricytes (*center*), rubricytes (*lower right*).

**Figure 15.** Rubricytes (early and late stages).

*Note:* All the peripheral smears are magnification ×1000 (oil immersion) and are stained with Wright's stain unless otherwise marked.

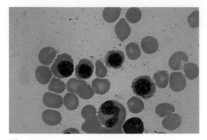

Fig. 16

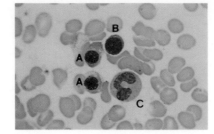

Fig. 17

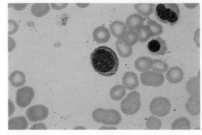

Fig. 18

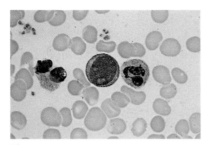

Fig. 19

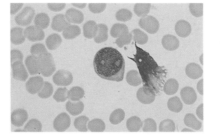

Fig. 20

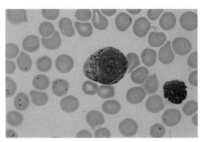

Fig. 21

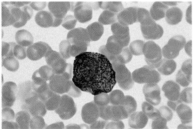

Fig. 22

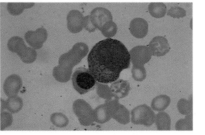

Fig. 23

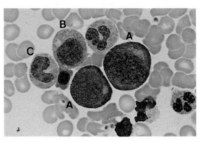

Fig. 24

**Figure 16.** Rubricytes *(center)*.

**Figure 17.** Rubricytes *(A)*, lymphocyte *(B)*, N. segmented *(C)*.

**Figure 18.** Prorubricyte *(center)*, metarubricyte *(right)*.

**Figure 19.** Myeloblast *(center)*, N. segmented *(right)*, disintegrated neutrophil *(left)*.

**Figure 20.** Myeloblast *(center)*, smudge cell *(right)*.

**Figure 21.** Progranulocyte.

**Figure 22.** Progranulocyte.

**Figure 23.** Progranulocyte *(center)*, rubricyte *(lower left)*.

**Figure 24.** Rubriblasts *(A)*, N. myelocyte *(B)*, N. metamyelocyte *(C)*.

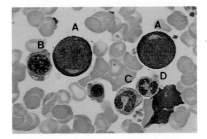

Fig. 25

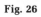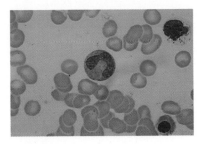

Fig. 26

Fig. 27

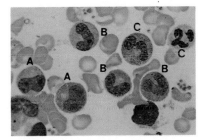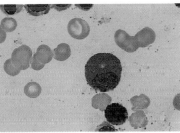

Fig. 28

Fig. 29

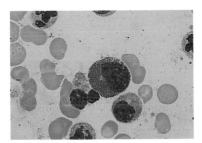

Fig. 30

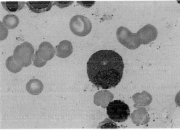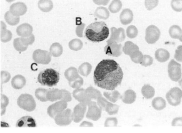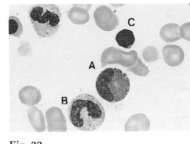

Fig. 31

Fig. 32

Fig. 33

**Figure 25.** Rubriblasts *(A)*, rubricyte *(B)*, N. band *(C)*, and segmented neutrophil *(D)*.

**Figure 26.** N. myelocyte *(A)*, N. metamyelocyte *(B)*, plasmocyte *(C)*, metarubricytes *(D)*, segmented neutrophils *(E)*.

**Figure 27.** N. band *(center)*, metarubricyte *(lower right)*.

**Figure 28.** Two N. metamyelocytes *(A)*, three N. bands *(B)*, two N. segmented *(C)*.

**Figure 29.** Two N. segmented.

**Figure 30.** Eosinophil myelocyte *(center)*, small N. myelocyte *(below right)*.

**Figure 31.** E. myelocyte *(center)*, basophil *(below)*.

**Figure 32.** E. metamyelocyte *(A)*, N. band *(B)*, rubricyte *(C)*.

**Figure 33.** E. band *(A)*, N. band *(B)*, lymphocyte *(C)*.

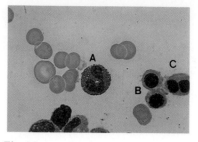

Fig. 34

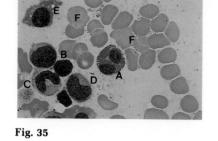

Fig. 35

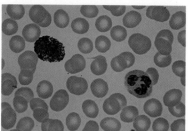

Fig. 36

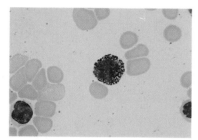

Fig. 37

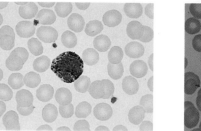

Fig. 38

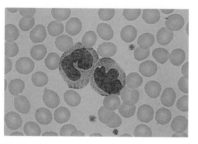

Fig. 39

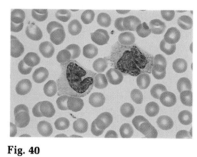

Fig. 40

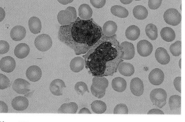

Fig. 41

Fig. 42

**Figure 34.** E. segmented *(A)*, two rubricytes *(B)*, and binucleated metarubricyte *(C)*.

**Figure 35.** E. segmented *(A)*, lymphocyte *(B)*, N. band *(C)*, N. metamyelocyte *(D)*, plasmocyte *(E)*, two diffusely basophilic red cells *(F)*.

**Figure 36.** Eosinophil (segmented).

**Figure 37.** Basophil *(center)*, lymphocyte *(lower left)*.

**Figure 38.** Basophil *(center)*.

**Figure 39.** Basophil *(left)*, N. segmented *(right)*.

**Figure 40.** Monocytes.

**Figure 41.** Monocytes.

**Figure 42.** Monocytes.

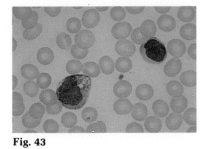 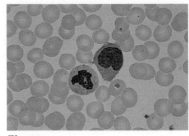 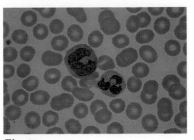

**Fig. 43**  **Fig. 44**  **Fig. 45**

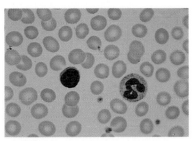 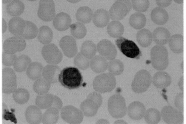 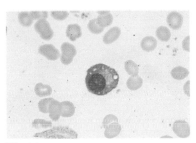

**Fig. 46**  **Fig. 47**  **Fig. 48**

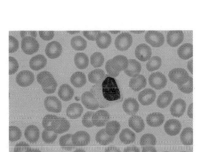

**Fig. 49**  **Fig. 50**  **Fig. 51**

**Figure 43.** Monocyte *(left)*, lymphocyte *(right)*.

**Figure 44.** Monocyte *(right)*, N. segmented *(left)*.

**Figure 45.** Monocyte *(center left)*, N. segmented *(right)*.

**Figure 46.** Lymphocyte *(left)*, N. segmented *(right)*.

**Figure 47.** Lymphocytes.

**Figure 48.** Lymphocytes, large *(left)* and small *(right)*.

**Figure 49.** Lymphocyte, large.

**Figure 50.** Lymphocyte, large.

**Figure 51.** Plasmocyte.

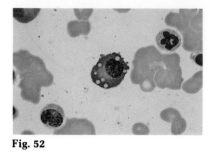

Fig. 52

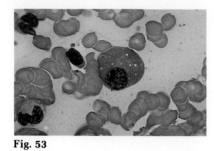

Fig. 53

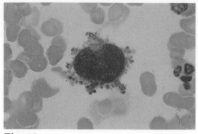

Fig. 54

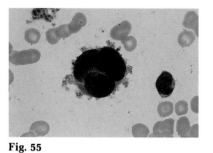

Fig. 55

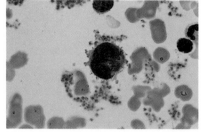

Fig. 56

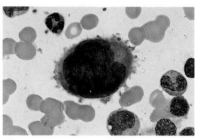

Fig. 57

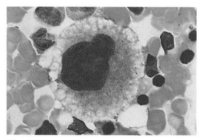

Fig. 58

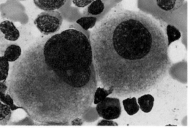

Fig. 59

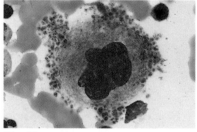

Fig. 60

**Figure 52.** Plasmocyte *(center)*, N. segmented *(upper right)*, resting monocyte *(lower left)*.

**Figure 53.** Plasmocyte *(center)*, small lymphocyte *(left center)*.

**Figure 54.** Early megakaryocyte.

**Figure 55.** Early megakaryocyte *(center)*, small lymphocyte *(right)*.

**Figure 56.** Early megakaryocyte.

**Figure 57.** Early megakaryocyte *(center)*.

**Figure 58.** Megakaryocyte without platelets.

**Figure 59.** Megakaryocytes without platelets.

**Figure 60.** Megakaryocyte with platelets.

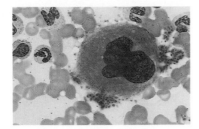

Fig. 61

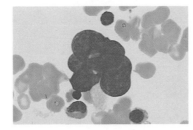

Fig. 62

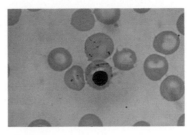

Fig. 63

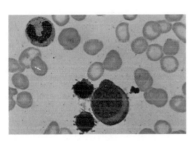

Fig. 64

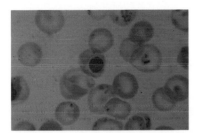

Fig. 65

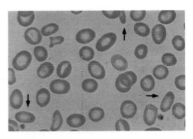

Fig. 66

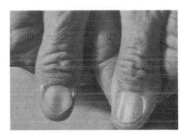

Fig. 67

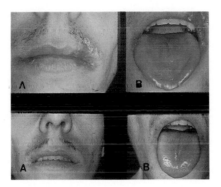

Fig. 68

Fig. 69

**Figure 61.** Megakaryocyte with platelets.

**Figure 62.** Naked nuclei, megakaryocyte.

**Figure 63.** Erythropoietic porphyria. Note the precipitated porphyrins in the cytoplasm. (From Listen, Look, and Learn. National Committee for Careers in the Medical Laboratory.)

**Figure 64.** Siderocyte/sideroblast *(center)*. (From Listen, Look, and Learn. National Committee for Careers in the Medical Laboratory.)

**Figure 65.** Ringed sideroblast *(center)*. (From Listen, Look, and Learn. National Committee for Careers in the Medical Laboratory.)

**Figure 66.** Peripheral blood smear in iron-deficiency anemia showing microcytosis and hypochromia and poikilocytosis. Note the occasional thin ovalocyte or pencil cell. (From Listen, Look, and Learn. National Committee for Careers in the Medical Laboratory.)

**Figure 67.** Bone marrow aspirate in iron-deficiency showing ineffective erythropoiesis, "ragged" erythroid precursors. (From Listen, Look, and Learn. National Committee for Careers in the Medical Laboratory.)

**Figure 68.** Clinical manifestations of iron-deficiency anemia: cheilitis *(A)*, and glossitis *(B)*, before and after therapy.

**Figure 69.** Koilonychia characteristic of iron deficiency: spooning of nails.

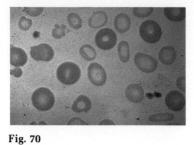 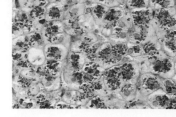 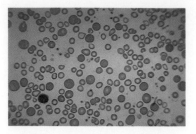

Fig. 70 Fig. 71 Fig. 72

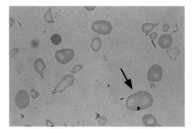 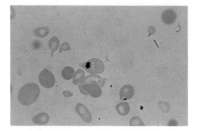 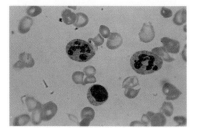

Fig. 73 Fig. 74 Fig. 75

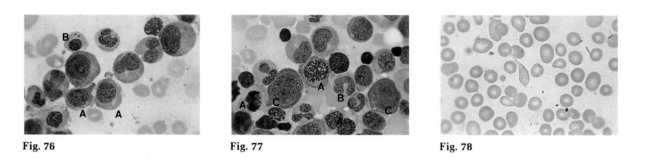

Fig. 76 Fig. 77 Fig. 78

**Figure 70.** Peripheral blood of patient with iron-deficiency anemia following therapy. Note the two populations of red cells.

**Figure 71.** Liver biopsy with micronodular cirrhosis in patient with idiopathic hemochromatosis. Note the deposits of iron.

**Figure 72.** Sideroblastic anemia (peripheral blood). Note the characteristic dimorphic blood picture. (500× magnification.)

**Figure 73.** Extreme degree of anisocytosis (+4) and poikilocytosis (+4) with oval macrocytosis *(arrow)* in a severe pernicious anemia case.

**Figure 74.** Howell-Jolly bodies in an oval macrocyte in pernicious anemia *(center)*.

**Figure 75.** Neutrophil hypersegmentation in pernicious anemia.

**Figure 76.** Polychromatophilic megaloblasts *(A)*; and orthochromic megaloblast with multiple Howell-Jolly bodies *(B)*. Bone marrow.

**Figure 77.** Mitotic figures in megaloblastic marrow *(A)*; large megaloblastic band neutrophil *(B)*; and megaloblastic pronormoblast with open, sieve-like chromatin *(C)*.

**Figure 78.** Cabot ring in pernicious anemia *(center)*.

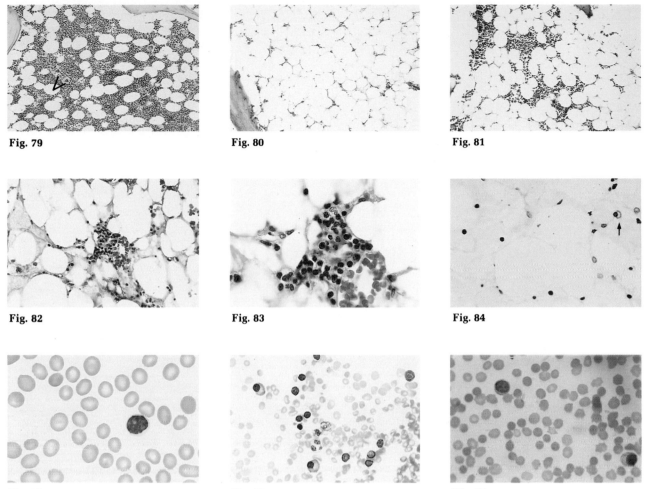

**Figure 79.** Normal bone marrow biopsy showing approximately 50 percent marrow cellularity. Note the megakaryocytes (low power).

**Figure 80.** Markedly hypocellular bone marrow biopsy as commonly seen in severe aplastic anemia (low power).

**Figure 81.** Bone marrow biopsy showing variable cellularity (low power).

**Figure 82.** Bone marrow biopsy showing small lymphoid aggregate or nodule (low power).

**Figure 83.** Higher magnification of lymphoid aggregate in Figure 82. (Magnification ×400.)

**Figure 84.** Bone marrow showing marked hypocellularity with scattered lymphocytes and a plasma cell *(arrow)* (low power).

**Figure 85.** Wright-stained peripheral blood smear. Red cells are normochromic, and slightly macrocytic with slight anisocytosis. No reticulocytes or platelets are present.

**Figure 86.** Wright-stained bone marrow touch preparation. Aspirate was a "dry tap." Present are a few scattered lymphocytes and plasma cells. (Magnification ×400.)

**Figure 87.** Hereditary spherocytosis (peripheral blood). Note the small condensed spherocytes with no central pallor.

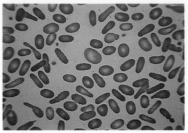

Fig. 88

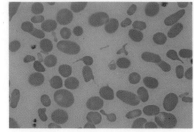

Fig. 89

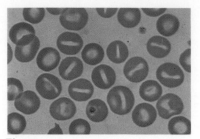

Fig. 90

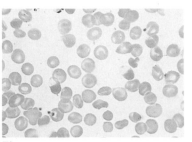

Fig. 91

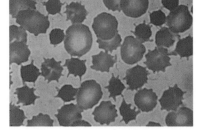

Fig. 92

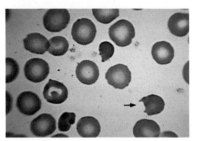

Fig. 93

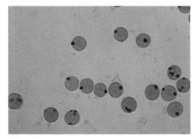

Fig. 94

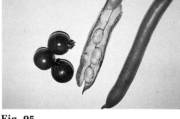

Fig. 95

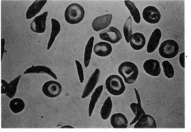

Fig. 96

**Figure 88.** Hereditary elliptocytosis (peripheral blood). Note the high percentage of elliptocytes or ovalocytes.

**Figure 89.** Hereditary pyropoikilocytosis (peripheral blood). Note the bizarre micropoikilocytosis, red cell budding, microspherocytes, and elliptocytes.

**Figure 90.** Hereditary stomatocytosis (peripheral blood). Note the high percentage of red cells with a central slit of pallor. (From Listen, Look, and Learn. National Committee for Careers in the Medical Laboratory.)

**Figure 91.** Hereditary xerocytosis (peripheral blood).

**Figure 92.** Acanthocytosis from a patient with abetalipoproteinemia. (From Hyun, BH, Ashton, JK, and Dolan, K: Practical Hematology. A Laboratory Guide With Accompanying Filmstrip. WB Saunders, Philadelphia, 1975.)

**Figure 93.** Peripheral blood smear from a patient with G-6-PD deficiency. Note the small condensed "bite" or "helmet" cells.

**Figure 94.** Heinz bodies. (From Listen, Look, and Learn. National Committee for Careers in the Medical Laboratory.)

**Figure 95.** Fava beans.

**Figure 96.** Sickle cell disease (peripheral blood). Note the sickle-shaped red cells and target cells. (From Listen, Look, and Learn. National Committee for Careers in the Medical Laboratory.)

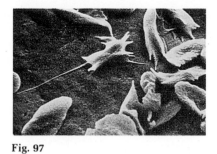

Fig. 97

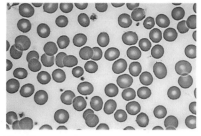

Fig. 98

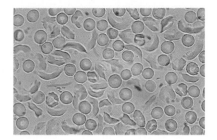

Fig. 99

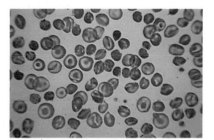

Fig. 100

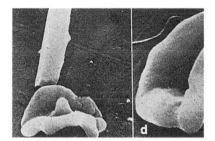

Fig. 102

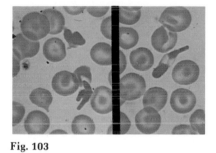

Fig. 100

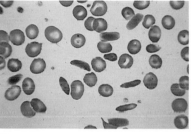

Fig. 101

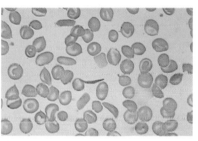

Fig. 102

Fig. 103

Fig. 104

Fig. 105

**Figure 97.** Scanning electron micrograph (SEM) of sickle cells. (From Listen, Look, and Learn. National Committee for Careers in the Medical Laboratory.)

**Figure 98.** Sickle trait (peripheral blood). Note the normal-appearing smear.

**Figure 99.** Sodium metabisulfite sickle preparation.

**Figure 100.** Hemoglobin C disease (presplenectomy). Note the numerous target and envelope forms.

**Figure 101.** Hemoglobin C disease (peripheral blood). Note the particular crystals: "bar of gold" and numerous target cells (post-splenectomy). (From Listen, Look, and Learn. National Committee for Careers in the Medical Laboratory.)

**Figure 102.** SEM of hemoglobin C crystals. (From Listen, Look, and Learn. National Committee for Careers in the Medical Laboratory.)

**Figure 103.** SC disease (peripheral blood). Note the type of "Washington Monument" crystals and target cells. (From Listen, Look, and Learn. National Committee for Careers in the Medical Laboratory.)

**Figure 104.** SC disease (peripheral blood).

**Figure 105.** Sickle thalassemia syndrome (peripheral blood).

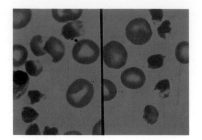

Fig. 106

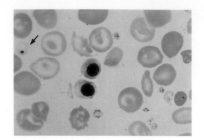

Fig. 107

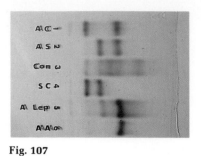

Fig. 108

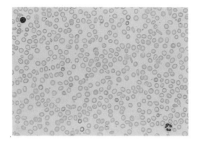

Fig. 109

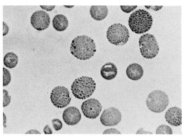

Fig. 110

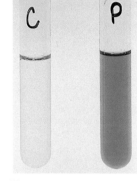

Fig. 111

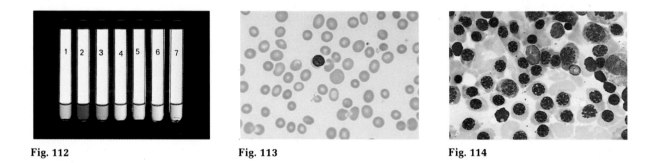

Fig. 112          Fig. 113          Fig. 114

**Figure 106.** Unstable hemoglobin: hemoglobin Zurich (peripheral blood). (From Listen, Look, and Learn. National Committee for Careers in the Medical Laboratory.)

**Figure 107.** Hemoglobin electrophoretic patterns. *1*, Hemoglobin (Hb) A/C; *2*, Hb A/S; *3*, commercial control; *4*, Hb S/C; *5*, HbA/Lepore; and *6*, Hb A/A normal control.

**Figure 108.** Peripheral smear in β thalassemia major. Note the nucleated red cells, the Howell-Jolly body in the hypochromic microcyte *(arrow)*, the numerous target cells and the moderate anisocytosis and poikilocytosis (Wright's stain). (From Listen, Look, and Learn. National Committee for Careers in the Medical Laboratory.)

**Figure 109.** Peripheral smear in thalassemia minor. Note the microcytosis and the hypochromia with mild anisocytosis and poikilocytosis. A few target cells are present. (Wright's stain, magnification ×400.)

**Figure 110.** Hemoglobin H inclusions (supravital stain). (From Listen, Look, and Learn. National Committee for Careers in the Medical Laboratory.)

**Figure 111.** Sugar water test. The tube on the left represents the control (C), and the tube on the right represents the patient (P) with a positive sugar water test. Ten to 80 percent hemolysis will be seen in PNH.

**Figure 112.** Ham's test. Positive results will occur in patients with PNH. A positive test is reported when hemolysis occurs in tube number 1 containing fresh normal serum and patient cells, tube number 2 containing acidified normal serum and patient cells, and tube number 3 containing acidified patient serum and patient cells.

**Figure 113.** Peripheral blood smear from a patient with paroxysmal nocturnal hemoglobinuria (magnification ×600).

**Figure 114.** Bone marrow aspirate smear from a patient with paroxysmal nocturnal hemoglobinuria demonstrating erythroid hyperplasia (magnification ×500).

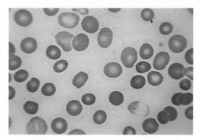

Fig. 115

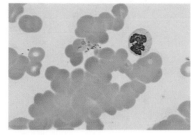

Fig. 116

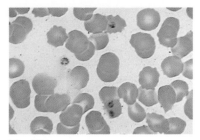

Fig. 117

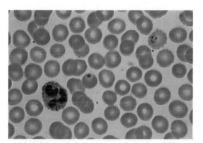

Fig. 118

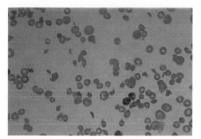

Fig. 119

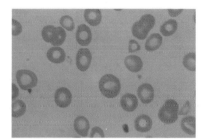

Fig. 120

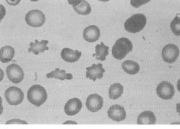

Fig. 121

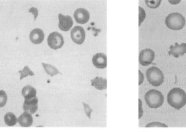

Fig. 122

Fig. 123

**Figure 115.** Autoimmune hemolytic anemia (peripheral blood). Note spherocytes and polychromasia.

**Figure 116.** Cold agglutinin disease (peripheral blood). Note the autoagglutination of red cells, polychromasia, anisocytosis, and poikilocytosis.

**Figure 117.** Ringed forms of Plasmodium falciparum in red blood cells (RBCs). Note that the same RBCs are infected with more than one ring.

**Figure 118.** Late stages of P. vivax malaria. Note and contrast the platelet on the RBC *(center)* and the ring form of malaria toward the periphery *(upper right)*.

**Figure 119.** Comparison of parasitemia of malaria *(left)* and babesiosis *(right)*.

**Figure 120.** Basophilic stippling in lead poisoning *(center)*.

**Figure 121.** Peripheral blood showing red cell fragmentation with thrombocytopenia and nucleated RBCs from a case of TTP. (Magnification ×500.)

**Figure 122.** RBC fragmentation in microangiopathic hemolysis from a patient with prosthetic cardiac valve (mechanical hemolysis). Note the presence of schistocytes.

**Figure 123.** Burr cells (peripheral blood).

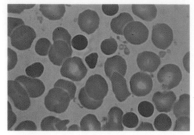
Fig. 124

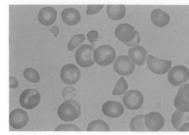
Fig. 125

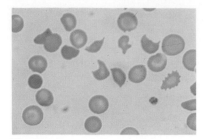
Fig. 126

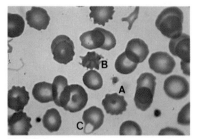
Fig. 127

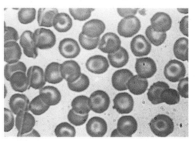
Fig. 128

Fig. 129

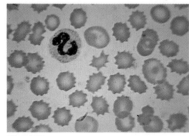
Fig. 130

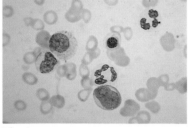
Fig. 131

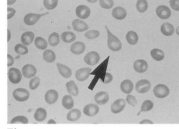
Fig. 132

**Figure 124.** Peripheral blood from a patient with extensive burns. Note typical microspherocytes and membranous fragments. (From Listen, Look, and Learn. National Committee for Careers in the Medical Laboratory.)

**Figure 125.** Peripheral blood from a patient with disseminated carcinoma. Note presence of schistocytes and helmet cells. (From Listen, Look, and Learn. National Committee for Careers in the Medical Laboratory.)

**Figure 126.** Peripheral blood from a patient with malignant hypertension. Note presence of schistocytes, helmet cells, and a burr cell. (From Listen, Look, and Learn. National Committee for Careers in the Medical Laboratory.)

**Figure 127.** Renal disease (peripheral blood). Note presence of burr cells (A), thorn cell (B), and blister cell (C). (From Listen, Look, and Learn. National Committee for Careers in the Medical Laboratory.)

**Figure 128.** Peripheral blood of a patient after kidney transplant and splenectomy. Note small, condensed, irregularly shaped cells and presence of a Howell-Jolly body. (From Listen, Look, and Learn. National Committee for Careers in the Medical Laboratory.)

**Figure 129.** Target cells seen on the peripheral blood smear of a patient with liver disease.

**Figure 130.** "Spur cell anemia" (acanthocytosis) associated with severe liver disease.

**Figure 131.** "Leukoerythroblastosis," a peripheral blood picture that often accompanies marrow infiltration by tumors (myelophthisic anemia). Note the presence of immature red and white cells.

**Figure 132.** Teardrop-shaped red cells (arrow). (From the American Society of Clinical Pathologists, with permission.)

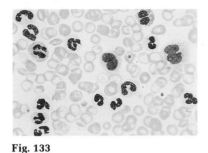 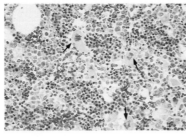 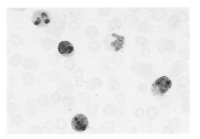

**Fig. 133**          **Fig. 134**          **Fig. 135**

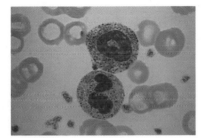 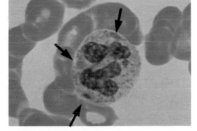 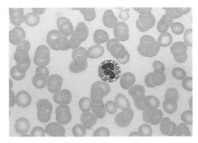

**Fig. 136**          **Fig. 137**          **Fig. 138**

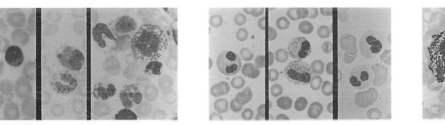

**Fig. 139**          **Fig. 140**          **Fig. 141**

**Figure 133.** Polycythemia vera (PV) (peripheral blood). Note hypochromia and increased cellularity. (Magnification ×400.)

**Figure 134.** Bone marrow showing panhyperplasia in PV. Note increased number of megakaryocytes *(arrow)*. Hematoxylin and eosin stain (low power).

**Figure 135.** LAP stain of peripheral blood showing increased activity in PV (red staining).

**Figure 136.** Toxic granulation (peripheral blood). Note the prominent dark-staining granules.

**Figure 137.** Döhle bodies *(arrows)*. Note the large bluish bodies in the periphery of the cytoplasm.

**Figure 138.** Vacuolated neutrophils suggesting the presence of infection or a severe inflammation.

**Figure 139.** Chédiak-Higashi. *Left*, lymphocyte in peripheral blood; *middle and right*, bone marrow eosinophil. (From Hyun, BH, Ashton, JK, and Dolan, K: Practical Hematology. A Laboratory Guide With Accompanying Filmstrip. WB Saunders, Philadelphia, 1975.)

**Figure 140.** Pelger-Huët anomaly. Peripheral blood. (From Hyun, BH, Ashton, JK, and Dolan, K: Practical Hematology. A Laboratory Guide With Accompanying Filmstrip. WB Saunders, Philadelphia, 1975.)

**Figure 141.** Alder-Reilly anomaly. *Left and middle*, note azurophilic granulation in cells from peripheral blood; *right*, bone marrow. (From Hyun, BH, Ashton, JK, and Dolan, K: Practical Hematology. A Laboratory Guide With Accompanying Filmstrip. WB Saunders, Philadelphia, 1975.)

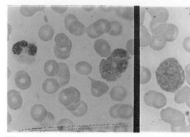
**Fig. 142**

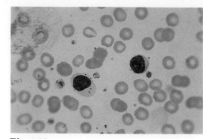
**Fig. 143**

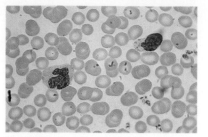
**Fig. 144**

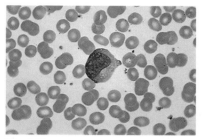
**Fig. 145**

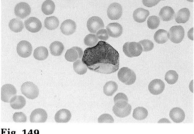
**Fig. 146**

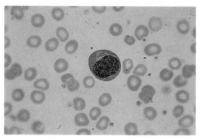
**Fig. 147**

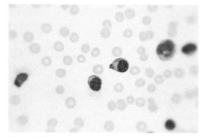
**Fig. 148**

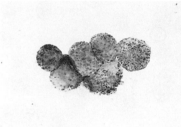
**Fig. 149**

**Fig. 150**

**Figure 142.** May-Hegglin anomaly. *Left*, Döhle body; *right*, giant platelet. (From Hyun, BH, Ashton, JK, and Dolan, K: Practical Hematology. A Laboratory Guide With Accompanying Filmstrip. WB Saunders, Philadelphia, 1975.)

**Figure 143.** Normal large lymphocyte with azurophilic granules *(left)* and normal small lymphocyte *(right)*.

**Figure 144.** Normal monocyte *(left)* and medium-size lymphocyte *(right)*.

**Figure 145.** Large reactive lymphocyte with prominent perinuclear halo in infectious mononucleosis.

**Figure 146.** Reactive lymphocytes in infectious mononucleosis.

**Figure 147.** Plasmacytoid reactive lymphocyte in a drug reaction.

**Figure 148.** Plasmacytoid lymphocytes. Note the red staining accumulation of immunoglobulin in the cytoplasm.

**Figure 149.** Auer rod in myeloblast.

**Figure 150.** Myeloperoxidase positivity in acute promyelocytic leukemia.

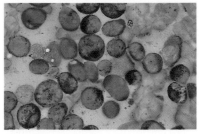

Fig. 151

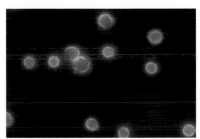

Fig. 152

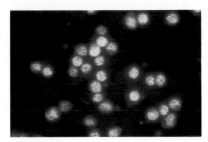

Fig. 153

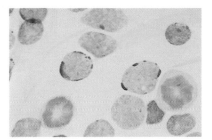

Fig. 154

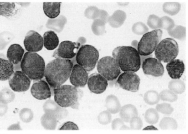

Fig. 155

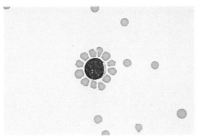

Fig. 156

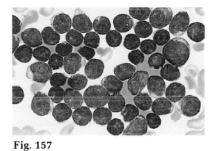

Fig. 157

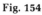

Fig. 158

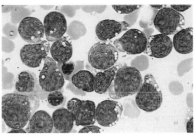

Fig. 159

**Figure 151.** Sudan black B positivity in AML (M2).

**Figure 152.** Nonspecific esterase (alpha-naphthyl butyrate) positivity in acute monocytic leukemia (M5).

**Figure 153.** TdT positivity in ALL using immunofluorescence method.

**Figure 154.** Periodic acid–Schiff positivity in ALL. Note the "block" staining pattern.

**Figure 155.** Surface immunoglobulin (SIg) positive cells in B-cell ALL (L3).

**Figure 156.** E-rosette formation in T-cell ALL.

**Figure 157.** Acute lymphoblastic leukemia, L1, bone marrow.

**Figure 158.** Acute lymphoblastic leukemia, L2, bone marrow.

**Figure 159.** Acute lymphoblastic leukemia, L3, bone marrow.

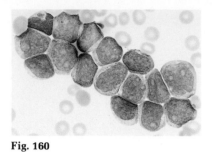

Fig. 160

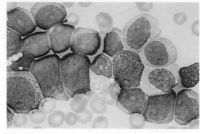

Fig. 161

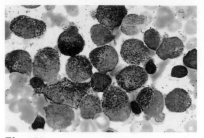

Fig. 162

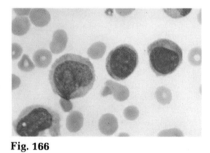

Fig. 163

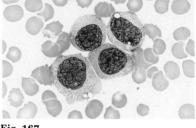

Fig. 164

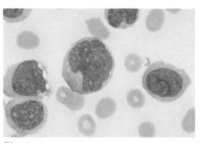

Fig. 165

Fig. 166

Fig. 167

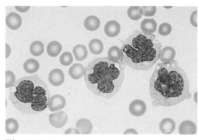

Fig. 168

**Figure 160.** Acute myeloblastic leukemia without maturation, M1, bone marrow.

**Figure 161.** Acute myeloblastic leukemia with maturation, M2, bone marrow.

**Figure 162.** Acute promyelocytic leukemia, M3, bone marrow.

**Figure 163.** Acute "microgranular" promyelocytic leukemia, M3m, peripheral blood.

**Figure 164.** Acute myelomonocytic leukemia, M4, bone marrow.

**Figure 165.** Acute myelomonocytic leukemia, M4, peripheral blood.

**Figure 166.** Acute myelomonocytic leukemia, M4, peripheral blood.

**Figure 167.** Acute monocytic leukemia, poorly differentiated, M5a, peripheral blood.

**Figure 168.** Acute monocytic leukemia, well differentiated, M5b, peripheral blood.

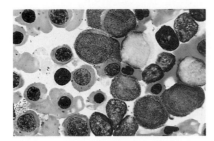

Fig. 169

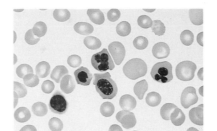

Fig. 170

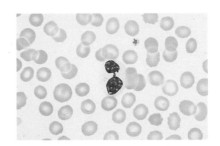

Fig. 171

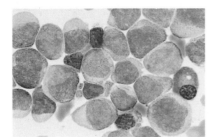

Fig. 172

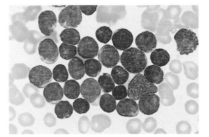

Fig. 173

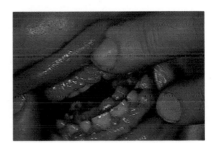

Fig. 174

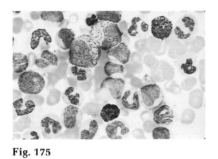

Fig. 175

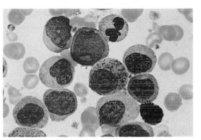

Fig. 176

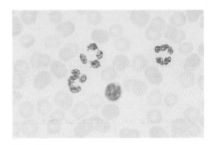

Fig. 177

**Figure 169.** Erythroleukemia, M6, bone marrow.

**Figure 170.** Erythroleukemia, M6, peripheral blood.

**Figure 171.** Pseudo–Pelger-Huët cell in peripheral blood of patient with myelodysplastic syndrome. Note that the cytoplasm is hypogranular.

**Figure 172.** Case study one: bone marrow (ALL).

**Figure 173.** Case study two: bone marrow (AML).

**Figure 174.** Gum hypertrophy: a clinical manifestation of acute leukemia.

**Figure 175.** Peripheral smear: chronic myelogenous leukemia (CML). (From Listen, Look, and Learn. National Committee for Careers in the Medical Laboratory.)

**Figure 176.** CML: bone marrow aspirate.

**Figure 177.** LAP stain of peripheral blood showing little or no activity in CML.

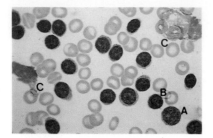

Fig. 178

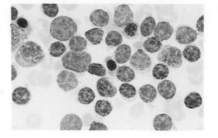

Fig. 179

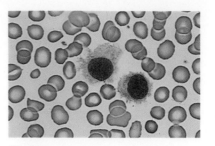

Fig. 180

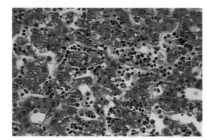

Fig. 181

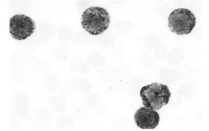

Fig. 182

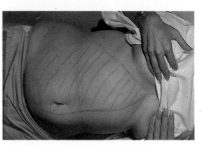

Fig. 183

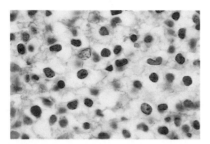

Fig. 184

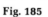

Fig. 185

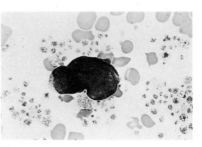

Fig. 186

**Figure 178.** Chronic lymphocytic leukemia (CLL). Note lymphoblast (*A*), lymphocytes (*B*), and smudge cells (*C*).

**Figure 179.** CLL: bone marrow aspirate.

**Figure 180.** Hairy cell leukemia (HCL): peripheral blood. (From the American Society of Clinical Pathologists, with permission.)

**Figure 181.** HCL: bone marrow aspirate.

**Figure 182.** Leukemoid reaction: increased LAP activity.

**Figure 183.** Hepatomegaly: a characteristic finding in patients with myelofibrosis with myeloid metaplasia (MMM).

**Figure 184.** Extramedullary hematopoiesis in the liver of a patient with MMM.

**Figure 185.** Tear drops: peripheral blood in a patient with myelofibrosis.

**Figure 186.** Essential thrombocythemia: peripheral blood megakaryocyte and numerous platelets. (From the American Society of Clinical Pathologists, with permission.)

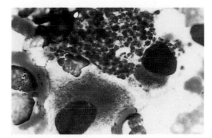

Fig. 187

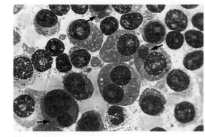

Fig. 188

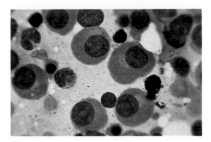

Fig. 189

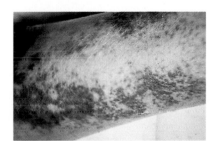

Fig. 190

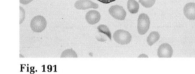

Fig. 191

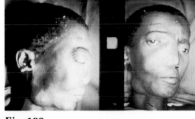

Fig. 192

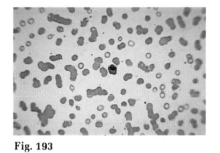

Fig. 193

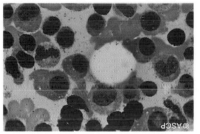

Fig. 194

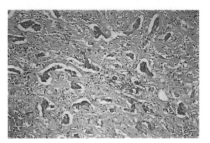

Fig. 195

**Figure 187.** Essential thrombocythemia: bone marrow. Note increased megakaryocytes. (From the American Society of Clinical Pathologists, with permission.)

**Figure 188.** Bone marrow aspirate showing atypical and binucleate plasma cells and Russell bodies *(arrows).*

**Figure 189.** Bone marrow biopsy showing replacement of marrow by plasma cells.

**Figure 190.** Patient with cryoglobulinemic purpura. Note the skin manifestations.

**Figure 191.** Peripheral blood in plasma cell leukemia showing presence of circulating plasma cells. (From Listen, Look, and Learn. National Committee for Careers in the Medical Laboratory.)

**Figure 192.** Plasmacytomas of the face and jaw in a patient with multiple myeloma.

**Figure 193.** Peripheral blood showing marked rouleaux formation. Note the "stacked-coin" appearance of the red cells.

**Figure 194.** Plasmacytoid lymphocytes in marrow aspirate from a patient with Waldenström's macroglobulinemia. (From the American Society of Clinical Pathologists, with permission.)

**Figure 195.** Amorphous amyloid deposits replacing normal liver architecture.

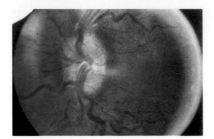

Fig. 196

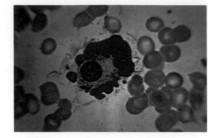

Fig. 197

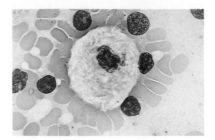

Fig. 198

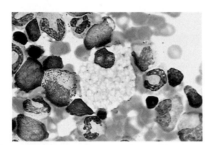

Fig. 199

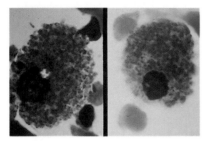

Fig. 200

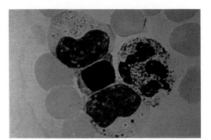

Fig. 201

Fig. 202

Fig. 203

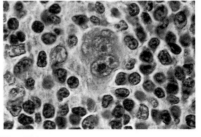

Fig. 204

**Figure 196.** Tortuous veins with "sausage-linked" appearance present in the fundus of the eye (hyperviscosity syndrome).

**Figure 197.** Flame cell: sometimes associated with IgA myeloma.

**Figure 198.** Gaucher's cell: bone marrow aspirate.

**Figure 199.** Neimann-Pick cell: bone marrow aspirate.

**Figure 200.** Tay-Sachs disease: vacuolated lymphocytes.

**Figure 201.** Hurler's anomaly. Note the abnormally coarse azurophilic granules present in neutrophils, lymphocytes, and monocytes.

**Figure 202.** Sea-blue histiocytes. (From the American Society of Clinical Pathologists, with permission.)

**Figure 203.** Gross anatomy of a kidney involved in metastatic lymphoma. Note the white nodular lymphocytic infiltration. (Courtesy of Dr. John Sutherland.)

**Figure 204.** Reed-Sternberg cell *(center)* (×100): Hodgkin's disease, mixed cellularity. Lymphocytes are reduced in number with the presence of numerous eosinophils and reticular cells.

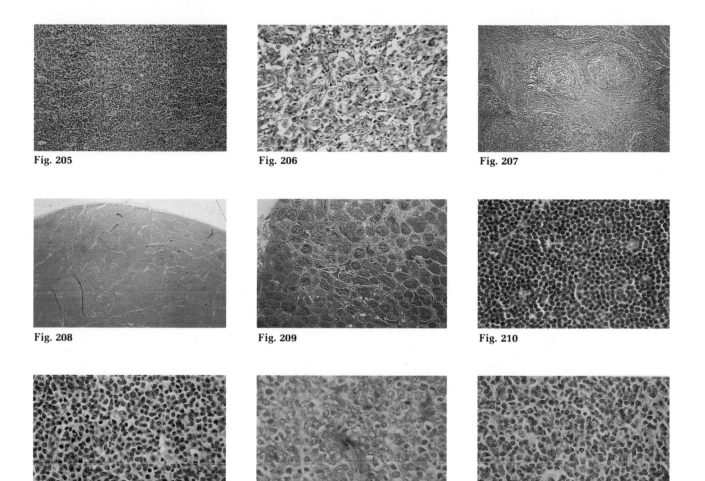

Fig. 205　　Fig. 206　　Fig. 207

Fig. 208　　Fig. 209　　Fig. 210

Fig. 211　　Fig. 212　　Fig. 213

**Figure 205.** Lymph node in Hodgkin's disease: lymphocyte predominance. Note the abundance of dark-staining lymphocytes. (Low power ×10.) (Courtesy of Dr. John Sutherland.)

**Figure 206.** Hodgkin's disease: lymphocyte depleted. Anaplastic reticular cells with few lymphocytes present. (High power ×40.) (Courtesy of Dr. John Sutherland.)

**Figure 207.** Hodgkin's disease: nodular sclerosing. Islands of nodal tissue are separated by collagen bands giving the lymph node a nodular characteristic. (Power ×2.5.)

**Figure 208.** Diffuse lymphoma. Note infiltration throughout the lymph node overshadowing normal architecture. (Courtesy of Dr. John Sutherland.)

**Figure 209.** Follicular or nodular lymphoma. Note identifiable nodules within lymph nodes. (Courtesy of Dr. John Sutherland.)

**Figure 210.** Non-Hodgkin's lymphoma: well-differentiated lymphocytic lymphoma. Note monotonous sheet of infiltrating lymphocytes. (Courtesy of Dr. John Sutherland.)

**Figure 211.** Non-Hodgkin's lymphoma: poorly differentiated lymphocytic lymphoma. Note increased number of pale-staining immature lymphocytes. (Courtesy of Dr. John Sutherland.)

**Figure 212.** Non-Hodgkin's lymphoma: histiocytic lymphoma. Note large pale-staining nuclei of the infiltrating histiocytes. (Courtesy of Dr. John Sutherland.)

**Figure 213.** Non-Hodgkin's lymphoma: mixed histiocytic lymphocytic lymphoma. Note pale-staining histiocytes and the darker-staining lymphocytes. (Courtesy of Dr. John Sutherland.)

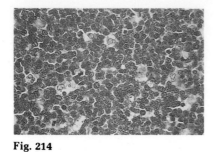
Fig. 214

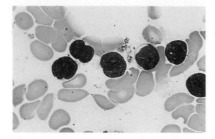
Fig. 215

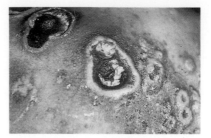
Fig. 216

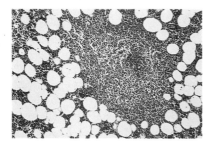
Fig. 217

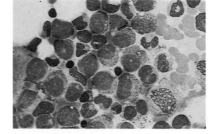
Fig. 218

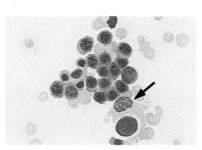
Fig. 219

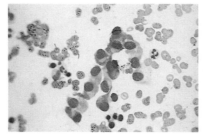
Fig. 220

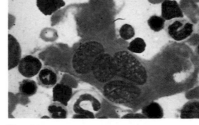
Fig. 221

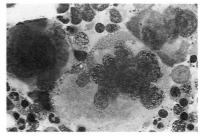
Fig. 222

**Figure 214.** Undifferentiated lymphoma: Burkitt's type. Note that prominent histiocytes give a "starry sky" pattern. (Courtesy of Dr. John Sutherland.)

**Figure 215.** Sézary cells in peripheral blood. Note large abnormal T lymphocytes with prominent nuclear folds and clefts giving the nucleus a cerebriform shape. (From the American Society of Clinical Pathologists, with permission.)

**Figure 216.** Mycosis fungoides (skin).

**Figure 217.** A lymphocytic nodule (follicle) in bone marrow as shown here may alter very significantly the marrow differential count when aspirated and gives false impression of lymphocytic malignancy. (Magnification ×250.)

**Figure 218.** Compartment of granulopoiesis. A reticular cell with open reticulated chromatin and light blue cytoplasm containing dust-like fine granules *(right lower corner)* is situated among numerous granulocytic precursors, especially myelocytes. (Magnification ×640.)

**Figure 219.** Erythropoietic island composed mainly of polychromatophilic normoblasts. The nutrient-histiocyte *(arrow)* is slightly displaced of its central position by smearing of the particle. Its cytoplasmic slender processes envelop a basophilic normoblast establishing intimate contact with the maturing red cell precursor. (Magnification ×640.)

**Figure 220.** Group of osteoblasts *(center)* aspirated from the marrow of a child. (Magnification ×640.)

**Figure 221.** Osteoclast usually is seen as a single giant cell with multiple and separated nuclei and basophilic granular cytoplasm *(center)*. (Magnification ×640.)

**Figure 222.** In comparison the megakaryocytes tend to be in small groups with multilobated single nuclei. Mature megakaryocytes have numerous fine cytoplasmic granules and occasionally platelet units can be seen at their periphery. (Magnification ×640.)

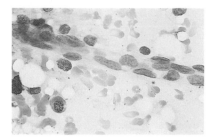
Fig. 223

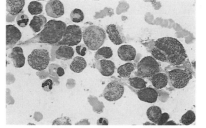
Fig. 224

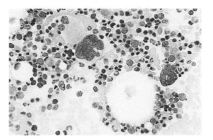
Fig. 225

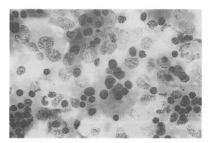
Fig. 226

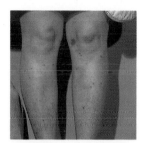
Fig. 227

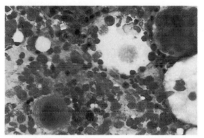
Fig. 228

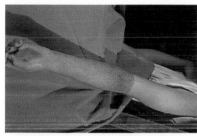
Fig. 229

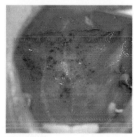
Fig. 230

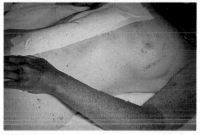
Fig. 231

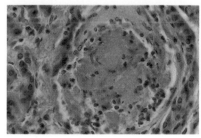
Fig. 232

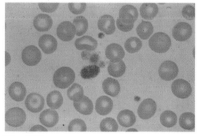
Fig. 233

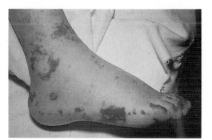
Fig. 234

**Figure 223.** A string of endothelial cells aspirated from hypocellular marrow. The nuclei are elongated and slightly tapered. The cytoplasm is transparent and barely visible. (Magnification ×640.)

**Figure 224.** Metastatic tumor to the bone marrow. The tumor cells are usually pleomorphic and in groups with large nuclear: cytoplasmic ratios. (Magnification ×640.)

**Figure 225.** Smear of normal cellular marrow with normal maturation of erythropoietic, granulocytic, and megakaryocytic cells. (Magnification ×250.)

**Figure 226.** Iron stain of bone marrow smear showing the processes of the nutrient-histiocytes surrounding the erythrocyte precursors. (Magnification ×640.)

**Figure 227.** Petechial bleeding of the lower extremities in a patient with idiopathic thrombocytopenic purpura (ITP).

**Figure 228.** ITP: bone marrow aspirate. Note increased number of megakaryocytes with normal cellularity (M/E 3:1).

**Figure 229.** Positive tourniquet test in a patient with ITP.

**Figure 230.** Oral cavity, patient with ITP.

**Figure 231.** Post-transfusion purpura (PTP).

**Figure 232.** Renal biopsy from a case of thrombotic thrombocytopenic purpura (TTP) showing glomerular deposits of platelet-fibrin microvascular occlusion.

**Figure 233.** Giant platelet from a patient with myeloproliferative disease with thrombocytosis.

**Figure 234.** Anaphylactoid (Henock-Schönlein) purpura. Purpuric lesions of the foot.

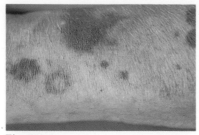

Fig. 235

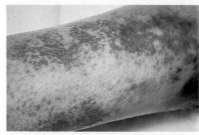

Fig. 236

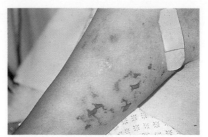

Fig. 237

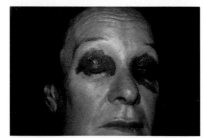

Fig. 238

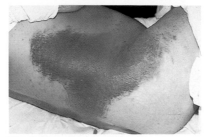

Fig. 239

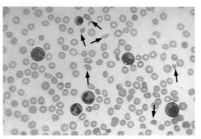

Fig. 240

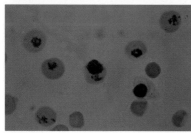

Fig. 241

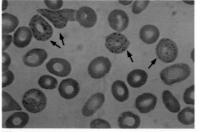

Fig. 242

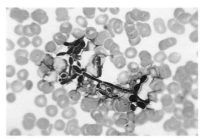

Fig. 243

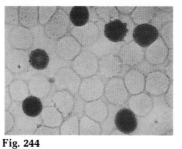

Fig. 244

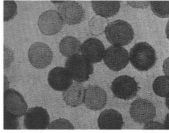

Fig. 245

**Figure 235.** Senile purpura (skin manifestations).

**Figure 236.** Steroid purpura (skin manifestations).

**Figure 237.** Cryoglobulinemic purpura (skin manifestations).

**Figure 238.** Amyloid purpura. Note characteristic periorbital distribution.

**Figure 239.** Diffuse hemorrhage: a clinical manifestation of a patient with disseminated intravascular coagulation (DIC). Note the multiple cutaneous ecchymoses.

**Figure 240.** DIC (peripheral blood). Note presence of schistocytes (*arrows*) and nucleated red cell (*top border*).

**Figure 241.** Reticulocytes. New methylene blue stain of peripheral blood. Note *non-nucleated* reticulocytes with varying amounts of stained reticulum (RNA). Reticulocytosis is associated with increased erythropoietic activity reflected by polychromasia on the Wright's stain of the peripheral smear (see Figure 115). (From Listen, Look, and Learn. National Committee for Careers in the Medical Laboratory.)

**Figure 242.** Coarse basophilic stippling. Compare this with fine diffuse basophilic stippling in Figure 120. (From Listen, Look, and Learn. National Committee for Careers in the Medical Laboratory.)

**Figure 243.** Candidemia: peripheral blood. Candida albicans in the peripheral blood demonstrating both hyphae, pseudohyphae, and yeast forms. Note that some of the organism has broken out of the cytoplasm of disintegrating monocytes of which nuclear remnants are still visible.

**Figure 244.** Kleihauer-Betke stain of newborn blood. Red-staining cells contain hemoglobin F; clear staining cells contain hemoglobin A. (From Listen, Look, and Learn. National Committee for Careers in the Medical Laboratory.)

**Figure 245.** Kleihauer-Betke stain of blood from a patient with hereditary persistence of fetal hemoglobin (HPFH). Note that all the red cells stain red, owing to the varying amounts of hemoglobin F. (From Listen, Look, and Learn. National Committee for Careers in the Medical Laboratory.)

# Hematopoiesis

"Hematopoiesis" refers to the formation and development of the various types of blood cells from the marrow hematopoietic stem cell. During the first weeks of embryonic life, hematopoiesis begins in the yolk sac with mesenchymal stem cells forming so-called blood islands. Yolk sac stem cells from the central area of the blood islands dislodge and are swept into the primordial plasma. These nucleated cells differentiate into primitive erythroid cells that contain embryonic hemoglobins but do not mature into circulating erythrocytes.[1-4]

Yolk sac stem cells migrate first to the liver and then to the spleen during the third month of fetal life, thus making the liver and spleen early sites of blood cell formation (Fig. 1-1). Erythropoiesis begins in the marrow about the 12th week of embryogenesis and is soon followed by granulopoiesis and megakaryopoiesis. Eventually the marrow becomes the major site of blood cell development in the fetus.[1-4]

At the time of birth, the liver and spleen have ceased cell development and the active sites of hematopoiesis are in bone cavities, since bone seems to provide the proper environment for proliferation and differentiation. The change from fetal to adult hemoglobin proceeds slowly over the next few months. Hematopoiesis gradually decreases in the shaft of the long bones and, after age 4, fat cells begin to appear in the long bones. Around age 18, hematopoietic marrow is found in the sternum, ribs, pelvis, vertebrae, and skull. Generally, hematopoiesis is sustained in a steady state, as production of mature cells equals blood cell loss. When there is increased demand for blood cells, active marrow may again be found in the spleen, liver, and other tissues.[1-4]

In the healthy adult, blood cell formation (with the probable exception of lymphocyte production) takes place in the bone marrow, which maintains an environment appropriate for proliferation and mat-

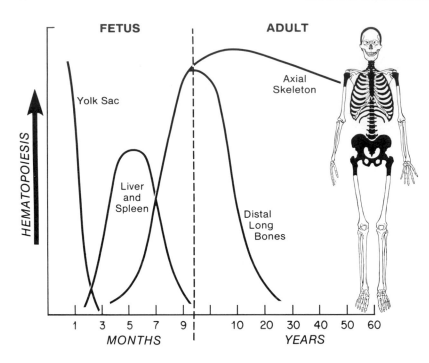

**Figure 1–1.** Location of active marrow growth in the fetus and adult. During fetal development, hematopoiesis is first established in the yolk sac mesenchyme, later moves to the liver and spleen, and finally is limited to the bony skeleton. From infancy to adulthood, there is a progressive restriction of productive marrow to the axial skeleton and proximal ends of the long bones, shown as the shaded areas on the drawing of the skeleton. (From Hillman and Finch,[3] p. 2, with permission.)

uration of cells. Hematopoiesis occurs in the extravascular part of the red marrow. A single layer of epithelial cells separates the extravascular marrow compartment from the intravascular compartment (venous sinuses). When blood cells produced in the marrow are almost mature and ready to circulate in the peripheral blood, the cells leave the marrow parenchyma by passing through fenestrations in endothelial cells and emerge into the venous sinuses.[1–4]

The various cell lineages in bone marrow originate from pluripotent hematopoietic stem cells (Fig. 1-2). The pluripotential stem cell provides a cellular reserve for the stem cells committed to the lymphoid stem cell line for lymphopoiesis and to the nonlymphoid stem cell line for producing the other hematopoietic cells. The nonlymphoid (or myeloid) committed stem cell produces the erythrocytic, granulocytic (neutrophilic, eosinophilic, basophilic), monocytic-macrophage, and megakaryocytic-platelet lines. The lymphoid committed stem cell produces lymphocytic and plasmocytic cells. The pluripotential hematopoietic stem cells are not identifiable as such in marrow smears, but when isolated in cell culture systems they have been observed to be small round cells with fine chromatin, nucleoli, and blue nongranular cytoplasm (similar to an early lymphoid cell).[1–3]

The hematopoietic stem cell has been defined as a colony-forming unit (CFU) in experimental methods which assay stem cells. In a classic experiment, Till and McCullock[21] irradiated mice and then injected suspensions of marrow cells intravenously. About 10 days later, nodules of injected marrow could be observed on the surface of the spleen and in microscopic study of splenic tissue. The nodules were named "spleen colonies," and the progenitor cells that formed these colonies were called colony-forming unit–spleen (CFU-S).[1–4]

Under the influence of the splenic microenvironment, an injected stem cell from a suspension of marrow cells proliferates and differentiates into a large colony. Enumeration of the colonies allows for an indirect method of quantitation of the number of injected CFU-S. Each colony is derived from a single stem cell. Proof of the clonality of the nodules is substantiated by using cells with chromosome markers induced by radiation when 95 percent or more of the metaphases in the colonies are observed. In addition, if a colony is removed cautiously from the spleen two weeks after injection and a suspension of cells is made and injected into irradiated mice, numerous colonies are observed. Such evidence demonstrates the self-renewal capability of CFU-S in the colonies.[1,2]

Spleen colonies observed at first were primarily composed of erythroid cells with a few megakaryocytes and granulocytes, but later the colonies were noted to be mixtures of these cell lines. Thus, the committed myeloid (pertaining to marrow) stem cell (CFU-S) is considered to be multipotent and to give rise to granulocytes, erythrocytes, monocytes, and megakaryocytes (see Fig. 1-2). Hence, the term "CFU-GEMM" (granulocytic erythrocytic myelocytic monocytic) has been suggested and may be substituted for "CFU-S."

In vitro culture methods now provide another assay system for hematopoietic stem cells. Progenitor stem cells (CFU-S) have been identified by their activity to form large in vitro colonies on semisolid

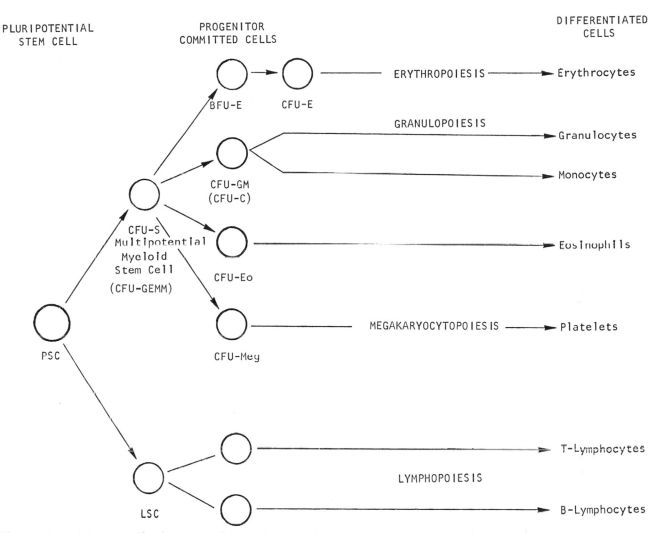

**Figure 1 – 2.** Hematopoiesis. The pluripotential stem cell (PSC) produces the multipotential myeloid stem cell needed for erythropoiesis, granulopoiesis, and megakaryocytopoiesis and the lymphoid stem cell (LSC) for lymphopoiesis. BFU-E, burst-forming unit – erythroid; CFU-E, colony-forming unit – erythroid; CFU-GM, colony-forming unit – granulocyte-monocyte; CFU-C, colony-forming unit – culture; CFU-Eo, colony-forming unit – eosinophil; CFU-Meg, colony-forming unit – megakaryocyte.

culture media which contains growth factor or colony-stimulating factor (CSF) for sustained growth. CSF consists of cell extracts from monocytes, macrophages, endothelial cells, fat cells, and other cellular elements. In the presence of CSF, colonies of granulocytes and monocytes are formed in 7 to 10 days. These colonies of granulocytes and monocytes have been named CFU-C (C for culture) or CFU-GM (GM for granulocytes and monocytes), indicating that they are committed to the production of granulocytic and monocytic cells (see Fig. 1-2; Table 1-1).[1–5]

## ERYTHROPOIESIS (see Color Figure 1)

Mature erythrocytes are derived from committed erythroid progenitor cells through a series of mitotic divisions and maturation phases. Erythropoietin, a humoral agent produced largely by the kidney,

stimulates erythropoiesis by acting on stem cells to induce proliferation and differentiation of erythrocytes. Tissue hypoxia is the main stimulus for the production of erythropoietin by the kidney.[1–4,9]

Following the introduction of the assays for CFU-S, in vitro assays using plasma clots or methyl cellulose culture techniques defined two classes of erythroid stem cells (see Fig. 1-2). The committed myeloid stem cell differentiates in vitro into a primitive erythroid cell called burst-forming unit – erythroid (BFU-E), which requires large amounts of erythropoietin and long culture times to form large erythroid colonies (or "bursts"). The BFU-E differentiates into an erythroid stem cell called colony-forming unit – erythroid (CFU-E), which gives rise to tiny erythroid colonies and requires low levels of erythropoietin and short culture times. The clonal culture method is an important in vitro development in designating the compartment com-

Table 1–1. KNOWN HEMATOPOIETIC PROGENITOR CELLS

| Term | Required stimulus | Detected by | Postulated role |
|------|-------------------|-------------|-----------------|
| CFU-S (CFU-GEMM) | HIM* of certain mouse tissues | Spleen colony assay | Pluripotent stem cell |
| CFU-Ct | CSA from "feeder cells," tissue extracts, leukocyte extracts, urine, etc. | Colony formation in agar medium | Committed progenitor of granulopoiesis |
| BFU-E | Erythropoietin, helper T lymphocytes | Colony formation in plasma clot culture | Committed progenitor of erythropoiesis (early) |
| CFU-E | Erythropoietin | Colony formation in plasma clot culture | Committed progenitor of erythropoiesis (late) |

*Hemopoietic inductive microenvironment.
†The synonym CFU-GM is a more suitable term because it indicates that these are granulocytic-monocytic progenitor cells. It also parallels the term CFU-E.
From Beck,[1] p. 5, with permission.

mitted to erythropoiesis. Under ordinary conditions the BFU-E and CFU-E compartments replenish erythroid cells to the storage compartment (Fig. 1-3).[1-3]

"Erythron" is the term used to describe the total population of mature erythrocytes and their precursors in blood, bone marrow, and other sites. This term indicates that the widely distributed red cells function as a unit. Erythrocytes function as an intermediary in the exchange of respiratory gases, oxygen and carbon dioxide, between the lungs and tissues. Hemoglobin, the oxygen transport protein

within the red cell, binds reversibly to oxygen and constitutes 33 percent of the red cell contents. The hemoglobin molecule, with a molecular weight of nearly 65,000 daltons,[1] is a tetramer with two pairs of polypeptide chains. Attached to each of the four polypeptide chains is a heme group, a complex of iron (ferrous) and protoporphyrin. Globin is the protein portion of the hemoglobin molecule. For effective red cell production (erythropoiesis), 85 percent or more of marrow erythroid activity requires the balanced incorporation of heme and globin to form hemoglobin. The immature nucleated red cell must

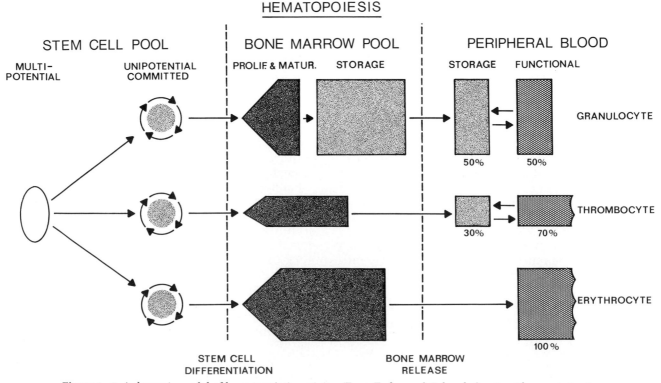

Figure 1–3. A dynamic model of hematopoietic activity. (From Erslev and Gabuzda,[2] p. 5, with permission.)

have an adequate supply of iron, as well as normal production of porphyrin and globin polypeptide chains for adequate synthesis of hemoglobin. Folic acid and vitamin $B_{12}$ are also needed in adequate amounts to maintain proliferation and maturation. Defects may occur at any stage of development in the marrow, causing death of cells. Under normal conditions, 10 to 15 percent of nucleated red cells die in the marrow during maturation. Failure to deliver an appropriate number of erythrocytes to the blood is termed "ineffective erythropoiesis.[1-3]

Erythropoiesis occurs in the marrow over a period of about four to five days through successive morphologic alterations in the nucleated cells (Fig. 1-4) from rubriblast (proerythroblast) to metarubricyte (orthochromatic erythroblast), followed by a non-nucleated polychromatophilic erythrocyte that is released into blood to mature into a hemoglobin-containing erythrocyte in one to two days. Four successive mitotic divisions occur in the early phases, but in the latest nucleated stage (metarubricyte) cells are no longer able to divide. Fourteen to 16 erythrocytes are produced from one rubriblast (see Fig. 1-4).[1-3] During the early maturational stages, mitochondria, Golgi apparatus, and polyribosomes are developed. In the later nucleated stages there is increasing hemoglobin synthesis. The presence of hemoglobin is usually not evident in Wright's stain of normal nucleated red cells until the rubricyte (polychromatic erythroblast) stage. With successive developmental stages, there is reduction in the size of the nucleated cells, condensation of chromatin, absence of nucleoli, decrease in ribonucleic acid (RNA) in the cytoplasm, decrease in mitochondria, and gradual increase in synthesis of hemoglobin.

## Rubriblasts (Pronormoblasts, Proerythroblasts)

The rubriblast, the earliest cell of the erythrocytic series, has a round primitive nucleus with visible nucleoli and chromatin strands that are indistinct and dispersed. There is no evidence of clumped chromatin. The nucleus stains a reddish-blue with

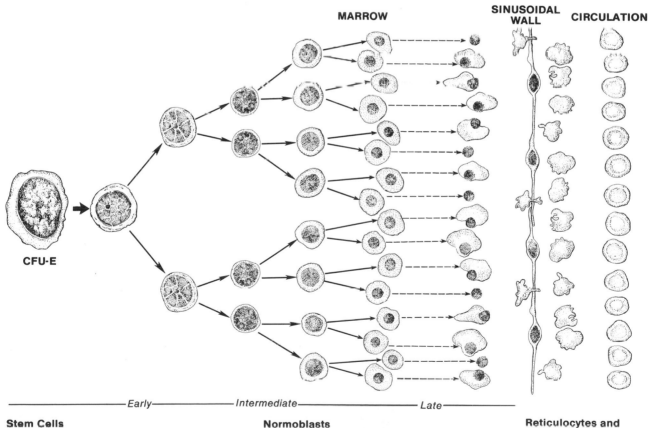

**MARROW**  **SINUSOIDAL WALL**  **CIRCULATION**

CFU-E

Early ———— Intermediate ———— Late

**Stem Cells**  **Normoblasts**  **Reticulocytes and Mature Red Cells**

**Figure 1–4.** Proliferation and maturation of the CFU-E to form adult red cells. Each primitive erythroid cell undergoes four mitoses, during which time there is a progressive increase in hemoglobin content. These steps in proliferation and maturation are divided into early, intermediate, and late stages of normoblast development. From each red cell precursor are produced 14 to 16 progeny, which then lose their nuclei to become marrow reticulocytes and subsequently, circulating reticulocytes, and adult red blood cells. Red cells normally enter circulation as reticulocytes, containing a small amount of residual RNA for approximately another 24 hours. (From Hillman and Finch,[3] p. 4, with permission.)

Wright's stain. The cytoplasm stains a royal or larkspur blue owing to the presence of RNA and to the superimposed pinkish tint of hemoglobin over the blue; this imparts to the cytoplasm a dark and royal blue color similar to that seen in some plasmocytes **(see Color Figures 1 and 7 to 10)**.[9]

Rubriblasts range in size between 18 and 25 $\mu$m. Frequently a rubriblast is slightly larger than a myeloblast and has more cytoplasm that is a deeper blue. One percent or less rubriblasts are observed in normal bone marrow (Table 1-2).

### Prorubricytes (Basophilic Normoblasts, Basophilic Erythroblasts)

In the prorubricyte the nuclear chromatin pattern has coarsened and the nucleoli are absent or ill defined. The cytoplasm contains varying amounts of hemoglobin, which may rarely impart a pinkish tinge but whose overall predominant color is blue **(see Color Figures 1, 11 to 14, and 18)**.[9]

A prorubricyte is normally smaller than a rubriblast. One to 4 percent of prorubricytes are found in normal marrow.

### Rubricytes (Polychromatic Normoblasts, Polychromatic Erythroblasts)

Nuclear chromatin is thickened and irregularly condensed in the rubricyte. Light-staining parachromatin areas are visible among the dark-blue staining, pyknotic areas. Nucleoli are no longer visible **(see Color Figures 1, 8, 12, 14 to 17, 25, 32, and 34)**.

A rubricyte is smaller than a prorubricyte. It has relatively more cytoplasm with a smaller nucleus than a prorubricyte. The cytoplasm contains varying mixtures of blue (RNA) and pink (hemoglobin) stain, but in the later rubricytes the pinkish stain is usually predominant.

There are 10 to 20 percent of rubricytes in the marrow of a healthy adult. Rubricytes are not present in normal blood of adults but may appear in that of newborns.[9]

### Metarubricytes (Orthochromatic Normoblasts, Orthochromatic Erythroblasts)

The nucleus of a metarubricyte is relatively small in relation to the cytoplasm and is destined to be extruded. A metarubricyte has a solid blue-black degenerated nucleus with a nonlinear clumped chromatin structure. The cytoplasm is predominantly pinkish (reddish) due to increasing hemoglobin synthesis, but there remain minimal amounts of residual blue (RNA) **(see Color Figures 1, 8, 18, 26, and 27)**.

The number of metarubricytes in normal marrow varies between 5 and 10 percent. Metarubricytes are not observed in adults with normal peripheral blood but can be found in the blood of normal newborns.[9]

### Diffusely Basophilic Erythrocytes (Polychromatophilic Erythrocytes)

The nucleus of a metarubricyte is ultimately extruded from the erythrocyte, leaving a diffusely basophilic or polychromatophilic cell. Some of the bluish staining color remains, owing to the presence of RNA. The erythrocyte contains approximately two thirds of its total hemoglobin content by the time the nucleus is lost. RNA together with the remaining mitochondria aid in synthesis of the remainder of the hemoglobin. RNA content and mitochondria decrease as hemoglobin synthesis continues.[2,9]

A diffusely basophilic erythrocyte is larger than a mature red cell. It is released in two or three days from the marrow and circulates for one or two days before maturing into an erythrocyte. There rarely or never are diffusely basophilic erythrocytes in the blood of healthy adults, but frequently polychromatophilic cells occur in the blood of healthy newborns.

When stained with new methylene blue, diffusely basophilic cells reveal granulofilamentous structures and are classified as reticulocytes **(see**

### Table 1-2. BLOOD CELLS

| | Hematopoietic Tissues | | | | | Circulating Blood |
|---|---|---|---|---|---|---|
| Stem Cell | Myeloblast | Promyelocyte | E. Myelocyte | | | Eosinophil |
| | | | N. Myelocyte | N. Metamyelocyte | Neutrophil Band | Neutrophil Segmented |
| | | | B. Myelocyte | | | Basophil |
| | Monoblast | Promonocyte | | | | Monocyte |
| | Megakaryoblast | Promegakaryocyte | Megakaryocyte | Megakaryocyte | | Thrombocyte |
| | Rubriblast | Prorubricyte | Rubricyte | Metarubricyte | Diffusely Basophilic Erythrocyte | Erythrocyte |
| | Lymphoblast | Prolymphocyte | | | | Lymphocyte |
| | Plasmoblast | Proplasmocyte | | | Plasmocyte | |

From Diggs,[9] p. 1, with permission.

**Color Figures 1 and 35)**. With anemia or hypoxia, erythropoietin stimulates erythroid precursors to proliferate and increase the number of early erythroid cells. An increased number of polychromatophilic cells are delivered early from the marrow, and, therefore, the reticulocyte count is increased.

### Erythrocytes (Discocytes)

A normal erythrocyte is a biconcave disc that is 7 to 8 $\mu$m in mean diameter, 1.5 to 2.5 $\mu$m thick, and has a volume of 90 fl. In Wright-stained smears, an erythrocyte appears as a circular cell with a distinct and smooth margin. In the central portion where the cell is thinnest, the intensity of the stain is less than at the marginal area creating an area of normal central pallor. At the thin end of the smear, red cells are flattened out, lack central pallor, and do not reveal their biconcavity.

A mature erythrocyte is not able to synthesize protein since it is without a nucleus and mitochondria, but it has a unique yet limited metabolism to sustain life while traversing the microvasculature. Erythrocytes are pliable or flexible and are capable of making unusual changes in shape. The structure of the cell membrane and the metabolism within the cell are intimately related to a properly functioning and normally surviving red cell in the circulation.[3]

Red blood cells have an average lifespan of approximately 120 days. Most senescent or damaged red cells are removed by the spleen from the circulation. This process is referred to as extravascular destruction. Upon disruption of the membrane, cellular components, such as iron and amino acids, are broken down, recovered, stored, and reused to support erythropoiesis. Less than 10 percent of senescent red cells may also be destroyed normally in the circulation (intravascular destruction).[3]

The essential characteristics required by the erythron for normal erythropoiesis are adequate proliferation, maturation, storage, production, metabolism, oxygen supply, hemoglobin, and breakdown.

## GRANULOPOIESIS (see Color Figure 2)

### Neutrophils

Granulopoiesis or myelopoiesis refers to the production of neutrophils, monocytes, eosinophils, and basophils. Neutrophils are produced in the bone marrow from committed myeloid (pertaining to marrow) stem cell precursors. They are stored in the bone marrow, released to enter the peripheral blood for a few hours, and then leave the blood to enter tissues and body cavities. Under normal circumstances the rate that neutrophils enter the blood and the rate that these cells egress to tissue are in equilibrium. Neutrophils remain in blood approximately 7 to 10 hours. The half disappearance time of labeled neutrophil segmented cells is reported to be about seven hours.[1-3] As these cells exit the blood for the tissues, they are replaced by other neutrophils from the marrow. There is no evidence that neutrophils return from tissue to blood or marrow.

Neutrophils leave the marrow by moving through transiently formed pores in endothelial cells that separate marrow parenchyma from venous sinuses; when leaving blood (diapedesis) for tissue, neutrophils migrate between endothelial cells. Neutrophils leave blood when there is demand from tissues, inflammatory sites, or body cavities. Chemotactic factors from infectious or inflammatory tissue direct the migration of neutrophils. These factors combine with receptors on the surface of granulocytes and then direct neutrophils to inflamed areas.[1,2,5]

Granulocytes share with monocytes a common progenitor cell that is designated in marrow agar cultures as CFU-GM. With exposure to colony-stimulating factor from monocytes or macrophages, CFU-GM will grow colonies of granulocytes and monocytes.[1,2,5]

The earliest cell of the neutrophilic series in marrow is the myeloblast, and there is a continuum of differentiation and maturation from the blast to the most mature cell (neutrophil segmented) requiring from seven to eleven days. Myeloblasts, promyelocytes, and myelocytes are capable of mitosis and compose the mitotic pool. There is no mitotic division beyond the myelocyte stage. Myelocytes mature into metamyelocytes, bands, and segmented neutrophils, which are designated as the postmitotic maturation and storage pool. The large storage pool of bands and segmented cells remain in the marrow for about 10 days and can be called upon when needed (see Fig. 1-3). Once in the blood, half of the neutrophils are freely circulating, while an equal number are in a marginating pool on the walls of blood vessels, particularly in lungs, liver, and spleen.[1,2,5]

Maturation of the granulocytic series of cells is characterized by the development of primary blue-staining granules that are later replaced by secondary granules that differ in their affinity for various dyes. Cells with an affinity for basic dyes are basophils; those cells that stain reddish-orange with the acid dye eosin are eosinophils; the cells that do not stain intensely with either acid or basic dyes are called neutrophils. As these motile cells mature, the nucleus undergoes progressive changes from round to multilobular forms.

The events involved in the primary function of neutrophils in host defense are migration to area of infection, recognition, phagocytosis, and killing and digestion of invading microorganisms; neutrophils are particularly efficient in phagocytizing bacteria coated with antibody.[1,2,4,5] These events are discussed in Chapter 16.

## Myeloblasts

A myeloblast has a round nucleus that stains predominantly reddish-blue. The interlaced chromatin strands are delicate, finely dispersed, and evenly stained, but are not clumped. One or more nucleoli are usually demonstrable. There is a slight to moderate amount of bluish nongranular cytoplasm that stains lighter next to the nucleus than at the periphery of the cell **(see Color Figures 2, 19, and 20)**. A myeloblast is smaller and has less blue cytoplasm than a rubriblast. After about three to five mitotic divisions, the myeloblast matures into a progranulocyte.[9]

Myeloblasts vary in size from 15 to 20 $\mu$m. They are not observed in normal peripheral blood. There is 1 percent or less of myeloblasts in normal bone marrow (Table 1-3).

## Promyelocytes (Progranulocytes)

A committed stem cell is no longer identified as a myeloblast when it develops distinct granules. These early primary granules stain dark blue or reddish-blue and may be round or irregular in shape. The granules may appear over the nucleus, as well as in the cytoplasm. These primary granules are lysosomes and contain myeloperoxidase, acid phosphatase, bactericidal cationic proteins, neutral proteases, and lysozyme.[1,2,5,6]

The nucleus of a promyelocyte is usually round and is large in relation to the cytoplasm. The chromatin structure is slightly coarser than that in a myeloblast. Nucleoli may be visible but are not usually distinct **(see Color Figures 2 and 21 to 23)**.[9]

The cytoplasm is blue with a relatively light zone adjacent to the nucleus. The periphery of the cytoplasm is smooth and is not indented by neighboring cells.

### Table 1-3. BONE MARROW CELLS: NORMAL ADULT VALUES

| | |
|---|---|
| Stem cell | 0–0.01% |
| Myeloblast | 0–1 |
| Promyelocyte | 1–5 |
| N. Myelocyte | 2–10 |
| N. Metamyelocyte | 5–15 |
| N. Band | 10–40 |
| N. Segmented | 10–30 |
| Eosinophil | 0–3 |
| Basophil | 0–1 |
| Lymphocyte | 5–15 |
| Plasmocyte | 0–1 |
| Monocyte | 0–2 |
| Other cells | 0–1 |
| Megakaryocyte | 0.1–0.5 |
| Rubriblast | 0–1 |
| Prorubricyte | 1–4 |
| Rubricyte | 10–20 |
| Metarubricyte | 5–10 |

WBC:Nucleated RBC Ratio 4:1

From Diggs,[9] p. 4, with permission.

The size of a promyelocyte may be variable depending on the stage of a given cell in the mitotic cycle, but this cell may be larger than a myeloblast. Progranulocytes do not appear in normal peripheral blood. One to 5 percent of progranulocytes are observed in normal bone marrow.[9]

## Neutrophilic Myelocytes

A promyelocyte becomes a myelocyte when the granules differentiate to such a degree that one can identify secondary neutrophilic granules. The first sign of neutrophilic differentiation has been called the "dawn of neutrophilia" or "beginning neutrophilia," which refers to a relatively light island of ill-defined reddish (or pinkish) secondary lysosomal granules that develop adjacent to the nucleus and in proximity to the remaining primary granules. As myelocytes divide and age, the primary granules become fewer and the secondary neutrophilic granules predominate. Secondary granules are called specific granules and they contain lactoferrin, lysozyme, and alkaline phosphatase.[7-13]

The nuclei of myelocytes may be round, oval, or flattened on one side. Chromatin strands are unevenly stained and thickened. Nucleoli are absent or indistinct in myelocytes **(see Color Figures 2, 24, 26, and 30)**.

Neutrophilic myelocytes are often smaller than progranulocytes and have relatively larger amounts of cytoplasm. Normal peripheral blood does not contain neutrophilic myelocytes. There are 2 to 10 percent of myelocytes in normal bone marrow.[9]

## Neutrophilic Metamyelocytes

As maturation proceeds, the nucleus becomes slightly indented (or bean-shaped), which serves to identify the cell as a metamyelocyte. The indentation is less than half the width of the arbitrary round nucleus. There is noticeable clumping of the chromatin, but the chromatin structure is not as dense as that of neutrophilic segmented cells.

Small, pinkish secondary granules fill the cytoplasm and there may be a few darker primary granules remaining **(see Color Figures 2, 24, 26, 28, and 35)**. These maturing cells remain in marrow and form a granulocytic reserve.

Metamyelocytes are smaller than myelocytes and are rare or absent in normal peripheral blood. There are approximately 5 to 15 percent of metamyelocytes in normal bone marrow.[9]

## Neutrophilic Bands (N. Nonsegmented, N. Nonfilamented)

When the stage is reached in which the nuclear indentation is greater than half the width of the hypothetical round nucleus, the cell is identified as a neutrophilic band. The opposite edges of the nucleus become almost parallel for an appreciable distance giving the appearance of a horseshoe or a curved link of sausage. The nucleus shows degenerative changes, and there is usually a dark pyknotic mass at each pole where the lobe is destined to be. The secondary neutrophilic granules are small, are evenly distributed, and stain various shades of pink. There may be an occasional dark primary granule (see Color Figures 1, 25, and 27).

Neutrophilic bands are often slightly smaller than metamyelocytes. Band forms constitute from 1 to 6 percent of the leukocytes in the peripheral blood of healthy individuals and from 10 to 40 percent of the nucleated cells in bone marrow (see Tables 1-3, 1-4).[9]

### Neutrophilic Segmented (N. Filamented, N. Polymorphonuclear Leukocyte, PMN)

In a neutrophilic segmented cell the nucleus is separated into definite lobes with a narrow filament or strand connecting the lobes. Nuclear chromatin is heavily clumped or pyknotic. The cytoplasm in an ideal stain is light pink and the small, numerous, and evenly distributed secondary granules have a pink color or take a "neutral" stain. Neutrophil secondary granules are lysosomes which contain hydrolytic enzymes. There may also be a few darkly stained primary granules (see Color Figures 2, 25, 26, 28, 29, and 39).[9]

Mature neutrophils are approximately twice the size of normal erythrocytes. Fifty to 70 percent of segmented neutrophils are found in the peripheral blood of older children and adults, and 10 to 30 percent are found in normal bone marrow. Approximately 5 percent of the neutrophils have one lobe, 35 percent have two lobes, 41 percent three lobes, 17 percent four lobes, and 2 percent five lobes.[9]

There is a gradual transition among the various stages of granulocytes. The division of neutrophils into developmental stages is somewhat arbitrary but is necessary for morphologic evaluation. Borderline cells that are difficult to distinguish from each other may be present. The major difficulty arises in differentiating between band and segmented cells and deciding if the link connecting the lobes is narrow enough to be called a filament or wide enough to be identified as a band. A filamented or segmented cell has a thread-like connection between two lobes and there is no visible chromatin in the connection. A band nucleus reveals two distinct margins with nuclear chromatin material visible between the margins. Lobes of nuclei often touch or are superimposed and it is impossible to see the connecting filaments. If the margin of a lobe can be traced as a definite and continuing line from one side of the nucleus across the isthmus to the other side, it may be assumed that a filament is present although it is not visible. In attempting to differentiate between a segmented and a band cell, identification should be made not on a single morphologic characteristic but on combined features. In case of doubt in identifying a borderline cell, the questionable cell should be placed in the most mature category.[9]

## Eosinophils

Eosinophils are usually easily recognizable because of the large, round secondary granules that have an affinity for the acid eosin stain. With Wright's stain, normal eosinophil granules stain orange to reddish-orange. The granules are spherical, uniform in size, and evenly distributed. Because of the nature of the granule, eosinophils may be recognized in unstained moist preparations of blood in light and phase microscopy. These secondary granules contain an electron-dense core with an oblong structure characterized in crystalline lines when observed in the electron microscope. This crystalloid structure is composed of cationic proteins and of major basic protein that binds to acid aniline dyes and that may help to explain the staining qualities of the granule.[4,5,9,14,15]

The granules of eosinophils contain various hydrolytic enzymes including peroxidase, acid phosphatase, aryl sulfatase, beta-glucuronidase, phospholipase, and ribonuclease, but they lack lysozyme.[4,8]

Eosinophils are produced in the bone marrow and have been considered to arise from the multipotential myeloid stem cell committed to form granulocytes (see Fig. 1-2). However, recent in vitro culture studies of granulopoiesis have shown that eosinophils and neutrophils form separate colonies when stimulated by a specific CSF. These culture results suggest that eosinophils are under separate genetic control and may be produced separately from the neutrophils by the committed myeloid stem cell (CFU-Eo) (see Fig. 1-2).[1,3]

Eosinophils pass through the same developmental stages of myelocyte, metamyelocyte, band, and segmented as do neutrophils (see Table 1-2 and Color Figures 2 and 30 to 36). The earliest eosinophil has a few dark-bluish primary granules intermingled with the specific reddish-orange granules. During development, the bluish granules become less visible and disappear and the specific secondary granules fill the cytoplasm.[9]

Mature eosinophils are stored in marrow for several days before appearing in peripheral blood. Transit time of the eosinophil in blood of humans has been reported to be somewhat longer than that of neutrophils. Eosinophils migrate from blood to tissue, with most eosinophils residing in tissue. Eosinophils may return from tissue into blood and marrow.

The roles of the eosinophil in host defense, metazoal infections, and immediate-type hypersensitivity are under investigation. The function of eosinophils is similar to that of neutrophils in that eosinophils can migrate into tissue or to an area of inflammation. These cells are able to ingest bacteria, but their ability to phagocytize and kill bacteria is less efficient than that of neutrophils.[4,6,8,14,15]

Normal adult peripheral blood contains 1 to 3 percent of eosinophils and approximately the same number are seen in normal bone marrow (see Tables 1-3, 1-4). In normal blood, eosinophils are about the size of or slightly larger than neutrophils and usually have a band or a two-lobed nucleus; rarely does an eosinophil have three segments.[9]

## Basophils

Although basophils constitute less than 2 percent of normal blood cells (see Table 1-4), the dark violet-blue granules aid in the immediate recognition of this cell. These granules are visible over the nucleus as well as lateral to the nucleus. They vary in size from 0.2 to 1.0 $\mu$m. The granules are coarse, unevenly distributed and vary in number, size, shape, and color. With Wright's stain the granules appear deep purplish-blue to dark purple-red. Basophil granules are water soluble. In cells that are poorly fixed during staining, the center of the granule may disappear, or the entire granule may be washed away, leaving a small, colorless cytoplasmic area.[9]

Basophils are produced in the marrow in a similar manner to that of neutrophil production, in that they arise from a multipotential precursor stem cell and develop along the same stages as the other granulocytes. Based on the shape of their nuclei, they may be identified as basophilic myelocytes, metamyelocytes, bands, and segmented cells. However, because of their granulation, the shape of the nucleus is often masked by the granules **(see Color Figures 2 and 37 to 39)**. Mature basophils rarely have more than two segments.[9]

Basophils differ from neutrophils in that they are not phagocytic. Basophilic granules contain histamine and heparin, and thus these cells have a significant role in acute systemic allergic reactions. If granule contents of basophils are released in massive amounts, anaphylactic shock occurs. The function of basophils has been stated to be secretion, by which the contents of the granules are released from the cytoplasm into the environment following

appropriate stimulus. The granules also contain a substance called eosinophil chemotactic factor, which attracts eosinophils when it is released during immediate hypersensitivity reactions (see Chapter 16).[8,16]

Basophils in all stages of maturation are smaller than promyelocytes and myelocytes. Their size is approximately the same as that of neutrophils.

Blood basophils and tissue basophils (mast cells) are closely related in their functions and biochemical characteristics.[16,17]

## Monocytes (see Color Figure 3)

Monocytes are phagocytic leukocytes that play a major role in defense against pathogenic organisms and foreign cells. In thin areas of the peripheral blood smear, the monocyte is larger than a neutrophil. Monocytes have abundant cytoplasm in relation to the nucleus. The monocytic cytoplasm in a Wright-stained smear is dull gray-blue in contrast to the pink-staining cytoplasm of neutrophils. The granules are usually fine, lightly stained, numerous, and evenly distributed, giving to the cell a ground-glass appearance. There may be varying numbers of prominent granules in addition to the small granules. Digestive vacuoles may be observed in the cytoplasm, as well as phagocytized erythrocytes, nuclei, cell fragments, bacteria, fungi, and pigment.[9]

The nuclei of monocytes frequently are kidney-shaped but may be deeply indented and may appear to have two or more lobes. One of the distinctive features of the monocyte is the appearance of brain-like convolutions of the nucleus. Another characteristic is the coarse, linear pattern of the chromatin with light spaces between the chromatin strands, which contrasts with the clumped chromatin of the lymphocyte.

The shape of the monocyte is variable. Many cells are round. Other cells reveal blunt pseudopods, which are manifestations of their slow mobility. These ameboid cells continue to move while the blood film is drying and become fixed before the cytoplasmic extensions are retracted. These pseudopods vary in size and number; the outer portion of the outstretched cytoplasm may have a hyaline appearance without granules in contrast to the inner granular cytoplasm.[9]

The three most helpful characteristic features of the monocyte are brain-like nuclear convolutions, blunt pseudopods, and dull gray-blue cytoplasm **(see Color Figures 3 and 40 to 45)**.

As monocytes grow, they become too large to pass readily through capillaries. Monocytes then migrate into tissue and mature into activated macrophages in many organs (e.g., alveolar macrophages, splenic macrophages, Kupffer's cells). Macrophages do not normally re-enter the bloodstream.

The monocyte-macrophage system plays a key

**Table 1–4. PERIPHERAL BLOOD CELLS: NORMAL ADULT VALUES**

|  | Percent | Per mm³ |
|---|---|---|
| N. Band | 1–5 | 50–500 |
| N. Segmented | 50–70 | 2500–7000 |
| Eosinophil | 1–3 | 50–300 |
| Basophil | 0–1 | 0–100 |
| Lymphocyte | 20–40 | 1000–4000 |
| Monocyte | 1–6 | 50–600 |

From Diggs,[9] p. 4, with permission.

role in host defense. Phagocytes entrap and kill pathogenic microorganisms, ingest and degrade noxious external agents, engulf and process antigens, and pass on processed antigenic substances to cells of the lymphocytic-plasmocytic system responsible for the synthesis of antibodies and for cell-mediated immunity. Phagocytic cells remove from the circulating blood hemoglobin-containing red cells, injured and dead cells, hemosiderin granules, white and red cell fragments, insoluble particles, activated clotting factors, and antigen-antibody complexes. Motile macrophages, escaping between epithelial cells of respiratory tracts and gastrointestinal and genitourinary organs, perform a scavenger function by clearing the body of unneeded debris. When activated, macrophages are able to kill some types of tumor cells in culture. Macrophages also serve as secretory cells by releasing interleukin-1, a soluble factor that induces T-cell proliferation, and by elaborating prostaglandins, which are mediators of inflammation. Monocytes and macrophages are a source of CSF and interferon.[1,2,4,8,18]

Monocytes account for 1 to 6 percent of normal blood leukocytes and for less than 2 percent of normal marrow cells (see Tables 1-1, 1-2). There is no large reserve pool of monocytes in marrow. Monocytes leave the marrow when mature and enter the bloodstream where they circulate for about 14 hours before entering tissue.[8,9,10]

### Monoblasts and Promonocytes (see Color Figure 4)

Similar to granulocytes, monocytes are derived from precursor committed hematopoietic stem cells in the marrow (CFU-GM) (see Fig. 1-2). The earliest cells produced by the committed stem cell are monoblasts and promonocytes, which eventually mature into monocytes. Promonocytes and monoblasts are not identifiable in bone marrow or peripheral blood smears except in disorders in which there is marked proliferation of monocytic cells. The identification of early monocytic cells is based on slightly indented or folded early nuclei and on association with more mature cells that have pseudopods and brain-like convolutions in the nucleus (see Color Figure 4).

## LYMPHOPOIESIS (see Color Figure 4)
## Lymphocytes (see Color Figure 5)

The second most numerous cells in the blood are lymphocytes, with a range of 20 to 40 percent. There are 5 to 15 lymphocytes in bone marrow smears (see Tables 1-3, 1-4). The majority of the lymphocytes are small in size, varying from 7 to 10 $\mu$m but there are also variable numbers of large lymphocytes which have diameters comparable to monocytes

(see Color Figures 5 and 48 to 50). Between the small- and large-sized lymphocytes are lymphocytes of many intermediate sizes. Size is not a reliable basis for determining the age or metabolic activity of lymphocytes, because the size varies with the thickness of the smear. Lymphocytes tend to become spherical and small in thick areas of the smear; in the thinnest end of the smear, lymphocytes may be spread out and appear large.[7-9]

Small lymphocytes usually are round with smooth margins (see Color Figures 46 to 48). Rarely a lymphocyte may have a spindle form with an oval nucleus and with cytoplasmic filaments extending outward at each end (see Color Figure 47). The margins of large lymphocytes frequently are indented by neighboring erythrocytes, causing them to have serrated (holly-leaf) shapes.[9]

When stained with Wright's stain, the color of the cytoplasm is blue with the intensity of the blue varying from light to dark in different cells. The color is evenly distributed in some cells and uneven in other cells. The intensity of the blue stain is greater at the periphery of the cell than near the Golgi area adjacent to the nucleus. The cytoplasm of some large lymphocytes that stain a pale sky blue have a structureless appearance; other large cells may reveal fine bluish interlacing fibrils with critical illumination.[9]

The majority of lymphocytes do not have granules. In some large cells there may be a variable number of a few well-defined granules that vary in size, are unevenly distributed, and are easily counted. These granules are purplish-red and have been called "azurophilic," a term that is misleading, as these granules are predominantly red rather than blue.[9]

The diameter of the nucleus of the smallest lymphocyte in peripheral blood is slightly smaller than or the same size as a normal erythrocyte in the same microscopic field. The nucleus in relation to the cytoplasm is large, and the nuclei of lymphocytes are round or slightly indented. Chromatin structure is lumpy or clumped and stained dark purple with lighter bluish-purple areas between chromatin aggregates.

Nucleoli are present in some lymphocytes but are not visible in light microscopy, for they are obscured by the darkly stained chromatin masses. The fact that nucleoli may be present in small lymphocytes is evidence that these cells are capable of growth and replication.[5,9]

### Large Lymphocytes Versus Monocytes

A monocyte is often mistaken for a large lymphocyte (see Color Figure 43) because its cytoplasm may be blue, granules may be indistinct, nucleus is round, and blunt pseudopods and digestive vacuoles are missing. To distinguish monocytes from large lymphocytes, nuclear structure, character of the cytoplasm, and shape of the cells are useful. The nucleus of a lymphocyte tends to be clumped rather than linear as it is in a monocyte (see Color Figures 48 to 50). There is a greater tendency for the nuclear chromatin to be condensed at the periphery of the nucleus in the lymphocyte. Brain-like convolutions present in a monocyte are not observed in a lymphocyte.[9]

Large lymphocytes and monocytes may have distinct bluish-red granules. In a monocyte the large bluish-red granules are interspersed with numerous fine granules in the cytoplasm and cannot be enumerated. In a lymphocyte these large granules are prominent and can be counted easily, as there are no other granules. Because of the finely granular cytoplasm, the monocyte has a ground-glass appearance, whereas the cytoplasm of the lymphocyte has a relatively clear nongranular background. Large lymphocytes are often deeply indented by neighboring red cells. Monocytes tend to project blunt pseudopods between cells or to compress cells rather than be indented by them.[9]

### Activated and Reactive Lymphocytes

When stimulated by appropriate antigen, lymphocytes have been shown to transform into cells that are immunologically competent. The size of activated lymphocytes varies, but usually these cells are large. The increase in size is due to an increase in DNA in the nucleus and of RNA in the cytoplasm. Nuclei may be oval or indented with an intermediate chromatin pattern. Nuclei of some lymphocytes have blast-like nuclei with nucleoli. Varying degrees of cytoplasmic basophilia may be present. There may be distinctive reddish granules. The cytoplasm may have a bubbly appearance, and vacuoles may be seen.[9]

Lymphocytes that respond to antigenic stimuli constitute a wide spectrum of morphologic variants. The most striking variants are observed in infectious mononucleosis, but reactive lymphocytes are present in lesser numbers in other virus-related diseases and conditions such as post-transfusion reactions, organ transplants, and serum sickness.

### Lymphoblasts and Prolymphocytes (see Color Figure 5)

Lymphocytes originate from a lymphoid stem cell committed to lymphopoiesis (see Fig. 1-2). The earliest lymphocytes are identified as lymphoblasts and prolymphocytes. Lymphoblasts contain a large round nucleus with a small or moderate amount of basophilic cytoplasm. The nuclear chromatin strands in lymphoblasts are thin, evenly stained, and not clumped. One or several nucleoli are usually demonstrable (see Color Figure 5).

Prolymphocytes have an intermediate chromatin pattern that has begun to clump in some areas of the nucleus but does not appear as clumped as in mature lymphocytes. Nucleoli are less distinct than in lymphoblasts. Differences are subtle and in case of doubt, the cell should be called a lymphocyte.

### Additional Information

Lymphocytes are primarily concerned with maintaining the immune defense system. Lymphoid stem cells are not able to initiate immune responses until they have been processed either in the thymus or the bursa-equivalent organs. Lymphocyte precursors mature into T (thymus-derived) and B (bursa-related) cells under the influence of particular microenvironments. T cells are responsible for cell-mediated immune responses. B cells after antigenic stimulation respond by transforming into plasmoblasts and maturing into plasmocytes, which manufacture and secrete various types of immunoglobulins (humoral antibodies). It is not possible on the basis of morphologic characteristics as revealed by light microscopy to differentiate between T and B lymphocytes. Distinction between the two cell types relies on membrane marker studies.[4-7,9,18]

## Plasmocytes (see Color Figure 4)

Lymphocytes and plasmocytes are closely related cells. Progenitor cells of plasma cells, as well as lymphocytes, live in lymphoid organs. These two types of cells have morphologic features and immunologic functions that are distinct from those of non-lymphoid cells. Lymphocytes and plasmocytes are essential in body defense against bacteria, viruses, and other microorganisms.[5,9]

Plasmocytes are not observed in peripheral blood smears of normal individuals but constitute about 1 percent of the nucleated cells in normal marrow. Plasmocytes may be present in peripheral blood of patients with viral infections. Mature plasmocytes range in size from 15 to 25 $\mu$m. They may be round or oval with slightly irregular margins. The cytoplasm is nongranular and usually stains a deep or vibrant blue, which has been described as "cornflower" or "larkspur" blue. The cytoplasm adjacent to the nucleus is pale with a perinuclear clear zone containing the Golgi apparatus. Fibrillar structures that stain blue may be demonstrable in the cytoplasm. One or several small vacuoles may be observed. There is no evidence of phagocytosis.[9]

The nucleus of a plasmocyte is relatively small, round, or oval and is eccentrically placed in the cell. The nuclear chromatin is heavily clumped or coarse and lumpy as that of a lymphocyte (see Color Figures 4, 9, 13, 35, and 51 to 53).[9]

Plasmocytes in marrow can be torn in the process of aspiration and may have irregular spiculate margins. Plasmocytes may cluster around large, nongranular tissue cells, representing a manifestation of the immune response in which antigenic material, processed by macrophages, is transferred to plasma cells, which will then manufacture immune globulins.[2,9]

After stimulation by antigen, some lymphocytes of B-cell lineage transform into cells with basophilic cytoplasm and blast-like chromatin structure. These plasmocytoid cells develop into functioning plasma cells that manufacture and secrete immunoglobulins.[1,2]

Immune globulins manufactured by plasma cells produce unusual morphologic variants. The proteinaceous material is in the form of round globules that may be red ("Russell bodies"), pink, blue, or colorless. The globules may fill the cytoplasm, giving the appearance of a bunch of grapes. In some cells, the red color has a diffuse distribution producing so-called flame cells.[9] This red color is probably due to glycoprotein, which is particularly abundant in plasma cells producing IgA.

### Plasmoblasts and Proplasmocytes (see Color Figure 4)

Cells designated as plasmoblasts are similar to blast cells of other series. The nuclei are large in relation to the cytoplasm, appear round with linear chromatin strands, and have a nucleolus. The cytoplasm is dark blue and nongranular. Plasmoblasts are identified primarily in the presence of proplasmocytes and plasmocytes but cannot be differentiated from stem cells on the basis of size, shape, color, and structure. The major differences between a plasmoblast and a proplasmocyte are a relatively light area near the nucleus, an intermediate chromatin structure, an eccentric nucleus, and an ill-defined or absent nucleolus in proplasmocytes (see Color Figure 4). Plasmoblasts and plasmocytes are not observed in normal bone marrow but may appear in conditions associated with abnormal immunoglobulin production.

## MEGAKARYOCYTOPOIESIS (see Color Figure 6)

The megakaryocyte is one of the largest cells in the bone marrow and arises from the same multipotential stem cell as do the granulocytes and erythrocytes (see Fig. 1-2). The megakaryocyte is derived from a committed progenitor cell (CFU-Meg) following stimulation by a hormone, thrombopoietin, which is believed to control platelet production. CFU-Meg, the committed progenitor of thrombopoiesis, is detected by colony formation in plasma clot culture. A megakaryoblast undergoes a sequence of maturation stages to differentiate into a promegakaryocyte and megakaryocyte without platelets (see Color Figures 6 and 54 to 61). The nucleus of the megakaryoblast undergoes DNA synthesis rapidly with multiple mitotic divisions (endomitosis) forming two, four, eight, or more nuclei, but without cytoplasmic division, thus producing giant polyploid cells. These multiple nuclei remain attached to each other usually and frequently are superimposed on each other. The nuclei maintain a linear chromatin pattern while the cytoplasm increases in volume and reveals maturation changes characterized by granule development resulting in platelet formation.[9,19,20]

Masses of platelets appear at the edge of the megakaryocyte in the four to eight nuclear stage, but occasionally platelets form in earlier cells with one or two nuclei. In marrow smears of normal individuals, there are one to four megakaryocytes per 1000 nucleated cells, and these cells are in the latest stages of maturation.[9]

### Megakaryoblasts

Megakaryoblasts are moderately large cells in the range of 20 to 45 μm with primitive chromatin structure, one or two nucleoli, basophilic nongranular cytoplasm, and high nuclear-cytoplasmic ratio. Cytoplasmic basophilia indicates an abundance of ribosomes ultrastructurally. Blunt cytoplasmic protrusions that stain blue and contain chromophobic globules are characteristic.[2,9,19]

Pathologic alterations in megakaryoblasts are observed in myeloproliferative disease. Micromegakaryoblasts are noted in chronic myelocytic leukemia, preleukemic states, and the blast crisis of chronic granulocytic leukemia. Such cells are small (8 to 15 μm) and difficult to distinguish from myeloblasts, but cytoplasmic blebs or budding platelets help in identification of micromegakaryoblasts. The presence of a specific peroxidase in the nuclear envelope in electron micrographs is diagnostic.[2,9]

### Promegakaryocytes

A promegakaryocyte differs from a megakaryoblast in that the nucleus is divided into two or four lobes, there may be reddish-blue granules in the cytoplasm, and the cytoplasm is less basophilic (see Color Figures 54 to 57). There may be cytoplasmic protrusions that have a homogeneous or bubbly appearance. With electron microscopy an elaborate membrane network connected with the plasma membrane of the cell gives evidence of the beginning of a demarcating membrane system.[9,19]

A variant of the promegakaryocyte is a large cell with granular cytoplasm adjacent to the nucleus, a collar of vacuolated cytoplasm, and a third distinct marginal zone with cytoplasmic protrusions often containing colorless globules.[9]

### Megakaryocytes Without Platelets

In the third stage of maturation, megakaryocytic cells have increased in volume with an abundant amount of cytoplasm and polyploid nuclei. The chromatin is linear and coarse with spaces between the strands. There are numerous small, uniformly distributed granules that stain reddish-blue (see

Color Figures 58 and 59). The demarcation membrane system has begun to appear as narrow channels.[2,9]

## Megakaryocytes With Platelets

The final stage of maturation of megakaryocytes is characterized by a large multilobular nucleus and an aggregation of the granular cytoplasm into masses of platelets separated from the granular cytoplasm by demarcation membranes. Individual platelets are attached to the cytoplasm by a narrow strand (see Color Figures 60 and 61).

Mature megakaryocytes are located adjacent to marrow sinuses and extend portions of their cytoplasm through the basement membrane and between endothelial cells of the marrow sinusoids in order to get platelets into the sinus. Membrane-bound platelets are swept into the flowing bloodstream from these cytoplasmic projections. Further fragmentation to form individual platelets occurs after release into the sinus. One megakaryocyte can release several thousand platelets. After platelets are released, there remains a bare nucleus that is often lobulated and that may have a narrow rim of cytoplasm (see Color Figure 62).[9]

Distinctive features of differentiated megakaryocytes include large volume, nuclear ploidy, reddish granular cytoplasm, and a demarcation membrane system enabling platelet formation.

## Platelets (Thrombocytes)

Platelets are fragments of cytoplasm shed from the periphery of megakaryocytes. Platelets have no nuclei. In peripheral smears of normal adults, platelets vary in size from 1 to 4 $\mu$m. Platelets stain light blue and contain a variable number of small reddish-blue granules.

Platelets tend to adhere to each other, and there may be small aggregates of platelets in a well-made normal smear. In the thin area of the smear where erythrocytes are not overlapping each other, the number per oil immersion field varies from 7 to 25. A blood smear report is not complete unless the platelet number and morphology are given.[9]

Megakaryopoiesis and platelet formation are stimulated by a decrease in thrombocytes and are suppressed with an increase in thrombocytes.[1,2]

## References

1. Beck, WS: Hematology, ed 4. MIT Press, Cambridge, 1985.
2. Erslev, AJ and Gabuzda, TG: Pathophysiology of Blood, ed 3. WB Saunders, Philadelphia, 1985.
3. Hillman, RS and Finch, CA: Red Cell Manual, ed 5. FA Davis, Philadelphia, 1985.
4. Spivak, JL: Fundamentals of Clinical Hematology, ed 2. Harper & Row, Philadelphia, 1984.
5. Boggs, DR and Winkelstein, A: White Cell Manual, ed 4. FA Davis, Philadelphia, 1983.
6. Williams, WW, et al: Hematology, ed 3. McGraw-Hill, New York, 1984.
7. Wintrobe, MM, et al: Clinical Hematology, ed 8. Lea & Febiger, Philadelphia, 1981.
8. Zucker-Franklin, D, et al: Atlas of Blood Cells, Function and Pathology, Vol 1. Lea & Febiger, Philadelphia, 1981.
9. Diggs, LW, Sturm, D, and Bell, A: The Morphology of Human Blood Cells. Abbott Laboratories, Abbott Park, IL, 1985.
10. Bainton, DF and Farquher, MG: Origin of granules in polymorphonuclear leukocytes; two types derived from opposite faces of the Golgi complex of developing granulocytes. J Cell Biol 28:277, 1966.
11. Boggs, DR: Physiology of neutrophil proliferation, maturation and circulation. Clin Haematol 4:535, 1975.
12. Murphy, P: The Neutrophil. Plenum Press, New York, 1976.
13. Stossel, TP and Cohen, HJ: Neutrophil function normal and abnormal. In Gordon, AS, et al (eds): The Year in Hematology. Plenum Press, New York, 1977.
14. Zucker-Franklin, D: Eosinophil function and disorders. Adv Intern Med 19:1, 1974.
15. Beeson, PB and Bass, DA: The eosinophil. In Smith, LH (ed): Major Problems in Internal Medicine, Vol 14. WB Saunders, Philadelphia, 1977.
16. Dvorak, HF and Dvorak, AM: Basophilic leukocytes: Structure, function and role in disease. Clin Haematol 4:651, 1975.
17. Parwaresch, MR: The Human Blood Basophil. Springer-Verlag, Berlin, 1976.
18. Metcalf, D: Detection and analysis of human granulocyte-monocyte precursors using semi-solid cultures. Clin Haematol 8:263, 1979.
19. Zucker-Franklin, D, et al: Atlas of Blood Cells, Function and Pathology, Vol 2. Lea & Febiger, Philadelphia, 1981.
20. Ebbe, S: Megakaryocytopoiesis and platelet turnover. Ser Hematol 1:65, 1968.
21. Till, JE and McCullock, EA: A direct measurement of the radiation sensitivity of normal mouse bone marrow cells. Radiat Res 14:213, 1961.

## Bibliography

Marcus, AJ and Zucker MB: The Physiology of Blood Platelets. Grune & Stratton, New York, 1965.
Wright, JH: The origin and nature of blood platelets. Boston Med Surg J 154:643, 1906.
Zucker-Franklin, D: The ultrastructure of megakaryocytes and platelets. In Gordon, AS (ed): Regulation of Hematopoiesis. Appleton-Century-Crofts, New York, 1970.

# CHAPTER 2

D. HARMENING PITTIGLIO, Ph.D., M.T.(ASCP)

# Red Cell Metabolism

Three areas of red blood cell (RBC) metabolism are crucial for normal erythrocyte survival and function: the RBC membrane, hemoglobin structure and function, and cellular energetics. Defects or problems associated with any of these areas will result in impaired RBC survival.[1] A thorough working knowledge of these areas of RBC physiology will ensure basic understanding of the various complex erythrocyte functions.

## RED CELL MEMBRANE

The actual biochemical structure and organization of the RBC membrane still remains to be elucidated. However, our general knowledge of all plasma membranes has been expanded. The RBC membrane viewed by transmission electron microscopy (TEM) appears as a trilaminar structure consisting of a dark-light-dark band arrangement of layers (Fig. 2-1). These layers represent (1) an outer hydrophilic portion chemically composed of glycolipid, glycoprotein, and protein; (2) a central hydrophobic layer containing protein, cholesterol, and phospholipid; and (3) an inner hydrophilic layer containing protein.

The RBC membrane represents a semipermeable lipid bilayer supported by a protein mesh-like cytoskeleton structure (Fig. 2-2). This fluid lipid matrix contains equal amounts of cholesterol and phospholipids with a mosaic of proteins interspersed throughout at various intervals. Those proteins that extend from the outer surface and traverse the entire membrane to the inner cytoplasmic side of the RBC are termed "integral" membrane proteins. The other class of RBC membrane proteins, called "peripheral" proteins, is limited to the cytoplasmic surface of the membrane, which is beneath the lipid bilayer and forms the RBC cytoskeleton. Both the protein and the lipids are organized asymmetrically

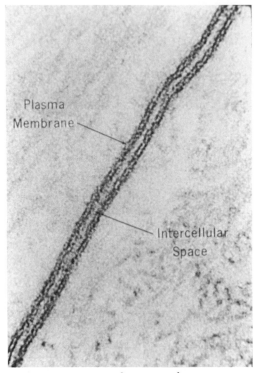

**Figure 2-1.** TEM plasma membrane.

within the RBC membrane. The chemical composition of the membrane mass is approximately 42 percent lipids, 50 percent proteins, and 8 percent carbohydrates.[2]

## Red Cell Membrane Lipids

### Phospholipids

The erythrocyte membrane lipid consists of a bilayer of phospholipids interspersed with molecules of unesterified cholesterol and glycolipids. Two groups of phospholipids are known to possess a distinct asymmetry within the bilayer matrix of the RBC: choline phospholipids and amino phospholipids.[3]

Choline phospholipids, consisting of phosphatidyl choline and sphingomyelin, are primarily located on the outer half of the lipid bilayer readily accessible to the external environment.[3] Due to their outward orientation in the lipid bilayer, the choline phospholipids may represent controlling points in the major pathways of lipid renewal as there is an exchange between plasma fatty acids and the RBC membrane. Fatty acids are incorporated through an energy-dependent process into membrane phospholipid. Therefore, changes in body lipid transport and metabolism may cause abnormalities in the plasma phospholipid concentration, which may alter the RBC membrane composition, resulting in a decreased RBC survival in circulation.

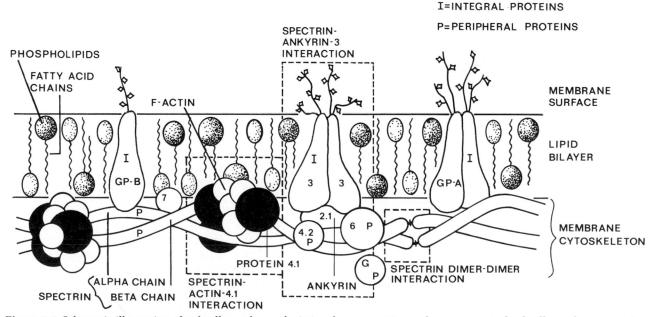

**Figure 2-2.** Schematic illustration of red cell membrane depicting the composition and arrangement of red cell membrane proteins. GP-A = glycophorin A; GP-B = glycophorin B; G = globin. Numbers refer to pattern of migration on SDS polyacrylamide gel pattern stained with Coomassie blue. Relations of protein to each other and to lipids are purely hypothetical; however, the positions of the proteins relative to the inside or outside of the lipid bilayer are accurate. Note that proteins are not drawn to scale and that many minor proteins are omitted.

In addition it is suggested that the interaction of these phospholipids with cholesterol may play a role in cholesterol homeostasis in the RBC membrane.[4]

In contrast, amino phospholipids, consisting of phosphatidylethanolamine and phosphatidylserine, are located almost exclusively on the inside half or cytoplasmic side of the RBC membrane along with phosphatidylinositol.[5] This specific orientation of these phospholipids maintains a precise lipid pattern that is critical to normal RBC survival in circulation. Alteration of this arrangement leading to the abnormal appearance of these amino phospholipids on the outer surface of the lipid bilayer promotes activation of the clotting cascade and may result in extravascular hemolysis.[2,6] Stabilization of this phospholipid asymmetry in the erythrocyte membrane is maintained through the interaction with specific peripheral proteins (see section on RBC membrane proteins).[7]

### Glycolipids and Cholesterol

The majority of the glycolipids are located in the outer half of the lipid bilayer and interact with glycoproteins to form many of the RBC antigens. Cholesterol is approximately equally distributed, being located on both sides of the lipid bilayer inserted between the choline and amino phospholipids.[4] Cholesterol comprises 25 percent of the RBC membrane lipid and is present in a 1 : 1 molar ratio with phospholipids. Red blood cell membrane cholesterol is in continual exchange with plasma cholesterol and is therefore affected by changes in body lipid transport. Accumulation of cholesterol results in morphologic changes in the RBC, such as target cells, and may cause RBC membrane damage (Fig. 2-3).

Acanthocytes, RBCs with irregular, spiny projections called spicules (Fig. 2-4), have also been associated with an excess accumulation of membrane cholesterol in association with liver disease and particular lipid disorders, such as abetalipoproteinemia. All of these RBCs have a decreased survival because the excess lipid makes the cell membrane less deformable.

Another example, the congenital deficiency of the plasma enzyme LCAT (lecithin: cholesterol acyltransferase), leads to an excess of free cholesterol in both the plasma and RBC membrane, resulting in, among other problems, a chronic hemolytic anemia.[1] In general, all of these lipids are mobile within the plane of the erythrocyte membrane; and as a result of this phenomenon, the RBC membrane is characteristically a viscous, two-dimensional fluid. This lipid bilayer also acts as an impenetrable barrier. Consequently, most transport across the RBC membrane is to occur through transport protein globules.

### Red Cell Membrane Proteins

It is estimated that 10 major and 200 minor proteins are asymmetrically organized within the RBC membrane. After solubilization of the RBC membrane with the detergent sodium dodecyl sulfite (SDS), membrane proteins can be separated by polyacrylamide gel electrophoresis and stained. The separated RBC membrane proteins are numbered 1 through 8 when stained with Coomassie blue and 1 through 4 when stained with periodic acid–Schiff (PAS) stain, which is the basis of their nomenclature (Fig. 2-5). The proteins range in molecular weight from 16,000 to 240,000 daltons.[2]

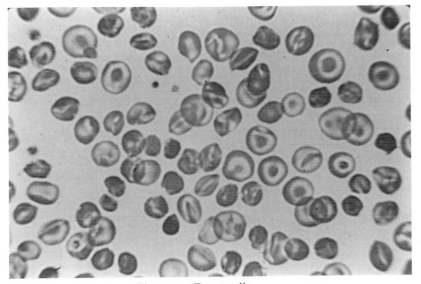

**Figure 2-3.** Target cells.

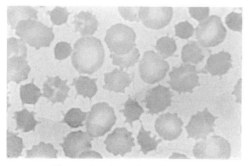

**Figure 2-4.** Acanthocytes.

Two of the most important protein constituents include glycophorin, an "integral" membrane protein, and spectrin, a "peripheral" membrane protein.

### Integral Membrane Proteins

Glycophorin, the major integral membrane protein, is the principal RBC glycoprotein, representing approximately 10 percent of the total membrane protein. The molecule contains approximately 60 percent carbohydrate and accounts for most of the membrane sialic acid, which gives the erythrocyte its negative charge. Glycophorin, similar to other

integral membrane proteins, spans the entire thickness of the lipid bilayer, and appears on the external surface of the RBC membrane, accounting for the location of many RBC antigens. Three types of glycophorins have been described—glycophorin A, B, and C (see PAS bands 1, 2, and 3).[7] In addition, all glycoproteins are exposed on the outer RBC membrane surface and migrate primarily in band 3 of the SDS gel electrophoretic pattern stained with Coomassie blue (see Fig. 2-5).[8] The majority of these proteins, as mentioned previously, carry RBC antigens and are receptors (such as the glycophorins) or are transport proteins (such as band 3, the anion exchange channel glycoprotein). It is speculated that band 3 and the glycophorins play a major role in anchoring the RBC membrane cytoskeleton to the lipid bilayer. As a result, lateral mobility of these integral proteins within the lipid bilayer is relatively restricted.

### Peripheral Proteins

Spectrin, the principal "peripheral" protein, is a large molecule that represents approximately 75 percent of the peripheral protein and 25 percent of the total membrane protein.[10]

Spectrin is composed of a helix of two polypeptide

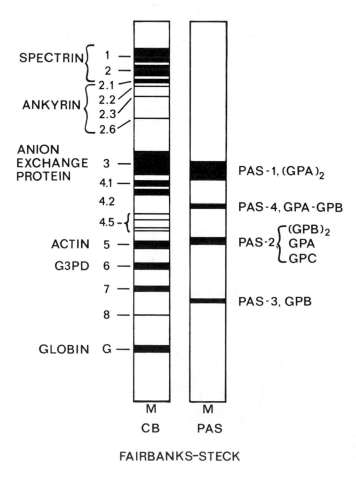

**Figure 2-5.** Schematic illustration of SDS polyacrylamide gel electrophoresis patterns of red cell membrane proteins stained with Coomassie blue (CB) and sialoglycoptroteins astained with periodic acid – Schiff (PAS) stain. GPA, GPB, and GPC refer to glycophorins A, B, and C, respectively. $(GPA)_2$ and $(GPB)_2$ are the dimers, and GPA-GPB is the heterodimer of GPA and GPB.

chains, an alpha chain (band 1, molecular weight 240,000) and a beta chain (band 2, molecular weight 225,000 daltons).[11] These chains form dimers which link together with other alpha-beta chains to form tetramers.[12] Spectrin is intimately related to RBC membrane integrity as it binds with other peripheral proteins such as actin (band 5), ankyrin (band 2.1), and band 4.1 to form a "skeleton" of microfilaments on the inner surface of the RBC membrane (see Fig. 2-2). These microfilaments strengthen the membrane, protecting the cell from being broken by circulatory shear forces, and also control the biconcave shape and deformability of the cell.[13] Two sets of spectrin complexes tie the RBC cytoskeleton network together: a spectrin-actin-band 4.1 complex, and a spectrin-ankyrin complex which binds to the integral protein, band 3, to anchor the skeleton to the overlaying lipid bilayer (see Fig. 2-2).[14,15] In addition, spectrin is also linked to the RBC lipid bilayer through the bonding between band 4.1 and the integral protein, glycophorin C.[16-17] The preservation of the spectrin-actin-band 4.1 and spectrin-ankyrin network, and thus the integrity of the RBC membrane, requires phosphorylation of spectrin by a protein kinase present in the membrane, which is energy-dependent, being catalyzed by ATP.[18] Other peripheral membrane proteins which lack carbohydrates and are confined to the cytoplasmic membrane surface include certain enzymes such as glyceraldehyde-3-phosphate dehydrogenase (band 6), and structural proteins such as hemoglobin.

As mentioned previously, the normal chemical composition as well as structural arrangement and molecular interactions of the erythrocyte membrane are crucial to the normal red cell survival in circulation of 120 days. In addition, they play a critical role in two important RBC characteristics: deformability and permeability.

## Deformability

As mentioned previously, a loss of ATP (energy) levels leads to a decrease in the phosphorylation of spectrin and, in turn, a loss of membrane deformability. An accumulation or increase in deposition of membrane calcium also results, causing an increase in membrane rigidity and loss of pliability. These cells are at a marked disadvantage when they pass through the small (3 to 5 $\mu$ diameter) sinusoidal orifices of the spleen, one of whose functions is extravascular sequestration and removal of aged, damaged, or less deformable RBCs or fragments of their membrane (see Fig. 2-6).[19] The loss of RBC membrane is exemplified by the formation of spherocytes (Fig. 2-7), cells with a reduced surface-to-volume ratio, and "bite cells" (Fig. 2-8), in which the removal of a portion of membrane has left a permanent indentation in the remaining cell membrane. The survival of these forms is also shortened.

## Permeability

The RBC membrane is freely permeable to water and anions; chloride ($Cl^-$) and bicarbonate ($HCO_3^-$) traverse the membrane in less than a second. It is speculated that this massive exchange of $HCO_3^-$ and $Cl^-$ ions occurs through a large number of exchange channels formed by the integral membrane protein, band 3, a glycoprotein previously described (see section on RBC membrane integral proteins).[3] In contrast, the RBC membrane is relatively impermeable to cations, with a half-time exchange of sodium ($Na^+$) and potassium ($K^+$) of over 30 hours. It is primarily through the control of the sodium and potassium intracellular concentrations that the RBC maintains its volume and water homeostasis. The erythrocyte intracellular:extracellular ratios

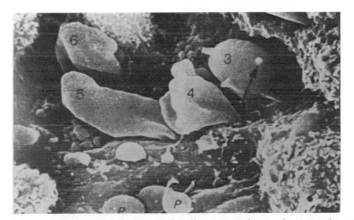

**Figure 2-6.** SEM of red cells (1 to 6) squeezing through fenestrated wall in transit from splenic cord to sinus. Epithelial lining of sinus wall, to which platelets (P) adhere, along with "hairy" white cells, probably macrophages, are shown. (From Weiss, L: A scanning electron microscopic study of the spleen. Blood 43:665, 1974, with permission.)

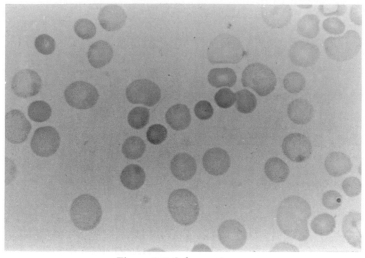

**Figure 2-7.** Spherocytes.

for sodium and potassium are 1:12 and 25:1, respectively. The passive influx of sodium and potassium is controlled by as many as 300 cationic pumps, which actively transport sodium out of the cell and potassium into the cell. Like other cationic pumps, these sodium-potassium pumps are energy-dependent requiring ATP. The functional active transport of these particular cations by these cationic pumps also requires the membrane enzyme, sodium-potassium ATPase. It is interesting to note that full activation of the sodium-potassium ATPase pumps requires the presence of the RBC membrane aminophospholipid, phosphatidyl serine.[3] Similarly, calcium ($Ca^{++}$) is also actively pumped from the interior of the RBC through the energy-dependent calcium-ATPase cationic pump. Calmodulin, a cytoplasmic calcium-binding protein, is speculated to control these calcium-ATPase pumps, preventing excessive intracellular calcium buildup, which is deleterious to the RBC, resulting in shape changes and loss of deformability. The permeability properties of the RBC membrane, as well as active cation transport, are crucial to preventing colloid osmotic hemolysis and controlling the volume of the red cell. In addition, ATP-depleted cells allow the accumulation of excess intracellular calcium and sodium, followed by potassium and water loss, resulting in a dehydrated, rigid cell subsequently sequestered by the spleen. The energy required for active transport and maintenance of membrane electrochemical gradients is provided by ATP. Any abnormality that increases membrane permeability or alters cationic transport may lead to a decrease in RBC survival.

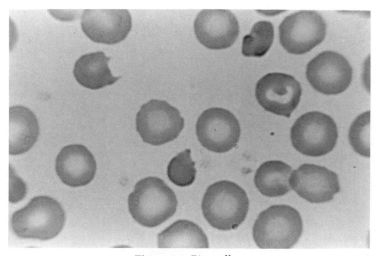

**Figure 2-8.** Bite cells.

## HEMOGLOBIN STRUCTURE AND FUNCTION

Hemoglobin, a conjugated protein with a molecular weight of approximately 68,000, comprises 95 percent of the RBC's dry weight, or 33 percent of the RBC's weight by volume.[20] Approximately 65 percent of the hemoglobin synthesis occurs during the nucleated stages of RBC maturation, and 35 percent occurs during the reticulocyte stage. Normal hemoglobin consists of globin (a tetramer of two pairs of polypeptide chains) and four heme groups, each of which contains a protoporphyrin ring plus iron $(Fe^{++})$.

### Hemoglobin Synthesis

Normal hemoglobin production is dependent on three processes (Fig. 2-9):

1. Adequate iron delivery and supply
2. Adequate synthesis of protoporphyrins (the precursor of heme)
3. Adequate globin synthesis

### Iron Delivery and Supply

Iron is delivered to the membrane of the RBC precursor by the protein carrier transferrin. The majority of the iron that crosses the membrane and enters the cytoplasm of the cell is committed to hemoglo-

bin synthesis and thereby proceeds to the mitochondria for insertion into the protoporphyrin ring to form heme. Excess iron in the cytoplasm aggregates as ferritin, the amount of which is dependent on the ratio between the level of plasma iron and the amount of iron required by the erythrocyte for hemoglobin synthesis. Two thirds of the total body iron supply is bound to heme in the hemoglobin molecule (see Chapter 4 for a discussion of iron kinetics).[20]

### Synthesis of Protoporphyrins

Protoporphyrin synthesis begins in the mitochondria with the formation of delta aminolevulinic acid ($\delta$ALA) from glycine and succinyl CoA, which is the major rate-limiting step in heme biosynthesis. The mitochondrial enzyme $\delta$ALA synthetase, which mediates this reaction, is influenced by erythropoietin and requires the presence of the cofactor pyridoxal posphate (vitamin $B_6$).[21]

In the cytoplasm, condensation of two molecules of $\delta$ALA, catalyzed by $\delta$ALA dehydrase, produces the pyrrole porphobilinogen (PBG). Uroporphyrinogen (UPG) is formed by the condensation of four molecules of porphobilinogen. Because four molecules are involved in this reaction, the formation of four types of isomers is theoretically possible. However, only two types of isomers have occurred

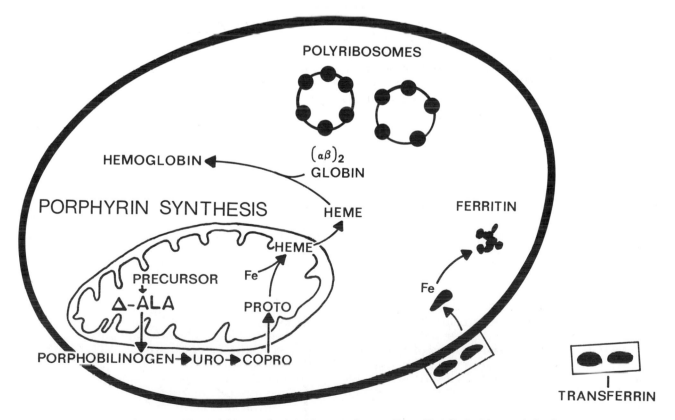

**Figure 2-9.** Hemoglobin synthesis in the reticulocyte. (From Pittiglio,[1] with permission.)

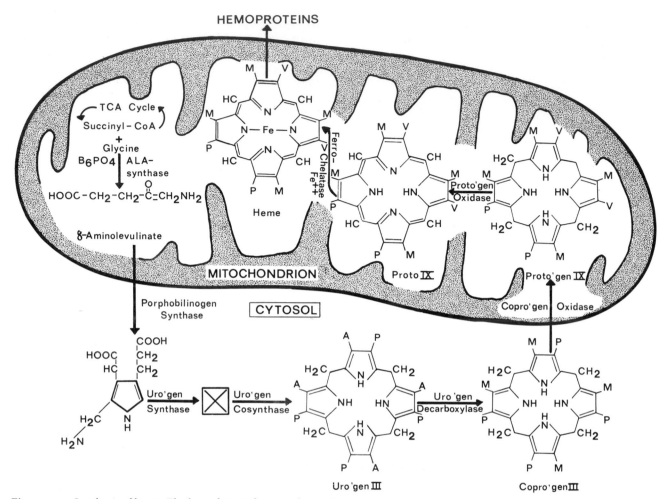

**Figure 2-10.** Synthesis of heme. The heme biosynthetic pathway showing the distribution of enzymes between the mitochondria and the cytoplasm. Intermediates between uroporphyrinogen and coproporphyrinogen, designated by $\boxed{X}$, remain unidentified. $B_6PO_4 =$ pyridoxal phosphate. (From Tietz, NW: Textbook of Clinical Chemistry. WB Saunders, Philadelphia, 1986, with permission.)

physiologically—UPG I and III—and virtually all of the UPG is the type III isomer. (The formation of UPG type I isomer represents an enzymatic "dead-end" pathway; heme can only be derived from UPG III (Fig. 2-10). This abnormal pathway is associated with a rare inherited disorder known as "congenital erythropoietic porphyria," resulting from large amounts of UPG I accumulating in the RBCs, bone marrow, and urine **(see Color Figure 63).**

Coproporphyrinogen (CPG) is next formed via decarboxylation reactions from UPG III. The final steps of heme synthesis are carried out in the mitochondria and involve the formation of protoporphyrinogen (PP) from CPG III. Because PP chemically has three types of side chains, 15 possible isomers of PP can form, compared with four possible UPG and CPG isomers. However, normal mitochondrial physiology leads to the formation of only one of these isomers, PP-IX, from CPG III. After further conversion of protoporphyrin IX, the incorporation of iron results in heme (ferroprotoporphyrin IX) formation (see Fig. 2-10).

Porphyrinogens, not porphyrins, are the intermediates of heme synthesis. Porphyrinogens are unstable tetrapyrroles that are readily and irreversibly oxidized to form porphyrins. In contrast, porphyrins are highly stable resonating molecules that are normally found in small quantities in the urine as the result of normal RBC catabolism.[21]

Excessive formation of porphyrins can occur if any one of the normal enzymatic steps in heme synthesis is blocked and can result in one of a number of metabolic disorders collectively called the porphyrias.

## Porphyrias

The porphyrias represent inherited metabolic abnormalities. There are two general types of porphyrias: erythropoietic porphyria, previously described, and hepatic porphyrias. Both of these represent inherited biochemical defects leading to excessive production of porphyrins in the two major sites of heme synthesis, the bone marrow and the liver, respectively.

One of the more common hepatic porphyrias, acute intermittent porphyria, is an autosomal dominant disorder characterized by acute attacks of abdominal pain, neurologic problems, hypertension, constipation, and psychiatric disturbances.[21]

General clinical manifestations of erythropoietic porphyria include photosensitivity and dermatitis, which results from the deposition of porphyrins in the skin, as well as hemolytic anemia associated with splenomegaly.[21] The mode of inheritance for congenital erythropoietic porphyria is autosomal recessive.

Two *acquired* conditions that need to be mentioned also lead to the excessive production of porphyrin precursors. These include lead intoxification and porphyria cutanea tarda, which develops most often as a result of chronic alcoholic liver disease.[16] Lead interferes with protoporphyrin synthesis, leading to a condition that mimics erythropoietic porphyria and is characterized by abdominal pain, neuropathy, and hypochromic anemia with basophilic stippling of RBCs and signs of hemolysis (Fig. 2-11). Lead intoxification does not produce photodermatitis characterized by other erythropoietic porphyrias.[17] Patients with chronic alcoholic liver disease may develop porphyria cutanea tarda, a condition resembling a hepatic porphyria and characterized by photodermatitis.

## Globin Synthesis

Globin chain synthesis occurs on RBC-specific cytoplasmic ribosomes, which are initiated from the inheritance of various structural genes. Each gene results in the formation of a specific polypeptide chain. Each somatic diploid cell, including the RBC, contains four alpha ($\alpha$) genes, two beta ($\beta$) genes, two delta ($\delta$) genes, and four gamma ($\gamma$) genes. The alpha genes are located on chromosome 16, and the beta, delta, and gamma genes are located on chromosome 11. The resulting gene products formed have been called alpha, beta, delta, and gamma chains. In the fetus, it should be noted that during the first few weeks of life, a different polypeptide chain, epsilon ($\epsilon$), is synthesized forming tetramer molecules that are designated "embryonic" hemoglobin ($\epsilon_4$ or $\alpha_2\epsilon_2$).[22] Figure 2-12 depicts the time sequence of globin chain synthesis during fetal development, birth, and infancy.

All adult normal hemoglobins are formed as tetramers consisting of two alpha chains plus two (non-alpha) globin chains. Normal adult RBCs contain the following types of hemoglobin:

92–95% of the hemoglobin is HbA, which consists of $\alpha_2\beta_2$ chains

3–5% of the hemoglobin is HbA$_{1c}$ (glycosylated), which consists of $\alpha_2$ ($\beta$-NH-glucose)$_2$ chains

2–3% of the hemoglobin is HbA$_2$, which consist of $\alpha_2\delta_2$ chains

1–2% of the hemoglobin is HbF (fetal hemoglobin), which consists of $\alpha_2\gamma_2$ chains

Each synthesized globin chain links with heme (ferroprotoporphyrin 9) to form hemoglobin, which primarily consists of two alpha chains, two beta chains, and four heme groups. Normal alpha chains consist of 141 amino acid residues linked together in a linear fashion, while normal beta chains consist of 146 amino acid residues. The precise order of amino acids is critical to the hemoglobin molecule's structure and function. The substitution of even one amino acid, such as valine, for the normal glutamic acid at the sixth position on the beta chain, can result in such functional abnormalities as a hemoglobin that tends to polymerize when deoxygenated (sickle hemoglobin). An adequate amount of globin chain synthesis is also important since decreased production of one of the polypeptide chains leads to a group of disorders known as thalassemia. Beta thalassemia, the more common form, refers to a decrease in beta chain production and alpha thalasse-

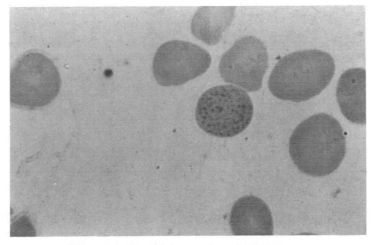

**Figure 2-11.** Basophilic stippling of red cells.

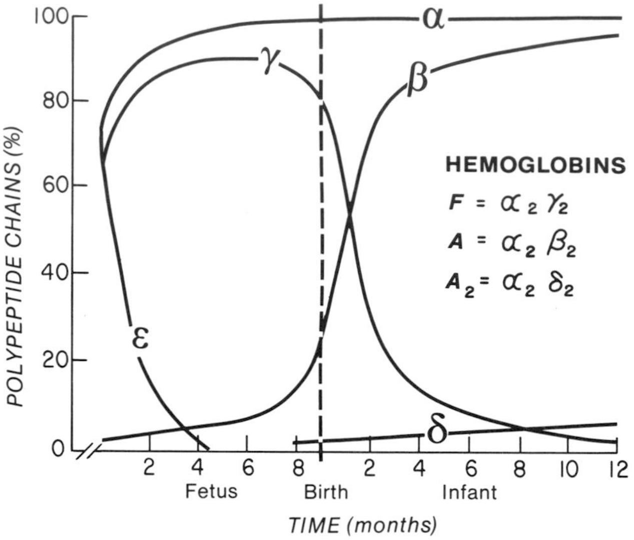

**Figure 2-12** Changes in globin chain synthesis during fetal development, birth, and infancy. (From Hillman, RS and Finch, CA: Red Cell Manual, ed 5. FA Davis, Philadelphia, 1985, with permission.)

mia refers to a decrease in alpha chain production (see Chapter 10).

The rate of globin synthesis is directly related to the rate of porphyrin synthesis, and vice versa; protoporphyrin synthesis is reduced when globin synthesis is impaired. There is, however, no such relationship with iron uptake when either globin or protoporphyrin synthesis is impaired; iron accumulates in the RBC cytoplasm as ferritin aggregates. The iron-laden, nucleated RBC is termed a "sideroblast," and the anucleated form a "siderocyte," when stained with Prussian blue for visualization of iron **(see Color Figure 64)**. When protoporphyrin synthesis is impaired, the mitochondria become encrusted with iron, which is visible around the nucleus of the RBC precursor when stained with Prussian blue. Such an RBC is termed a "ringed sideroblast" and is diagnostic for indicating a pathogenesis linked to deficient protoporphyrin synthesis **(see Color Figure 65)**.[21]

## Hemoglobin Function

Hemoglobin's primary function is gas transport (oxygen and carbon dioxide): delivery and release of oxygen to the tissues and facilitation of carbon dioxide excretion. Owing to hemoglobin's multichain structure, the molecule is capable of a considerable amount of allosteric movement as it loads and unloads oxygen. One of the most important controls of hemoglobin affinity for oxygen is the RBC organic phosphate 2,3-diphosphoglycerate (2,3-DPG). The unloading of oxygen by hemoglobin is accompanied by the widening of the space between beta chains and the binding of 2,3-DPG, on a mole-for-mole basis, with the formation of anionic

salt ridges between the beta chains. The resulting conformation of the deoxyhemoglobin molecule is known as the tense ("T") form, which has a lower affinity for oxygen. When hemoglobin loads oxygen and becomes oxyhemoglobin, the established salt bridges are broken and beta chains are pulled together, expelling 2,3-DPG. This is the relaxed ("R") form of the hemoglobin molecule and has a higher affinity for oxygen.

These allosteric changes that occur as the hemoglobin loads and unloads oxygen are referred to as the "respiratory movement." The dissociation and binding of oxygen by hemoglobin are not directly proportional to the $pO_2$ of its environment, but instead exhibit a sigmoid-curve relationship, the hemoglobin-oxygen dissociation curve depicted in Figure 2-13. The shape of this curve is very important physiologically, as it permits a considerable amount of oxygen to be delivered to the tissues with a small drop in oxygen tension. For example, in the environment of the lungs, where the partial pressure of oxygen (oxygen tension), measured in millimeters of mercury (Hg), is nearly 100 mmHg, the hemoglobin molecule is almost 100 percent saturated with oxygen (Fig. 2-13, point A). As the red cells travel to the tissues where the partial pressure of oxygen drops to an average 40 mmHg (mean venous oxygen tension), the hemoglobin saturation drops to approximately 75 percent saturation, releasing approximately 25 percent of the oxygen to the tissues (point B).

This is the normal situation of oxygen delivery at basal metabolic rate. In situations such as hypoxia, a compensatory "shift to the right" of the hemoglobin-oxygen dissociation curve (Fig. 2-14) occurs to alleviate a tissue oxygen deficit. This rightward shift of the curve, mediated by increased levels of 2,3-DPG, results in a decrease in hemoglobin's affinity for the oxygen molecule and an increase in oxygen delivery to the tissues. Note that the oxygen saturation of hemoglobin in the environment of the tissues (40 mmHg $pO_2$ [see Fig. 2-13, point B]) is now only 50 percent; the other 50 percent of the oxygen is being released to the tissues. The RBCs thus have become more efficient in terms of oxygen delivery.

Therefore, a patient who is suffering from an anemia due to loss of RBCs may be able to compensate by shifting the oxygen dissociation curve to the right, making the RBCs, while few in number, more efficient. Some patients may be able to tolerate anemia better than others because of this compensatory mechanism. A shift to the right may also occur in response to acidosis or a rise in body temperature. The shift to the right of the hemoglobin-oxygen dissociation curve is only one way in which patients may compensate for various types of hypoxia. Other ways include an increase in total cardiac output and increases in erythropoiesis.

A "shift to the left" of the hemoglobin-oxygen

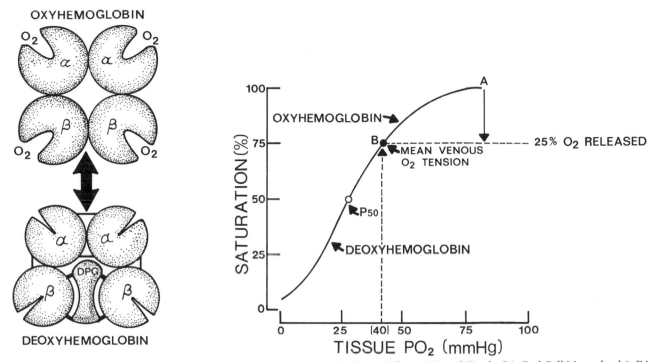

OXYHEMOGLOBIN

DEOXYHEMOGLOBIN

**Figure 2-13.** Normal hemoglobin-oxygen dissociation curve. (Modified from Hillman, RS and Finch, CA: Red Cell Manual, ed 5. FA Davis, Philadelphia, 1985.)

dissociation curve results, conversely, in an increase in hemoglobin-oxygen affinity and a decrease in oxygen delivery to the tissues (Fig. 2-15). With such a dissociation curve RBCs are much less efficient since only 12 percent of the oxygen can be released to the tissues (point B). Among the conditions that can shift the oxygen dissociation curve to the left are alkalosis; increased quantities of abnormal hemoglobins, such as methemoglobin and carboxyhemoglobin; increased quantities of hemoglobin F; or multiple transfusions of 2,3-DPG–depleted

stored blood (attesting to the importance of 2,3-DPG in oxygen release).

Hemoglobin-oxygen affinity can also be expressed by $P_{50}$ values, which designate the partial pressure of oxygen at which hemoglobin is 50 percent saturated with oxygen under standard in vitro conditions of temperature and pH. The $P_{50}$ of normal blood is 26 to 30 mmHg. An increase in $P_{50}$ represents a decrease in hemoglobin-oxygen affinity, or a shift to the right of the oxygen dissociation curve. A decrease in $P_{50}$ represents an increase in hemoglo-

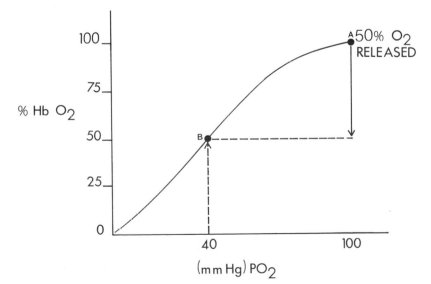

**Figure 2-14.** Right-shifted hemoglobin-oxygen dissociation curve. (From Pittiglio,[1] with permission.)

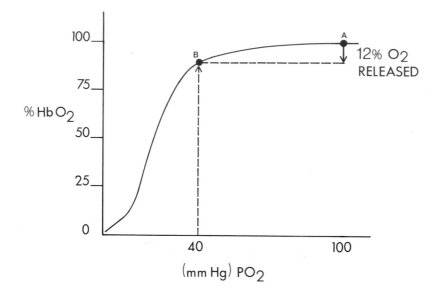

**Figure 2-15.** Left-shifted hemoglobin-oxygen dissociation curve. (From Pittiglio,[1] with permission.)

bin-oxygen affinity, or a shift to the left of the oxygen dissociation curve. In addition to the reasons listed previously for shifts in the curve, inherited abnormalities of the hemoglobin molecule can result in either situation; these abnormalities are described by the $P_{50}$ measurements. Abnormalities in hemoglobin structure or function can therefore have profound effects on the RBC's ability to provide oxygen to the tissues.

## Abnormal Hemoglobins of Clinical Importance

The hemoglobins previously described, oxyhemoglobin and reduced hemoglobin, are physiologic hemoglobins, because they function in the transport and delivery of oxygen within the circulation. Abnormal hemoglobins of clinical significance that are unable to transport or deliver oxygen include the following:

1. Carboxyhemoglobin
2. Methemoglobin
3. Sulfhemoglobin

In carboxyhemoglobin, the oxygen molecules bound to heme have been replaced with carbon monoxide (CO). This replacement process is relatively slow and dependent upon the concentration of carbon monoxide in the blood. Once attached, however, the binding of carbon monoxide to the heme of the hemoglobin molecule is 200 times tighter than the binding of oxygen to heme.[22] The concentration of carbon monoxide can be increased in a number of conditions, including chronic heavy smokers.

Methemoglobin is formed when the iron of the hemoglobin molecule is oxidized to the ferric ($Fe^{+++}$) state. In order to carry oxygen iron must be in the reduced ferrous ($Fe^{++}$) state. Normally, less than 1 percent of the total circulating hemoglobin is in the methemoglobin form. Increased formation of methemoglobin can occur as a result of an overload of oxidant stress owing to the ingestion of strong oxidant drugs, or as a result of an enzyme deficiency (see the section on RBC metabolic pathways).

Sulfhemoglobin is formed when a source of sulfur, such as a sulfur-containing drug or chronic constipation, builds up the sulfur content of blood. Sulfhemoglobin is incapable of carrying oxygen and represents an irreversible change of the hemoglobin molecule that persists until the RBCs are removed from the circulation. Both carboxyhemoglobin and methemoglobin, however, can be reverted back to oxyhemoglobin through the use of oxygen inhalation and the administration of strong reducing substances, respectively.

Table 2-1 lists the toxic levels for each abnormal hemoglobin at which cyanosis, anemia, and death may occur owing to a tissue oxygen deficit and increased concentration of circulating abnormal hemoglobin.

## MAINTENANCE OF HEMOGLOBIN FUNCTION: ACTIVE RED CELL METABOLIC PATHWAYS

Active erythrocyte metabolic pathways are necessary for the production of adequate ATP levels. Such generated energy is crucial to RBC survival and function in that it is necessary for maintaining

**Table 2-1. TOXIC LEVELS FOR ABNORMAL HEMOGLOBINS OF CLINICAL IMPORTANCE**

| Abnormal Hemoglobin | Toxic Level |
| --- | --- |
| 1. Carboxyhemoglobin | 5.0 g% |
| 2. Methemoglobin | 1.5 g% |
| 3. Sulfhemoglobin | 0.5 g% |

(1) hemoglobin function, (2) membrane integrity and deformability, (3) RBC volume, and (4) adequate amounts of reduced pyridine nucleotides.

Red blood cells generate energy almost exclusively through the anaerobic breakdown of glucose since the metabolism of the anucleated erthrocyte is more limited than that of other body cells. The adult RBC possesses little ability to metabolize fatty acids and amino acids. Additionally, mature RBCs contain no mitochrondrial apparatus for oxidative metabolism (see Table 2-2, which compares RBC metabolism during various stages of maturation). The RBCs metabolic pathways are mainly anaerobic, fortunately, since the function of the RBC is to deliver oxygen and not to consume it. Four pathways of RBC metabolism will be considered: the anaerobic glycolytic pathway and three ancillary pathways that serve to maintain the function of hemoglobin (Fig. 2-16). All of these processes are essential if the RBC is to transport oxygen and maintain those physical characteristics required for its survival in circulation.

Ninety percent of the ATP needed by RBCs is generated by the Embden-Meyerhof glycolytic pathway, the RBC's main metabolic pathway. Here, the metabolism of glucose results in the net generation of two molecules of ATP. Although this ATP synthesis is inefficient when compared with cells that use the Krebs' cycle (aerobic metabolism), it provides sufficient ATP for the RBC's requirements. Glycolysis also generates NADH from $NAD^+$, important in some of the RBC's other metabolic pathways (see further on).

Another 5 to 10 percent of glucose is metabolized by the hexose monophosphate shunt (also called the phosphogluconate pathway), which produces the pyridine nucleotide NADPH from $NADP^+$.[1] NADPH, together with reduced glutathione, provides the main line of defense for the RBC against oxidative injury. Oxidant drugs, as well as infections, can cause the accumulation of hydrogen peroxide and other oxidants, which can be toxic to cell proteins. The sequence of biochemical reactions shown in Figure 2-17 occurs within the normal RBC with adequate levels of appropriate enzymes and substrate to prevent the accumulation of these agents.

When the hexose monophosphate pathway is functionally deficient, the amount of reduced glutathione becomes insufficient to neutralize intracellular oxidants. This results in globin denaturation and precipitation as aggregates (Heinz bodies) within the cell. If this process sufficiently damages the membrane, cell destruction occurs. Inherited defects in the pentose phosphate glutathione pathway, the most common of which is G-6-PD deficiency, result in the formation of Heinz bodies with subsequent extravascular hemolysis. (It should be noted that glutathione not only is crucial to keeping hemoglobin in a functional state but also is important in maintaining RBC integrity by reducing sulfhydryl groups of hemoglobin, membrane protein, and enzymes subsequent to oxidation.)

The methemoglobin reductase pathway is another important component of RBC metabolism. Two methemoglobin reductase systems are important in maintaining heme iron in the reduced ($Fe^{++}$, ferrous), functional state. Both pathways are dependent on the regeneration of reduced pyridine nucleotides and are referred to as the NADH and NADPH methemoglobin reductase pathways. In the absence of the enzyme methemoglobin reductase and the reducing action of the pyridine nucleotide NADH, there is an accumulation of methemoglobin, resulting from the conversion of the ferrous iron of heme to the ferric form ($Fe^{+++}$). Methemoglobin is a nonfunctional form of hemoglobin, having lost oxygen transport capabilities as the metheme portion cannot combine with oxygen. Normal efficiency of the methemoglobin reductase pathway is exemplified by the fact that usually no more than 1 percent of RBC hemoglobin exists as methemoglobin in the RBCs of healthy individuals.

Another important pathway that is crucial to RBC function is the Leubering-Rapoport shunt. This pathway causes an extraordinary accumulation of

**Table 2–2. COMPARISON OF RED CELL METABOLIC ACTIVITIES DURING VARIOUS STAGES OF MATURATION**

|  | Nucleated RBC | Reticulocyte | Adult RBC |
|---|---|---|---|
| Replication | + | 0 | 0 |
| DNA synthesis | + | 0 | 0 |
| RNA synthesis | + | 0 | 0 |
| Lipid synthesis | + | + | 0 |
| RNA present | + | + | 0 |
| Heme synthesis | + | + | 0 |
| Protein synthesis | + | + | 0 |
| Mitochondria | + | + | 0 |
| Krebs' tricarboxylic acid cycle | + | + | 0 |
| Embden-Meyerhof pathway | + | + | + |
| Pentose phosphate pathway | + | + | + |
| Maturation and/or senescence | + | + | + |

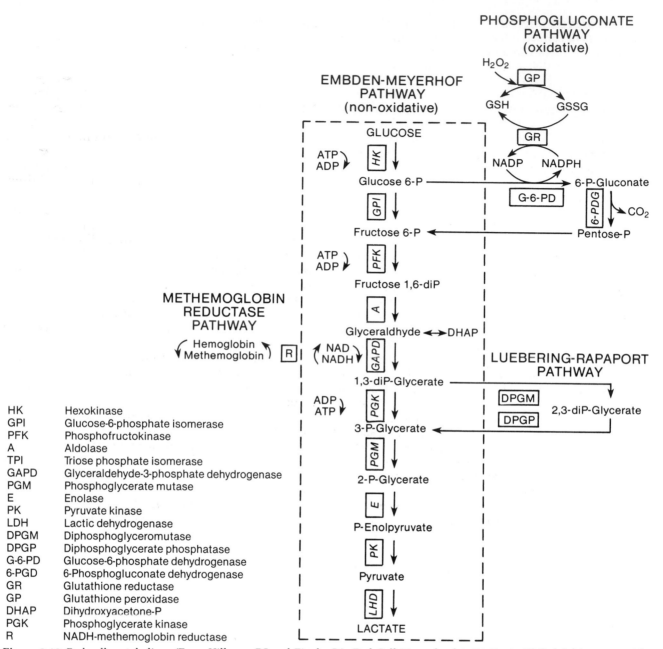

| | |
|---|---|
| HK | Hexokinase |
| GPI | Glucose-6-phosphate isomerase |
| PFK | Phosphofructokinase |
| A | Aldolase |
| TPI | Triose phosphate isomerase |
| GAPD | Glyceraldehyde-3-phosphate dehydrogenase |
| PGM | Phosphoglycerate mutase |
| E | Enolase |
| PK | Pyruvate kinase |
| LDH | Lactic dehydrogenase |
| DPGM | Diphosphoglyceromutase |
| DPGP | Diphosphoglycerate phosphatase |
| G-6-PD | Glucose-6-phosphate dehydrogenase |
| 6-PGD | 6-Phosphogluconate dehydrogenase |
| GR | Glutathione reductase |
| GP | Glutathione peroxidase |
| DHAP | Dihydroxyacetone-P |
| PGK | Phosphoglycerate kinase |
| R | NADH-methemoglobin reductase |

**Figure 2-16.** Red cell metabolism. (From Hillman, RS and Finch, CA: Red Cell Manual, ed 4. FA Davis, Philadelphia, 1974, with permission.)

Reaction A.    $RBC$ + infection or oxidant $\longrightarrow H_2O_2$

Reaction B.    $H_2O_2 + 2GSH$ (reduced glutathione) $\xrightarrow{\text{Glutathione peroxidase}}$ $GSSG$ (oxidized glutathione) $+ 2H_2O$

Reaction C.    $GSSG + NADPH$ (reduced form) $+ H^+ \xrightarrow{\text{Glutathione reductase}}$ $2GSH + NADP^+$ (oxidized form)

Reaction D.    $G\text{-}6\text{-}P$ (glucose-6-phosphate) $+ NADP^+ \xrightarrow{\text{Glucose-6-Phosphate dehydrogenase}}$ $6\text{-}PG$ (6-phosphogluconate) $+ NADPH + H^+$

**Figure 2-17.** Reactions within erythrocytes to prevent accumulation of oxidants.

the RBC organic phosphate 2,3-DPG, important because of its profound effect on hemoglobin's affinity for oxygen and also because its stores can serve as a reserve for additional ATP generation.

## Erythrocyte Senescence

The RBC, a 6 to 8 micron biconcave disc, travels 200 to 300 miles during its lifespan of 120 days. During this time circulating RBCs undergo the process of senescence or aging. Various metabolic and physical changes associated with the aging of RBCs are listed in Table 2-3. Each day 1 percent of the old RBCs in circulation are taken out by a system of fixed macrophages in the body known as the reticuloendothelial system (RES). These RBCs are replaced by the daily release of 1 percent of the younger RBCs, reticulocytes, from the bone marrow storage pool.[23] As erythrocytes become old, certain glycolytic enzymes decrease in activity, resulting in a decrease in the production of energy and a loss of deformability. At a certain critical point the RBCs are no longer able to traverse the microvasculature and are phagocytized by the RES cells. Although RES cells are located in various organs and throughout the body, those of the spleen, called "littoral cells," are the most sensitive detectors of RBC abnormalities. This is primarily due to the microanatomic arrangement of the spleen and its characteristic microvasculature, which reduces the plasma volume and flow of blood exposing the RBCs to the phagocytic action of the RES cells of the spleen for a longer time. Ninety percent of the destruction of senescent RBCs occurs by the process of extravascular hemolysis (Fig. 2-18). During this process, old or damaged RBCs are phagocytized by the RES cells and digested by their lysosomes. The hemoglobin molecule is disassembled, being broken down into its various components. The iron recovered is salvaged, and returned by the plasma protein carrier, transferrin, to the erythroid precursors in the marrow for synthesis of the new hemoglobin. Globin is broken down into amino acids and redirected to the amino acid pool of the body. Finally, the protoporphyrin ring of heme is broken down, exhaling its alpha carbon as carbon monoxide. The opened tetrapyrrole, biliverdin, is converted to bilirubin and carried by the plasma protein albumin to the liver. In the liver, bilirubin is conjugated to bilirubin glucuronide and excreted along with bile into the intestines. Here it is further converted through bacterial action into urobilinogen (stercobilinogen) and excreted in the stool. A small amount of urobilinogen is reabsorbed through enterohepatic circulation, filtered by the kidneys, and excreted in small amounts in the urine. Both unconjugated (prehepatic) and conjugated (posthepatic) bilirubin can be measured in the plasma as "indirect" and "direct" bilirubin, respectively, and used to monitor the amount of hemolysis.

Only 5 to 10 percent of normal RBC destruction occurs through the process of intravascular hemolysis (Fig. 2-19). During this process, RBC breakdown occurs within the lumen of the blood vessels. The RBC ruptures, releasing hemoglobin directly into the bloodstream. The hemoglobin molecule dissociates into alpha-beta dimers and is picked up by the protein carrier, "haptoglobin." The haptoglobin-hemoglobin complex prevents renal excretion of hemoglobin and carries the dimers to the liver cell for further catabolism. The hepatocyte uptake and processing is identical at this point to the process previously described for extravascular hemolysis (see Fig. 2-18). Haptoglobin levels, therefore, fall in plasma as it is removed as the hemoglobin-haptoglobin complex. It is estimated that as little as 1 to 2 ml of RBC intravascular hemolysis can totally deplete the amount of plasma haptoglobin. Normally, 50 to 200 mg/dl of plasma haptoglobin is available and represents the hemoglobin-dimer binding capacity. As haptoglobin is depleted, unbound hemoglobin dimers appear in the plasma (hemoglobinemia) and are filtered through the kidneys and reabsorbed by the renal tubular cells. The renal tubular uptake capacity is approximately 5 grams per day of filtered hemoglobin. Beyond this level, free hemoglobin appears in the urine (hemoglobinuria).

Hemoglobinuria is always associated with hemoglobinemia. Normal plasma hemoglobin levels are approximately 2 to 5 mg/dl, which is exceeded when free hemoglobin is released as a result of excessive intravascular hemolysis. Depending on the amount of hemolysis and type of hemoglobin, the plasma may be pink, red, or brown. Likewise, in hemoglobinuria the urine may also be pink, red, brown, or black. Two hemoglobin pigments, oxyhemoglobin and methemoglobin, are produced by auto-oxidation of the hemoglobin in the urinary tract when the urine is acidic. Oxyhemoglobin is bright red, and methemoglobin is dark brown. The

## Table 2–3. CHANGES OCCURRING DURING AGING OF RBC

| Increases | Decreases |
| --- | --- |
| Membrane-bound IgG | Several enzyme activities |
| Density | Sialic acid |
| Spheroidal shape | Deformability |
| MCHC* | MCV† |
| Internal viscosity | Phospholipid |
| Agglutinability | Cholesterol |
| Na+ | K+ |
| Methemoglobin | Protoporphyrin |
| Oxygen affinity | |

From Garratty, G: Basic mechanisms of in vivo cell destruction. In Bell, C (ed): A Seminar in Immune-Mediated Cell Destruction. American Association of Blood Banks, 1981, with permission.

*MCHC = mean cell hemoglobin concentration.
†MCV = mean cell volume.

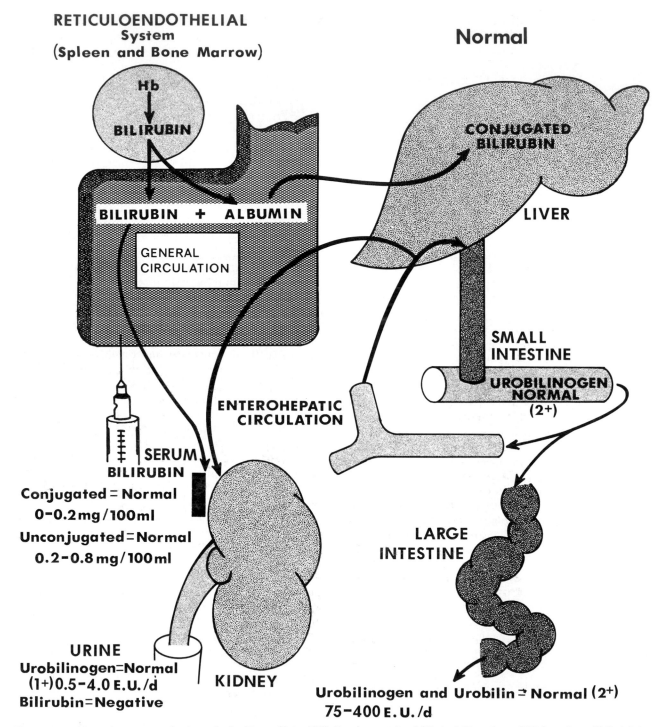

**RETICULOENDOTHELIAL**
System
(Spleen and Bone Marrow)

**Normal**

Hb

**BILIRUBIN**

**BILIRUBIN + ALBUMIN**

GENERAL CIRCULATION

**CONJUGATED BILIRUBIN**

**LIVER**

**SMALL INTESTINE**

**UROBILINOGEN NORMAL (2+)**

**ENTEROHEPATIC CIRCULATION**

**SERUM BILIRUBIN**

Conjugated = Normal
0-0.2 mg/100ml

Unconjugated = Normal
0.2-0.8 mg/100ml

**LARGE INTESTINE**

**URINE**
Urobilinogen = Normal
(1+)0.5-4.0 E.U./d
Bilirubin = Negative

**KIDNEY**

Urobilinogen and Urobilin ⇌ Normal (2+)
75-400 E.U./d

**Figure 2-18.** Normal extravascular hemolysis. (From Tietz, NW: Fundamentals of Clinical Chemistry. WB Saunders, Philadelphia, 1982, with permission.)

color of the urine, therefore, depends on the amount of hemolysis and concentration and relative proportions of these two pigments. Oxyhemoglobin predominates in alkaline urine, and methemoglobin predominates in acidic urine.

Hemoglobin, which is neither processed by the kidneys nor bound to haptoglobin, is oxidized to methemoglobin, which is further disassembled as metheme groups are released and globin degradated. Free metheme is quickly bound by another transport protein, "hemopexin," and carried to the liver cell to be catabolized as previously described. The heme binding capacity of hemopexin is approximately 50 to 100 mg/dl, and when this is exceeded

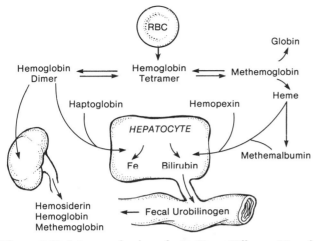

**Figure 2-19.** Intravascular hemolysis. (From Hillman, RS and Finch, CA: Red Cell Manual, ed 4. FA Davis, Philadelphia, 1974, with permission.)

the metheme groups combine with albumin to form methemalbumin. Albumin cannot transfer the metheme across the membrane of the hepatocyte for subsequent degradation. As a result, the methemalbumin circulates until additional hemopexin is produced by the liver to serve as the protein carrier. It is this circulating methemalbumin that imparts a brown tinge to the plasma or blood. (Table 2-4 provides a review of the various protein carriers discussed regarding hemolysis.) Intravascular hemolysis, as a result of RBC senescence, is so minimal that it is limited to the involvement of only haptoglobin, which is rarely depleted. Hemoglobinemia and hemoglobinuria, as well as the other processes discussed, come into play only with excessive intravascular hemolysis, which can occur in various hemolytic anemias (refer to Chapters 11 and 12).

## CONCLUSION

This chapter has outlined and described three important areas of RBC structure and metabolism. An understanding of these aspects of the RBC is important in appreciating the development and pathogenesis of the many forms of inherited and acquired RBC defects that result in hemolytic anemias.

**Table 2–4. PROTEIN CARRIERS**

| Protein | Substance Carried |
| --- | --- |
| Transferrin | Iron |
| Haptoglobin | Hemoglobin dimers |
| Hemopexin | Metheme |
| Albumin | Bilirubin |

## References

1. Pittiglio, DH: Red cell structure and function. In Clinical Hematology and the Blood Bank: Hemolytic Anemias. American Association of Blood Banks, 1982, p 1.
2. Wolfe, LC: Red cell membrane storage lesions. Transfusion 25:185, 1985.
3. Schrier, SL: The red cell membrane and its abnormalities. In Hoffbrand, AV (ed): Recent Advances in Hematology, Vol 3. Blackwell Scientific Publications, Oxford, England, 1982, pp 69–93.
4. Demel, RA, Jansen, JW, Van Dijck, PWM, et al: The preferential interaction of cholesterol with different classes of phospholipids. Biochim Biophys Acta 465:1, 1977.
5. Cohen, CM: The molecular organization of the red cell membrane skeleton. Semin Hematol 20:141, 1983.
6. Jain, SK, Mohandas, N, Clark, MR, et al: The effect of malonyldialdehyde, a product of lipid peroxidation, on the deformability, dehydration and $^{51}Cr$-survival of erythrocytes. Br J Hematol 53:247, 1983.
7. Tanaka, Y and Schroit, AJ: Insertion of fluorescent phosphatidylserine into the plasma membrane of red blood cells. J Biol Chem 258:11335, 1983.
8. Fairbanks, G, Steck, TL, and Wallach, DFH: Electrophoretic analysis of the major polypeptides of the human erythrocyte membrane. Biochemistry 10:2606, 1971.
9. Scamurra, D and Davey, FR: Anemias associated with spherocytic erythrocytes. Lab Med 16(2):83, 1985.
10. Sheetz, MP: Membrane skeletal dynamics: Role in modulation of red cell deformability, mobility of transmembrane proteins, and shape. Semin Hematol 20:175, 1983.
11. Knowles, W, Marchesi, SL, and Marchesi, VT: Spectrin: Structure, function, and abnormalities. Semin Hematol 20:159, 1983.
12. Coetzer, T and Zail, S: Spectrin tetramer-dimer equilibrium in hereditary elliptocytosis. Blood 59:900, 1982.
13. Mohandas, N, Chasis, JA, and Shohet, SB: The influence of membrane skeleton on red cell deformability, membrane material properties and shape. Semin Hematol 20:225, 1983.
14. Haest, CWM, Plasa, G, Kamp, D, et al: Spectrin as a stabilizer of the phospholipid asymmetry in the human erythrocyte membrane. Biochim Biophys Acta 509:21, 1978.
15. Lubin, B, Chiu, D, Schwartz, RS, et al: Abnormal membrane phospholipid organization in spectrin-deficient human red cells. Blood 62(Suppl 1):34a, 1983.
16. Wolfe, LC, John, KM, Falcone, JC, et al: A genetic defect in the binding of protein 4.1 to spectrin in a kindred with hereditary spherocytosis. N Engl J Med 307:1367, 1982.
17. Becker, P, Donner, S, and Lux, S: Evidence for a defect in spectrin thiols in the type of hereditary spherocytosis associated with defective spectrin-4.1 binding. Blood 62(Suppl 1):43a, 1983.
18. Palek, J and Lux, SE: Red cell membrane skeletal defects in hereditary and acquired hemolytic anemias. Semin Hematol 20:189, 1983.
19. Ferrant, A: The role of the spleen in hemolysis. Clin Hematol 12:489, 1983.
20. Perutz, MF: Hemoglobin structure and respiratory transport. Sci Am 239, 1978.
21. Robinson, SH and Glass, J: Disorders of heme metabolism: Sideroblastic anemia and the porphyrias. In Nathan, DG and Oski, FA (eds): Hematology of Infancy and Childhood, ed 2. WB Saunders, Philadelphia, 1981, pp 336–391.
22. Miale, JB: Laboratory Medicine Hematology, ed 6. CV Mosby, St. Louis, 1982.
23. Kapff, CT and Jandl, JH: Blood Atlas and Sourcebook of Hematology, ed 1. Little, Brown, Boston, 1981.

# CHAPTER 3

ARMAND B. GLASSMAN, M.D.

# Anemia: Diagnosis and Implications

## Definition of Anemia

Anemia in its broadest sense is a functional inability of the blood to supply the tissue with adequate oxygen for proper metabolic function.[1] Clinically, the diagnosis of anemia is made by patient history, physical examination, signs and symptoms, and hematologic laboratory findings. Determining the specific etiology of an anemia is of importance to the physician so that the appropriate therapy and prognosis related to the natural history of the disease can be applied for the patient. Anemia is usually associated with decreased levels of hemoglobin, or a decreased packed red blood cell (RBC) volume, also known as the hematocrit. There are rare circumstances in which abnormal hemoglobin levels have very strong oxygen-binding capacities or oxygen is not released normally to tissue, resulting in all the clinical signs and symptoms of anemia and yet a normal or raised level of hemoglobin or hematocrit. From a practical laboratory standpoint, the usual diagnostic criterion for a patient with "anemia" is a decreased hemoglobin (Hb), hematocrit (HCT), or RBC count.

Since the majority of patients with anemia have lowered hemoglobin levels, the status of anemia may be classified arbitrarily as moderate (10 g of hemoglobin/100 ml) or severe (less than 7 g of hemoglobin/100 ml).[2] Moderate anemias are not usually accompanied by clinically evident signs or symptoms. However, depending on the age of the patient or the cardiovascular condition, even moderate amounts of anemia can be associated with exertional dyspnea (difficulty breathing), light-headedness, vertigo, muscle weakness, headache, or general lethargy.

**Table 3–1. NORMAL VALUES FOR HEMOGLOBIN**

| | |
|---|---|
| Newborns (less than 1 wk old) | 14.0–22.0 g/dl |
| 6 months old | 11.0–14.0 g/dl |
| Childhood (1–15 yr old) | 11.0–15.0 g/dl |
| Adult Men | 13.0–17.0 g/dl |
| Adult Women | 12.0–16.0 g/dl |

## Considerations by Age, Gender, and Other Factors

Newborns (less than 1 week of age) have a hemoglobin of $18 \pm 4$ g/dl as a reference range. At approximately 6 months of age the reference range is $12.5 \pm 1.5$ g/dl. Childhood levels from the ages of 1 to 15 cover a reference range of approximately $13.0 \pm 2$ g/dl. Adult hemoglobin reference ranges are approximately $15.5 \pm 1.2$ g/dl for men and $14 \pm 2$ g/dl for women (Table 3–1). Reference ranges for individual laboratories reflecting the patient population served should be obtained. In the geriatric age group, the difference between hemoglobin levels of men and women is narrowed. Hemoglobin levels of geriatric men usually decrease slightly and begin to approach those of the postmenopausal woman. Many other factors enter into individual "normal" hemoglobin levels, including the geographic elevation at which one lives. Persons living in elevations above 8000 ft can have a persistent increase of their hemoglobin secondary to decreased oxygen saturation in the ambient atmosphere.[3] Diseases of the lung may alter oxygen diffusion at the lung alveolar membranes resulting in increased hemoglobin levels (secondary polycythemia) as an attempt to compensate for this.[4] Various diseases and disorders are associated with lower than usual hemoglobin levels and can include nutritional deficiencies, external or internal loss of blood, accelerated destruction of RBCs, ineffective or decreased production of RBCs, abnormal hemoglobin synthesis or bone marrow replacement by infection, suppression by toxins, chemicals, or radiation.[5]

## Causes of Anemia

The causes of anemia are multiple. They are generally classified as nutritional deficiency, blood loss, accelerated destruction, bone marrow replacement, infection or toxicity, hematopoietic stem cell arrest or damage, and hereditary or acquired.

## SIGNIFICANCE OF ANEMIA AND COMPENSATORY MECHANISMS

### Red Blood Cell and Hemoglobin Production

In a healthy ambulatory individual 1 percent of the circulating RBCs are replaced daily, and approximately 1 percent of these RBCs are reticulocytes.[6] In order to produce this number of RBCs with normal RBC maturation processes, one needs a bone marrow with adequate functioning stem cells and the ability to release mature RBCs from the bone marrow. Proper hemoglobin and RBC production requires a variety of nutritional factors including iron, vitamin $B_{12}$, folic acid, and normal hemoglobin synthesis pathways. The role of hemoglobin synthesis in anemias is covered in greater detail in the chapter on hemoglobinopathies.

In severe anemias (less than 7 g/dl) symptoms of functional impairment of a number of organ systems may be very evident. With minimal exercise, the patient's cardiac, pulmonary, and vasomotor rates may increase dramatically. If the anemia is secondary to blood loss and decreased intravascular volume, the patient's blood pressure may drop significantly when he or she is raised from the reclining to a sitting or standing position. The heart rate will be increased in order to elevate the cardiac output to keep pace with peripheral tissue oxygen demands in the face of a decreased oxygen-carrying capacity of the lowered hemoglobin level. Respiratory symptoms including dyspnea on exertion also may occur with anemia. An interesting compensatory mechanism that occurs is an increase in the 2,3-diphosphoglycerate (2,3-DPG) levels. This compound is a remarkable physiologic regulator of normal hemoglobin as it relates to its oxygen-carrying capacity and tissue oxygen delivery.[7] In the presence of 2,3-DPG, hemoglobin can more readily release the oxygen it is carrying to peripheral tissues. This enhanced release of oxygen occurs regardless of pH or blood arterial oxygen level.

Rapid blood loss of large volumes (greater than 10 percent total blood volume) may result in the aforementioned symptoms as well as hypotension and syncope. When there is a decreased hemoglobin level without blood loss to the external environment, there is a compensatory increase in plasma in order to maintain the intravascular volume. A person can have a moderately low hemoglobin and yet have few of the effects of the depleted intravascular volume because of these fluid shift mechanisms.

A normal individual responds to anemia with elevated levels of erythropoietin (see Chapter 2). Erythropoietin levels are sometimes used as ancillary diagnostic aids in the differential diagnosis of anemia. Responses of the bone marrow to produce new RBCs when given proper nutrients, vitamins, and other factors may be evaluated by the reticulocyte count.

## CLINICAL DIAGNOSIS OF ANEMIA

The clinical diagnosis of anemia is made by a combination of factors including patient history, physical signs, and changes in the hematologic profile. The signs and symptoms of anemia are generally nonspecific, such as fatigue and weakness, and may include gastrointestinal symptoms such as nausea, constipation, diarrhea, or increased gas. The patient may complain of dypsnea after a level of exertion that previously had not caused any problems. For example, an individual who previously could climb two flights of stairs without difficulty or significant shortness of breath, might report that he now must stop after climbing one flight of stairs and is then very short of breath. Subsequent information might indicate that he has passed very dark stools (melena), and measurement of his hemoglobin may reveal a level of 8 g/dl. The suggestion from the clinical information is that the patient's anemia is being caused by gastrointestinal bleeding.

Physical signs of anemia are usually not specific for the underlying disease. Occasionally, in patients who have specific physical findings, the underlying diagnosis may be suspected. One example would be signs of malnutrition and neurologic changes with loss of proprioception and vibration sense in a patient with vitamin $B_{12}$ deficiency.[8] Another example would be severe pallor, smooth tongue, and an esophageal web seen in a patient with severe iron-deficiency anemia.[9] Patients who are anemic may appear to have pale coloration of mucosal membranes, nailbeds, and skin in light-skinned individuals. Occasionally, a mild temperature elevation may be present, particularly in patients having certain types of hemolytic anemia. In the presence of anemia, heart murmurs may be heard, sometimes secondary to the cause of the anemia, owing to increased cardiac work load. Patients with bacterial endocarditis will have fever, heart murmurs, and anemia.[10]

## CLASSIFICATION OF ANEMIA

The individual types of anemias can be classified according to several different methods. Anemias are often classified according to their causes, such as blood loss, iron deficiency, hemolysis, or folate deficiency. Anemias can also be classified systematically by using hematocrit, hemoglobin, blood cell indices, and/or the reticulocyte count.[11] The laboratorian most frequently is involved in these quantitative measurements and subsequent evaluations.

The RBC indices are the mean cell volume (MCV), mean cell hemoglobin (MCH), and mean cell hemoglobin concentration (MCHC). The MCV is used as an estimation of the average size of the RBC, and may be either calculated by dividing the hematocrit by the number of RBCs, or directly measured using most automated cell counters (see further on). If the MCV is in the reference range, then the RBCs are referred to as being normocytic RBCs. When the MCV is less than normal, the RBCs are referred to as being microcytic; when greater than normal, mac-

rocytic. Both MCH and the MCHC are used to determine the content of hemoglobin in RBCs. The MCHC is said to be more reliable than the MCH, because it considers the entire blood volume rather than a single cell.[12] The MCH is not dependable when RBCs vary markedly in size. If there is a normal MCHC, then the RBCs are referred to as normochromic. Hypochromic RBCs have a less than normal MCHC; there are no truly hyperchromic RBCs.

The red blood cell indices are accurately calculated by the automated blood profiling machines. These instruments provide precise numerical values of the Hb, the numbers of RBCs, and the MCV. Although less accurate, careful microscopic examination of a peripheral blood smear can tell the examiner whether the RBCs are normocytic, microcytic, macrocytic, normochromic, or hypochromic. Red blood cell index calculations and reference ranges are:

MCV equals HCT (%) × 10, divided by RBC count (millions/mm³); reference range: $90 \pm 10 \ \mu^3$.

$$MCV = \frac{HCT \times 10}{(RBC \ count \ in \ millions)} \ or$$
$$(RBC \ in \ millions/mm^3)$$

MCH equals Hb (g/dl) × 10, divided by RBC count (millions/mm); reference range: $29 \pm 2$ g.

$$MCH = \frac{Hb \ (in \ grams) \times 10}{(RBC \ count \ in \ millions)} \ or$$
$$(RBC \ in \ millions/mm^3)$$

MCHC equals Hb (g/dl) × 100 divided by HCT (%); reference range: $34 \pm 2\%$.

$$MCHC = \frac{Hb \ (g/dl) \times 100}{HCT}$$

Use of the RBC indices in the differential diagnosis of anemia can provide a general idea as to what is occurring (Table 3–2). A normocytic normochromic anemia may be the result of bone marrow failure, hemolytic anemia, or some subset of either of these conditions. The differential diagnosis of bone marrow failure includes the concern for whether there was normal or decreased RBC production. Under consideration for hemolytic anemia, a reticulocyte count is usually of use and indicates that there is bone marrow capacity for increased RBC production while RBC destruction exceeds the amount of production. The reticulocyte count measures *effective* RBC production. Hemolytic anemia occurs when there is decreased RBC survival and may be the result of extracorpuscular, intracorpuscular, or a combination of extracorpuscular and intracorpuscular elimination.

Macrocytic normochromic anemias usually

Table 3–2. CLASSIFICATION OF ANEMIA BY RBC INDICES

| Size (MCV) ($\mu^3$ or fl) | Hgb Content (MCHC) (g/dl) | May be associated With |
|---|---|---|
| Normocytic 80–100 | Normochromic 32–36 | Bone marrow failure, hemolytic anemia, chronic renal disease, leukemia, metastatic malignancy |
| Macrocytic >100 | Normochromic 32–36 | Megaloblastic, nonmegaloblastic macrocytic anemias (e.g., liver disease, myelodysplasias) |
| Microcytic <80 | Hypochromic <32 | Iron deficiency, sideroblastic anemia, thalassemia, lead poisoning, chronic diseases, chronic infection or inflammation, unstable hemoglobins |

occur in association with folate or vitamin $B_{12}$ deficiency. The most commonly encountered anemias are the microcytic hypochromic anemias usually related to iron-deficiency anemia. Thalassemia, a hemoglobinopathy, is also a common cause of microcytosis. Less frequently seen are the sideroblastic anemias which are also associated with decreased mean corpuscular volume.

## DIFFERENTIAL DIAGNOSIS OF ANEMIA

The differential diagnosis of anemia is based on a combination of the clinical and laboratory findings, as shown in Table 3–2 and Figure 3-1.

## GENERAL COMMENTS ON TREATMENT OF ANEMIAS

The treatment of anemia should be dependent on its etiology. Anemias must be evaluated as to their cause before either supportive (e.g., transfusion therapy) or replacement therapy (e.g., iron for iron-deficiency anemia) is begun. Table 3–2 and Figure 3-1 represent only some of the possible causes for anemia. It is obvious that more than one cause of anemia can coexist in a patient. Obtaining the proper diagnostic studies in the shortest and most cost-effective manner is the responsibility of the attending physician and the professionals in the clinical laboratory sciences. More details concerning the appropriate treatment of anemias will be discussed in specific chapters.

The natural history of anemia depends on its etiology. For example, an iron-deficiency anemia associated with carcinoma of the colon may present first as simply an iron-deficiency anemia resulting from blood loss from the tumor. Later, with more extensive tumor involvement and possible replacement of the bone marrow, there may be a bone marrow failure component to the anemia because of bone marrow replacement (a myelophthisic anemia). Patients with pernicious anemia will require a lifetime of parenteral vitamin $B_{12}$ supplementation. Patients with megaloblastic anemia may require only a balanced diet and replacement of folic acid.

Transfusions may obscure and confuse the findings of necessary diagnostic tests in patients with anemia. Transfusions can suppress erythropoiesis; alter vitamin $B_{12}$, folate, and iron levels; and thwart the interpretation of diagnostic tests looking for the specific etiology of the anemia.

## TESTS IN DIAGNOSIS OF ANEMIA
### Hemoglobin

Hemoglobin is the main component of the RBC. It is the physiologic carrier of oxygen to tissues and acts as a buffer to handle carbon dioxide formed in metabolic activities. There are three common methods for measuring hemoglobin: the cyanmethemoglobin method, the oxyhemoglobin method, and the method in which iron content is measured. The cyanmethemoglobin method is the one recommended by the International Committee for Standardization in Hematology as modified in 1978 and will be the only one discussed here at any length. In this technique, blood is diluted in a solution of potassium ferricyanide and potassium cyanide. The hemoglobin is oxidized to methemoglobin and subsequently in the presence of the potassium cyanide forms hemoglobincyanide. The absorption maximum is at wavelength 540 nm. The absorbance of the solution is read in a spectrophotometer at 540 nm and compared with a standard cyanmethemoglobin solution. The advantages of this method are that most forms of hemoglobin are measured, the sample can be directly compared with a standard, the solutions are stable, and the coefficient of variation for the method is less than 2 percent at physiologic ranges.

Errors that can occur in the measurement of hemoglobin include improperly obtaining a specimen, improper handling of the sample, and difficulties with the reagents, equipment, or operator.

### Hematocrit

The hematocrit, or packed RBC volume, is the ratio of the volume of RBCs to the volume of whole blood. Hematocrit is usually expressed as a percentage (e.g., 42 percent) but may be expressed as a decimal fraction (e.g., 0.42). The venous hematocrit agrees closely with the central blood hematocrit but is greater than the total body hematocrit. Anticoagulants—usually EDTA, oxalate, or heparin—are used in order to keep the blood from clotting.

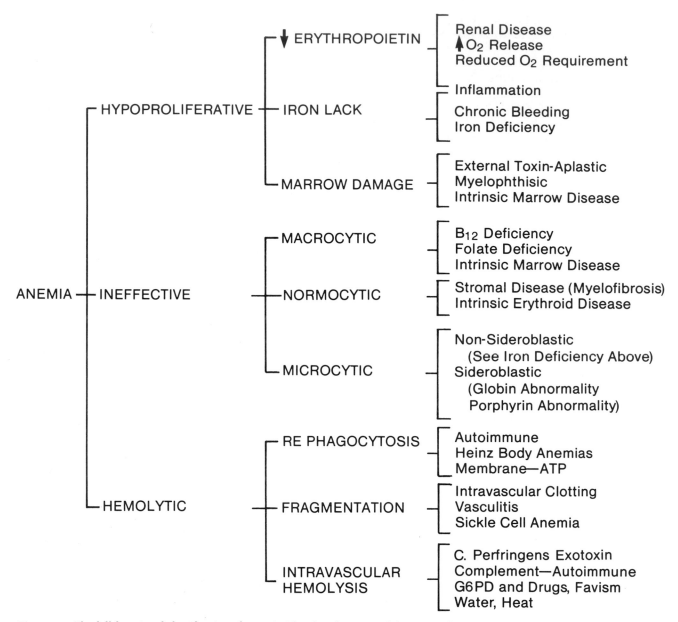

**Figure 3-1.** The full functional classification of anemia. The classification and diagnosis of an anemia are based on clinically recognizable abnormalities in erythron function. Initially, anemias can be subdivided as hypoproliferative, ineffective, or hemolytic. Each of these categories can then be further analyzed to reach a more specific diagnosis. (From Hillman, RS and Finch, CA: Red Cell Manual, ed 5. FA Davis, Philadelphia, 1985, p 58, with permission.)

Measurement of the hematocrit may be done by centrifugation or through calculations as done on many automated hematology instruments. The calculated hematocrit is the result of the mean corpuscular volume (MCV) times the RBC count.

The reference range for hematocrit is 40 to 51 percent in men and 37 to 47 percent in women. Different reference ranges are required, particularly for neonatal and early pediatric age groups.

Problems in the measurement of hematocrit can include incorrect centrifugation calibration, poor sample site, alteration of proper anticoagulant to blood ratio owing to amount of blood drawn, and reading error particularly for centrifuged hematocrits. The coefficient of variation for hematocrit, within the reference range, in our laboratory, is approximately 2 percent. With centrifuge hematocrit techniques, the lower hematocrit values are associated with the higher coefficients of variation.

## Red Blood Cell Indices

Red blood cell indices have been introduced briefly earlier. The mean cell volume (MCV) is the average volume of red cells and is measured directly or calculated from the hematocrit and RBC count (MCV equals the hematocrit times 1000 divided by the RBC count in millions per microliter) expressed in femtoliters or cubic micrometers.

The mean cell hemoglobin (MCH) is the content of hemoglobin in the average RBC. MCH is calculated from the hemoglobin concentration and the RBC count (MCH equals hemoglobin in grams per deciliter divided by the RBC count in millions per microliter).

Mean cell hemoglobin concentration (MCHC) is the average concentration of hemoglobin in a volume of packed RBCs. MCHC is calculated from the hemoglobin concentration and the hematocrit (MCHC equals hemoglobin [grams per deciliter] divided by the hematocrit and is expressed in grams per deciliter).

Red blood cell indices are readily available from the newer automated hematology counting devices. In those devices where the MCV is derived from the voltage changes formed during the RBC count and the hemoglobin is measured by spectrophotometric determination of the cyanomethemoglobin, the values are calculated as follows. The hematocrit equals the MCV times the RBC count, the MCH is measured by the hemoglobin divided by the RBC count, and the MCHC is measured by the hemoglobin divided by the hematocrit. The reference range for MCV in our institution is 80 to 94 fl; for the MCHC 27 to 33 pg; and for the MCHC 32 to 36 g/dl.

In various anemic states, the indices may be altered as follows. Microcytic anemia: MCV less than 80 down to a low of approximately 50 fl; MCH less than 25 pg down to a low of approximately 15 pg; and an MCHC of less than 30 down to 22 g/l. MCV values in the macrocytic anemias are usually greater than 100 fl and may be as high as or higher than 120 fl. The MCHC may be normal or decreased even in a macrocytic anemia. The MCHC may increase only in spherocytosis, if at all.

## Peripheral Smear

Much information concerning the etiology of an anemia can be determined from a peripheral smear. The size and shape of the red cells can be noted. Alteration in size of the RBCs results in anisocytosis; alterations in their shape results in poikilocytosis. The hemoglobin (chromatic) content of the red cells can be inspected visually on the peripheral smear. In addition, the peripheral smear may provide a clue to the etiology of the anemia or the bone marrow response, or both. The white cells may be evaluated. For example, lobulations of the polymorphonuclear leukocytes are seen in the hypersegmented granulocytes of macrocytic anemias. Coexistent neutropenia, thrombocytopenia, and anemia may indicate that there is bone marrow failure or a lack of a nutritional substances to provide adequate bone marrow production.

The presence of basophilic stippling in the RBCs may suggest the presence of increased bone marrow reduction and reticulocytosis. Basophilic stippling of RBCs indicates remnants of ribonucleic acid and may be associated with lead poisoning and some malignancies. Howell-Jolly bodies are small, round, blue inclusions seen in RBCs that are the result of leftover fragments of deoxyribonucleic acid. Howell-Jolly bodies are often seen in hyposplenism or asplenism, pernicious anemia, and some hemoglobinopathies, particularly thalassemia.[13] The Pappenheimer body is a purplish-blue granule when stained by Wright's stain and a coarse blue granule when stained with the Prussian blue iron stain. Pappenheimer's bodies are iron or siderotic granules. The clinical disorders associated with Pappenheimer's bodies include sideroblastic anemia, alcoholism, thalassemia, and some preleukemic states.[14] Iron granules found in nucleated RBCs are known as sideroblasts. Those found in RBCs without a nucleus are referred to as siderocytes. In ringed sideroblasts, there are more than five granules in a ring around the nucleus of an orthochromatic normoblast. Ringed sideroblasts are indicative of ineffective erythropoiesis.

A thread-like blue ring entirely contained within an abnormal RBC, which may or may not have a "figure 8" as well as a round or oval configuration, is known as a Cabot ring.[15] This is a remnant of the nuclear membrane. This may be seen in several clinical disorders including severe anemia. Heinz bodies are small, rounded, angular inclusions about 1 micron in diameter that are aggregates of denatured hemoglobin and are negative when stained with Prussian blue or other iron stains. Heinz bodies can be demonstrated only by using supravital stains (e.g., methylene blue) and are not visible with the usual Wright's stain. The clinical disorders that have been associated with the Heinz bodies include postsplenectomy, glucose-6-phosphate dehydrogenase deficiency after exposure to oxidizing drugs, a variety of unstable hemoglobinopathies, and alpha thalassemia.

## Reticulocyte Count

The reticulocyte count is of great use in determining the response and potential of the bone marrow. Reticulocytes are non-nucleated RBCs that still contain ribonucleic acid (RNA).[16] Reticulocytes may be visualized after incubation with a variety of so-called supravital dyes, including new methylene blue or brilliant cresyl blue. RNA is precipitated as a dye protein complex. Reticulocytes under normal circumstances lose their RNA a day or so after reaching the bloodstream from the marrow. A reticulocyte can be expressed as an absolute count, production index, or a percentage.

Interpretation of the reticulocyte count must take into account the age of the patient and nutritional status. Normal adults have a reticulocyte count of between 0.5 and 1.5 percent, or from 24 to 84 times $10^9$ reticulocytes per liter. The newborn has a higher reticulocyte count, which falls to the adult range usually by the second to third week of life. Sources of error in the reticulocyte count are associated with the sampling error of counting relatively few reticulocytes in a large number of erythrocytes. The 95 percent confidence level for counting 100 percent RBCs where the reticulocyte count is 1 percent ranges from 0.4 to 1.6 percent — obviously a very high coefficient of variation.

## Bone Marrow Smear and Biopsy

Bone marrow aspiration and biopsy are important diagnostic tools in determination of anemia. Bone marrow interpretation and evaluation will be covered later in this book. Factors to be evaluated in interpretation of a bone marrow aspirate smear and biopsy include maturation of the red and white cell series, presence of megakaryocytes, ratio of myeloid to erythroid series, abundance of iron stores, presence or absence of granulomas, tumor cells, and overall estimate of bone marrow activity (bone marrow biopsy).

Interpretation requires a differential count of the myeloid and erythroid series, an iron stain, and other appropriate stains if a differential diagnosis of lymphoproliferative or myeloproliferative disorders is entertained. Other appropriate specific stains may be indicated if metastatic tumor or infection is suspected or being evaluated.

## Hemoglobin Electrophoresis

Hemoglobin electrophoresis is used to identify hemoglobinopathies and thalassemia syndromes. There are a variety of techniques in hemoglobin electrophoresis, including standard cellulose acetate and barbital buffer methods and specific isoelectric focusing techniques. A minimum of a cellulose acetate and starch agar gel techniques using both barbital and citrate buffers should be available. Additional identification such as column separation of fetal and hemoglobin $A_2$ can be extremely useful. Interpretation of hemoglobin electrophoresis will be discussed further in the chapters on hemoglobinopathies.

## Antiglobulin Testing

The presence or absence of immune globulin, immune globulin fragments as well as complement and complement products on the RBC may be useful in the differential evaluation of hemolytic anemias. These techniques and reagents are often available in immunohematology (blood banking) laboratories. The presence of immune globulin or complement or both on the RBC surface in the proper clinical context can be supportive of a diagnosis of autoimmune hemolytic anemia.

## Osmotic Fragility

The osmotic fragility test is used to determine whether RBCs are more sensitive to lysis when they are introduced to solutions of hypotonic saline. A series of tubes containing solutions of saline from 0.0 to 0.9 percent are incubated at room temperature. Percent hemolysis is measured and plotted for each concentration. Spherical cells have a limited capacity to expand in these hypotonic solutions and lyse at a higher concentration of sodium chloride than do either the normal RBCs or cells from patients with a hemoglobinopathy or iron-deficiency anemia. In hereditary spherocytosis, RBCs have an increased osmotic fragility. This also may be seen in acquired spherocytic anemias. Patients with hereditary spherocytosis have increased autohemolysis as well.

Sucrose hemolysis is a related test. It is used to aid in the differential diagnosis of paroxysmal nocturnal hemoglobinuria (PNH) (see Chapter 11). Sucrose provides a low ionic strength solution that promotes the binding of complement to the RBCs. In PNH and some hypoplastic anemias, as well as in some preleukemic states, the RBCs are abnormally sensitive to this kind of complement-mediated hemolysis. Some overlap in positives is occasionally seen in megaloblastic anemias and some autoimmune hemolytic anemias. If a serum lacks complement activity, a false-negative test result can occur. The acidified serum test (Ham's test) is the definitive test in the diagnosis of PNH. In acidified serum, the complement is activated by the alternate pathway, binds to the RBCs and lyses the abnormal cells of paroxysmal nocturnal hemoglobinuria. Ten to 50 percent of the cells in PNH may be lysed in acidified serum. A positive test also occurs in congenital dyserythropoietic anemia type II (CDA-II) (see Chapter 7). Lysis occurs in CDA-II not with the patient's own serum but with the addition of other normal serum (with some, but not all, normal sera) and the sucrose hemolysis test result is negative.

## Red Blood Cell Enzymes and Metabolic Activities

Evaluation of a variety of enzymes in the carbohydrate aerobic and anaerobic metabolic pathways is possible. These enzyme deficiencies are associated with hemolytic anemias. The mature RBC lacks a nucleus and mitochondria. Ninety percent of the energy production occurs through the Embden-Meyerhof pathway.[17] Abnormalities in this pathway result in impaired high-energy phosphate generation and a chronic hemolytic anemia. Heinz bodies are usually not seen. The most common RBC enzyme deficiency is glucose-6-phosphate dehydrogenase deficiency, which is present in about 10 percent of black American men and which is also found in whites and orientals. The deficiency exists in X-linked and non–X-linked varieties. Pyruvate kinase (PK) deficiency is the most common RBC enzyme deficiency involving the Embden-Meyerhof glycolytic pathway.[18] It can result in a mild to moderately severe hemolytic anemia and splenomegaly. Inheritance is autosomal recessive, but PK mutants are thought to occur relatively frequently. A fluorescent spot test, in which the blood is mixed with the proper substrate plus coenzyme and buffer, can be used for qualitative identification of enzyme cellular deficiencies. Quantitative assays can be performed on a variety of spectrophotometric instruments. Other enzyme and metabolic abnormalities of RBCs do occur but tend to be much rarer. (For a more detailed discussion of enzyme deficiences, see Chapter 8).

## Red Blood Cell Protein and Membrane Studies

There are a variety of emerging techniques that can evaluate the lipid and protein makeup of the RBC membrane, but at present, they are not readily available as routine clinical laboratory tests. These techniques may be of great value in the differential diagnosis of some of the dyserythropoietic anemias. Assays of RBC membranes and proteins such as spectrin may aid in the understanding of spherocytic anemias and other related hemolytic anemias. Chapter 7 discusses the hemolytic anemias caused by membrane defects.

## Other Tests

Erythropoietin levels may be useful in determining a proper response of the bone marrow in disorders in which a high reticulocyte count is expected. A high erythropoietin level in the presence of a high hemoglobin level may indicate that there is an abnormal hemoglobin binding oxygen and not releasing it at the level of the tissues, or some other oxygen transfer abnormality. Deficient levels of erythropoietin may indicate a congenital absence of erythropoietin, or changes that cause decreased production of erythropoietin, or both.

## Bone Marrow Cultures

This is an emerging technology in which the attempt is made to grow bone marrow precursor cells in culture to determine the viability of stem cells.[19] The use of this technique for differential diagnosis of aplastic anemias and anemias of bone marrow failure is yet to be fully exploited. It is apparent that some of the aplastic anemias may be associated with either bone marrow stem cell failure, suppression of bone marrow stem cells by cells of the lymphocyte series or humoral antibody, or alterations in the bone marrow milieu that prevent maturation of the precursor cells.[20]

## Haptoglobin

Haptoglobin is an indirect test to measure the capability of circulating haptoglobin to bind released hemoglobin. It is of questionable use in the evaluation of hemolytic anemias.

## Serum Iron and Iron-Binding Capacity

Iron and iron-binding capacity tests are extremely important for differential diagnosis and definitive evaluation of iron in patients who have iron-deficiency anemia. The usual ratio of serum iron to iron-binding capacity is roughly 30 percent. Levels below 20 percent for serum iron in relation to serum iron-binding capacity are indicative of iron-deficiency anemia. Reference ranges for serum iron are approximately 50 to 150 mg/dl with an iron-binding capacity of 200 to 300 mg/dl. Transferrin and ferritin levels, which can be measured by enzyme-linked immunoassays or radioimmunoassays, can be useful in evaluation of iron-deficiency states. Ferritin level measurement is recommended for following bone marrow iron stores and can be a helpful test, particularly when there is severe iron deficiency or iron overload. Transferrin level measurement is not usually as useful.

The direct measurement of folate and vitamin $B_{12}$ levels by either radioimmunoassays or bioassays is useful for definitive diagnosis in assessing the differential diagnosis of megaloblastic anemias. Controversy continues as to whether one should measure folate and vitamin $B_{12}$ levels in the serum alone or whether there would be more sensitive testing in measuring intra-erythrocytic levels.

## Summary

Anemia has physiologic, functional, and quantitative parameters that may be related to hemoglobin or hematocrit levels. The differential diagnosis of anemia requires careful consideration of a wide variety of marrow, extramedullary, and inter-relating disease states. A broad and deep armamentarium of tests is available to aid in the differential diagnosis of the wide variety of anemias. In many respects, to know anemia is to know a great deal about clinical laboratory techniques and the practice of medicine.

## PATIENT STUDIES IN ANEMIA

Individual patient studies of anemia will be addressed in Chapters 4 through 14.

## References

1. Beck, WS: Hematology, ed 3. MIT Press, Cambridge, MA, 1981, p 16.
2. Wintrobe, M, Lee, BR, Boggs, DR, et al: Clinical Hematology, ed 8. Lea & Febiger, Philadelphia, 1981, pp 529–558.
3. Isselbacher, KJ, Adams, RD, Braunwald, E, et al: Harrison's Principles of Internal Medicine. McGraw-Hill, New York, 1980, pp 262–263.
4. Erslev, AJ: Polycythemia. In Wyngaarden, JB and Smith, LH (eds): Cecil's Textbook of Medicine. WB Saunders, Philadelphia, 1982, pp 937–943.
5. Rifkind, RA, Bank, A, Marks, PA, et al: Fundamentals of Hematology, ed 2. Year Book Medical Publishers, Chicago, 1980, pp 19–22.
6. Woodson, RD, Shahedi, NT, MacKinney, AA, Jr, et al: Introduction to hemopoiesis. In MacKinney, AA, Jr, (ed): Pathophysiology of Blood. John Wiley & Sons, New York, 1984, pp 12–15.
7. Wintrobe, MM, Lee, GR, Boggs, DR, et al: Clinical Hematology, ed 8. Lea & Febiger, Philadelphia, 1981, pp 94–95.
8. Kupp, MA, and Chatton, MJ: Current Medical Diagnosis and Treatment. Lange Medical Publications, California, 1980, p 293.
9. Nelson, DA and Davey, FR: Erythrocytic disorders. In Henry, JB (ed): Todd, Sanford, and Davidsohn, Clinical Diagnosis and Management by Laboratory Methods, ed 17. WB Saunders, Philadelphia, 1984, p 665.
10. Kaye, D: Infective endocarditis. In Kaye, D and Rose, LF (eds): Fundamentals of Internal Medicine. CV Mosby, St. Louis, 1983, pp 168–172.
11. Ravel, R: Clinical Laboratory Medicine: Clinical Application of Laboratory Data, ed 3. Year Book Medical Publishers, Chicago, 1978, pp 1–8.
12. Miale, JB: Laboratory Medicine Hematology, ed 6. CV Mosby, St. Louis, 1982, pp 379–380.
13. Williams, WJ, Beutler, E, Erslev, AJ, et al: Hematology, ed 3. McGraw-Hill, New York, 1983, pp 270–271.
14. Miale, JB: Laboratory Medicine Hematology, ed 6. CV Mosby, St. Louis, 1982, pp 488–489, 582.
15. Henry, JB (ed): Todd, Sanford, and Davidsohn: Clinical Diagnosis and Management by Laboratory Methods, ed 17. WB Saunders, Philadelphia, 1984, pp 609–610.
16. Wintrobe, MM, Lee, GR, Boggs, D, et al: Clinical Hematology, ed 8. Lea & Febiger, Philadelphia, 1981, p 112.
17. Nelson, DA, and Davey, FR: Erythrocytic disorders. In Henry, JB (ed): Todd, Sanford, and Davidsohn: Clinical Diagnosis and Management by Laboratory Methods, ed 17. WB Saunders, Philadelphia, 1984, p 687.
18. Wintrobe, MM, Lee, GR, Boggs, D, et al: Clinical Hematology, ed 8. Lea & Febiger, Philadelphia, 1981, p 773.
19. Nelson, DA and Davey, FR: Erythrocytic disorders. In Henry, JB (ed): Todd, Sanford, and Davidsohn: Clinical Diagnosis and Management by Laboratory Methods, ed 17. WB Saunders, Philadelphia, 1984, pp 626–629.
20. Erslev, AJ and Weiss, L: Structure and function of hemopoietic organs. In Williams, WJ, Beutler, E, Erslev, AJ, et al (eds): Hematology, ed 3. McGraw-Hill, New York, 1983, pp 78–81.

# CHAPTER 4

RICHARD P. JUNGHANS, Ph.D., M.D., AND
RONALD A. SACHER, M.D., F.R.C.P.(C)

# Iron Metabolism and Hypochromic Anemias

Iron is an important element in the biologic world. It is crucial to oxygen transport and functions as a central cofactor in catalytic energy transfer and reactions. Its absorption and storage are the focus of complex biologic mechanisms to ensure its continued availability to the needs of the body.

Iron is abundant in nature, and iron absorption is closely regulated to prevent iron overload. Paradoxically, however, iron-deficiency anemia constitutes the major disorder of iron metabolism.

This chapter focuses on the mechanisms responsible for iron balance in humans and reviews some of the metabolic functions in which iron participates. A discussion of the clinical syndromes of iron deficiency, iron overload, and defective iron utilization will be presented.

## NORMAL IRON METABOLISM

Iron is the most abundant trace element in the body. It is primarily used for hemoglobin synthesis, and approximately two thirds of the total body iron (2500 mg) is bound to heme. One milligram of iron is required for each milliliter of red cells (RBCs) produced. Each day 20 to 25 mg of iron are needed for erythropoiesis. Ninety-five percent of this required iron is recycled iron salvaged from normal RBC turnover and hemoglobin catabolism. Only 1 mg per day (representing only 5 percent of the iron turnover) is newly absorbed to balance minimal iron losses incurred by fecal and urinary excretion, as well as through sweating and desquamated skin. Figure 4-1 illustrates the continuous process of daily iron turnover. The remaining body iron representing one third of the total iron content is stored within the liver, spleen, and bone marrow or is carried in myoglobin and coenzymes of the cytochrome electron transport proteins.

**Distribution of Iron-Containing Compounds.** Iron-containing proteins are classified as heme and nonheme. The heme iron moieties contain a porphyrin-iron complex (Fig. 4-2) and include the oxygen carriers hemoglobin and myoglobin, certain catalases and peroxidases, and the cytochrome electron transport proteins. The nonheme iron-containing proteins include a large number of sulfur-iron bonding compounds such as the flavo-metalloproteins, xanthine oxidase, aldehyde dehydrogenase, and others that are frequently respir-

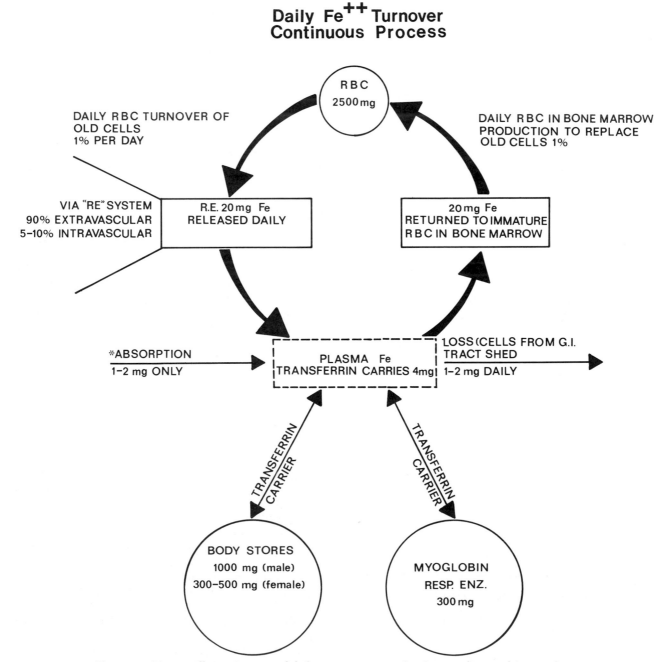

**Figure 4-1.** Diagram illustrating normal daily iron turnover and pathways of internal iron exchanges.

## PROTOPORPHYRIN IX

## HEME

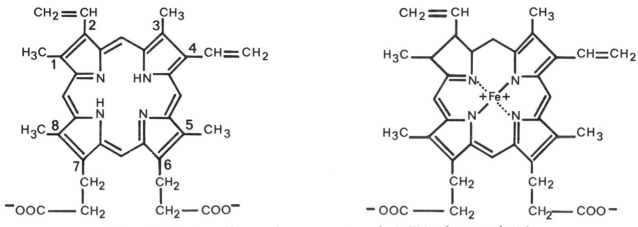

**Figure 4-2.** Structure of heme and precursor protoporphyrin IX (nonheme-porphyrin).

atory chain–linked. This group also includes the iron transport proteins transferrin and lactoferrin and the iron-storage protein ferritin.[1] Table 4–1 shows the distribution of iron-containing compounds in an average human adult.

## IRON ABSORPTION

Absorption of iron is regulated by a natural intestinal mechanism whereby the gastrointestinal (GI) mucosal cells admit just enough iron to cover losses, without permitting excessive absorption. An average absorption of 10 percent of the total dietary intake of 10 to 20 mg of iron per day is normal for a healthy individual. The amount of iron absorbed from the diet varies greatly depending upon the fol-

lowing: (1) the amount and type of iron ingested, (2) the presence or absence of other foodstuffs, (3) gastric acidity, (4) pancreatic secretion, (5) the state of the iron stores of the body, (6) the activity of the bone marrow, and (7) the state of the intestinal mucosa. Although the entire GI tract has the capacity to absorb iron, maximum absorption of iron occurs in the duodenum and upper jejunum, owing to the presence of optimum conditions of pH and redox potential. In the state of a severe iron deficiency, the body can increase absorption up to 30 percent to try to compensate for the depletion.

Elemental iron is biologically active in the ferrous ($Fe^{++}$) and ferric ($Fe^{+++}$) states. In general, an acidic condition, or lower pH, favors the ferrous state and iron absorption, whereas neutral and alkaline pHs favor the ferric state and decreased iron absorption.

## Table 4–1. DISTRIBUTION OF IRON IN HUMANS

| | Protein (g) | Iron Content (g) | Percent Total Body Iron |
|---|---|---|---|
| Hemoglobin | 750 | 2.5 | 65 |
| Myoglobin | 45 | 0.15 | 4 |
| Catalase | 5 | 0.005 | 0.13 |
| Cytochrome C | 0.8 | 0.003 | 0.08 |
| Transferrin | 10 | 0.006 | 0.15 |
| Ferritin, tissue | 5 | 1.0 | 30 |
| serum | 0.0004 | —* | |
| | | 3.7 g total | |

Values for a 70 kg man; differences with women are primarily in ferritin and ferritin iron, which may be only 20% of male levels in menstruating women. Catalase and cytochrome C are the major iron-containing catalytic proteins; other enzymes and cytochromes account for smaller proportions of iron use.

*Ferritin accounts for 0.2% of serum iron, or about 0.01 mg total.

## Iron Requirements

In an adult man, the average daily iron requirement is 1 mg/day. Most of this iron is necessary to replace intracellular iron that is lost as a result of shedding superficial epithelial cells from the GI tract and the skin. Since heme iron is the most abundant source of iron, RBC loss as a result of bleeding is the major source of iron depletion. In menstruating women, the average blood loss is 60 to 80 ml/month, representing approximately 30 to 40 mg of iron lost per month; an additional 1 to 1.5 mg of iron daily is therefore needed to maintain iron balance. Increased need above replacement also occurs during the first two years of infancy and during the period of peak growth phases of adolescence in boys and in women during pregnancy (Table 4–2). During pregnancy, iron absorption increases up to 20 percent.[6]

Table 4–2. RECOMMENDED DAILY ALLOWANCE (RDA) BALANCED AGAINST DAILY IRON LOSS

| | Urine, Skin, Feces | LOSS Growth (mg) | LOSS Menstruation (mg) | Pregnancy (mg) | INTAKE RDA mg (10% absorption) |
|---|---|---|---|---|---|
| Infants | 0.5–1.0 | 0.5 | | | 10–15 |
| Children | 0.5–1.0 | 0.5 | | | 10–15 |
| Adolescent male | 0.5–1.0 | 0.5 | | | 10–15 |
| Adolescent female | 0.5–1.0 | 0.5 | 1.0–1.5 | | 20–30 |
| Menstruating female | 0.5–1.0 | | 1.0–1.5 | | 15–25 |
| Pregnant female | 0.5–1.0 | | | 1.0–2.0 | 15–30 |
| Adult male | 0.5–1.0 | | | | 5–10 |
| Postmenopausal female | 0.5–1.0 | | | | 5–10 |

Modified from Hoffbrand, AV and Lewis, SM (eds): Tutorials in Postgraduate Hematology. Heinemann, London.

## Dietary Iron

Iron exists in foods in the form of ferric hydroxide compounds, ferric protein complexes, and heme protein complexes. The best sources of dietary iron are liver (as a repository of major body iron stores), red meat, egg yolk, enriched flour products, molasses, dried fruits, dark green vegetables, and legumes. Although spinach is rich in iron, it is a poor dietary source, because in this food iron is complexed with phosphates and phytates which render iron less soluble and therefore less available for absorption. Most food iron is complexed in the ferric form, and to be split from the protein or prosthetic group carriers it must first be reduced to the ferrous form before it is absorbed. This conversion is facilitated by gastric acidity and dietary ascorbic acid (vitamin C) found in fruit or fruit juices. Chelation of iron with low molecular weight compounds such as amino acids and fructose also promotes the solubility of iron, facilitating absorption. Cooking of foodstuffs helps to generate free iron by disrupting complex iron compounds.[1]

A normal diet in Western countries contains approximately 10 to 20 mg of elemental iron, and under ordinary circumstances only about 10 percent of this is absorbed. The recommended daily allowance (RDA) of iron for men, women, and children can be found in Table 4–2. It is difficult, however, to design a diet that contains more than 7 mg of iron per 1000 kcal in the absence of dietary supplements. Hence some programs have advocated requiring major supplementation of iron in all wheat flour, as is the custom in Sweden. Because there is a potential for iron overload and hemochromatosis in susceptible persons, however, this approach has been modified in most other countries.[8,14]

## Iron Transport and Storage

Iron is transported from the mucosal cells to the blood in the ferrous state, where it is converted to the ferric state by serum ferroxidases. It is then incorporated into a specific iron-transport protein, transferrin, a plasma betaglobulin, which binds up the two atoms of ferric iron per protein molecule. (Saturation averages 30 percent for each site, and both sites are occupied only in about 10 percent of the molecules. These numbers vary widely in iron-deficiency and iron-overload states.) Transferrin is a glycoprotein with a molecular weight of 80,000 daltons that is synthesized in the liver and has a half-life of 8 to 10 days. The transferrin capacity to bind iron in normal plasma is 240 to 280 mg/dl. Transferrin is also widely distributed in the extravascular fluid. The binding and release of ferric iron to transferrin is a dynamic process and transferrin readily releases its iron to the developing erythroid precursors. It attaches to receptors on the developing erythrocyte membrane, and free transferrin is then available to bind more iron.[1]

Following absorption, iron enters the portal circulation and is then delivered to the body tissues, where it is utilized. Transferrin unloads its iron to erythroid precursors for hemoglobin synthesis or to a wide variety of other tissues, most notably the liver, where it is bound to the major body storage protein, ferritin (Fig. 4-3). Approximately 10 to 15 percent of total body iron is stored as ferritin, constituting 0.5 to 1.0 g.

Ferritin is a large, multisubunit protein that exists in different forms (isotypes) in different tissues. The apoprotein apoferritin is a sphere-shaped molecule with a hollow core that is occupied by a ferric hydroxyphosphate complex. Each ferritin molecule has a capacity of about 4500 iron atoms, but occupancy averages 3000 or less.[10,12]

The amount of apoferritin produced by the body is influenced by the storage needs and by the iron available from the diet. In iron deficiency, very little is produced. When iron is absorbed in excess of the ferritin storage capacity, denatured ferritin and excess iron is deposited in lysozomal membranes to form a pseudocrystalline complex. This amorphous iron, termed hemosiderin, is visible on light microscopy by Prussian blue staining. A Prussian blue stain of bone marrow normally demonstrates approximately 25 percent of developing erythroid cells with cytoplasmic hemosiderin granules (sideroblasts).

All tissues synthesizing ferritin also release ferritin into the blood. This ferritin contains little or no iron and is partially glycosylated. Circulating ferri-

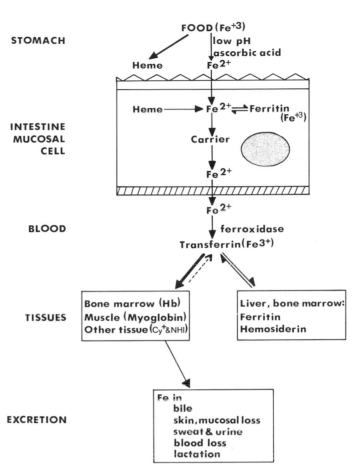

**Figure 4-3.** Iron balance in humans. Cy = cytochromic enzymes; NHI = nonhemoglobin iron.

tin is only a tiny fraction of the tissue stores (see Table 4–1), but this quantity of ferritin is in dynamic equilibrium with total body iron stores. Serum ferritin, however, may be elevated in acute inflammatory conditions or with liver injury (acute phase reactant), and therefore evaluation of iron stores in these patients may be more difficult.

When the body needs iron immediately in response to blood loss or during periods of dietary insufficiency, iron is released from tissue ferritin and transported via transferrin to sites of erythropoiesis. Approximately 40 mg of iron can be mobilized per day in individuals with average iron stores of 1 g. With stores of 0.2 g, only 20 mg per day can be mobilized and then only for a few days (see Fig. 4-1). Consequently, the ability to respond to iron need is greatly influenced by the magnitude of iron stores.

## Iron Recycling

The major biosynthetic demand for iron is in the production of hemoglobin for new erythrocytes. Red cells have a lifespan of approximately 120 days, implying a turnover of about 1 percent per day and accounting for 20 to 25 mg of iron, well in excess of the daily dietary requirements. This iron is virtually quantitatively recovered by the body for reuse. Senescent RBCs are phagocytized by macro-

phages of the mononuclear phagocytic system (MPS), also called the reticuloendothelial system (RES); hemoglobin is denatured; and heme is released into the cell cytoplasm (see Fig. 4-1). Catabolism of heme is achieved by microsomal enzymes. Released iron is then transported from the macrophage by transferrin, which makes it available for reuse in biosynthetic processes. Approximately 80 percent of the exchanged iron cycles directly between the erythroid marrow and the MPS. Hence, most of the iron used in synthesizing new hemoglobin is directly derived from the breakdown of hemoglobin released from effete cells (see Fig. 4-1).

Any free (ferrous state) iron released from hemoglobin will be converted to ferric iron by serum ferroxidases and bound to transferrin to re-enter the cycle of iron utilization.

## CLINICAL SYNDROMES

### Iron Deficiency

#### Etiology

Iron deficiency is a state in which body iron stores are depleted. The severity of the depletion dictates the degree of clinical disorder, if any. The causes of iron deficiency are related to poor dietary supplementation, diminished absorption, distribution defects, increased requirements, and excessive iron (blood) loss (Table 4-3).

Clinical iron deficiency as a result of decreased iron intake is rarely the primary reason for the deficiency. Since iron is present in low levels in a wide variety of foods, it may take many years to deplete body iron stores purely on the basis of decreased oral intake. However, iron depletion from decreased dietary intake can occur in infancy, as it is compounded by increased iron requirements. This is rarely a problem in Western countries, where iron fortification in food is common.

Diminished iron absorption is encountered in the presence of general malabsorption states such as celiac disease, or as a result of defective gastric function in achlorhydria or pernicious anemia or following gastrectomy.

Clinical iron deficiency, however, is most commonly produced by blood loss. As such, iron deficiency is a symptom of a disorder rather than a primary disease. Menstruating women account for the largest group of iron-deficient individuals. Laboratory evidence of iron depletion may be present in up to 30 percent of this group, and clinical iron deficiency may be found in 15 percent. The average menstrual cycle is associated with 60 to 80 ml of blood loss per month, and consequently menstruating women require 1 to 1.5 mg of additional iron over and above their usual body iron needs in order to maintain iron balance. In men and postmenopausal women, GI blood loss represents the major cause of iron deficiency. Conditions such as bleeding peptic ulcer, diverticulosis, inflammatory bowel disease, and hemorrhoids represent common causes of GI bleeding. Other causes of iron loss include coughing and expectoration of blood (hemoptysis), including idiopathic pulmonary hemosiderosis and Goodpasture's syndrome; blood loss in the urine (hematuria); blood donation (200 mg of iron lost per unit of blood donated); and hemodialysis.

Iron deficiency as a result of increased demand occurs most commonly in infancy when the demands for growth may be greater than the dietary supply.[6] Other situations of increased demand (without blood loss) may occur during the adolescent growth spurt in boys (but deficiency is rare), and during pregnancy. The greatest physiologic demands for iron may occur during the second and third trimesters of pregnancy. Expansion of the mother's RBC mass requires approximately 400 mg of iron, and the requirements of the fetus and placenta require an additional 400 mg of iron. The lack of bleeding as a result of amenorrhea occurring with pregnancy saves approximately 200 mg of iron, but the blood losses occurring following pregnancy account for as much as 250 to 350 mg of iron. Approximately 1 g of iron can be lost with each pregnancy. With total body iron stores representing only 0.5 to 1.5 g, rapid successive pregnancies in the absence of iron supplementation can easily deplete body iron and lead to clinically significant iron-deficiency anemia.

A rare but severe iron-deficiency state may occur with congenital deficiency of the iron-binding protein transferrin, called atransferrinemia. In this condition, total body iron stores may be normal.

## Anemia

Iron deficiency is the most common iron-related disorder, and anemia is its most prominent clinical manifestation. The clinical manifestations of iron-deficiency anemia are similar to those of anemia in other hematologic syndromes and depend on the degree of anemia present. Fatigue, lethargy, and dizziness are common. The elderly tolerate the anemia less well and may complain of palpitations, marked shortness of breath, and even chest pain with effort in the face of coronary artery disease. General clinical signs include pallor of the mucous membranes when the hematocrit is below 30 percent and evidence of a hyperdynamic circulation with bounding pulse and systolic flow murmurs.

Classically, the hematologic indices show a hypochromic (MCHC less than 30 g/dl), microcytic (MCV less than 80 fl) picture with an anemia of moderate to severe degree (hemoglobin less than 8 g/dl; hematocrit less than 30) (see Color Figure 66, and Table 4-4).[2,9] These numbers are usual for individuals who present with symptoms secondary to their anemia, but a wide range of findings is compatible with inadequate iron supplies. Most individuals with iron deficiencies have milder anemias and are asymptomatic.

Iron deficiency occurs in three phases (see Table 4-4):

1. Iron depletion: Ferritin and hemosiderin iron stores are depleted.
2. Iron-deficient erythropoiesis: Serum iron levels fall, and iron-binding capacity rises.
3. Iron-deficiency anemia: Hemoglobin falls, and anemia develops as the iron deficiency affects heme synthesis.

The anemia itself also proceeds in stages. The anemia is first normochromic and normocytic; then

## Table 4-3. CAUSES OF IRON-DEFICIENCY DISORDERS

| | |
|---|---|
| Dietary inadequacy | Increased iron loss |
| Malabsorption | Menstruation |
|   Gastrectomy | Gastrointestinal bleeding |
|   Achlorhydria | Hemoptysis |
|   Duodenal bypass | Hematuria |
|   Steatorrhea | Hemodialysis |
|   Celiac disease | Blood donation |
|   Pica | Increased iron requirements |
| Maldistribution | Pregnancy |
|   Atransferrinemia | Lactation |
|   Copper deficiency | Infancy |

**Table 4–4. SEQUENTIAL CHANGES IN DEVELOPMENT OF IRON DEFICIENCY***

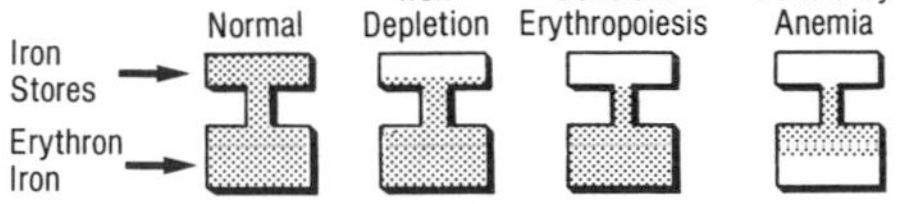

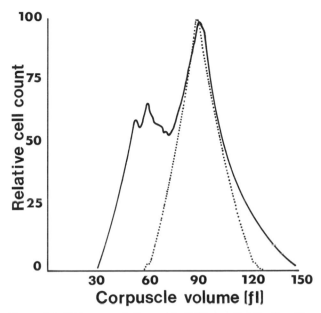

| | Normal | Iron Depletion | Iron Deficient Erythropoiesis | Iron Deficiency Anemia |
|---|---|---|---|---|
| RE Marrow Fe | 2-3+ | 0-1+ | 0 | 0 |
| Transferrin IBC ($\mu$g/100 mL) | 330±30 | 360 | 390 | 410 |
| Plasma ferritin ($\mu$g/mL) | 100±60 | 20 | 10 | <10 |
| Iron absorption (%) | 5-10 | 10-15 | 10-20 | 10-20 |
| Plasma iron ($\mu$g/100 mL) | 115±50 | 115 | <60 | <40 |
| Transferrin saturation (%) | 35±15 | 30 | <15 | <10 |
| Sideroblasts (%) | 40-60 | 40-60 | <10 | <10 |
| RBC Protoporphyrin | 30 | 30 | 100 | 200 |
| Erythrocytes | Normal | Normal | Normal | Microcytic/ Hypochromic |

*From Hillman, RS and Finch, CA: Red Cell Manual, ed 5. FA Davis, Philadelphia, p 60, with permission.

microcytosis gradually becomes evident; and finally the cells become hypochromic and microcytic as the anemia becomes more severe **(see Color Figure 66).** One of the early findings concealed in the "normal" MCV calculations is anisocytosis evident on the smear exam, which reflects the accumulation of smaller microcytic cells as they are added to the larger, older cell population that was produced when iron availability was better. At this stage the hemoglobin may still be within the acceptable range; however, the serum iron may be low and total iron-binding capacity elevated. Automatic counters capable of plotting size distributions clearly reveal the presence of these two populations (Fig. 4-4), until the anemia has become chronic and the microcytic cells predominate.[2] As the anemia progresses, severely hypochromic cells will appear as small hemoglobin rings with clear centers. The more severe anemias also accumulate bizarre forms (poikilocytosis) and nucleated RBCs showing decreased hemoglobinization and ragged cytoplasm **(see Color Figure 67).**

Iron-deficiency anemia (IDA) is an example of "ineffective erythropoiesis" due to a deficiency of iron that results in a decreased ability to make hemoglobin within the RBC. This is the most common type of anemia routinely encountered within the laboratory.

Hemoglobin formation requires not only adequate iron supply and delivery, but also adequate protoporphyrin synthesis to form heme and adequate globin synthesis (see Chapter 2).[1,11] A defect in any of these areas results in a hypochromic microcytic red cell due to the inability to form hemoglobin (Table 4–5). It is hypothesized that a smaller

**Figure 4-4.** Histogram of dimorphic RBC size distribution. Two populations of RBCs were present with MCV of 64 fl (microcytes) and 90 fl (normocytes), with a "normal" aggregate MCV of 81 fl. *Dotted line* shows profile of normocytic subject. (Adapted from Bessman, D: Erythropoiesis during recovery from iron deficiency: Normocytes and macrocytes. Blood 50:987, 1977.)

RBC occurs in these disorders, because deficient or decreased hemoglobinization of the cytoplasm at the correct stage of RBC maturation fails to signal the precursor RBCs to stop dividing. As a result, the RBC divides a greater number of times than normal, resulting in a nuclear-to-cytoplasmic maturation asynchrony. The cytoplasmic maturation lags behind the nuclear maturation, which leads to "ineffective erythropoiesis." Table 4–5 lists the various disorders of ineffective hemoglobin formation that lead to a microcytic hypochromic anemia.

## Other Clinical Consequences of Iron Deficiency

Although depletion of hemoglobin is the most important consequence of iron deficiency, depletion of iron-containing enzymes in other tissues may produce a wide range of other clinical disorders (Table 4–6). These manifestations of iron deficiency are rare, however, except when dietary iron is endemically poor or when severe and chronic deficiencies develop for other reasons.[4]

The iron enzyme myeloperoxidase is essential to

**Table 4–5. DIFFERENTIAL DIAGNOSIS OF HYPOCHROMIC MICROCYTIC ANEMIA**

1. Iron-deficiency anemia
2. Thalassemia syndromes
3. Sideroblastic anemias
4. Anemia of chronic disease

**Table 4–6. MANIFESTATIONS OF IRON DEFICIENCY**

Hematologic
   Anemia
   Immune deficiency
   Splenomegaly
Neurologic
   Pica
   Headaches
   Paresthesias
   Retinal hemorrhage
Epithelial
   Koilonychia (spoon nails)
   Lingual papillae atrophy
   Angular stomatitis
   Plummer-Vinson syndrome (hypopharyngeal-esophageal
      webs and dysphagia)
   Gastric atrophy
   Gastritis
   Achlorhydria
   Ozena (nasal mucosa atrophy)
Skeletal

neutrophil phagocytosis and bacterial killing, and both functions may be diminished with iron depletion. Cell-mediated immunity (a T-cell function) can be impaired, but antibody production (a B-cell function) is normal. However, clinical studies have not translated these findings into effects on susceptibility to infection. Splenomegaly may be encountered in association with the severest anemias (hemoglobin less than 7 g/dl) and probably reflects the greatly increased turnover of large numbers of poikilocytes produced. Other tissue manifestations of iron depletion may be found, such as cheilitis **(see Color Figure 68)**. In addition, depletion of cytochrome enzymes may produce early muscle fatigue and headaches.

Neurologic manifestations can include headaches, paresthesias, irritability, retinal hemorrhage (as in any severe anemia), and very rarely, papilledema and cerebral edema. Severe iron-deficiency anemia has reportedly been associated with benign intracranial hypertension. One relatively common and curious manifestation of tissue iron depletion is pica, a habitual craving most commonly expressed as ice eating (pagophagia) or as habitual eating of a crunchy food (such as pickles) or of starch. The symptoms generally resolve with iron therapy. (When pica is a primary disorder and involves clay or starch eating, iron deficiency may be the result.)

Iron deficiency can also express itself in the rapidly replaced epithelial tissues of the body, although the mechanisms involved are unknown. Koilonychia (flattened or "spoon" nails) is now relatively rare although once a "classic" manifestation **(see Color Figure 69)**. Tongue and oral lesions (glossitis, cheilitis) are far more common and are reversed with iron therapy **(see Color Figure 68)**. However, esophageal webs are not reversible and must be broken or dilated if symptomatic. The association of iron-deficiency anemia and esophageal webs—particularly postcricoid esophageal webs—has been called the Plummer-Vinson syndrome (Fig. 4-5). Forms of atrophy of the gastric mucosa are common and may be associated with gastritis or, in severe cases, with gastric atrophy and achlorhydria. This may perpetuate the blood loss and exaggerate the iron deficiency. Most gastric changes are asymptomatic. The presence of a secondary achlorhydria of course would diminish the body's ability to absorb iron necessary to relieve the condition. In some cases the gastric atrophy is permanent.

Bony changes are rare but may present in children with chronic iron deficiency as widened diploic spaces of the skull and medullary expansion with cortical thinning of linear bone.

## Therapy

It should be emphasized that iron-deficiency anemia is a symptom and not the cause of a disease process. Therefore, therapy is directed primarily toward treatment of the underlying disease (e.g., correction of cause of bleeding) and then toward treatment of the iron deficiency. In severe iron deficiency, the RBC mass is approximately half normal size and the recycled iron approximates 10 mg/day. When therapy is instituted, the maximal iron that can be utilized to make new hemoglobin is only modestly in excess of 20 mg. In iron-deficiency ane-

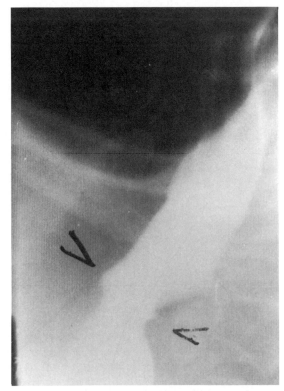

**Figure 4-5.** Esophageal webs in Plummer-Vinson syndrome (barium swallow roentgenogram).

mia, the number of developing RBCs within the marrow is usually not decreased. However, neither is the erythroid marrow greatly expanded (as in pernicious anemia or chronic hemolytic states) and iron therapy consequently will result only in a modest increase in production of new cells. However, iron incorporation will be much greater when available iron is present. The implication then is that much larger amounts of absorbed iron will not hasten recovery from the anemia any sooner than the additional 20 mg/day required to meet erythron needs. The excess will instead move into tissue storage, replenishing iron stores, which is the second major goal of therapy.[3]

Iron stores are created by slow accumulation over a period of years, and unsupplemented diet alone cannot be used therapeutically to correct iron deficiency. For example, even a half pound of steak each day would provide only 8 mg of iron. Therapy is directed at providing 150 to 200 mg of elemental iron per day. This is usually administered in the form of supplemental ferrous sulfate tablets or elixir. Parenteral therapy is available but infrequently indicated. Each tablet (hydrated ferrous sulfate) contains 300 mg of the salt and 60 mg of elemental iron. Ferrous sulfate in an iron-deficient patient is 10 to 20 percent absorbed on an empty stomach. The therapeutic goal of providing 150 to 200 mg of elemental iron is met with three to four tablets of ferrous sulfate.

Absorption of ferrous sulfate is best when taken at least 1 hour before meals, but gastric side effects may occur in many patients—including GI irritability, nausea, diarrhea, and/or constipation—and may dictate that the medicine be taken with meals. The dose may be decreased to two tablets if necessary to ensure patient compliance and still obtain a therapeutic effect. One study compared doses of 100 mg and 400 mg of iron per day in iron-deficient patients. At the end of four weeks, the anemia in each group had resolved and the excess that had been absorbed and consequently moved into storage differed only marginally; 70 mg and 125 mg, respectively.[3]

The response to therapy occurs in three stages. The first is an improvement in the feeling of well-being, with disappearance of pica and reversal of oral and tongue lesions over the first to the seventh day of treatment. The second stage begins with a modest reticulocytosis of 5 to 10 percent occurring one week after instituting therapy (see **Color Figure 70**). A patient with appropriately responding iron-deficiency anemia should be at least one half corrected by 18 days. All should be fully normalized by one to two months. The third phase, which begins concurrent with the first two, is replenishment of the storage iron. Throughout therapy, iron is absorbed in excess of what can be used for producing new RBCs and meeting other metabolic needs of the body. As previously indicated, even these iron stores must accumulate gradually and cannot be "forced" by higher doses of oral iron.

Following two months of therapy and correction of anemia (a sign of adequate absorption), there should have been a modest replenishment of iron stores (to a level of approximately 100 to 200 mg). At this time it is reasonable to reduce the iron supplementation to one tablet daily, and subsequently to reduce it to one tablet three to four times per week as chronic therapy. If an underlying pathologic lesion has been corrected (e.g., bleeding polyps), it may be possible to discontinue iron therapy altogether after the initial two-month period of treatment and to rely on diet alone for gradual replenishment of iron stores. One tablet (60 mg/day) is adequate supplementation for prophylaxis during pregnancy.

Many iron formulations are available, but none offer significant advantages over ferrous sulfate and nearly all are far more expensive.[5] Ferrous gluconate and ferrous fumarate yield equivalent absorption and response per milligram of iron. Contrary to manufacturer claims, however, it is doubtful that gastric effects are any less. Enteric-coated and prolonged-release forms of iron can reduce iron absorption, and combination pills containing ascorbic acid or other marginal "enhancers" often increase side effects and costs when a small increase in non-enteric ferrous sulfate would do just as well at a much lower cost. In any case, as discussed earlier, there is limited clinical value in "pushing" iron doses to very high levels.

When patients cannot tolerate the GI side effects of ferrous sulfate, when patient's compliance is poor, or in conditions when malabsorption states are present, parenteral iron in the form of iron dextran can be substituted. Parenteral iron is given either intramuscularly or intravenously. The intramuscular administration can be given in divided doses over an extended period of time after calculating the amount of iron needed to correct the anemia and to replenish iron stores. The intravenous dose can be administered in a bolus infusion. Anaphylaxis is an infrequent consequence of either method of parenteral administration, but the risks associated with intravenous use are considered less.

## Iron Overload

### Hemosiderosis

Hemosiderosis is the accumulation of iron to supranormal levels, producing gross hemosiderin deposition in macrophages of the spleen, liver, bone marrow, and other tissues.[0,14] In hemosiderosis iron deposition is predominantly in reticuloendothelial cells, whereas the iron overload in hemochromatosis leads to deposition in parenchymal cells. The most important causes of hemosiderosis are hemolytic anemias, multiple blood transfusions, and disorders of erythropoiesis (megaloblastic anemia, sideroblastic anemia, and thalassemias). Chronic exposures to high dietary iron and increased iron absorption caused by chronic alcohol abuse can also generate systemic iron overload. In general, the reticuloendothelial iron deposition in hemosiderosis is not usually accompanied by organ damage but may lead to hemochromatosis, in which such damage can occur.

There is a direct relationship between the percentage of saturation of transferrin and the level of iron within the reticuloendothelial stores. An increase in iron stores is usually associated with a high percentage saturation of transferrin, except in situations of chronic disease (Table 4–7). Desferrioxamine-induced urinary iron excretion is generally greater than 4 mg/day (normal is less than 2 mg/24 hr) and is a good measure of the existence of iron overload. Desferrioxamine may also be used in the therapeutic management of the iron overload states (see further on).[13]

## Hemochromatosis

Hemochromatosis is a more severe form of iron accumulation that has progressed over a long period of time to involve widespread parenchymal iron deposition and organ injury (see Color Figure 71).[8,14] It presents classically as a triad of skin pigmentation, diabetes mellitus, and hepatomegaly (often cirrhosis), with or without heart disease and hypogonadism. This has led to the classic terms "bronze diabetes" and "pigment cirrhosis." The bronze skin discoloration is due primarily to an effect on the melanin synthesis and is not due to frank iron deposition in the skin. Morbidity is most commonly related to the cirrhosis and diabetes when the dis-

order is advanced, and there is an elevated incidence of hepatocellular carcinoma. Heart failure and arrhythmias may also develop. Hematologic consequences of hemochromatosis are few.

All causes of hemosiderosis when taken to extreme can result in iron deposition within parenchymal cells and potentially parenchymal damage. Idiopathic hemochromatosis is a recessively inherited syndrome in which regulation of iron absorption is defective and abnormally high levels of iron accumulate within the parenchymal cells with relatively minimal deposition within the reticuloendothelial system (see Color Figure 71).[14] Full expression of the syndrome is rare in the United States and occurs almost exclusively in middle-aged men. There has been some association with the presence of this gene and the HLA-A3 phenotype. Although the gene is thought to be present in 10 percent of the population and homozygous in 1 percent, there is an effect on iron intake and chronic losses (e.g., menstruation) that can limit its expression. In Sweden, where flour has been fortified with iron for 30 years, 5 percent of men have persistent iron elevations and 2 percent have increased iron stores consistent with early hemochromatosis. This type of data has produced caution when wider use of such supplementation has been considered. Secondary hemochromatosis with parenchymal iron overload is also common in anemic states requiring frequent blood transfusions.

Serum irons may be elevated 10-fold or more, with transferrin saturations approximating 100 percent, and total body iron stores may be 20 to 100 g. Desferrioxamine-induced urinary excretion ranges from 5 mg/24 hr to more than 20 mg/24 hr.[13]

The standard of therapy is frequent and periodic phlebotomy in an attempt to induce iron depletion, except when iron overload is secondary to transfusions for anemic conditions. In the latter case, chelation therapy with desferrioxamine is used to reduce iron deposition. Most morbidity is related to cirrhosis and diabetes when the disorder is advanced and there is a high incidence of hepatocellular carcinoma.

## Disorders of Iron Metabolism

### Sideroblastic Anemias

The sideroblastic anemias are a group of disorders characterized by abnormalities of heme metabolism, although the precise nature of the defects are often not understood. The hallmark of this group of disorders is the presence of "ringed sideroblasts" in the marrow and the appearance of a dimorphic peripheral blood picture (see Color Figure 72). These cells result from an inability to utilize available iron that is delivered to erythroblasts, which becomes "trapped" in the mitochondria of the developing

Table 4–7. SERUM IRON, TIBC,* AND PERCENT SATURATION IN VARIOUS CLINICAL CONDITIONS

| Normal | Serum Iron (60–150) (g/dl) | TIBC (300–360) (g/dl) | Saturation (20–50) (%) |
|---|---|---|---|
| Iron deficiency | ↓ | ↑ | ↓ |
| Chronic infections | ↓ | ↓ | ↓ |
| Malignancy | ↓ | ↓ | ↓ |
| Menstruation | ↓ | N | ↓ |
| Iron poisoning | ↑ | ↓ | ↑ |
| Hemolytic anemia | ↑ | N | ↑ |
| Hemochromatosis | ↑ | N | ↑ |
| Pyridoxine deficiency | ↑ | N | ↑ |
| Lead poisoning | ↑ | N | ↑ |
| Thalassemia | ↑ | ↓, N | ↑ |

↓ = decrease; ↑ = increase; N = normal.
*TIBC = total iron-binding capacity
Adapted from Henry, JB: Clinical Diagnosis and Management by Laboratory Methods, ed 17. WB Saunders, Philadelphia, 1984.

cells. The distribution of these iron-choked mitochondria is usually a "ring" or halo around the nucleus **(see Color Figure 65)**. Other disorders of iron metabolism may be associated with the appearance of abnormally granulated sideroblasts. See Table 4–4 for classification of sideroblastic anemias.

Sideroblastic anemia is generally associated with more than 15 percent ringed sideroblasts and may be classified as (1) congenital sideroblastic anemia or (2) acquired idiopathic sideroblastic anemia. Acquired sideroblastic anemia may be associated with certain secondary states, but in many cases no secondary cause is found and the disorder is termed primary (idiopathic) sideroblastic anemia (Table 4–8). This disorder represents a disturbance of erythropoiesis, characterized by (1) abnormal erythroid maturation (dyserythropoiesis) and (2) abnormal iron utilization, the hallmark of which is the presence of typical ringed sideroblasts. This disorder is classified under the myelodysplastic syndromes (see Chapter 19) but has also been considered a preleukemic disorder since one third of patients may transform to acute leukemia.

Acquired idiopathic sideroblastic anemia is a disease of middle-aged and elderly patients. The usual clinical presenting symptoms are those of anemia. Occasionally, patients may present with other symptoms of marrow compromise with infections or bleeding manifestations. The liver is usually not enlarged, and splenomegaly is uncommon.

Peripheral blood characteristically shows two RBC populations (dimorphic), with one population of normochromic erythrocytes that may be macrocytic and the other population of obviously hypochromic microcytic cells reflecting the disturbed iron utilization. The RBC indices show which cell population predominates. Consequently, the MCV may be low normal or even occasionally increased. Erythrocytes usually show marked morphologic variations with a spectrum of cells including diffuse polychromatophilia, oval macrocytes, microcytes, and teardrop and pencil poikilocytes.The reticulocyte count may be low, normal, or elevated, reflecting the degree of ineffective erythropoiesis. The MCH and MCHC are often low but may be normal. The white cells are usually normal but may show the Pelger-Huët phenomenon. The polymorphonuclear leukocytes are often agranular. Platelet count is variable but is usually normal.

The bone marrow is usually hypercellular and most often shows a megaloblastoid dyserythropoiesis. Abnormal megakaryocytes, including micromegakaryocytes, are further evidence of a dysplastic state. The iron stain characteristically shows excessive iron deposition with greater than 15 percent ringed sideroblasts. There is further evidence of iron overload in the macrophages. Chromosomal studies performed on the marrow often show aneuploidy.

Other laboratory tests are reflective of an ineffective erythropoiesis with an elevated lactic dehydrogenase and uric acid. The leukocyte alkaline phosphatase (LAP) is usually normal. With the defects in synthesis of porphyrin or the ring insertion of iron, regulation of iron absorption is disturbed and systemic accumulation of iron ensues. The serum iron is usually greater than normal with a high percentage of transferrin saturation (see Table 4–7) and the serum ferritin levels are likewise elevated. The serum vitamin $B_{12}$ and folic acid levels are normal.

Initial therapy usually involves an attempt to ascertain responses to folic acid and pyridoxine treatment. One third of patients may temporarily respond to pyridoxine or pyridoxal-5-phosphate treatment. Most commonly, patients fail to respond to any specific therapy and become transfusion dependent. Transfusion compounds the iron-overload syndrome. Approximately 30 percent of patients may undergo acute leukemic transformation; however, this population cannot be characterized at the initial presentation. Patients with chromosomal abnormalities may be more likely to develop leukemia.

Sideroblastic anemia may occur in other myeloproliferative diseases and has been reported in patients with pernicious anemia and hemolytic anemias.

Other conditions associated with sideroblastic anemia in which a definable cause is present are included in the category of secondary sideroblastic anemias and are listed in Table 4–8.

### Anemia of Chronic Disorders

Anemia of chronic disorders is discussed in Chapter 14 but is mentioned here because of the frequent need to distinguish this anemia from that of iron deficiency. A wide range of disorders can give rise to this condition and include chronic infections, chronic noninfectious inflammatory processes, and malignant neoplasms. The anemias are typically modest with hemoglobins usually in the 7 to 11 g/dl

**Table 4–8. CLASSIFICATION OF SIDEROBLASTIC ANEMIAS**

| | |
|---|---|
| Inherited: | Rare sex-linked |
| Acquired: | Primary (idiopathic) (see myelodysplasias) |
| | Secondary |
| | 1. Associated with other myeloproliferative syndromes (viz., leukemias, polycythemia vera) |
| | 2. Pyridoxine-deficient or responsive anemias |
| |    a. Vitamin $B_6$ deficiency |
| |    b. Drugs: isoniazid, cycloserine |
| |    c. Alcoholism |
| | 3. Disorders of hemoglobin synthesis |
| |    a. Folate deficiency, $B_{12}$ deficiency |
| |    b. Lead poisoning |
| |    c. Alcoholism |
| |    d. Erythropoietic porphyria |

range. Usually the peripheral blood smear shows a normochromic/normocytic picture, but with advanced states the cells may be hypochromic and slightly microcytic or slightly macrocytic. Microcytosis is usually not as severe as in pure iron deficiency and mean cell volume values of less than 70 to 75 fl are rare.[9]

Laboratory studies typically show low or low-normal serum iron and iron-binding capacity. Transferrin saturation overlaps significantly with iron deficiency with values of 7 to 15 percent, but values of 5 percent or less are found only in iron deficiency (see Table 4–7). Free erythrocyte protoporphyrin levels are elevated in chronic disease anemias and cannot be used to separate this disorder from iron deficiency.[11] The serum ferritin is increased in chronic disease anemia, with values of 50 to 2000 ng/ml, and can be a useful discriminator that spares the need for bone marrow studies. Serum ferritin values are rarely above 10 ng/ml in iron-deficiency anemia.[10,12] When infection or inflammation occurs together in a patient with iron deficiency, serum ferritin levels may infrequently rise to 50 to 100 ng/ml but are generally less. In such cases when the picture is still ambiguous, a bone marrow aspirate will reveal ample iron stores in chronic disease anemia and distinguish it finally from iron deficiency. The chronic disease marrow shows hemosiderin iron deposition in reticuloendothelial cells reflecting a defect in the release of iron to erythrocyte precursors.[7]

Much speculation has been generated to explain the mechanism of anemia of chronic disease, but data are often contradictory or incomplete. Research has been focused on erythropoietin levels in this disorder and marrow responsiveness, either or both of which can be depressed. Other studies have suggested a role for a leukocyte pyrogen produced during inflammatory responses by neutrophils and macrophages with a marrow depressant activity. See Chapter 16 for further discussion.

Therapy is directed at correcting the underlying disorder. The anemia is rarely significant enough to warrant transfusion.

## LABORATORY EVALUATION OF IRON STATUS
### Peripheral Blood Smear

Although many sophisticated methods exist to assess iron utilization and kinetics, examination of a Wright-stained peripheral smear is a simple, cost-effective method of characterizing iron status and consequently hypochromic, microcytic anemias.[9] The differential diagnosis of the causes of these anemias has been discussed. Most notably, in this context, the RBCs are examined for their relative size, shape, hemoglobinization, and morphologic variations. They are termed hypochromic when they

stain unusually pale and the central area of pallor is increased (see Color Figure 66). Hypochromic cells result from reduced hemoglobin synthesis or abnormally thin RBCs. Abnormal hemoglobin synthesis may occur in iron deficiency, disturbances in iron metabolism, and disorders of globin and porphyrin synthesis.

Microcytosis results from the production of abnormally small RBCs that may occur in many conditions associated with abnormal erythropoiesis and, in particular, the conditions previously mentioned. The relative size of the normal RBC is approximately that of a small lymphocyte. A combined deficiency of iron and folate or vitamin B$_{12}$ may produce a dimorphic blood film in which a dual population of cells may be present.[2] One population is normally hemoglobinized, whereas the other is underhemoglobinized. A dimorphic cell population may also occur in sideroblastic anemias as well as following transfusions.

Automated cell counters provide the most accurate method of quantitation of cell size and cell hemoglobinization. The mean corpuscular volume (MCV), mean corpuscular hemoglobin (MCH), and mean corpuscular hemoglobin concentration (MCHC) will confirm the existence of a hypochromic/microcytic profile (see Chapter 31).[2] However useful these data may be, they are no substitute for direct visualization of the blood smear.

Combined deficiencies and disorders may coexist, which may be apparent only on evaluation of the peripheral blood film. Moreover, the presence of schistocytes, burr cells, teardrops, target cells, or nucleated RBCs is another important hematologic abnormality that may give a clue to the etiology of the hypochromic/microcytic anemia and that would be inapparent from electronic data alone.

Erythrocytes on a peripheral blood smear may also be stained by the Prussian blue reaction for the presence of intracellular iron particles. These iron particles, if present, consist of nonheme iron and when found in non-nucleated RBCs are called "siderocytes." (Developing erythroid precursors in the bone marrow containing iron are termed sideroblasts, as previously discussed.) These siderotic granules may also be detected on Giemsa staining and are then termed "Pappenheimer bodies" (see Color Figure 64). This nonheme iron consists of ferritin granules that have been degraded into hemosiderin. Ordinarily, siderocytes are not present in the normal peripheral blood smear; however, they may be found in situations of iron overload, such as hemochromatosis, hemolytic anemias, and post-splenectomy.

### Chemical Tests
#### Serum Iron

Measurement of serum iron can be accomplished by various techniques. In most instances, the iron is separated from serum proteins and coupled with a chromogen to develop a colored complex that can be read spectrophotometrically. Total serum iron is obtained by this test, but virtually all of it is transferrin-bound.[15]

Blood levels for iron estimation should routinely be drawn in the morning after a 12-hour fast and after having taken no iron-containing medications for 12 to 24 hours. The body experiences a diurnal variation in serum iron that may be one-quarter lower in the evening than early in the day. The normal range for serum iron is 50 to 150 $\mu$g/dl, averaging 125 $\mu$g/dl in men and 100 $\mu$g/dl in women. In the elderly, the serum iron levels decrease to 40 to 80 $\mu$g/dl. Serum iron levels vary in response to various physiologic disorders: decreased in iron deficiency, chronic infections and malignancy; increased in iron poisoning, intravascular hemolysis, hepatic necrosis, pernicious anemia, hemochromatosis, and other disorders listed in Table 4–7.

## Total Iron-Binding Capacity (TIBC)

The capacity of serum transferrin to bind iron is obtained by this test; it is an indirect measure of the serum transferrin concentration. The assay is performed as in serum iron, except that excess iron is added to the sample to saturate all transferrin binding sites, and the unbound iron is removed prior to assay. Therefore, the total ability of transferrin to bind iron is assessed by the determination of the total amount of iron bound. This assay does not measure the serum transferrin (protein) level.

The normal range for TIBC in adults is 300 to 360 $\mu$g/dl and tends to decrease with age to approximately 250 $\mu$g/dl in persons greater than 70 years old. Unlike serum iron, there is no diurnal variation in TIBC. Classically, transferrin, and hence TIBC, is increased in the presence of iron deficiency but may be normal or low in chronic disease states, malnutrition, and nephrosis, when transferrin and iron may be lost in the urine (see Table 4–7).[15]

## Transferrin Saturation

Transferrin saturation is not directly measured but is obtained as a ratio:

$$\text{Percentage saturation} = \frac{\text{Serum iron}}{\text{TIBC}} \times 100$$

It is more useful than serum iron as a measure of body iron stores and ranges from 20 to 45 percent. In iron deficiency, values are typically below 16 percent, but diagnosis in children requires concurrent findings of hypochromia and microcytosis as well. Chronic disorders also have low transferrin saturation, but any saturation (in children or adults) of 5 percent or less is specific for iron deficiency. In sideroblastic anemia, iron poisoning, and intravascular hemolysis, transferrin saturation may reach 100 percent.

## Serum Ferritin

In otherwise healthy individuals, the presentation of a typical hypochromic, microcytic anemia and low serum iron (with or without obtaining a TIBC and transferrin saturation) is adequate for diagnosis of iron deficiency, rendering further tests unnecessary. However, when the clinical setting is less obvious (see Table 4–3), a more direct assessment of body iron stores may be needed.

As discussed in a preceding section, ferritin enters the serum from virtually all ferritin producing tissues but is present devoid of iron in its glycosylated form and also in a very low concentration relative to the tissue ferritin. (Total serum ferritin approximates 0.3 mg versus 2 g or more in the tissues; see Table 4–1.) However, since it is in equilibrium with tissue ferritin, it can be a very good indicator of iron stores.[10,12]

Serum ferritin is measured conveniently by a radioimmunoassay. Normal levels average 90 $\mu$g/l in men and 30 $\mu$g/l in children and premenopausal women with ranges of 20 to 250 and 10 to 200 $\mu$g/l, respectively. Throughout childhood, boys and girls have blood levels that are equal at about 30 $\mu$g/l, but then boys begin to show a rise in their late teens that continues until the age of 30 when the 90 $\mu$g/l level is obtained. When women reach menopause, a similar rise occurs and eventually approaches levels seen in men. Each 1 $\mu$g/l of ferritin is taken to represent 8 to 10 mg of storage iron, but a more precise representation is 0.14 mg of storage iron per kilogram of body weight.[15]

The measurement of serum ferritin can be particularly useful in distinguishing iron deficiency from hypochromic, microcytic anemia of chronic disease. In the latter, serum iron and transferrin saturation may frequently be ambiguous. Serum ferritins are generally below 10 $\mu$g/l in iron deficiency, but are usually normal or elevated in chronic disease. Serum ferritin levels are also elevated in inflammation, liver disease, and leukemias, which may lead to a relative over-representation of body iron stores. In the presence of these disorders, normal serum ferritin levels may mask an iron-deficiency state. In these situations and when the peripheral smear is also ambiguous yet the clinical suspicion of an iron-deficiency state is high, direct visualization of bone marrow iron stores must be undertaken. In iron overload, serum ferritin may increase to as much as 10,000 $\mu$g/l. Serum ferritin levels remain low for as long as 2 to 3 weeks following initiation of oral iron therapy. However, intravenous iron promotes a rapid increase in the serum ferritin to normal levels within 24 hours of administration.

## Free Erythrocyte Protoporphyrin (FEP)

The erythrocyte enzyme, ferrochelatase, inserts the ferrous iron into the protoporphyrin IX molecule in the final step of heme synthesis (see Fig. 4-2).[1] Protoporphyrin without iron is not incorporated into hemoglobin. Erythrocytes normally produce a slight excess of protoporphyrin over what is needed for heme synthesis; but when iron is deficient, protoporphyrin increases several-fold. Ferrochelatase represents a rate-limiting enzyme step in the heme synthetic pathway and the insertion of iron into protoporphyrin facilitates a negative feedback (see Chapter 2).

Measurement of free erythrocyte protoporphyrin (FEP) provides one of the most sensitive early indicators of iron deficiency.[11] It is abnormal in a high proportion of patients with deficient iron stores but in whom the hemogram is still normal. The FEP is elevated in patients with chronic disease states and lead poisoning, both of which produce disturbances in iron metabolism. FEP is usually increased also in patients with idiopathic refractory sideroblastic anemia, but it may be reduced in patients with other forms of anemia. In disorders of hemoglobin (as opposed to heme) synthesis, FEP levels are normal and therefore this is a useful method in distinguishing the hypochromic/microcytic anemia of thalassemia from iron deficiency.

FEP is measured by extraction and fluorescence or direct assessment by a hemofluorometer. Normal values depend on the method and laboratory, but nominal ranges are 15 to 80 $\mu$g/dl of RBCs. The value may also be expressed as a ratio of FEP to hemoglobin. In the presence of iron deficiency and chronic disease states, FEP levels increase approximately fivefold. FEP remains with the RBC for its entire lifespan. Hence, iron deficiency can be diagnosed even after iron therapy has been instituted and the serum iron and ferritin have normalized.

## Miscellaneous Tests

A number of more specialized procedures are available for assessing iron uptake and storage.

Cobalt (Co) is absorbed via iron pathways but, unlike iron, is excreted in the urine. The cobalt excretion test will reflect increased uptake in persons with iron deficiency, in those having recent blood loss, or in those who are prone to hemochromatosis. It is in this latter diagnosis that this test can be used.

Drugs such as desferrioxamine can be injected into patients to determine the amount of labile iron that can be excreted by binding with this chelator. This drug is a high-affinity, low molecular weight compound that complexes serum iron and markedly increases urinary iron excretion. The iron excretion correlates roughly with iron stores and is greatly increased in iron overload states such as hemochromatosis and sideroblastic anemia.[13]

As a rule, these more specialized tests add little information that cannot be obtained by the more standard techniques described earlier and are reserved primarily for research purposes.

## Tissue Iron Determination

When the clinical setting and laboratory studies are inconclusive, direct estimation of iron stores must be obtained. This may be achieved by biopsy of the liver or, more commonly, of the bone marrow.[7]

Bone marrow iron can be appreciated directly in unstained preparations of aspirates as the golden refractile granules of hemosiderin. More reproducible assessments are obtained with Prussian blue staining, which renders the hemosiderin blue. Histologic grading (0 to 6+) correlates reasonably well with iron content of the sample (Table 4–9). Grades 1+ to 3+ are considered normal, 0 is considered iron deficient, and grades 4+ to 6+ are present in iron overload states. Anemia of chronic disease shows normal or elevated marrow iron (2+ to 5+), and marrow studies therefore readily separate this diagnosis of hypochromic, microcytic anemia from that of iron deficiency. Iron stores are normal or increased (2+ to 4+) in thalassemia minor and in many hemoglobinopathies. They are consistently high (5+ to 6+) in thalassemia major, sideroblastic anemias, and hemochromatosis. Grading criteria for liver iron are also available.

Morphologically, hemosiderin in small granules reflects intracytoplasmic aggregates of ferritin. Erythroblasts containing such granules are termed sideroblasts. In normal marrow, approximately 30 percent of the erythroblasts contain such granules and the percentage of sideroblasts in the marrow corresponds closely to the percent saturation of transferrin. These granules are extruded by the mature erythrocytes prior to discharge from the marrow, but they may occur peripherally as "siderocytes" with a "stress marrow" and, as already mentioned, in iron-overload states. The so-called ringed sideroblasts of the sideroblastic anemias are different: granules are larger and represent abnormal deposits of iron (probably as insoluble ferric phosphate) within mitochondria, which are swollen with their iron burden. Defects in heme biosyn-

**Table 4–9. CRITERIA FOR GRADING IRON STAINS IN BONE MARROW ASPIRATES**

| Grade | Criteria | Iron Content ($\mu$g/g)* |
|---|---|---|
| 0 | No iron granules observed | 43 ± 23 |
| 1+ | Small granules in reticulum cells seen only with oil-immersion lens | 130 ± 50 |
| 2+ | Few small granules visible with low-power lens | 223 ± 75 |
| 3+ | Numerous small granules in all marrow particles | 406 ± 131 |
| 4+ | Large granules in small clumps | 767 ± 247 |
| 5+ | Dense, large clumps of granules obscuring marrow detail | 1618 ± 464 |
| 6+ | Very large deposits, obscuring marrow cells | 3681 ± 1400 |

thesis in the mitochondria appear to be responsible for this overload of iron within in the organelle (see section on sideroblastic anemias).

There is such variation in marrow morphology with any stage of iron deficiency that it is not useful to try to characterize the range of possible findings here. The principal value of the marrow study is for direct assessment of iron stores and for ruling out other disorders. Usually, however, the marrow does show microblastic erythroid maturation with erythroid hyperplasia and defective hemoglobinization ("ragged erythropoiesis") **(see Color Figure 67)**. Granulopoiesis is most often normal but does, on occasion, show hypersegmented polymorphonuclear leukocytes. In certain conditions of iron deficiency, megakaryocytes may be increased.

Marrow evaluation of iron stores can yield falsely normal iron estimates in patients who have received parenteral iron therapy or blood transfusions prior to evaluation. In such cases, the FEP levels may be the best measure of an antecedent iron deficiency.

## Test Expense

Table 4–10 provides a list of approximate charges for laboratory tests and procedures in 1986. Costs vary for individual practitioners and laboratories.

An automated hemogram with RBC indices, reticulocyte count, and iron and TIBC studies—the basic workup for iron deficiency—runs approximately $31. Transferrin saturation is left for the physician to calculate. If interpretation is ambiguous, addition of a serum ferritin determination will make the cost of the workup close to $53. Addition of FEP could increase the total cost to $72 when used to show an antecedent iron deficiency when iron therapy has been initiated (inappropriately) prior to workup. The major use of the FEP remains to distinguish thalassemia trait from iron deficiency.

Bone marrow biopsy adds a more invasive dimension to the workup but also provides a more definitive measure of iron stores. Although the procedure is simple enough, additional charges including bone marrow performance, interpretation, and

Table 4–10. COSTS OF LABORATORY TESTS, 1986

| Test | Cost |
| --- | --- |
| Hematocrit | $ 6 |
| Complete blood count (CBC) with RBC indices | 10 |
| Reticulocyte count | 6 |
| Serum iron | 10 |
| Serum iron and TIBC | 15 |
| Serum ferritin | 22 |
| Free erythrocyte protoporphyrin (FEP) | 19 |
| Haptoglobin | 26 |

consultation by a hematologist must be included, which may add $150 to $250 to the expense.

Clearly, the clinical setting should have a strong influence in the choice of tests, both for economy of workup and for sparing the patient unneeded discomfort and expense. A 26-year-old, menstruating woman needs only a hemogram and an iron level test (with or without a TIBC) to begin iron therapy. While iron deficiency remains the *only* indication for iron therapy, in some instances a therapeutic trial (which costs less than $5 per month of treatment) may be considered when uncertainty remains in spite of a reasonable clinical suspicion. Follow-up hemogram and reticulocyte count after two weeks to one month will provide an indication of appropriateness of therapy.

## ILLUSTRATIVE CASE HISTORIES

### Case 1

A 40-year-old white woman presented to her doctor with weakness, fatigue, and dizziness of three weeks' duration. On further inquiry, it was apparent that the symptoms had been present for three months previously but had gradually become worse. The patient denied having abdominal pain, change in bowel habits, or gastrointestinal bleeding. Her weight had been constant, and she had no difficulty swallowing. She gave a past history of having had anemia 25 years previously. Ten years ago she had also been found to be anemic. Evaluation at that time included a negative GI radiology series. More recently, she had also noted that her nails were brittle and that she had been experiencing recurrent headaches.

She had started menstruating at the age of 11, with 30 to 31 day cycles, bleeding for six days during each cycle. Recently, the bleeding had been more severe, with the passage of clots. She used up to 80 tampons per cycle. She denied recurring infections, fever, or other bleeding manifestations.

**Dietary History.** She ate all foods, including red meat; but more recently she had developed a strong desire for ice and pickles.

**Medications.** She had recently taken aspirin for headaches, consumed alcohol socially, and received iron therapy in the past for her anemia. She experienced marked GI discomfort, including abdominal pain, diarrhea, and severe cramps with oral iron therapy.

**Family History.** Her mother and sister were anemic in the past. She has five children, the oldest of whom is age 15.

**Physical Examination.** Her weight was 165 lbs, with a height of 5'5½". Her pulse was 86 per min (regular); and her blood pressure 120/80.

Her nails were soft but did not exhibit any koilonychia. There was no clinical jaundice. The rest of the examination was essentially unremarkable. Specifically, there was no lymphadenopathy or hepatosplenomegaly. Her heart sounds were normal, and no murmurs were audible. No evidence of clinical bleeding was noted.

**Laboratory Data.** Her hematocrit level was 25 percent; hemoglobin was 8.2 g/dl. The MCV was 64 fl, MCH 20 pg/dl, and MCHC 31 g/dl. Reticulocyte count was 2.5 percent. White cell count was 5000/mm³ with a normal differential, and platelet count was 498,000/mm³ and the sedimentation rate was normal. Her urinalysis was normal. The serum iron was 14 μg/dl with a total iron-binding capacity 486 μg/dl. Her serum ferritin was less than 4 g/ml. Her routine chemistry was normal. Stool guaiac times three was negative.

**Clinical Course.** She was diagnosed as having iron-deficiency anemia resulting from excessive menstrual blood loss and was referred to her gynecologist for evaluation. Gynecologic examination showed a slightly bulky uterus with normal ovaries. A diagnostic dilation and curettage was performed. Histology of the curetting showed normal proliferative endometrium with no evidence of endometrial inflammation or abnormal pathology. In view of her past history of severe intolerence of oral iron treatment, she was given parenteral iron therapy. Her dosage was calculated sufficient to replete the iron stores and replenish the iron needed for optimal hemoglobinization. She received weekly iron injections over the following four months. During that time, she showed a good reticulocyte response with an hematocrit of 36 percent, six weeks after initial treatment was started. After three months her MCV was 79 fl, MCH 26 pg/dl, and MCHC 32 percent. Her serum iron was 52 μg/dl and TIBC was 350 μg/dl. Ferritin was normal. She continued, however, to have heavy menstrual periods but was lost to follow-up for nine months. She again presented with a hematocrit of 26.5 percent, MCV 62 fl, MCH 19.3 pg/dl, and MCHC 31.1 g/dl. Her serum iron was 15 μg/dl, and TIBC 592 μg/dl. She was seen by her gynecologist and a hysterectomy was performed. The uterus showed intramural fibroids. Prior to surgery she was given several injections of parenteral iron treatment to increase her hematocrit level prior to surgery.

**Comment.** There are several typical manifestations of this patient's clinical course.

1. The history of anemia from an early adulthood probably relates to excessive menstrual bleeding. One large series from Glasgow showed 25 percent of healthy young women were found to be iron deficient. This patient's iron depletion was aggrevated by five successive pregnancies. This was also compounded by continued excessive menstrual bleeding, which necessitated her seeking attention. She had been studied for iron deficiency in the past with a workup including evaluation for GI bleeding. In men, the most common cause of iron-deficiency anemia is GI blood loss, whereas in women it is menstrual blood loss. The history of aspirin intake for this patient's headaches also warranted exclusion of GI bleeding. However, her history was so significant for menstrual blood loss that this was almost certainly the cause.

2. A most important evaluation of any patient with anemia includes a detailed history. This is particularly evident in iron-deficiency anemia, when a history of bleeding needs to be evaluated as was done in this case. Note also her dietary history, specifically the presence of pica — for ice and pickles. This is a fairly common manifestation of tissue iron depletion.

3. This patient's intolerance to oral iron therapy is not uncommon. Many patients experience difficulties while on oral iron treatment. If this is the case, parenteral iron can be administered.

4. Iron deficiency, as already mentioned, is a symptom rather than a disease. This patient's problems resulted from gynecologic pathology. Severe iron deficiency requiring parenteral iron therapy failed to correct the anemia, owing to a persistence of bleeding. Consequently, a hysterectomy was performed. In all cases of iron deficiency, a search must be made for the cause and primary treatment instituted.

### Case 2

A 33-year-old white woman presented to a doctor because of central abdominal pain. The pain occurred 20 minutes after eating and was relieved by antacids. She experienced some nausea; however, there was no fatty food intolerance. She also experienced an abdominal distention and had been evaluated for this disorder previously. The diagnosis of an irritable colon was made. The rest of her systematic history was unremarkable. Specifically, she denied any history of jaundice or hepatitis.

**Medications.** These included occasional acetaminophen and antacids. She formerly consumed four to five glasses of wine per night but had had no alcohol since the onset of abdominal pain. She had smoked cigarettes for 10 years but had not done so in the last five.

**Family History.** She was one of four siblings, two of whom were investigated for similar symptoms and were found on routine testing to have elevated liver transaminases.

**Physical Examination.** This proved unremarkable. There was no clinical jaundice, and her skin did not reveal any bronze discoloration. She had no spider angiomata, cutaneous ecchymoses, petechiae, or clubbing of the digits. Her pulse rate was 80 per min (regular), her blood pressure 115/65, and the rest of the physical examination was normal.

**Laboratory Data.** Hematocrit was 39 percent, hemoglobin 13.3 g/dl with normochromic, normocytic indices. The reticulocyte count was 2 percent, the white cell count 4600/mm³ with a normal differential count. The platelet count was 214,000/mm³ with normal platelet morphology. The patient's urinalysis was normal. Liver function tests showed a serum glutamic oxaloacetic transaminase of 73 I.U./ml (normal range 7 to 40) and a serum glutamic pyruvate transaminase of 97 I.U./ml (normal 10 to 40). Her alkaline phosphatase was 183 I.U./ml (normal 30 to 100), and gammaglutamyl transpeptidase was 195 I.U./ml (normal up to 25). Her serum bilirubin, LDH, and the rest of her chemistry screen were all normal.

She was evaluated for abnormal liver function. Workup included a serum iron test, which was 150 µg/ml, a TIBC of 300 µg/ml, and a serum ferritin of 170 mg/ml (normal 10 to 150). She was initially referred to a gastroenterologist, who performed a liver biopsy. The biopsy demonstrated excessive iron in the liver parenchymal cells and Kupffer cells but no evidence of cirrhosis.

**Comment.** The abnormal liver function studies including the definitive test, a liver biopsy, clearly indicated an iron-overload syndrome. (A liver biopsy need not be performed in most cases.) Her family history was also significant for the fact that two siblings had abnormal liver function studies, probably also caused by iron deposition. Additional studies were performed, including HLA phenotyping, and she was shown to have HLA A3 and B7, phenotypes that are highly associated with familial hemochromatosis. Her major manifestations included liver cell function derangement. There was no evidence of any glucose intolerance, a feature also seen in this disorder. The symptoms that promoted her to go and seek medical attention were vague, but fortunately laboratory evaluation revealed the liver iron-overload.

She was put onto a therapeutic phlebotomy program and was initially phlebotomized one unit of blood weekly until her hematocrit dropped into the 33 range. At this point in time her liver function had shown improvement to the extent that her transaminase levels were normal. She was subsequently phlebotomized monthly. A recent serum iron measured 138 µg/ml, TIBC 445 µg/ml, and a serum ferritin of less than 4 mg/ml. The rest of the liver function tests are all within the normal range. She will require lifelong phlebotomy to maintain her in a negative iron balance state. Currently, she exhibits biochemical evidence of iron depletion; however, hematologically she is asymptomatic and perfectly healthy.

## References

1. Awad, WM and Wells, MS: Iron and heme metabolism. In Devlin, TM (ed): Textbook of Biochemistry with Clinical Correlations. John Wiley & Sons, New York 1982, pp 1061–1085.
2. Bessman, D: Erythropoiesis during recovery from iron deficiency: Normocytes and macrocytes. Blood 50;987, 1977.
3. Crosby, WH: The rationale for treating iron deficiency anemia. Arch Intern Med 144:471, 1984.
4. Dallman, PR, Beutler, E, and Finch, CA: Effects of iron deficiency exclusive of anemia. Br J Haematol 40:179, 1978.
5. Fairbanks, VF and Beutler, E: Iron deficiency. In Williams, WJ (ed): Hematology. McGraw-Hill, New York, 1983, pp 466–493.
6. Finch, CA and Huebers, H: Perspectives in iron metabolism. N Engl J Med 206:1520, 1982.
7. Gale, E, Torrance, J, and Bothwell, T: The quantitative estimation of total iron stores in human bone marrow. J Clin Invest 42:1076, 1963.
8. Halliday, JW and Powell, LW: Iron overload. Sem Hematol 19:42, 1982.
9. Kellermeyer, RW: General principles of the evaluation and therapy of anemias. Med Clin North Am 68:533, 1984.
10. Lipschitz, DA, Cook, JD, and Finch, CA: A clinical evaluation of serum ferritin as an index of iron stores. N Engl J Med 290:1213, 1974.
11. Marsh, WL, Nelson, DP, and Koenig, HM: Free erythrocyte protoporphyrin (FEP). I. Normal values for adults and evaluation of the hematofluorometer. II. The FEP test is clinically useful in classifying microcytic RBC disorders in adults. Am J Clin Pathol 79:655, 1983.
12. Munro, HN and Linder, MC: Ferritin: Structure, biosynthesis, and role in iron metabolism. Phys Rev 58:317, 1978.
13. Schafer, AI, Rabinowe, S, LeBoff, MS, et al: Long-term efficacy of desferoxamine iron chelation therapy in adults with acquired transfusional iron overload. Arch Intern Med 145:1217, 1985.
14. Simon, M: Secondary iron overload and the haemachromatosis alleles. Br J Haematol 60:1, 1985.
15. Woo, J and Cannon, DC: Metabolic intermediates and inorganic ions. In Henry, JB (ed): Clinical Diagnosis and Management by Laboratory Methods, ed 17. WB Saunders, Philadelphia, 1984.

## Bibliography

Bothwell, TH, Charlton, RW, Cook, JD, et al: Iron Metabolism in Man. Blackwell, Oxford, 1979.

# CHAPTER 5

MICHELE LYNNE BEST, B.S., M.T.(ASCP)

# Megaloblastic Anemias

## HISTORY AND DEFINITIONS

Megaloblastic anemia is a term used to describe an anemia associated with defective DNA synthesis and abnormal red cell maturation in the bone marrow. This abnormal maturation pattern is sometimes called "megaloblastic change," in contrast to normal or "normoblastic" maturation. It is also appropriate to use the term "megaloblastic change" to describe the characteristic morphology in the absence of anemia. Furthermore, megaloblastic maturation also affects granulocytic and megakaryocytic maturation. Megaloblastic dyspoiesis and megaloblastosis are other terms used to describe the same maturation defect. A similar term, megaloblastoid, has been used to describe changes in the bone marrow that are morphologically similar yet etiologically different from megaloblastic change.

The term "megaloblast" was first used by Ehrlich[1] in 1880 to describe a distinctly abnormal cell seen in the bone marrow of a patient with pernicious anemia. This extremely large, deeply basophilic, immature erythroid cell was thought by Ehrlich and others to represent a cell type unique to the disease process rather than a morphologically and functionally abnormal counterpart of the normal erythroid precursor cell that it is known to represent today. For years, the terms "megaloblast" and "normoblast" have been used to describe these abnormal and normal counterparts. Specific members of the normoblastic series are called pronormoblast, deeply basophilic normoblast, polychromatophilic normoblast, and orthochromic normoblast. The counterparts in megaloblastic maturation are described similarly by substituting the term "megaloblast" for "normoblast" (i.e., polychromatophilic megaloblast).

Pernicious anemia, the prototype of the megaloblastic anemias, was initially described in 1855 by Addison,[2] who described a patient with an idiopathic persistent anemia that progressed to death. The term "Addisonian anemia" was used for many years to describe this disorder. The name "pernicious anemia" was first used by Biermer[3] in 1872.

"Macrocytic anemia" is a term used to describe *any* anemia associated with an elevated mean corpuscular red cell volume (MCV). This is a morphologic category of anemia that includes but is not restricted to megaloblastic anemia. Unfortunately, "macrocytic anemia" is sometimes used as a synonym for "megaloblastic anemia." One term denotes a morphologic category of anemia (macrocytic) with several different causes; the other denotes an etiologic category (megaloblastic).

## BIOCHEMICAL BASIS OF MEGALOBLASTIC DYSPOIESIS

Megaloblastic dyspoiesis is the result of a slowdown in DNA synthesis in the developing cells of the bone marrow and other rapidly proliferative cells in the body. The primary defect is in DNA replication owing to a depletion of thymidine triphosphate, an immediate DNA precursor.[4] This deficiency causes retarded nuclear maturation and mitosis, which is responsible for both the enlargement of cells and the morphologic abnormalities observed. The ratio of RNA:DNA in megaloblastic cells is higher than normal, since RNA synthesis and therefore cytoplasmic maturation are not affected.

Impaired DNA synthesis can be caused by a variety of conditions, among them vitamin $B_{12}$ deficiency, folic acid deficiency, and administration of drugs that interfere with DNA metabolism. The most common categories of drugs involved are chemotherapeutic agents and anticonvulsants. The exact role that vitamin $B_{12}$ and folic acid play in DNA synthesis will be examined in the next section.

## Absorption and Metabolism of Vitamin $B_{12}$ and Folic Acid

Vitamin $B_{12}$ and folic acid must be present in adequate dietary amounts and effectively absorbed to be available for DNA synthesis in the bone marrow.

Vitamin $B_{12}$, also called cyanocobalamin, has the chemical structure similar to that shown in Figure 5-1. There are also a number of other cobalamin compounds in which the –CN atom is replaced

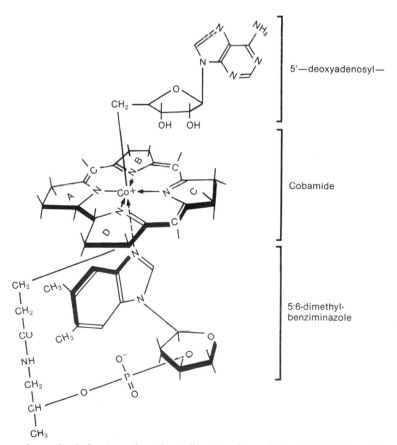

**Figure 5-1.** Structure of deoxyadenosyl cobalamin, a physiologically active form of vitamin $B_{12}$. (From Chanarin, I: The Megaloblastic Anemias. Blackwell Scientific, Boston, with permission.)

with other types of side chains. The term "vitamin $B_{12}$" is also often used collectively to describe cyanocobalamin and its analogues.

The richest dietary sources of vitamin $B_{12}$ are meats, eggs, dairy products, and liver. The minimum daily requirement is thought to be approximately 1 to 3 $\mu$g. Vitamin $B_{12}$ is absorbed via a binding protein called intrinsic factor, a glycoprotein produced by the gastric parietal cells. This intrinsic factor (IF) binds vitamin $B_{12}$, producing an IF-$B_{12}$ complex that attaches to receptors on the ileal mucosal cells allowing for its absorption (Fig. 5-2). Vitamin $B_{12}$ is then released from the ileal cell and bound to a transport protein in the bloodstream, transcobalamin II. Transcobalamin II, like IF, is a fairly selective binder of cyanocobalamin and does not bind the other vitamin $B_{12}$ analogues.[5]

Two other vitamin $B_{12}$–binding proteins, transcobalamin I and III, appear to play a minor role in transporting true vitamin $B_{12}$ (cyanocobalamin) but a major role in transporting the other vitamin $B_{12}$ analogues.[6]

As Figure 5-2 illustrates, transcobalamin II and other binders transport vitamin $B_{12}$ to the bone marrow and other tissues to be utilized or to the liver to be stored. The quantity of vitamin $B_{12}$ stored in the liver of the average person is large enough to last for approximately three years.

"Folic acid," "folate," and "pteroylglutamic acid" are synonyms for the compound shown in Figure 5-3. Pteroylglutamic acid is the parent compound of

a large number of closely related compounds often referred to as folates.

Folic acid is present as folate polyglutamate in high concentration in leafy green vegetables, liver, meats, and certain fruits. The minimum daily adult requirement for folate is approximately 50 $\mu$g.[7] Folate is absorbed in the mucosal cells of the duodenum and jejunum, where three biochemical reactions (hydrolysis, reduction, and methylation) convert the ingested polyglutamates to 5-methyltetrahydrofolate (Fig. 5-4). This monoglutamate form is readily and completely absorbed into portal circulation where it is transported by $\alpha_2$-macroglobulin, albumin, and transferrin[5] to the tissues and the liver. Folate stores in the liver are minimal. This explains why it takes only a few months of inadequate dietary intake to become folate deficient.

Once effectively absorbed and transported, vitamin $B_{12}$ and folic acid become available to the actively dividing cells of the body to perform their key roles in DNA synthesis.

Vitamin $B_{12}$ and a group of folic acid derivatives are required as cofactors in several key reactions leading to the synthesis of thymidine triphosphate and subsequently to DNA. A simplified diagram of these reactions is presented in Figure 5-5. Vitamin $B_{12}$ is required for the conversion of homocysteine to methionine, during which a methyl group is transferred from 5-methyltetrahydrofolate (5-methyl THF) to yield tetrahydrofolate (THF).[8] Folic acid and related folate compounds including THF participate in the conversion of deoxyuridine monophosphate to thymidine monophosphate, which eventually converts to thymidine triphosphate, one of the pyrimidine building blocks of DNA. It is evident from this diagram that a deficiency of either vitamin $B_{12}$ or folate has a serious impact on DNA synthesis.

## CAUSES OF MEGALOBLASTIC ANEMIA

When the normal cycle of adequate diet, absorption, transport, and cellular utilization of these vitamins is broken, a cellular deficiency and megaloblastic dyspoiesis result. Despite the fact that both deficiencies have very similar cellular consequences, the conditions that lead to these deficiencies are quite different. Folic acid deficiency will be discussed first, because it is the more common deficiency.

### Folic Acid Deficiency

By far, the leading cause of folic acid deficiency is dietary. The four major etiologic categories of folic acid deficiency are outlined in Table 5-1. Dietary deficiency results from a poor diet usually owing to alcoholism, poverty, old age, or chronic overcooking of vegetables. In the alcoholic, folate deficiency

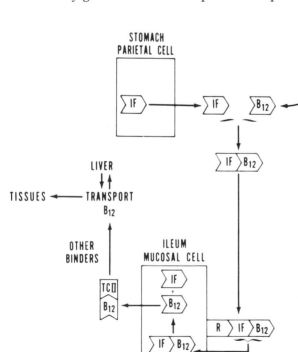

**Figure 5-2.** Absorption, transport, and storage of vitamin $B_{12}$. IF = intrinsic factor; R = tissue binders; TC II = transcobalamin II. (From Miale, JB: Laboratory Medicine: Hematology, ed 6. CV Mosby, St. Louis, 1982, p 425, with permission.)

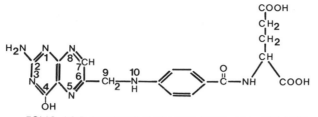

FOLIC ACID (PTEROYLGLUTAMIC ACID, PGA, FOLACIN)

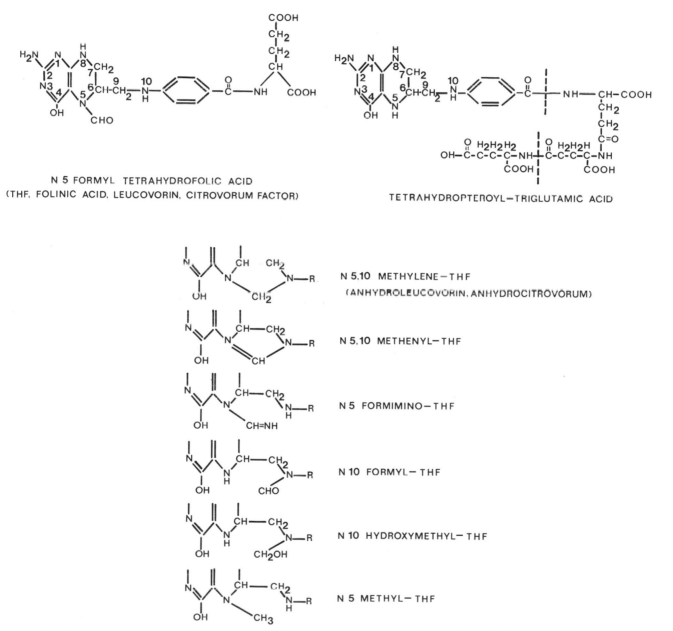

N 5 FORMYL TETRAHYDROFOLIC ACID
(THF, FOLINIC ACID, LEUCOVORIN, CITROVORUM FACTOR)

TETRAHYDROPTEROYL—TRIGLUTAMIC ACID

N 5,10 METHYLENE—THF
(ANHYDROLEUCOVORIN, ANHYDROCITROVORUM)

N 5,10 METHENYL—THF

N 5 FORMIMINO—THF

N 10 FORMYL—THF

N 10 HYDROXYMETHYL—THF

N 5 METHYL—THF

**Figure 5-3.** Structure of folic acid and its derivatives. THF = tetrahydrofolate. (From Harris, JW and Kellermeyer, RW: The Red Cell. Harvard University Press, Cambridge, 1970, p 395, with permission.)

## ERYTHROCYTES

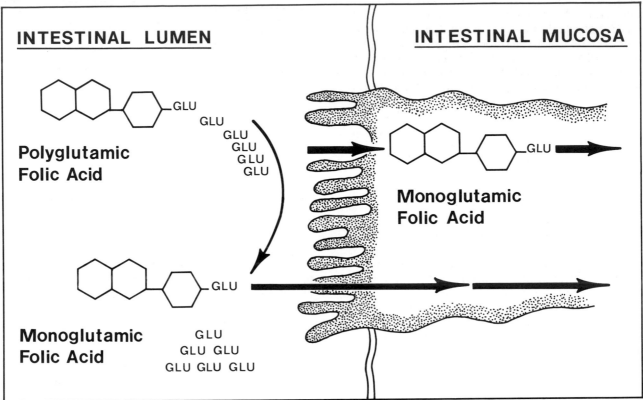

**Figure 5-4.** Intestinal absorption of the folate derivatives of food. (From Streiff, RR: JAMA 214:105, 1970, with permission.)

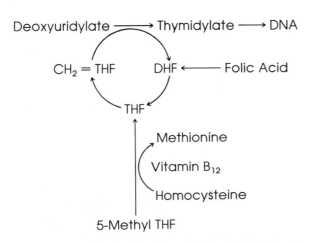

**Figure 5-5.** The roles of vitamin $B_{12}$ and folic acid in DNA synthesis. THF = tetrahydrofolate; DHF = dihydrofolate; $CH_2 =$ THF = methylene tetrahydrofolate. (Adapted from Waxman, Metz, and Herbert.[24])

## Table 5–1. CAUSES OF FOLIC ACID DEFICIENCY

**Inadequate intake**
  Alcoholism
  Poor diet
  Overcooking vegetables
**Increased utilization**
  Pregnancy
  Infancy
  Hemolytic anemia
  Acute leukemia
  Metastatic cancer
  Multiple myeloma
  Hyperthyroidism
  Exfoliative dermatitis
**Impaired absorption**
  Tropical and nontropical sprue
  Drug-related
  ?Alcohol
  Anatomic and functional intestinal abnormalities
**Increased loss**
  Hemodialysis
**Drug-related**
  Folate antagonists (e.g., methotrexate)
  Isoniazid
  Cycloserine
  Phenytoin
  Oral contraceptives

is the number one cause of anemia.[9] Inadequate dietary intake has usually been regarded as the primary cause; however, a study by Sullivan and Herbert[10] suggests that alcohol has a direct antagonistic effect on folic acid metabolism. In this study, patients with untreated megaloblastic anemia were given folic acid together with alcohol. The alcohol prevented a hematologic response to folate in these patients.

Inadequate dietary intake in the face of increased physiologic need occurs in young infants and pregnant women. Good vitamin supplementation in infancy and pregnancy can eliminate this cause of folate deficiency.

Increased utilization and consumption of folate occurs in the bone marrow itself if a chronic proliferation of cells such as hemolytic anemia, leukemia, or multiple myeloma is present. Although rarely the cause of the anemia seen in these patients, folate deficiency can cause a megaloblastic change in the cellular morphology of the bone marrow and peripheral blood.

The third major reason for folic acid deficiency is malabsorption syndromes; the most notable of which are tropical sprue and nontropical sprue. The term "sprue" referred originally to a chronic wasting disorder common in the tropics and associated with diarrhea, idiopathic steatorrhea ("fatty" stools), and glossitis.[9] The cause of sprue in the tropics remains a mystery, since it may respond simply to antibiotic treatment. Nontropical sprue is a similar clinical syndrome associated with a sensitivity of the intestinal tract to gluten, a wheat protein. It is sometimes called "gluten-induced enteropathy" and "adult celiac disease." Childhood celiac disease is a related malabsorption syndrome seen in children. These malabsorption syndromes can result in a combined deficiency of folate plus vitamin $B_{12}$ or iron deficiency.

Certain drugs such as methotrexate are used in cancer chemotherapy because they act as folate antagonists and inhibit pyrimidine synthesis. Other drugs associated with depressed serum folate levels for unclear reasons include certain anticonvulsants[11] and antituberculosis agents.[12]

## Vitamin $B_{12}$ Deficiency

Vitamin $B_{12}$ deficiency is almost always due to malabsorption.[13] Table 5–2 summarizes the causes of vitamin $B_{12}$ deficiency. As one can readily see, pernicious anemia represents one cause of malabsorption of vitamin $B_{12}$. Unfortunately, the term "pernicious anemia" has often been used as a synonym for vitamin $B_{12}$ deficiency and even for megaloblastic anemia, which is clearly incorrect. A resection of the stomach will result in a situation similar to that seen in pernicious anemia, i.e., lack of intrinsic factor production. Less common causes of vitamin $B_{12}$

**Table 5–2. CAUSES OF VITAMIN $B_{12}$ DEFICIENCY**

**Impaired absorption**
 Lack of intrinsic factor (pernicious anemia)
 Gastrectomy
 Chronic gastritis
 Tropical and nontropical sprue
 Inflammatory bowel disease (e.g., regional ileitis)
 Ileal resection
**Microorganism competition**
 Diphyllobothrium latum (fish tapeworm)
 Bacteria in blind loop syndrome
**Transport protein defects**
 Hereditary lack of transcobalamin II
 Abnormal transcobalamin II
 Abnormal $B_{12}$-binding protein
**Dietary deficiency**
 Strict veganism

deficiency include fish tapeworm infection and abnormalities in the major vitamin $B_{12}$ transport protein in the blood, transcobalamin II. Dietary deficiency of vitamin $B_{12}$ is extremely rare and occurs only in very strict vegetarians who eat no meat, eggs, or dairy products.

### Pernicious Anemia

Pernicious anemia was named by Biermer[3] because of its persistent, inevitably fatal nature. It was originally felt to be a dietary deficiency of vitamin $B_{12}$, which might be corrected by feeding liver to patients. Castle[14] in 1929 described the presence of an intrinsic factor in gastric contents, which was required for the absorption of vitamin $B_{12}$. It is now known that deficient production of this IF by the parietal cells of the stomach is the cause of pernicious anemia. Without this substance, vitamin $B_{12}$ cannot be absorbed into the body. The exact cause of the IF deficiency in pernicious anemia is still unknown, but a combination of genetic predilection and autoimmune factors is probably involved. The evidence for an autoimmune etiology centers on the fact that these patients produce autoantibodies to parietal cells and, to a lesser extent, to IF. It is felt that the antibody to parietal cells causes an atrophy of these cells, resulting in deficient production of both hydrochloric acid and IF. The discovery of these autoantibodies led to the advent of new tests for pernicious anemia based on the detection of anti-IF and antiparietal cell antibodies.

Pernicious anemia is most common in persons of Scandinavian and northern European ancestry but is also seen in a variety of other races and nationalities. The peak age at diagnosis is 60 years.[5] The clinical manifestations of pernicious anemia are the same as those seen in other types of vitamin $B_{12}$ deficiency and will be discussed subsequently. Fortunately, pernicious anemia is no longer "pernicious" and can be treated with lifelong injections of vitamin $B_{12}$. Pernicious anemia is also associated with autoimmune syndromes involving other tissues and organs (e.g., hypothyroidism, "Hashimoto" disease, and diabetes).

## CLINICAL MANIFESTATIONS

The clinical manifestations of megaloblastic anemia are grouped into two categories: (1) those seen in both vitamin $B_{12}$ and folate deficiency and (2) those seen only in vitamin $B_{12}$ deficiency.

Clinical manifestations common to both vitamin deficiencies include pallor, weakness, lightheadedness, and shortness of breath due to anemia; a lemon yellow pallor (slight jaundice) due to increased bilirubin; and epithelial abnormalities such as a smooth, sore tongue. The anemia in both cases is usually insidious in onset and well compensated for by the patient.

The neurologic manifestations (Table 5–3) seen in pernicious anemia are unique to vitamin $B_{12}$ deficiency and distinguish it from folate deficiency. These manifestations cause the numbness and tingling of extremities, gait abnormality, and difficulty with fine motor coordination that these patients experience. If left untreated, these abnormalities can progress to permanent neurologic damage.

Clinical signs and symptoms, although helpful in distinguishing vitamin $B_{12}$ from folic acid deficiency, cannot differentiate with certainty the exact etiology without the aid of the laboratory.

## MORPHOLOGY OF PERIPHERAL BLOOD AND BONE MARROW

Megaloblastic anemia is a classic example of how the deficiency of a single vitamin ($B_{12}$ or folic acid) can cause a cascade of destructive events affecting different cell types and tissues in the body. These events, although thought of as mainly affecting hematopoietic cells, affect all rapidly dividing cells in the body. The bone marrow in a megaloblastic anemia reveals the actual abnormality in maturation, whereas the peripheral blood reflects the effects of that abnormal maturation on the differentiated cells.

This section will focus on the morphologic effects on hematopoiesis seen in these two deficiencies. It is important to remember that the exact same abnormalities are seen in both vitamin $B_{12}$ and folic acid deficiency and that they cannot be distinguished

### Table 5–3. THE "P's" OF NEUROLOGIC MANIFESTATIONS IN PERNICIOUS ANEMIA

Peripheral neuropathy
Pyramidal tract signs
Posterior spinal column degeneration
Psychosis ("megaloblastic madness")

morphologically. Morphologic examination only determines that the anemia is megaloblastic in type; further laboratory tests are required to determine the specific etiology.

The peripheral blood finding most commonly associated with megaloblastic anemia is macrocytosis. In the years before the advent of the electronic particle counters, macrocytosis was detected by the enlargement of red cells on a peripheral blood smear. This was a very insensitive means of detecting slight increases in red cell size. The electronic counters provided the hematology laboratory with the first accurate and precise measurement of red cell size — the MCV. This electronically measured mean corpuscular red cell volume is a very sensitive means of detecting macrocytosis. Macrocytosis is important to establish since it is often one of the earliest peripheral blood abnormalities in vitamin $B_{12}$ or folate deficiency. Most patients with a megaloblastic anemia will have an MCV greater than 100 $\mu^3$ but rarely greater than 150 $\mu^3$; however, it must be remembered that the MCV is not *always* elevated in megaloblastic anemia. This is especially true for patients in whom striking anisocytosis or red cell dimorphism is present, as in the case of combined megaloblastic anemia and iron deficiency. As the MCV is an average value, these extremes in size can average out to give a normal MCV.

Examination of the peripheral smear is valuable in evaluating the etiology of an elevated MCV. Several types of macrocytes occur: (1) oval macrocytes, resulting probably from a megaloblastic process most commonly associated with $B_{12}$ and folate deficiency; (2) round, blue-grey macrocytes — polychromatophilic red cells due to reticulocytosis; and (3) round, pink macrocytes, most commonly associated with liver disease, alcoholism, and hypothyroidism.

The oval macrocyte is the most important red cell abnormality seen in megaloblastic anemia **(see Color Figure 73)**. Oval macrocytes are formed in the bone marrow as a result of megaloblastic or megaloblastoid erythropoiesis. The peripheral blood morphology in a severe case of megaloblastic anemia is depicted in **Color Figures 73, 74, and 75.** The severity of the red cell abnormalities in megaloblastic anemia correlates directly with the severity of anemia. In a severely anemic patient, striking anisocytosis and poikilocytosis are seen with an interesting mix of different types of poikilocytes, including oval macrocytes, target cells, schistocytes, spherocytes, and tailed red cells (teardrops). If the oval macrocytes are not recognized for their diagnostic importance, this mix of poikilocytes can be quite confusing. In a mild case, the oval macrocytosis may be very slight and hard to detect with minimal anisocytosis and poikilocytosis.

When anisocytosis is seen in megaloblastic anemia, it will result in an increased RDW (red cell distribution width) on the S-Plus series of Coulter instruments. The red cell histogram will reflect the wide disparity in red cell size in these cases, which at times show a perfectly normal MCV. The histogram will also reveal red cell dimorphism, which may be seen occasionally in megaloblastic anemia when iron deficiency coexists with a vitamin $B_{12}$ or folate deficiency. Red cell trimorphism may even be seen when these dimorphic patients get transfused with a third normal red cell population. These different-sized populations of red cells create very interesting red cell histograms in some cases of megaloblastic anemia.

Red cell inclusions are seen regularly in megaloblastic anemia. The most common is the Howell-Jolly body. The two major clinical situations in which Howell-Jolly bodies are seen on peripheral blood smears are megaloblastic anemia and postsplenectomy. The Howell-Jolly bodies seen in megaloblastic anemia are not numerous on the smear but are significant. There may be several Howell-Jolly bodies in a single red cell **(see Color Figure 74)**. These multiple Howell-Jolly bodies strongly suggest a megaloblastic etiology, because they are formed as a result of nuclear fragmentation or karyorrhexis in the bone marrow nucleated red cells. This fragmentation occurs readily in megaloblastic nucleated red cells, because their nuclei are defective. Other inclusions seen in megaloblastic anemia are basophilic stippling and Cabot rings. Cabot rings **(Color Figure 78)** are an extremely rare occurrence in the hematology laboratory; however, when seen, severe megaloblastic anemia is likely.

Occasionally, polychromatophilic red cells and nucleated red cells are seen in an untreated patient. The relative percentage of reticulocytes may be slightly increased owing to the severe decrease in the total red cells, but the absolute reticulocyte count is decreased, since erythropoiesis in these cases is ineffective in generating needed red cells. The absolute reticulocyte count is always a more accurate measure of red cell production by the bone marrow than the reticulocyte percentage. The nucleated red cells seen in the peripheral blood may exhibit the same abnormal nuclear features as the cells in the bone marrow and should be identified as megaloblastic nucleated red cells. With treatment, polychromatophilia and nucleated red cells become more numerous, and polychromatophilic oval macrocytes may be seen.

The triad of an elevated MCV, oval macrocytes, and hypersegmented neutrophils constitutes strong evidence of megaloblastic dyspoiesis. Hypersegmentation of polymorphonuclear neutrophils is defined as an increase in the average lobe number of the circulating neutrophils **(see Color Figure 75)**. It is reported as present in our laboratory when 5 percent of the neutrophils have five or more lobes. Rare numbers of neutrophils with six or more lobes and eosinophils with four or more lobes should also be reported as hypersegmented. Neutrophil lobe counts as high as 13 have been reported in megaloblastic anemia by Miale.[15] Hypersegmented neutrophils are often larger than normal (macropolycytes) and their lobes tend to look very detached with a longer, stringy-looking filamentation. This peculiar-looking lobulation often alerts the morphologist to the presence of hypersegmentation. Hypersegmentation is usually the first sign of megaloblastic dyspoiesis in the peripheral blood, and it is seen in 98 percent of the patients with megaloblastic anemia.[16] It is also the last smear abnormality to disappear in treated patients. Hypersegmented neutrophils may persist in the peripheral blood for about 10 days to two weeks after specific therapy has been initiated.[17]

The final key element of the peripheral blood in many cases is pancytopenia. Pancytopenia is defined as the combination of a decreased white cell count, a decreased red cell count, and a decreased platelet count. The diagnostic importance of pancytopenia in hematology cannot be overemphasized. Megaloblastic anemia is just one of a variety of hematologic disorders that present with a pancytopenia (see Chapter 6). Pancytopenia in megaloblastic anemia is the direct result of the megaloblastic dyspoiesis and ineffective cell production that occurs in all three cell lines produced in the bone marrow. The precursors of these cell lines are numerous in the marrow, yet their mature products — red cells, white cells (granulocytes), and platelets — are decreased in number in the peripheral blood. This is known as ineffective hematopoiesis and, specifically for red cells, ineffective erythropoiesis. Megaloblastic hematopoiesis is ineffective, because, despite the fact the bone marrow is actively producing nucleated precursors, mature cells are not effectively manufactured and released. This is thought to occur because the defective nucleated precursors die prematurely in the bone marrow.

The degree of cytopenia (cell reduction) is variable, but the white cell counts are usually between 2.0 and $4.0 \times 10^9/l$, with a relative lymphocytosis due to granulocytopenia. There may be a mild shift to the left with myelocytes noted on the smear in some cases. The platelet count is usually between 50 and $150 \times 10^9/l$, but platelet counts as low as $15 \times 10^9/l$ have been recorded. The red cell count, hemoglobin, and hematocrit are reduced to varying levels dependent on the severity of the deficiency. As already noted the MCV is increased, as is the MCH; however, the MCHC is normal in most cases.

The bone marrow morphology in a megaloblastic anemia **(see Color Figures 76 and 77)** reveals the actual abnormality in maturation which results from vitamin $B_{12}$ or folic acid deficiency. Although the morphology is very interesting and valuable from an educational standpoint, the examination of the bone marrow is not *required* to diagnose the ordinary case of megaloblastic anemia. If the peripheral smear reveals the characteristic abnormalities just described, testing the level of serum vitamin $B_{12}$, folic acid, and red cell folate will establish the diagnosis in most cases. However, since megaloblastic peripheral blood features can occur in myelodysplastic syndromes, a bone marrow aspirate is usually performed prior to the institution of therapy.

The term "megaloblastic change" is used to describe a morphologic abnormality in the bone marrow referred to as asynchrony, the lack of the normal coordinated nuclear and cytoplasmic development of hematopoietic cells in the bone marrow. This is also called nuclear-cytoplasmic dissociation. In normoblastic red cell development, the hemoglobinization and pinking of the cytoplasmic occur "in time" with nuclear maturation and changes in the nuclear chromatin clumping pattern. In megaloblastic red cell precursors, the nuclear maturation is lagging well behind the hemoglobinization in the cytoplasm, because of the impaired DNA synthesis. The cells are also visibly larger than normal, owing to the lag in DNA replication and cell division. Megaloblastic change is most noticeable in the later stages of red cell development—the polychromatophilic (rubricyte) and orthochromic (metarubricyte) stages. The orthochromic stage of normoblastic maturation normally shows a dense pyknotic nuclear chromatin with a very hemoglobinized pink cytoplasm. The orthochromic stage, if megaloblastic, shows the nuclear clumping pattern of a younger cell like a rubricyte with the cytoplasmic pinking expected of the orthochromic (metarubricyte) stage. A corresponding abnormality in maturation is seen at every stage of the red cell series. The megaloblast initially described by Ehrlich[1] was a pronormoblast with a much more open, sieve-like chromatin pattern than is normally seen. These very immature megaloblastic pronormoblasts are abundant in the more severe cases but not in mild cases of megaloblastosis. In milder cases, megaloblastic change in the orthochromic stage is much easier to identify. Other abnormalities seen in the later nucleated stages include multiple Howell-Jolly bodies and nuclear karyorrhexis.

Megaloblastic change is not restricted to the erythroid precursors. It is also seen in the other dividing cell lines of the bone marrow, especially the granulocytic precursors. The most typical granulocytic abnormalities are the giant band and giant metamyelocyte **(see Color Figure 77).** These cells, as in the case of the erythroid precursors, exhibit gigantism and a nuclear maturation lagging behind cytoplasmic maturation, i.e., the nuclear chromatin is not clumping as much as a band or metamyelocyte should. In some cases, megaloblastic change in

the granulocytes is more evident than in the erythroid cells. The megakaryocytes, when abnormal, are hyperlobulated and the lobes may appear somewhat detached and peculiar.

The bone marrow is hypercellular with erythroid hyperplasia and a reversed M : E ratio. The normal M : E ratio is 3 : 1 or 4 : 1, whereas in megaloblastic anemia it is often 1 : 1 or 1 : 3. The increased cellularity reflects the futile and ineffective attempt of the bone marrow to respond to the anemia by regenerating red cells. Increased numbers of mitoses and atypical-appearing mitoses are common in megaloblastic bone marrows. The bone marrow iron is normal to increased, and if increased, numerous macrophages laden with iron will be seen. Excess iron is present owing to the accelerated death of erythroid precursors in the marrow, a process that releases large amounts of heme iron.

## MEGALOBLASTIC CHANGES IN NONDEFICIENT PATIENTS

Megaloblastic dyspoiesis is not limited to situations in which vitamin $B_{12}$ or folic acid deficiency exist. It can sometimes be an indicator that the bone marrow is developing a clone of neoplastic cells. This is the case in myelodysplastic syndrome (preleukemia), in which a megaloblastic dyserythropoiesis is the most common finding in the bone marrow.[18] This dyserythropoiesis (abnormal erythropoiesis) will result in the exact same red cell abnormality seen in megaloblastic anemia: the oval macrocyte. Oval macrocytosis is seen in the peripheral blood in 74 percent of the patients with preleukemic syndrome.[18] Myelodysplastic syndrome frequently shows a pancytopenia that is more severe than that seen in megaloblastic anemia, i.e., the white cell counts are lower (in 1000 to 2000/mm³ range) and the platelet counts are lower (less than 50,000/mm³).

Another disease that shows marked megaloblastic dyserythropoiesis and that morphologically can resemble megaloblastic anemia is erythroleukemia (FAB class $M_6$). Erythroleukemia can look similar to myelodysplastic syndrome in the peripheral blood or can show a flagrant erythroblastosis with bizarre megaloblastic nucleated red cells and accompanying myeloblasts.

Myelodysplasia and erythroleukemia show a megaloblastic-like change in the erythroid precursors of the bone marrow that is often referred to as "megaloblastoid" to distinguish the very different malignant or premalignant etiology. Many hematologists dislike the term "megaloblastoid," because of the difficulty in morphologically determining megaloblastic versus megaloblastoid.

A more detailed discussion of myelodysplastic syndromes and erythroleukemia may be found in Chapter 21.

## NONMEGALOBLASTIC CAUSES OF MACROCYTOSIS

Macrocytosis is a common hematologic abnormality in a large hospital center. One study by Breedveld, Bieger, and van Wermeskerken[19] noted that an MCV greater than 100 $\mu^3$ was present in 2.3 percent of 10,000 blood counts performed at Bronova Hospital in the Netherlands. This percentage is probably somewhat higher (3 to 4 percent) in a large urban hospital center in the United States. Table 5–4 summarizes the causes of macrocytosis in 70 of the patients studied by Breedveld. This table illustrates that the causes of macrocytosis are quite variable, and very important diagnostically. Megaloblastic anemia is the most common cause of an elevated MCV, but the nonmegaloblastic causes such as alcoholism account for many of the increased MCVs seen in the laboratory. Patients receiving certain immunosuppressive agents consistently show elevated MCVs; these cases were excluded from the Breedveld study.

The two major causes of nonmegaloblastic macrocytosis are alcoholism and hematologic disease. Macrocytosis is such a common finding in alcoholics that the MCV has been recommended as a sensitive screening test for this condition. This form of macrocytosis in alcoholism appears to be related to a direct effect of alcohol on the red cell, rather than to folic acid deficiency. A patient history and liver function tests can be used to substantiate alcoholism as the cause of the elevated MCV.

Hematologic diseases associated with macrocytosis come under two major categories: (1) hematologic malignancy and (2) hemolysis. The most common hematologic malignancies involved are chronic myeloproliferative disorders, myelodysplastic syndromes, acute myelogenous leukemias, and multiple myeloma. Hemolysis can be associated with macrocytosis if the reticulocyte count is greater than 5 percent, because for each 1 percent increase in the reticulocyte count, the MCV increases by 1 $\mu$.[20] This is explained by the fact that the mean cell volume (size) of a reticulocyte is greater than that of a mature red cell. This cause of red cell

enlargement can also be detected on the peripheral blood smear as polychromatophilia.

Sideroblastic (refractory, idiopathic, or hereditary) and aplastic anemia can also result in macrocytosis. Sideroblastic anemia frequently shows a dimorphic red cell population, one population being macrocytic and one microcytic, hypochromic. This may result in a normal or slightly elevated MCV dependent on the size of cells in the particular case. Both sideroblastic and aplastic anemia require a bone marrow examination for diagnosis.

Occasionally, an elevated MCV is present as a laboratory artifact, i.e., not truly owing to increased red cell size. Two such situations are the presence of cold agglutinins and a very elevated white cell count. These two situations can easily be detected by looking carefully at the results of other instrument parameters and the peripheral smear.

## LABORATORY TESTS IN DIFFERENTIAL DIAGNOSIS OF MACROCYTOSIS

The presence of abnormal hematologic findings, usually an elevated MCV, necessitates a logical scheme of laboratory evaluation and testing. As mentioned before, peripheral blood morphology, especially the type of macrocyte seen on smear and the presence or absence of hypersegmented neutrophils, only helps to determine whether the anemia is megaloblastic or nonmegaloblastic in nature. The exact cause of the anemia must be determined by further laboratory testing owing to the many different causes of vitamin $B_{12}$ and folic acid deficiency. Figure 5-6 illustrates a logical scheme of laboratory testing in cases of macrocytosis.

The first determination to be made is whether the macrocytosis is strictly due to an increased reticulocyte count. If the reticulocyte count is sufficiently increased to cause the degree of MCV elevation seen, no other laboratory tests are required to evaluate the macrocytosis. Checking for a possible hemolytic state or blood loss is more appropriate in this case. If the macrocytes are not reticulocytes, a serum vitamin $B_{12}$ and folate level plus a red cell folate should be performed. These three tests must be performed simultaneously for correct interpretation of the results. The serum vitamin $B_{12}$ level and the red cell folate level are the tests that most accurately reflect tissue levels of these vitamins. The serum folate level is less reliable than the red cell folate in assessing tissue levels, because of its tendency to be falsely normal if the patient has had a recent intake of folate-rich foods. Nevertheless, the serum folate is important in the correct interpretation of serum vitamin $B_{12}$ results.

Prior to the 1970s, serum vitamin $B_{12}$ and folate levels were performed by microbiologic assay. The principle of the procedure was that if a certain bacteria requires either vitamin $B_{12}$ or folic acid for

**Table 5–4. CAUSES OF MACROCYTOSIS**

| Cause | Percentage of Patients |
|---|---|
| Vitamin deficiency ($B_{12}$ or folic acid) | 38.5 |
| Alcoholism | 27 |
| Chronic hepatitis | 0.03 |
| Hematologic disease | 18.6 |
|     Hematologic malignancy | 12.9 |
|     Hemolytic anemia | 5.7 |
| Hypothyroidism | 0.03 |
| Unknown | 0.085 |

Adapted from Breedveld et al.[19]

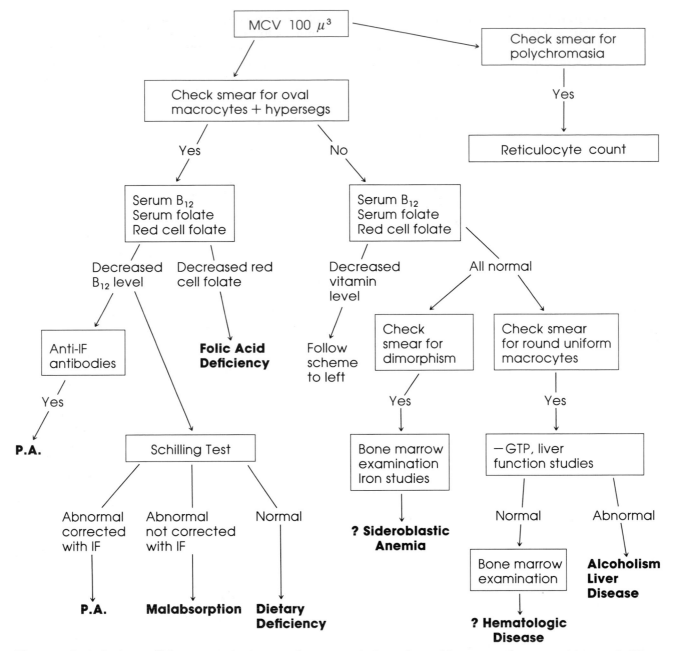

**Figure 5-6.** Logical scheme of laboratory testing in cases of macrocytosis. Boxes denote laboratory evaluations and/or tests; **boldface** type denotes diagnoses.

growth and this organism is incubated with patient's serum as the sole source of the vitamin, the amount of bacterial growth will directly correlate with the amount of the vitamin in the serum. Bacterial growth was measured spectrophotometrically by the turbidity produced and compared with serum standards with known amounts of vitamin $B_{12}$ or folic acid. These methods were accurate, but time-consuming, cumbersome, and impossible to use if the patient was taking antibiotics.

The radioisotope methods for vitamin $B_{12}$ and folate became the methods of choice in the 1970s,

because they were quick, precise, and presumably accurate procedures for determining serum levels as well as the red cell folate level. In retrospect, it is now felt that these new methods were introduced into routine clinical use too rapidly, with insufficient validation of their accuracy.[21] It was noted by various centers around the country that vitamin $B_{12}$ levels by isotopic methods were inappropriately high; i.e., patients had normal vitamin $B_{12}$ levels with obvious megaloblastic anemia due to vitamin $B_{12}$ deficiency. Isotope methods are based on the principle of competitive binding; i.e., the isotope-labeled vitamin competes with the unlabeled vitamin present in the patient's serum for a limited number of binding sites on a specific binding protein. The vitamin level in the patient's serum can be calculated based on the radiometrically measured amount of labeled vitamin bound to the binder or alternatively on the amount left unbound in the supernatant. The more labeled vitamin bound, the lower the patient's serum vitamin level, as less unlabeled vitamin was present in the patient's serum to compete for the sites.

The binding protein used in the vitamin $B_{12}$ assay currently is intrinsic factor. For accuracy, the binder used must specifically bind vitamin $B_{12}$ and no other substance. The binders initially used in many vitamin $B_{12}$ kits were neither purified nor specific enough and bound cobalamin analogues as well as vitamin $B_{12}$ itself. A 1978 study by Kolhouse and coworkers[22] demonstrated that 10 to 20 percent of patients with pernicious anemia showed false-normal vitamin $B_{12}$ levels by radioisotope methods. In recent years, these binders have been modified to correct this problem; however, kits to be used should be investigated carefully regarding their ability to differentiate normal from abnormal patients.

A variety of kits for performing serum and red cell folate levels by radioisotope methods have been introduced in recent years. These methods have also come under fire as being somewhat unreliable. It is uncertain whether any of these folate radioassay methods is superior or inferior to the microbiologic method.[21] There is no question, though, that the red cell folate level is a better test for tissue folate levels than the serum level. The serum folate level is useful in the interpretation of the results of the serum vitamin $B_{12}$ level. It is well known that the serum vitamin $B_{12}$ level will decrease in folic acid deficiency and that if both serum levels are decreased, the deficiency is either a folic acid deficiency or a rare combined vitamin $B_{12}$–folate deficiency. It is also true that patients with low serum vitamin $B_{12}$ levels tend to show increased levels of serum folic acid. These corresponding fluctuations are a result of the interrelationship of these two vitamins in normal metabolism.

Once vitamin $B_{12}$ deficiency has been established, the specific cause of the deficiency must be determined by further laboratory testing. Since pernicious anemia and other types of malabsorption are the leading causes of vitamin $B_{12}$ deficiency, laboratory testing has centered around the diagnosis of these states.

A new highly specific but somewhat insensitive test for pernicious anemia exists, the test for the "blocking" type of antibodies to intrinsic factor. Such antibodies are present in 50 to 60 percent of patients with pernicious anemia.[21] This test, if positive, is diagnostic of pernicious anemia and proba-

bly eliminates the need for the much more cumbersome Schilling test. However, if these antibodies are not present, a Schilling test must be performed. The other antibody detectable in the serum of patients with pernicious anemia is parietal cell antibody. Tests for parietal cell antibodies are rarely useful in pernicious anemia because of low specificity. These antibodies can be found in the serum of normal healthy patients and in those of patients with a variety of disorders other than pernicious anemia (particularly in other autoimmune syndromes).

The Schilling test is a procedure to evaluate the ability of the patient's intestinal tract to absorb vitamin $B_{12}$. It involves the oral administration of a standardized dose of $B_{12}$ labeled with $Co^{57}$ or $Co^{58}$. Simultaneously, an intramuscular flushing dose of unlabeled vitamin $B_{12}$ is given to the patient to bind all available storage sites for vitamin $B_{12}$. In this way, if intrinsic factor is present and normal absorption occurs, greater than 7 to 10 percent of the oral, labeled 1 $\mu$g dose will be excreted in the patient's urine collected over a 24-hour period. The excreted urine can then be assayed for radioactivity (part 1). If malabsorption of vitamin $B_{12}$ occurs, a decreased amount of labeled vitamin $B_{12}$ will be excreted. Intrinsic factor may then be given with the oral dose of vitamin $B_{12}$ and the Schilling test repeated to see if the Schilling test is corrected to normal with addition of IF (part 2). If so corrected, the patient has pernicious anemia. If the Schilling test does not correct with the addition of IF, other causes for the $B_{12}$ malabsorption must be investigated. It is important to remember that the accuracy of the Schilling test is dependent on (1) a complete urine collection and (2) normal renal function.

In the patient with a decreased red cell folate and documented folic acid deficiency, a careful evaluation of diet and drug history, alcohol intake, as well as tests for malabsorption will usually identify the cause.

Cases of macrocytosis with a normal vitamin $B_{12}$ and folate level require careful investigation. The major causes of nonmegaloblastic macrocytosis have been previously discussed. If the macrocytic red cells are round, pink, uniform, and possibly targeting, then liver function tests should be performed. These tests will confirm that alcoholism or liver disease is the cause. If no evidence of alcoholism or liver disease is present, a bone marrow examination is required, which will pinpoint the presence of various hematologic malignancies, of myelodysplastic syndrome, and of disease states such as sideroblastic anemia that can cause macrocytosis. It may also detect the presence of a mild megaloblastic anemia that had falsely normal vitamin $B_{12}$ and folate levels. If red cell dimorphism is noted on the smear, iron studies will complement the bone marrow iron stain in identifying the presence of sideroblastic anemia.

Two routine chemistry tests of special interest in the diagnosis of megaloblastic anemia are the serum lactic dehydrogenase and bilirubin level. The serum lactic dehydrogenase (LD) is often strikingly elevated in patients with a megaloblastic anemia regardless of the cause. The fractions responsible for the elevation are $LD_1$ and $LD_2$, with $LD_1$ greater than $LD_2$ (flipped pattern).[23] The serum bilirubin is usually only slightly elevated, owing to an increase in the indirect fraction. The results described for these two tests are usually associated with a hemolytic process. Megaloblastic anemia is in reality a hemolytic process, because of the massive intramedullary destruction of red cell precursors in the bone marrow. This destruction has the exact same chemical results as the destruction of red blood cells peripherally (i.e., hemolytic anemia).

## TREATMENT
### Vitamin $B_{12}$ Deficiency

The majority of patients who develop vitamin $B_{12}$ defiency are maintained with lifelong vitamin $B_{12}$ therapy. During treatment, all patients require initial saturation of the body stores with vitamin $B_{12}$. In the United States, generally a minimum of six intramuscular injections of 1000 $\mu$g of cyanocobalamin given at two- or three-day intervals is required for initial saturation. In situations where the underlying disease process is irreversible, as in pernicious anemia, lifelong maintenance therapy is administered following the replenishment of the body stores of vitamin $B_{12}$.

Maintenance therapy varies in concentration given and intervals administered from one institution to another, depending on the severity of the deficiency and preference of the clinician. It should be noted that hydroxocobalamin may be preferred over cyanocobalamin for treatment of vitamin $B_{12}$ deficiencies, because the former derivative is retained in the body three times as well as cyanocobalamin and binds more tightly to body proteins. Hydroxocobalamin, however, is a more expensive product and may not be justifiable in extra cost, in as much as both products correct the anemia.

A rise in the reticulocyte count can be seen several days following treatment. This is followed by a reversal of the clinical abnormalities to normal in the majority of patients. It should be noted that treatment with folic acid will also partially correct the anemia of a patient with vitamin $B_{12}$ deficiency if given in very large doses (5 mg/day). However, neurologic deterioration will still progress in vitamin $B_{12}$ deficiency if folate alone is given. As a result, simultaneous treatment of megaloblastic anemia with vitamin $B_{12}$ and folate is usually administered as a therapeutic trial if the exact pathogenesis has not been definitively established.

### Folic Acid Deficiency

Physiologic daily doses for the treatment of folic acid deficiency range from 100 to 400 $\mu$g of folate, which is most commonly administered orally for a given period of time, usually several months. Larger doses of folate (1 to 5 mg daily) are also used to treat this deficiency; however, it is necessary to confirm that vitamin $B_{12}$ deficiency is not present before these large doses are prescribed. Lifelong therapy is generally unnecessary, because it is often possible to correct the cause of the folate deficiency, thus preventing its reoccurrence. Table 5–5 compares the treatment of vitamin $B_{12}$ and folic acid deficiencies.

### CASE HISTORY

This 50-year-old white female was referred to the hospital from an outpatient clinic because her hematocrit was 13 percent. She felt fairly well at the time but had recently lost 40 pounds (18 kg). She had noted a lack of appetite (anorexia) and shortness of breath on exertion (dyspnea) in the past few weeks. She had a previous history of iron-deficiency anemia 10 years ago.

Physical examination revealed a thin, pale woman with a slightly yellow tinge to her skin color and icteric sclerae. Her tongue was very smooth and slightly reddened.

Table 5–5. TREATMENT OF MEGALOBLASTIC ANEMIA*

|  | Vitamin $B_{12}$ Deficiency | Folic Acid Deficiency |
|---|---|---|
| Initial | 1000 $\mu$g cyanocobalamin I.M., 6 times over 2–3 wk | 1 mg folic acid daily for 3–4 mo |
| Maintenance | 1000 $\mu$g cyanocobalamin I.M., once every mo | Correct underlying cause; 1 mg of folic acid daily or weekly |
| Indications for prophylactic treatment | Total gastrectomy, ileal resection | Pregnancy, chronic hemolytic anemias, autoimmune hemolytic anemia, myelodysplastic syndromes, dialysis, parenteral feeding |

*Other therapy that may be needed initially in severe megaloblastic anemia includes administration of diuretics, potassium supplements, and platelet concentrates. Blood transfusion is best avoided.

Laboratory Data:

CBC:

| | |
|---|---|
| WBC | = 7000/mm$^3$ |
| RBC | = 1,260,000/mm$^3$ |
| Hemoglobin | = 3.7 g/dl |
| Hematocrit | = 11.2% |
| MCV | = 87$\mu^3$ |
| MCH | = 29.8 $\mu\mu$g |
| MCHC | = 32.9% |
| Platelet count | = 37,000/mm$^3$ |
| Differential | = 60% segmented neutro- |
| | phils |
| | 37% lymphocytes |
| | 1% monocytes |
| | 2% eosinophils |
| Reticulocyte % | = 2.6% (0.5–1.5) |
| Serum LD | = 8700 U/l (60–250) |
| Total bilirubin | = 3.2 mg/dl (0.2–1.0) |
| Indirect fraction | = 2.6 mg/dl (0.2–0.8) |
| Serum iron | = 204 $\mu$g/dl (42–166) |
| TIBC | = 204 $\mu$g/dl (239–380) |
| % Saturation | = 100% (20–50) |
| Serum ferritin | = 400 ng/ml (10–100) |
| Serum vitamin B$_{12}$ | = <50 pg/ml (200–900) |
| Red cell folate | = 375 ng/ml (160–640) |

The peripheral blood and bone marrow morphology pertaining to this case may be seen in **Color Figures 73 through 78.**

1. What is the probable etiology of the anemia?
2. What are the morphologic abnormalities in the blood and bone marrow?
3. What is the correct interpretation of the reticulocyte count?
4. What further test(s) should be performed?
5. What is unusual about this case's clinical presentation or laboratory findings?
6. Are all chemistry test results compatible with the diagnosis?

This case represents a classic example of a severe degree of anemia, well compensated for by the patient because of its insidious onset. This patient had relatively few complaints despite having a 3.7 g/dl hemoglobin. Her physical signs pointed to the possibility of a hemolytic anemia or liver disease. In this particular case, the answer was indeed in the red cell. The red cell morphology was very striking, with a 4+ degree of anisocytosis and poikilocytosis. The types of poikilocytes were quite diverse and confusing, varying from spherocytes and schistocytes to tailed cells (teardrops) and ovalocytes. The diagnostically significant poikilocyte in this case was the oval macrocyte, which indicated a probable megaloblastic etiology. This was an important finding because, since the MCV was normal, a macrocytic anemia was not at all suggested by the CBC. Hypersegmented neutrophils were present on the smear, as were multiple Howell-Jolly bodies and rare Cabot rings **(see Color Figure 78).** The classic signs of megaloblastic anemia were all present on the smear even though the MCV was not elevated. The absence of an elevated MCV is a rare occurrence in megaloblastic anemia but can be seen in severely anemic patients, such as this woman, in whom the anisocytosis is very striking. The reticulocyte percentage in this case appears slightly elevated, but this is due to the very decreased red cell count. The absolute reticulocyte count is severely decreased at 32,760/mm$^3$.

Pancytopenia was not present in this case, because the WBC was normal, but the degree of thrombocytopenia was more severe than is usually seen. The patient had no hemorrhagic problems despite the thrombocytopenia.

The bone marrow aspiration was performed and predictably showed a flagrant megaloblastic dyspoiesis.

The chemistry results were entirely compatible with megaloblastic anemia. The LD level of 8700, although striking, is not at all unexpected. The iron studies and serum bilirubin level revealed results typical of chronic hemolysis (i.e., elevated serum iron, percent saturation, serum ferritin, and indirect bilirubin fraction). As explained in the text, megaloblastic anemia shows chemical findings identical to those seen in hemolytic anemia.

Based on the peripheral blood and bone marrow morphology, serum vitamin B$_{12}$ and red cell folate tests were performed. These results clearly pointed to a vitamin B$_{12}$ deficiency. One of two tests had to be performed at this point — the Schilling test or the anti-IF antibody test. In this case, the two-part Schilling was performed. The patient excreted a decreased amount of the labeled dose (2.66 percent) in 24 hours. The vitamin B$_{12}$ excretion increased to normal (12 percent) with the addition of IF. These results were diagnostic of pernicious anemia.

This case is somewhat unusual in that (1) the patient had no reported neurologic abnormalities and (2) the MCV was perfectly normal.

## References

1. Ehrlich, P: Farbenanalytische Untersuchungen zur Histologie und Klinik des Blutes. Hirschwald, Berlin, 1891.
2. Addison, T: On the constitutional and local effects of diseases of the suprarenal capsules. S Highly, London, 1855.
3. Biermer, A: Uker eine Form vow progressiver pernicioser anamie. Correspondenzbl Schweiz Anzte 2:15, 1872.
4. Hoffbrand, AV, et al: Megaloblastic anemia: Initiation of DNA synthesis in excess of DNA chain elongation as the underlying mechanism. Clin Haematol 5(3):727, 1976.

5. Hardisty, RM, Weatherall, DJ: Blood and Its Disorders. Blackwell Scientific, Boston, 1982, pp 206, 225.

6. Kolhouse, JT and Allen, RH: Absorption, plasma transport and cellular retention of cobalamin analogues in the rabbit. J Clin Invest 60:1381, 1977.

7. Hillman, RS and Finch CA: Red Cell Manual. FA Davis, Philadelphia, 1985, p 80.

8. Chanarin, I, et al: How vitamin $B_{12}$ acts. BJH 47(4):487, 1981.

9. Williams, W, et al: Hematology. McGraw-Hill, New York, 1983, p 448.

10. Sullivan, IW and Herbert, V: Suppression of hematopoiesis by alcohol. J Clin Invest 43:2048, 1964.

11. Dahlke, MB and Mertens-Roesler, E: Malabsorption of folic acid due to diphenylhydantoin. Blood 30:341, 1967.

12. Klipstein, FA, Berlinger, FG, and Reed, LJ: Folate deficiency associated with drug therapy for tuberculosis. Blood 29:697, 1967.

13. Castle, WB: Megaloblastic anemia. Postgrad Med 64:117, 1978.

14. Castle, WB: Observations on the etiologic relationship of achylia gastrica to pernicious anemia. The effect of administration to patients with pernicious anemia of the contents of the normal human stomach recovered after the ingestion of beef muscle. Am J Med Sci 178:784, 1929.

15. Miale, JB: Laboratory Medicine Hematology. CV Mosby, St Louis, 1982, 425, 432.

16. Lindenbaum, J: Folate and $B_{12}$ deficiencies in alcoholism. Semin Hematol 17:119, 1980.

17. Nath, BJ and Lindenbaum, J: Persistence of neutrophil hypersegmentation during recovery from megaloblastic granulopoiesis. Ann Intern Med 90:757, 1979.

18. Pierre, RV and Hoagland, HC: Preleukemic States: Differential Diagnosis of Refractory Anemia, Dysmyelopoietic States, and Early Leukemias. ASCP Workshop Publication, 1980.

19. Breedveld, FC, Bieger, R, and van Wermeskerken, RKA: The clinical significance of macrocytosis. Acta Med Scand 209:319, 1981.

20. Friedman, EW: Reticulocyte counts: How to use them, what they mean. Diagn Med (July):29, 1984.

21. Lindenbaum, J: Status of laboratory testing in the diagnosis of megaloblastic anemia. Blood 61(4):624, 1983.

22. Kolhouse, JF, Kondo, H, Allan, NC, et al: Cobalamin analogues are present in human plasma and can mask cobalamin deficiency because current radioisotope dilution assays are not specific for true cobalamin. N Engl J Med 299:785, 1978.

23. Winston, RM, Warburton, FG, and Stott, A: Enzymatic diagnosis of megaloblastic anemia. Br J Haematol 19:587, 1970.

24. Waxman, S, Metz, J, and Herbert, V: Defective DNA synthesis in human megaloblastic bone marrow: Effects of homocysteine and methionine. J Clin Invest 48:284, 1969.

# CHAPTER 6

JOE MARTY, M.S., M.T.(ASCP)

# Aplastic Anemia (Including Pure Red Cell Aplasia and Congenital Dyserythropoietic Anemia)

## DEFINITION

Aplastic anemia is a severe, life-threatening syndrome in which production of erythrocytes, platelets, and leukocytes has failed. Both genders and all age groups are affected. The disorder may result from a varied pathogenesis and etiology, and radiation, chemicals, drugs, infections, and autoimmune mechanisms are known to be associated with aplastic anemia. The incidence varies considerably but is approximately 1 per 100,000.

## HISTORY

The first reported case of aplastic anemia was described in 1888 by Ehrlich.[1] He described a fatal case of severe anemia and leukopenia with hemorrhage in a young woman. The autopsy findings showed little evidence of marrow development and led Ehrlich to conclude that the anemia was due to a depression of marrow function. A descriptive name was first applied in 1904 when Chauffard introduced the term "aplastic anemia."[2]

Reports and reviews increased in number, and in 1934, after a report by Thompson and colleagues, aplastic anemia was first considered a distinct clinical entity.[3] However, conceptual difficulties persisted, and only now are criteria for diagnosis becoming more clearly defined and accepted.

## PATHOPHYSIOLOGY

The primary defect in aplastic anemia is reduction or depletion of hemopoietic precursor cells with decreased production of erythrocytes, leukocytes, and platelets, resulting in peripheral pancytopenia **(see Color Figures 79 through 86)**. Most data suggest quantitative or qualitative damage to pluripotential stem cells as the primary event in bone marrow failure.[4] Information on these stem cells (CFU-S) has been obtained from murine studies.[5] If bone marrow is infused into a lethally irradiated mouse, hematopoietic colonies will form in the spleen. These colonies are formed from single progenitor cells capable of self-renewal and production of granulocytes, erythrocytes, and megakaryocytes. There is evidence that suggests the existence of a similar stem cell in humans, and, indeed, that a stem cell aberration is fundamental is suggested by the success of bone marrow transplantation in identical twins. Stem cell numbers, CFU-C and BFU-E, and/or their ability to replicate, is decreased in aplastic anemia. It is uncertain how stem cells are damaged. Direct damage by radiation, chemicals, drugs, and infections is suspected, particularly so when previous exposure has occurred. Recently, a number of observations have also suggested that marrow hypoplasia and aplasia may have an immunologic basis.[6]

Cellular and humoral abnormalities in hematopoietic regulation and an altered marrow microenvironment[7] have also been implicated as possible factors in aplastic anemia. Recent studies have suggested that in some cases T lymphocytes may suppress hematopoiesis.[8] Thomas and Storb[9] suggest an autoimmune mechanism in which a foreign agent attaches to a stem cell. The foreign substance acts as a "hapten," and the stem cell becomes an innocent bystander in an autoimmune reaction.

The influence of genetic factors in the pathogenesis of aplastic anemia is supported by the association with Fanconi's anemia, which has a familial basis.

## ETIOLOGY (TABLE 6-1)

Aplastic anemia may be (1) acquired due to exposure to ionizing radiation, chemical agents, drugs, and infections; (2) idiopathic; or (3) due to a congenital disorder such as Fanconi's anemia.

Evidence for determining the causative agents in aplastic anemia is often circumstantial. Even with agents that are known to cause aplastic anemia, the number of individuals affected is small in relation to

the number of individuals exposed. This makes epidemiologic studies difficult and results in ambiguity and inconclusiveness in determining the true cause of the illness. Why certain individuals are abnormally susceptible to agents and develop aplastic anemia is not known. No method for predicting individual sensitivity to drug or chemical exposure has been discovered. Metabolic defects, such as primaquine-induced hemolysis in glucose-6-phosphate dehydrogenase (G-6-PD)–deficient individuals, have not been identified. It is important to establish whether a causative agent may be present, so that continued exposure can be eliminated.

## Acquired

### Ionizing Irradiation

The acute results of radiation injury on cells have been well studied and documented. Radiation effects are consistent and predictable, depending on the dose of radiation received and the tissue involved. Hematopoietic cells are particularly sensitive to these effects. If the dosage is high, the marrow may become completely acellular. Whole-body irradiation with 300–500 rads can result in complete loss of hematopoietic activity. Sublethal exposure results in severe leukopenia, thrombocytopenia, and anemia. Aplasia in sublethal exposure lasts approximately four to six weeks, after which time the bone marrow recovers and cell counts return to normal. Only very penetrating forms of external radiation — x- and gamma rays — are likely to damage hematopoietic cells. Low-energy radiation — alpha and beta particles — may damage cells if ingested. The effects of continuous low-energy radiation became apparent in radium dial workers, who ingested radium when they wetted their brushes by mouth.[12] When exposure to radiation has been minimal or low, the immediate toxic effects on hematopoiesis are usually reversible. However, with both acute and chronic radiation exposure, the delayed or long-term effects are less predictable. Aplastic anemia can occur many years after initial exposure. The incidence of leukemia and carcinoma is increased in exposed individuals. Radiation exposure is common with cancer therapy.

### Chemical Agents

A variety of chemical agents have been associated with development of aplastic anemia, including benzene, trinitrotoluene, insecticides and weed killers, arsenic, and so on. Chemical agents containing a benzene ring with a nitro or nitroso group are particularly implicated. Benzene, an organic solvent obtained from coal and petroleum, was the first recognized and is the most common cause of aplastic anemia. It has been widely used as a solvent in

**Table 6-1. CAUSES OF APLASTIC ANEMIA**

| | |
|---|---|
| A. Acquired owing to exposure to: | Chemical agents |
| | Drugs |
| | Infections |
| | Ionizing irradiation |
| B. Idiopathic | |
| C. Congenital: Fanconi's anemia | |

many different industries. Exposure is primarily from inhalation of vapor, although absorption through the skin can occur.

Aplastic anemia may develop shortly after exposure or as much as 10 years afterward. Most cases of benzene toxicity are reversible after exposure has been eliminated. The reversible anemia may have a hemolytic component resulting in reticulocytosis. Benzene has been implicated also as a cause of leukemia. Animal studies have suggested that benzene may inhibit RNA and DNA synthesis and interfere with cell division and maturation.[13]

## Idiosyncratic Reaction to Drugs[14]

Idiosyncratic reactions to those drugs producing aplastic anemia are uncommon. Often the etiology is assumed on the basis of epidemiologic data and temporal relationship to exposure. The literature carries long lists of drugs that may be implicated in aplastic anemia. However, a true relationship has been established in only a small number of cases, and unfortunately, no definitive tests are available to predict or document the drug association. Drugs that have been implicated in idiosyncratic aplastic anemia include chloramphenicol, phenylbutazone, oxyphenbutazone, and others that are listed in Table 6–2.

Chloramphenicol and phenylbutazone are drugs that most frequently cause aplastic anemia. The effects of chloramphenicol have been well studied and documented.[15] Approximately 1 per 40,000 individuals exposed to chloramphenicol will develop aplastic anemia. This is about 20 times more frequent than the incidence of aplastic anemia in the general population. The effects of chloramphenicol are either reversible, dose-dependent and predictable, or irreversible, dose-independent and unpredictable. Reversible bone marrow suppression most commonly effects erythropoiesis and is due to decreased heme and hemoglobin formation. The morphologic finding of prominent cytoplasmic vacuolization in erythroblasts is commonly present.

In contrast, the irreversible effects of chloramphenicol are less predictable. The age of the individual and the dosage of the drug have no apparent relationship to the incidence or occurrence.

Another well-studied marrow depressant is quinacrine. During World War II, quinacrine was given routinely to soldiers in the South Pacific for malaria prophylaxis. Custer analyzed the cases of aplastic anemia occurring there during the years 1943 and 1944 and found the incidence of aplastic anemia to be 3 per 100,000.[16]

Table 6–2 lists other drug categories that are associated with aplastic anemia. Clearly, as new drugs are developed, the associations and incidences will

## Table 6–2. AGENTS ASSOCIATED WITH APLASTIC ANEMIA

**Those Regularly Producing Marrow Hypoplasia If Dose is Sufficient**

Ionizing irradiation
Benzene and derivatives (e.g., toluene),
Cytostatic agents (e.g., 6-mercaptopurine, busulfan, melphalan, vincristine)
Other poisons (inorganic arsenic)

**Those Occasionally Associated with Marrow Hypoplasia**

| Class | Relatively Frequent | Infrequent |
|---|---|---|
| Antimicrobial | Chloramphenicol<br>Organic arsenicals<br>Penicillin, tetracyclines | Streptomycin<br>Amphotericin B<br>Sulfonamides<br>Sulfisoxazole (Gantrisin) |
| Anticonvulsant | Methylphenylethylhydantoin (Mesantoin)<br>Trimethadione (Tridione) | Methylphenylhydantion<br>Diphenylhydantion (Dilantin)<br>Primidone |
| Analgesic | Phenylbutazone | Aspirin |
| Antithyroid | | Carbimazole<br>Tapazole<br>KClO$_4$ |
| Hypoglycemic | | Tolbutamide (Orinase)<br>Chlorpropamide (Diabinese) |
| Antianxiety | | Chlorpromazine (Thorazine)<br>Chlordiazepoxide (Librium) |
| Insecticide | | DDT<br>Parathion |
| Miscellaneous | | Colchicine<br>Acetazolamide (Diamox)<br>Hair dyes<br>CCl$_4$, Bi, SCN |

(From Beck, WS: Hematology, ed 3. MIT Press, Cambridge, 1982, p 39, with permission.)

change. It is obvious that indiscriminate use of drugs should be avoided. In particular, potentially toxic drugs should be used only when alternative therapy is unavailable. Table 6–3 lists some drugs implicated in hematopoietic suppression.

## Infections

Not infrequently, aplastic anemia is associated with hepatitis — in particular, types B and non-A, non-B. Other infections such as Epstein-Barr virus, cytomegalovirus, miliary tuberculosis, and dengue fever also have been associated with aplastic anemia. Reports of aplastic anemia following viral hepatitis have been increasing.[17] Possible mechanisms in viral hepatitis–associated aplastic anemia include (1) prolonged serum levels of drugs or their metabolites because of liver damage, (2) direct damage to stem cells by the virus, (3) depressed hematopoiesis by the viral genome, and (4) virus-induced "haptogenic" autoimmune damage. The possibility exists that subclinical viral infections may contribute to the incidence of aplastic anemia. Another possibility is that viral infections are secondary to marrow aplasia or dysfunction.

## Idiopathic

The majority of patients will give no history of exposure to any known or suspected causative agents. Detailed clinical histories have probably implicated many agents that have little to do with aplastic anemia. It is often difficult to determine the cause of aplastic anemia, because, by the time the damage is apparent, the causative agent may be absent or present in too small an amount to be detectable. It is hoped that in the future more specific environmental factors will be identified.

## Congenital Disorders

### Fanconi's Anemia

Assessment of family history and physical and hematologic abnormalities, as well as chromosome analysis, is helpful in making a diagnosis of congenital marrow aplasia. Fanconi's anemia is the most common and best described of these disorders.[10,11] The inheritance pattern is autosomal recessive. Disorders that may be confused with Fanconi's anemia include dyskeratosis congenita, pure red cell aplasia, Shwachman's syndrome, and thrombocytopenia–absent radius (TAR) syndrome. Patients with Fanconi's anemia have physical abnormalities including cutaneous hyperpigmentation, skeletal disorders (most common of which is aplasia or hypoplasia of the thumb), poor growth, renal anomalies, microcephaly, mental retardation, and strabismus. Not all of these disorders need be present. The most common findings are skin hyperpigmentation and short stature. Chromosome analysis

---

**Table 6–3. SOME DRUGS IMPLICATED IN HEMOPOIETIC SUPPRESSION***

| | | |
|---|---|---|
| Acetophenetidin (1, 3) | Cycloheximide (3) | Para-aminosalicylic acid (3, 4) |
| Acetylsalicylic acid (aspirin) (1, 2, 3) | Dextromethorphan HBr (2) | Penicillin (1, 2, 3, 4) |
| Acetyl sulfisoxazole (3) | Diethylstilbestrol (2) | Phenobarbital (1, 2, 3, 4) |
| Aminosalicylic acid (3, 4) | Diphenylhydantoin (Dilantin) (4) | Phenylbutazone (Butazolidin) (1, 2, 3) |
| Ammonium thioglycolate (3) | Dipyrrone (3) | Pipamazine (1) |
| Amodiaquin HCl (3) | Ethinamate (2) | Primidone (1) |
| Arsenicals (1, 2, 3, 4) | Fumagillin (3) | Prochlorperazine (Compazine) (2, 3) |
| Arsphenamine (1, 2) | Gamma benzene hexachloride (1, 3) | Pyrimethamine (Daraprim) (1, 2, 3) |
| Atabrine (1, 2) | Hair lacquer (3) | Quinidine (2) |
| β-Naphthoxyacetic acid (2) | Imipramine HCl (3) | Quinine (2, 3) |
| Benzene (1, 2, 3, 4) | Iproniazid (1) | Reserpine (2) |
| Bishydroxycoumarin (3, 4) | Isoniazid (1, 3, 4) | Stibophen (2) |
| Carbamide (2) | Lead (1) | Streptomycin (1, 2, 3) |
| Carbon tetrachloride (1) | Lithium carbonate (1) | Sulfamethoxypyridazine (Kynex) (2, 3, 4) |
| Carbutamide (Orabetic) (2) | Mephenytoin (Mesantoin) (1, 2) | Tetracycline (3) |
| Chloramphenicol (1, 2, 3, 4) | Meprobamate (1, 2, 3) | Thenalidine tartrate (3) |
| Chlordane (1) | Methaminodiazepoxide (Librium) (3) | Thioridazine HCl (3) |
| Chlorophenothane (DDT) (1, 2) | Methapyrilene HCl (4) | Tolazoline HCl (1, 2) |
| Chlorothiazide (3) | Methylpromazine (3) | Tolbutamide (1, 2, 3) |
| Chlorpheniramine maleate (3) | Mezapine (2) | Tolbutamide (Orinase) (2) |
| Chlorpromazine (Thorazine) (3) | Nitrofurantion (4) | Trifluoperazine (1, 3) |
| Chlorpropamide (2) | Novobiocin (4) | Trifluoperazine (Stelazine) (3) |
| Chlortetracycline (1, 3) | Nystatin (2) | Trimethadione (Tridione) (1, 2) |
| Cinophen (3) | Oxyphenabutazone (2) | |
| Coldricine (2, 3) | | |

*More than 500 are listed in the latest report of the American Medical Association Subcommittee on Blood Dyscrasias. The drugs listed in this table are those that have produced dyscrasias when given alone. 1 = pancytopenia; 2 = thrombocytopenia; 3 = leukopenia; 4 = anemia.
(From Miale, J: Laboratory Medicine: Hematology, ed 6. CV Mosby, St. Louis, 1982, with permission.)

usually reveals frequent chromatid breaks and exchanges. The extent of initial pancytopenia is variable but progressive and becomes symptomatic around age 5. Initially the bone marrow may show normal cellularity or hypercellularity, but eventually hypocellularity develops. These patients also have an increased incidence of acute myelogenous leukemia and hepatocellular carcinoma from anabolic steroid use. Early treatment consisted of chronic androgen therapy. The majority of patients die in the second decade of life, owing to hemorrhage or infection. More recently, some patients have been treated with bone marrow transplantation with some success.

## CLINICAL MANIFESTATIONS

The onset of aplastic anemia is often insidious. Symptoms include fatigue, dyspnea, palpitation, and, to a lesser extent, infection. Physical examination may reveal pallor, purpura, ecchymoses, petechiae, and mucosal bleeding. These symptoms are due to anemia, thrombocytopenia, and granulocytopenia. Splenomegaly is unusual. Mild lymphadenopathy may be present.

## LABORATORY EXAMINATION

Characteristically, the hemoglobin, white blood count, and platelet count are decreased to a varying extent in aplastic anemia. Criteria for severe aplastic anemia vary in different institutions, but the following figures have been given as guidelines for choosing patients for transplantation:

1. No significant improvement in blood values during three weeks following diagnosis, *and*
2. At least two of the following blood values (presence of which defines severe aplastic anemia):
   a. Platelet concentration of less than 20 × $10^9$/l (20,000/$\mu$l)
   b. Neutrophil concentration of less than 0.5 × $10^9$/l (500/$\mu$l)
   c. Reticulocyte counts of less than 1 percent[18] in the presence of anemia

An examination of the peripheral blood will reveal normochromic, normocytic red cells and decreased numbers of platelets and granulocytes **(see Color Figure 85)**. Some patients will have slightly macrocytic red cells. Occasionally normoblasts, small numbers of myelocytes and metamyelocytes, and a few reticulocytes may be seen. Prominent reticulocytosis, blasts, and abnormal platelets should *not* be seen. Relative lymphocytosis may be present. There is no peripheral morphologic abnormality that is diagnostic of aplastic anemia.

Table 6–4 lists diseases likely to be mistaken for aplastic anemia.

Bone marrow aspiration often results in a dry tap

**Table 6–4. DIFFERENTIAL DIAGNOSIS OF PANCYTOPENIA**

Anemia of pregnancy
Chronic renal disease
Overwhelming infection
Megaloblastic anemia
Leukemia
Lymphoma
Myelodysplastic syndrome
Myelofibrosis
Myelophthisic anemia
Paroxysmal nocturnal hemoglobinuria (PNH)
Hypersplenism
Autoimmune disease

**(see Color Figure 86)**. Bone marrow biopsy examination most commonly reveals a marked hypocellular marrow with a reduction in all myeloid and erythroid and megakaryocytic elements **(see Color Figure 80)**. Small numbers of scattered lymphocytes are usually present, and an occasional aggregate or nodule of lymphocytes may be seen **(see Color Figures 82 to 84)**. Other patients may have a foci of normocellular marrow, or even of hypercellular marrow.[19] Sheets or infiltrates of abnormal cells are absent and, if seen, represent indiscrete "leukemia aplasticus." In the presence of a hypercellular marrow, leukemia and myelodysplasia must be excluded. It is crucial to remember that there may be variations in cellularity within the same section and from one site to another **(see Color Figure 81)**. It is, therefore, important to make an overall assessment and perhaps obtain multiple biopsies when the diagnosis is uncertain. Ideally, the length of core biopsy should be 1 to 2 cm. It may be necessary to follow the patient's course of illness carefully to establish the diagnosis.

## TREATMENT, CLINICAL COURSE, AND PROGNOSIS

The prognosis of untreated aplastic anemia is poor.[20] Most patients will die if untreated. However, some patients may recover spontaneously, and this unpredictability complicates treatment decisions. Patients with low counts who fall into the "severe" aplastic anemia category have the poorest prognosis. In general, simple supportive transfusion therapy in these cases produces only a 20 percent survival at two years.

Treatment for aplastic anemia in the past was mainly supportive, with administration of steroids and androgens. These drugs have been shown to have limited value and undesirable toxic side effects. Today, the treatment of choice for severe aplastic anemia in patients under age 40 is bone marrow transplatation,[21] if an HLA-identical sibling is available. For other patients, immunosuppressive therapy is recommended. This might include cyclophosphamide and antilymphocyte or antithymocyte globulin. Reports from transplant centers have indicated survival rates on the order of 60 to 80 percent, with complete hematopoietic recovery. These encouraging results have occurred in selected patients. Important factors for survival are early transplantation and avoidance of blood products, especially products from potential marrow donors. There is a higher mortality in multiply transfused patients because of graft rejection, which reportedly is 25 to 60 percent in these patients.[22] If transfusions are necessary, leukocyte-poor red blood cells (RBCs) and platelets are recommended. The main complications of bone marrow transplantation are graft rejection and acute or chronic graft-versus-host disease (GVHD). Early transplantation, avoidance of transfusions, and immunosuppressive therapy have greatly decreased the occurrence of these complications.

The prognosis in aplastic anemia is variable and primarily depends on the severity of the anemia, supportive care, and method of treatment. Patients who do poorly often die from progressive deterioration due to repeated bleeding and infection. Intracranial hemorrhage with coma is common. Patients treated successfully with transplants may develop acute or chronic GVHD and interstitial pneumonitis. However, today the prospects for cure are good, a significant improvement over the last decade.

## RELATED DISORDERS

### Pure Red Cell Aplasia

Pure red cell aplasia is a disorder predominantly involving erythropoiesis. Leukocytes and platelets do not appear to be affected. Bone marrow examination usually reveals normal cellularity with absence of erythroid precursors. Reticulocytes and nucleated RBCs are not seen in the peripheral blood. RBCs are normocytic or slightly macrocytic. Evidence of hemolysis or hemorrhage is not present. Serum erythropoietin is usually increased.

This disorder can be acquired or constitutional. In some patients with hemolytic anemia, and during infection, erythropoiesis may suddenly halt. This has been termed an "aplastic crisis." An example is a patient with hereditary spherocytosis who has asymptomatic disease and develops a crisis with sudden reticulocytopenia. If recovery does not occur, severe anemia will develop.

Anemia may also be seen after administration of certain drugs. This anemia usually disappears after withdrawal of the drug. Other causes of acquired pure red cell aplasia include malnutrition and neoplasia. In about half of the adults with pure red cell aplasia, a thymoma (tumor of the thymus gland) has been found. Removal of this tumor has benefited some patients. Immune suppression of erythropoiesis is believed to have played a role in this form of red cell aplasia. The immune etiology is supported by the fact that some patients respond to steroid treatment and that infants born to mothers with the condition may be anemic at birth.

A congenital form of red cell aplasia was defined in 1938 by Diamond and Blackfan.[23] The syndrome was characterized by a slowly progressive and refractory anemia detected early in infancy. Leukocytes and platelets are normal. Other minor congenital abnormalities may be present, but renal abnormalities are not observed, in contrast to Fanconi's anemia. About 25 percent of these patients will show a spontaneous remission. This disorder is believed to be a result of a defective stem cell.

Limited success in this group of disorders has been observed by giving steroids, androgens, or immunosuppressive therapy.

Another condition, transient erythroblastopenia of childhood (TEC), occurs in early infancy and is usually self-limited. It is believed to be a result of inhibitors—either humoral antibody or viral—to late erythroid precursors in the marrow. Bone marrows in these patients show absence of late erythroblasts.

## Congenital Dyserythropoietic Anemia (CDA)

CDA was classified into three categories by Heimpel and Wendt.[24] A potential fourth type was described by Benjamin as associates.[25] All types are characterized by indirect hyperbilirubinemia, ineffective erythropoiesis, and bizarre multinuclear erythroblasts. Multinuclear erythroblasts are not unique to CDA and can occur in other situations in which ineffective erythropoiesis is a prominent feature, such as hemoglobinopathies, megaloblastic anemias, and leukemia.

CDA type 1 is characterized by a mildly macrocytic anemia with prominent anisocytosis and poikilocytosis. Bone marrow smears show erythroblasts with multilobated nuclei, megaloblastic changes, and thin internuclear chromatin bridges between two erythroblasts. The disease is apparent at birth but does not seem to affect longevity. The inheritance is autosomal recessive.

CDA type 2 is known as HEMPAS (hereditary erythroblast multinuclearity with positive acidified serum test). Erythrocytes are similar to those in paroxysmal nocturnal hemoglobinuria (PNH) in that they are susceptible to hemolysis in acidified normal serum. They differ from PNH erythrocytes by their failure to hemolyze in the "sugar water" test. Type 2 CDA cells carry increased amounts of blood group antigen i and are susceptible to hemolysis by anti-i alloantibodies. (For a review of PNH, see Chapter 11.) Erythroblasts show bizarre changes but differ from type 1 cells in that megaloblastic features are not present. Most patients have a normocytic anemia with a relatively benign course. Physical findings may reveal jaundice and hepatosplenomegaly. The inheritance is autosomal recessive.

CDA type 3 is similar to type 1 and frequently has giant multinucleated erythroblasts. Megaloblastic changes are not prominent, and the nuclear chromatin does not have a spongy appearance, as may be seen in CDA type 1. CDA type 3 cells are not susceptible to lysis by acidified normal serum. The anemia is normocytic or slightly macrocytic. Inheritance is autosomal dominant.

Cells in the proposed type 4 CDA are similar in appearance to cells in type 2 CDA but differ ultrastructurally and lack serologic abnormalities.

## CASE STUDY

A 3-year-old Caucasian boy was taken to the physician because of easy bruising, persistent black eyes, nose bleeds, and pallor.

Physical examination revealed oral ulcers, widespread petechiae, a few slightly enlarged lymph nodes, but no hepatosplenomegaly. The past history was noncontributory.

The laboratory data revealed a WBC of $2.2 \times 10^9/l$, hematocrit of 10 percent, platelet count of $5 \times 10^9/l$, reticulocytes of 1.8 percent, and absolute neutrophil count of $286/\mu l$. A differential of the peripheral blood showed 13 percent granulocytes, 85 percent lymphocytes, and 2 percent monocytes. Bone marrow biopsy examination revealed a hypocellular marrow with increased numbers of lymphocytes and some myeloid cells, but no megakaryocytes or blasts.

A search for an HLA-compatible marrow donor was unsuccessful. The patient was initially treated with platelets, RBCs, steroids, and androgens. The symptoms did not improve, and the patient developed resistance to platelet donors and needed HLA-matched platelets. Treatment with antithymocyte globulin was tried with no immediate success. The patient was maintained with blood products and antibiotics. He had had recurrent problems due to the pancytopenia, including cellulitis and an episode of major intracranial bleeding. After 14 months of careful supportive therapy, a gradual improvement was noted. This continued for several months and his counts stabilized with a hematocrit of 38.5 percent, platelets of $99 \times 10^9/l$, WBC $5.7 \times 10^9/l$, absolute neutrophil count of $1596/\mu l$. The differential showed 28 percent granulocytes, 61 percent lymphocytes, and 1 percent eosinophils.

This is an unusual but not rare example of a spontaneous remission in an individual with severe idiopathic aplastic anemia. Typically in those individuals who do improve, the counts never completely return to normal. It is believed that more individuals would experience remission if they could be maintained through their course of severe pancytopenia as this child was. Unfortunately, hemorrhage and infection are still major problems, and not all individuals will show improvement in their counts. Therefore, the treatment of choice is bone marrow transplantation when an HLA-compatible bone marrow donor is available.

## References

1. Ehrlich, P: Ueber einen fall von anämie mit bemerkungen uber regenerative veränderungen des khochenmarks. Charite Ann 13:300, 1888.
2. Chauffard, M: Un cas d'anémie pernicieuse aplastique. Bull Soc Med Hop 21:313, 1904.
3. Thompson, WP, Richter, MN, and Edsall, KS: An analysis of so-called aplastic anemia. Am J Med Sci 187:77, 1934.
4. Boggs, DR and Boggs, SS: The pathogenesis of aplastic anemia: A defective pluripotent hematopoietic stem cell with inappropriate balance of differentiation and self-replication. Blood 48:71, 1976.
5. Worton, RG, McCulloch, EA, and Till JE: Physical separation of hemopoietic stem cells from cells forming colonies in culture. J Cell Phys 74:171, 1969.
6. Parkinson R: The immunopathology of marrow failure. Clin Haematol 7:475, 1978.
7. Keating, A, Singer, JW, Killen, PD, et al: Donor origin of the in vitro haematopoietic microenvironment after marrow transplantation in man. Nature 298:280, 1982.
8. Good, RA: Aplastic anemia-suppressor lymphocytes and hematopoiesis. N Engl J Med 296:41, 1977.
9. Thomas, DE and Storb, R: Acquired severe aplastic anemia: Progress and perplexity. Blood 64:325, 1984.
10. Fanconi, G: Die familiäre panmyelopathie. Schweiz Med Wochenschr 94:1309, 1964.
11. Barosi, G, Cazzola, M, Marchi, A, et al: Iron kinetics and erythropoiesis in Fanconi's anaemia. Scand J Haematol 21:29, 1978.
12. Martland, HS: Occupational poisoning in manufacture of luminous watch dials. JAMA 92:466, 1929.
13. Moeschlin, S and Speck, B: Experimental studies on the mechanism of action of benzene on the bone marrow (radioautographic studies using ³H-thymidine). Acta Haematol 38:104, 1967.
14. Williams, DM, Lynch, RE, and Cartwright, GE: Drug-induced aplastic anemia. Semin Hematol 10:195, 1973.
15. Wallerstein, RO, Condit, PK, Kasper, CK, et al: Statewide study of chloramphenicol therapy and fatal aplastic aneia. JAMA 208:2045, 1969.
16. Custer, RP: Aplastic anemia in soldiers treated with atabrine. Am J Med Sci 212:211, 1946.
17. Hagler, L, Pastore, RA, Bergin, JJ, et al: Aplastic anemia following viral hepatitis: Report of two fatal cases and literature review. Medicine 54:139, 1975.
18. Thomas, DE, Fefer, A, Buckner, CD, et al: Current status of bone marrow transplantation for aplastic anemia and acute leukemia. Blood 49:671, 1977.
19. Frisch, B and Lewis, SM: The bone marrow in aplastic anaemia: Diagnostic and prognostic features. J Clin Pathol 27:231, 1974.
20. Lynch, RE, Williams, DM, Reading, JC, et al: The prognosis in aplastic anemia. Blood 45:517, 1975.
21. Storb, R, Thomas, ED, Buckner, CD, et al: Marrow transplantation for aplastic anemia. Semin Hematol 21:27, 1984.

22. Storb, R, Prentice, RL, Thomas, ED, et al: Marrow transplantation for treatment of aplastic anemia: An analysis of factors associated with graft rejection. N Engl J Med 296:61, 1977.
23. Diamond, LK, Allen, DM, and Magill, FB: Congenital (erythroid) hypoplastic anemia. Am J Dis Child 102:403, 1961.
24. Heimpel, H and Wendt, F: Congenital dyserythropoietic anemia with karyorrhexis and multinuclearity of erythroblasts. Helu Med Acta 34:103, 1968.
25. Benjamin, JT, Rosse, WF, Dalldorf, FG, et al: Congenital dyserythropoietic anemia — type IV. J Pediatr 87:210, 1975.

## Bibliography

Camitta, BM, Storb, R, and Thomas, ED: Aplastic anemia. Pathogenesis, diagnosis, treatment, and prognosis. N Engl J Med 306:645, 1982.
Geary, CG (ed): Aplastic anemia. Ballière Tindall, London, 1979.
Scott, JL, Cartwright, GE, and Wintrobe, MM: Acquired aplastic anemia: An analysis of thirty-nine cases and review of the pertinent literature. Medicine 38:119, 1959.
Wintrobe, MM: Clinical Hematology, ed 8. Lea & Febiger, Philadelphia, 1981.

# CHAPTER 7

S. ZAIL, M.B., B.Ch., M.D., FRCPath (Lond)

# Introduction to Hemolytic Anemias: Intracorpuscular Defects
## I. Hereditary Defects of the Red Cell Membrane

## CLASSIFICATION OF HEMOLYTIC ANEMIAS

A hemolytic state exists when the in vivo survival of the red cell is shortened. The presence of anemia in an individual patient is, however, dependent on the degree of hemolysis and the compensatory response of the erythroid elements of the bone marrow. Normal bone marrow is able to increase its output about six- to eight-fold, so that anemia is not manifest until this capacity is exceeded, corresponding to a red cell lifespan of about 15 to 20 days or less. Anemia may, however, occur with more moderate shortening of the red cell lifespan if there is an associated depression of bone marrow function, which may occur in certain systemic diseases or exposure to chemicals or drugs.

A useful classification of the hemolytic anemias entails their subdivision into those disorders associated with an intrinsic (intracorpuscular) defect of the red cell and those associated with an extracorpuscular abnormality. Red cells from a patient with an intracorpuscular defect have a shortened survival in both the patient and in a normal recipient, while normal donor red cells survive normally in the patient. In contrast, normal red cells when transfused into a patient with an extracorpuscular abnormality, are destroyed more rapidly. The patient's red cells, when transfused into a healthy recipient, have a normal survival, provided they have not been irreversibly damaged. Hemolytic states have also traditionally been regarded as being intravascular or extravascular, i.e., sequestration occurs in reticuloendothelial tissue. However, vigorous extravascular hemolysis may often be associated with signs of hemoglobin release into the plasma such as hemoglobinemia and decreased haptoglobin levels. The distinction is still useful from a clinical standpoint as certain hemolytic states are associated with predominantly intravascular hemolysis (e.g., paroxysmal nocturnal hemoglobinuria, infections due to Clostridia or Plasmodium falciparum).

Hemolytic anemias may be classified as follows:

1. Intracorpuscular defects
   A. Hereditary defects
      1. Defects in the red cell membrane
      2. Enzyme defects
      3. Hemoglobinopathies
      4. Thalassemia syndromes
   B. Acquired defects
      1. Paroxysmal nocturnal hemoglobinuria
2. Extracorpuscular defects
   A. Immune hemolytic anemias
   B. Infections
   C. Chemicals and toxins
   D. Physical agents
   E. Microangiopathic and macroangiopathic hemolytic anemias
   F. Splenic sequestration (hypersplenism)
   G. General systemic disorders (in which hemolysis is not the dominant feature of the anemia)

## APPROACH TO DIAGNOSIS OF A HEMOLYTIC STATE

The approach to diagnosis of a hemolytic state initially involves establishing that the rate of red cell destruction is increased and then determining the cause of hemolysis.

## Establishing the Presence of Hemolysis

Diagnostic tests used to establish the presence of hemolysis rely on the fact that hemolysis is characterized by both increased cell destruction and increased production.

### Tests Reflecting Increased Red Cell Destruction

The most frequently used tests in this category are the serum unconjugated (indirect) bilirubin and serum haptoglobin determinations. The serum unconjugated bilirubin level seldom exceeds 3 to 4 mg/dl in uncomplicated hemolytic states and reflects the catabolism of heme derived from red cells phagocytosed by the reticuloendothelial system (Fig. 7-1). The test is, however, relatively insensitive, as is the measurement of fecal stercobilinogen and urine urobilinogen that represents further stages in the disposition of unconjugated bilirubin by the liver (Fig. 7-1). As the unconjugated bilirubin is bound to albumin it cannot pass the glomerular filter, and the jaundice is said to be "acholuric." On the other hand, a decreased serum haptoglobin level is a very sensitive test of both intravascular and extravascular hemolysis, and reflects the rapid clearance by the reticuloendothelial system of a complex formed between liberated hemoglobin and circulatory haptoglobin. Drawbacks to the use of serum haptoglobin levels are that low levels may occur in hepatocellular disease, reflecting decreased synthesis by the liver, while some individuals, particularly in black populations may have a genetically determined deficiency of haptoglobin. Increased synthesis of haptoglobin in acute inflammatory states or malignancy may also mask depletion of serum haptoglobin owing to hemolysis.

Other tests that reflect increased red cell destruction, particularly if it is primarily intravascular, determine the presence of hemoglobinemia, hemoglobinuria, and hemosiderinuria. The assessment of hemoglobinemia requires stringent precautions in the prevention of hemolysis during blood collection. Once the hemoglobin-binding capacity of serum haptoglobin is exceeded, hemoglobin passes through the glomerulus as alpha-beta chain dimers, which reassociate to $\alpha_2\text{-}\beta_2$ tetramers in the tubule where the hemoglobin is reabsorbed and degraded. The liberated iron is conserved as ferritin and hemosiderin. When the tubular reabsortive capacity for hemoglobin is exceeded, hemoglobinuria ensues and is detectable either by spectroscopic examination or by commercially available dipsticks that detect heme. Staining of the urine sediment for iron (e.g., with Prussian blue) will detect the hemosiderin- and ferritin-containing renal tubular cells that are sloughed several days after a hemolytic episode.

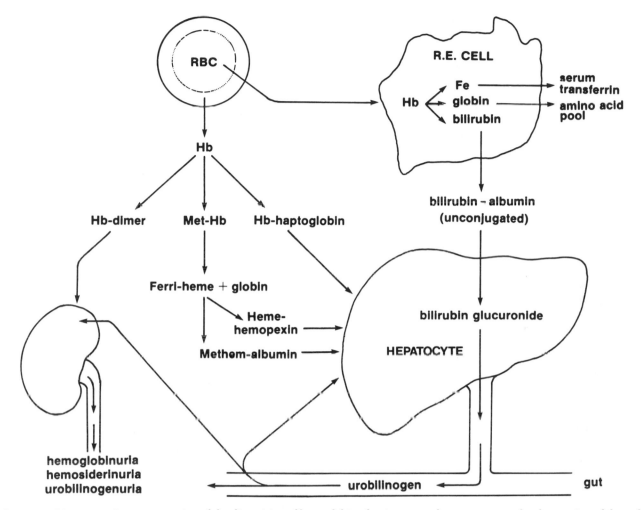

**Figure 7-1.** Diagrammatic representation of the disposition of hemoglobin after intravascular or extravascular destruction of the red cell.

Some of the free plasma hemoglobin may be oxidized to methemoglobin with subsequent dissociation of ferri-heme, which combines with albumin to form methemalbumin. Methemalbumin can be detected spectroscopically by the Schumm's test. This test is relatively insensitive and is seldom positive in mild hemolytic states. In routine practice, determination of red cell survival using $^{51}$Cr-labeled red cells is seldom required to document an increased rate of red cell destruction. The fate of hemoglobin when processed intravascularly or extravascularly is shown diagrammatically in Figure 7–1.

### Tests Reflecting Increased Red Cell Production

The compensatory bone marrow response to hemolysis results in the delivery of young red cells in the form of reticulocytes into the circulation. These young cells contain RNA, which stains supravitally with dyes such as new methylene blue or brilliant cresyl blue. The normal reticulocyte count is about 0.5 to 2.0 percent. This reflects the fact that each day approximately 1 percent of the red cell mass is destroyed and replaced by young red cells from the bone marrow, since red cell survival is approximately 120 days. The reticulocyte count is always elevated in a hemolytic state in which there is a normal compensatory bone marrow response. However, a more accurate assessment of red cell production is required, since the percentage of reticulocytes may be "spuriously" elevated as the reticulocytes may be diluted into a lesser number of total circulating red cells. In addition, in response to the anemia, reticulocytes may leave the bone marrow prematurely and mature in the circulation for longer than the normal maturation time of one day, again leading to a falsely elevated reticulocyte count. These cells (so-called shift reticulocytes) are recognizable as large bluish-grey erythrocytes on Romanowsky stains. The reticulocyte production index (RPI) corrects the hematocrit to a normal value of 45 percent and takes into account the maturation time of the reticulocyte at a particular hematocrit (approximately 1.0 day at a hematocrit of 45 percent, 1.5 days at 35 percent, 2.0 days at 25 percent, and 2.5 days at 15 percent).[1]

$$RPI = \frac{\% \text{ Reticulocytes}}{\text{Retic. maturation time}} \times \frac{\text{Hematocrit}}{45}$$

An RPI of greater than 2.5 to 3.0 is generally regarded as indicative of a hemolytic state, but it is very important to exclude the presence of hemorrhage in a particular patient, as this too may lead to an elevated RPI. Although the RPI is probably the single most useful test to detect a hemolytic state, a cautionary note is in order, as the test may not be sensitive enough to detect mild hemolytic states (see Chapter 31).

## Establishing Cause of Hemolysis

Once having documented the presence of hemolysis, it is our experience that the approach followed by Lux and Glader[2] in establishing the cause of hemolysis is pragmatic and logical and will be the technique followed in this chapter. The initial step consists of separating patients into Coombs test–positive (i.e., immunohemolytic anemias) and Coombs test–negative groups. The latter group is then further divided into "smear-positive" and "smear-negative" subgroups (Table 7–1). It is fundamentally important to assess morphology in peripheral smears that are free of artifact. On the basis of the classification according to the predominant morphologic criteria associated with a particular disease state (Table 7–1), it is possible to considerably narrow the differential diagnosis and then institute further appropriate tests to make a definitive diagnosis.

It is also worth emphasizing that many hemolytic states are associated with an underlying disease, as will become apparent in the ensuing chapters, and this should not be lost sight of in the assessment of the individual patient.

## HEREDITARY DEFECTS OF RED CELL MEMBRANE

## Biochemistry and Structure of Red Cell Membrane

An understanding of the etiology and pathophysiology of hemolytic states due to defects of the red cell membrane requires some knowledge of the structure and biochemistry of the red cell membrane. In particular, the properties of the membrane skeleton, which consists of a protein network connected to and lying just beneath the cell membrane, deserve special consideration, as several of the hemolytic states we shall discuss are associated with defective or absent membrane skeleton proteins. In its

**Table 7–1. PREDOMINANT RED CELL MORPHOLOGY COMMONLY ASSOCIATED WITH NONIMMUNE HEMOLYTIC DISORDERS**

Spherocytes
  Hereditary spherocytosis
  Acute oxidant injury (HMP shunt defects during hemolytic crisis, oxidant drugs, and chemicals)
  Clostridium welchii septicemia
  Severe burns, other red cell thermal injuries
  Spider, bee, and snake venoms
  Severe hypophosphatemia
Bizarre Poikilocytes
  Red cell fragmentation syndromes (microangiopathic and macroangiopathic hemolytic anemias)
  Hereditary elliptocytosis in neonates
  Hereditary pyropoikilocytosis
Elliptocytes
  Hereditary elliptocytosis
  Thalassemias
Stomatocytes
  Hereditary stomatocytosis and related disorders
  Stomatocytic elliptocytosis
Irreversibly Sickled Cells
  Sickle cell anemia
  Symptomatic sickle syndromes
Intraerythrocytic Parasites
  Malaria
  Babesiosis
  Bartonellosis

Prominent Basophilic Stippling
  Thalassemias
  Unstable hemoglobins
  Lead poisoning
  Pyrimidine-5-nucleotidase deficiency
Spiculated or Crenated Red Cells
  Acute hepatic necrosis (spur cell anemia)
  Uremia
  Infantile pyknocytosis
  Abetalipoproteinemia
  McLeod blood group
Target Cells
  Hemoglobins S, C, D, and E
  Thalassemias
  Hereditary xerocytosis
Nonspecific or Normal Morphology
  Embden-Meyerhof pathway defects
  HMP shunt defects
  Adenosine deaminase hyperactivity with low red cell ATP
  Unstable hemoglobins
  Paroxysmal nocturnal hemoglobinuria
  Dyserythropoietic anemias
  Copper toxicity (Wilson's disease)
  Cation permeability defects
  Erythropoietic porphyria
  Vitamin E deficiency
  Hypersplenism

Adapted from Lux and Glader.[2]

passage through the microcirculation and in its ability to withstand the strong shear forces in the circulation, the structural integrity of the red cell is to a large extent dependent on its ability to deform during flow. This important property of the red cell is dependent on three main factors: (1) membrane deformability, which is in turn largely dependent on the structural and functional integrity of the membrane skeleton; (2) the cell surface area–to-volume ratio; and (3) cytoplasmic viscosity. Alterations in these properties occur to various degrees in several of the hereditary defects of the red cell membrane and contribute to the ultimate destruction of the red cell.

The red cell membrane consists of a lipid bilayer that is associated in a complex way with a variety of proteins. Lipids constitute about half the mass of the membrane, while the proteins and glycoproteins constitute the other half. The lipids consist predominantly of cholesterol and phospholipid, with the polar head groups of the phospholipids oriented to each surface of the bilayer, and the hydrophobic fatty acyl side chains buried in the core of the bilayer (Fig. 7-2). The phospholipids are distributed asymmetrically in the bilayer, with the choline phospholipids (sphingomyelin and phosphatidyl choline) located in the outer half of the bilayer and the aminophospholipids (phosphatidylethanolamine and phosphatidylserine) located in the inner half.

Some of the proteins and glycoproteins associated with the membrane span the lipid bilayer and their intramembrane hydrophobic domains interact with the hydrophobic domains of the phospholipids. These are the integral membrane proteins (Fig. 7-2). Most of the remaining proteins are located on the cytoplasmic surface of the membrane and associate with the membrane by interacting with the integral membrane proteins or the polar head groups of the inner aminophospholipids. These are the peripheral membrane proteins, some of which are arranged in a specific way as a submembranous network called the membrane skeleton. The nomenclature of the membrane proteins is based on their separation by molecular weight by polyacrylamide gel electrophoresis in sodium dodecyl sulphate (SDS-PAGE) (Fig. 7-3). A schematic representation of the orientation of the proteins of the membrane skeleton in relation to the lipid bilayer and some integral proteins is shown in Figure 7–3. The membrane skeleton consists of a two-dimensional filamentous network consisting of spectrin, actin, and protein 4.1 (Fig. 7-3), Spectrin exists as a dimer of alpha and beta subunits of molecular weights 240,000 and 220,000, respectively, which forms tetramers by head-to-head associations through noncovalent interactions between a domain at one end of the alpha subunit and the phosphorylated end of the beta subunit.[3] There is some evidence that larger oligomers of spectrin may form by similar interactions. Spectrin forms the network by crosslinking and binding to short filaments of actin, this interaction being enhanced by association with protein 4.1. The skeleton is anchored to the membrane via ankyrin, which binds to one of the beta chains of the spectrin tetramer near the tetramer assembly site, as well as to a cytoplasmic portion of band 3, one of the major integral membrane proteins. Another major integral membrane protein, glycophorin A, is connected to the membrane skeleton through an interaction with protein 4.1.

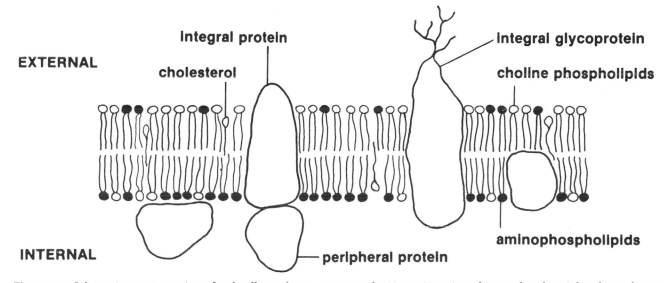

**Figure 7-2.** Schematic representation of red cell membrane structure showing orientation of integral and peripheral membrane proteins in relation to the lipid bilayer. (From Palek and Lux,[4] with permission.)

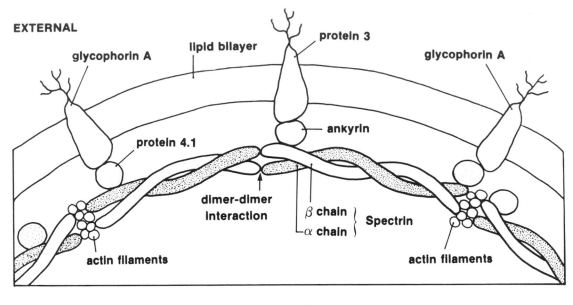

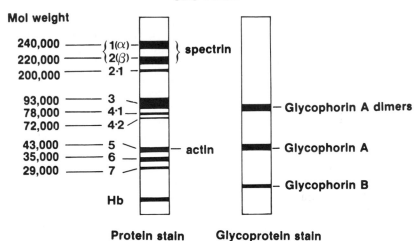

**Figure 7-3.** *Top,* schematic representation of the structure of the red cell membrane skeleton. *Bottom,* SDS-PAGE of red cell ghosts illustrating nomenclature of the membrane proteins and glycoproteins. (From Palek and Lux,[4] with permission.)

## Classification

Ideally, the classification of hereditary defects of the red cell membrane should be based on the delineation of specific defects of the membrane. The last few years have witnessed an explosive increase in knowledge in achieving this goal, particularly in the characterization of specific defects of the membrane skeleton. At present, however, all patients with clinical and morphologic evidence of a membrane defect cannot yet be categorized in this way, so that the classification used is still based on the prime morphologic features of the disorder (Table 7–2). Palek and Lux[4] have recently proposed the following nomenclature of known membrane skeleton defects, and these are shown also in Table 7–2. Skeletal protein deficiencies or defective protein associations are shown in brackets following the dis-

ease state. Superscripts $^+$ and $^\circ$ indicate a partial or complete protein deficiency, respectively. For example, HE [4.1°] denotes homozygous hereditary elliptocytosis associated with absence of protein 4.1. In the case of defective skeletal protein interactions, the defective protein (or its subunit if relevant) is underlined. For example, HS [Sp-4.1] represents hereditary spherocytosis with a defective spectrin-4.1 interaction, owing to a spectrin defect; HPP [Sp Dα-SpD] represents hereditary pyropoikilocytosis due to defective spectrin dimer-dimer interaction related to an abnormal alpha chain of spectrin.

## Hereditary Spherocytosis
### Mode of Inheritance

Hereditary spherocytosis is the most common hereditary hemolytic anemia in Caucasian people and

Table 7–2. HEREDITARY DEFECTS OF RED CELL MEMBRANE*

| Clinical Condition | Comments and Known Specific Defects |
| --- | --- |
| 1. Hereditary Spherocytosis (HS) | (a) Autosomal dominant inheritance—specific defect unknown in most cases, but all have a skeletal defect.<br>(b) Minority—HS (Sp-4.1).<br>(c) Very rare recessive variant HS (Sp+). |
| 2. Hereditary Elliptocytosis (HE) | Heterogeneous—at least eight clinical types have been delineated. Most common form is autosomal dominant mild HE (heterozygous and either asymptomatic or mild hemolysis). 20–40% have HE (SpDα-SpD). |
| 3. Hereditary Pyropoikilocytosis (HPP) | Relatively rare. Double heterozygous state. Most have HPP (SpDα-SpD), but at least two variants of alpha chain defects have been described. |
| 4. Hereditary Stomatocytosis | Heterogeneous. Specific defects unknown. |
| 5. Hereditary Xerocytosis | Specific defects unknown. Autosomal dominant. |

*Abetalipoproteinemia is a hereditary disorder (autosomal recessive) associated with abnormal red cell membrane lipid composition. However, the primary defect involves the plasma lipoproteins with secondary effects on the red cell membrane, and will not be considered here **(see Color Figure 92)**.

usually follows a classic autosomal dominant pattern of inheritance **(see Color Figure 87)**. However, for reasons not clear at present, in about a quarter of families there is no abnormality detectable in either parent. Although the latter finding might suggest a recessive type of inheritance in these families, the clinical findings are quite unlike those seen in the very rare examples of recessively inherited spherocytosis associated with deficient synthesis of spectrin, in which there is severe hemolysis and incomplete response to splenectomy.

### Etiology and Pathophysiology of Membrane Disorder

The fundamental expression of the membrane defect in hereditary spherocytosis (HS) is a loss of surface area of the red cell resulting in a decreased surface-to-volume ratio. This is manifested morphologically as spherocytosis and stomatocytosis (note that the majority of cells in HS are stomatocytic or spherostomatocytic rather than truly spherocytic). Such cells tolerate less swelling than normal red cells and are osmotically fragile. The decrease in surface-to-volume ratio also makes these cells less deformable than normal. This has a particularly deleterious effect on their survival in the spleen, and explains one of the hallmarks of HS, which is the excellent clinical response to splenectomy. The exact pathogenesis of the loss of surface area of the HS cell is still an enigma. Most authorities favor actual physical fragmentation of the membrane, but contraction of the membrane surface by other mechanisms is a possibility. One finding that seems certain, however, is that almost all cases have a defective membrane skeleton. In the minority of these cases a specific defect has been delineated— namely, a defect in spectrin affecting its interaction with protein 4.1 or, very rarely in recessively inherited HS, a partial deficiency (±50 percent) of spectrin. In an as yet unknown manner this skeletal instability leads to loss of membrane surface area. HS cells with a decreased surface-to-volume ratio are

selectively trapped and "conditioned" in the spleen, where the cells progressively lose more membrane surface and are ultimately destroyed. The exact mechanism of splenic conditioning and destruction of cells is again not clear. Previously held concepts that the HS cells undergo metabolic depletion with passive swelling and autohemolysis while they "stagnate" in the splenic cords are probably not correct, as it has been calculated that the average time HS cells spend in the spleen is too short for metabolic depletion to occur.[2] However, repeated metabolic stress in the "bywaters" of the spleen may contribute to the conditioning process. There is also indirect evidence that macrophage conditioning of HS cells may be of importance. In HS, peripheral red cells and particularly cells recovered from the splenic pulp are relatively dehydrated and have low concentrations of potassium and cell water, resulting in an elevated hemoglobin concentration ($\uparrow$ MCHC) and increased cytoplasmic viscosity. Some of the possible mechanisms of splenic conditioning and destruction of HS cells are summarized in Figure 7–4.

### Clinical Manifestations

The classic presenting features of patients with HS are the triad of jaundice, anemia, and enlarged spleen, but many patients do not show all these signs. The age of presentation can vary from within a day or two after birth to old age and sometimes may only be diagnosed during family studies or investigation for other reasons. About two thirds of HS patients present with a mild uncompensated hemolytic state manifesting with the aforementioned classic signs. Characteristically the jaundice is said to be "acholuric," as unconjugated bilirubin cannot pass the glomerular filter. Many of these patients have pigment gallstones, presumably due to increased concentrations of bilirubin in the bile. About a quarter of HS patients have a mild hemolytic state that is compensated for, and such patients are not anemic and are usually asymptomatic. A

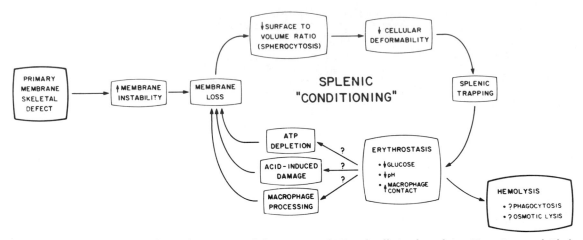

**Figure 7-4.** Postulated mechanisms of "conditioning" and destruction of HS red cells in the spleen. (From Lux and Glader,[2] with permission.)

minority of patients (about 10 percent) have a severe hemolytic anemia that may require blood transfusion. Aplastic crises, in which erythropoiesis is suppressed leading to more pronounced anemia, occurs particularly in this group but may supervene in patients with milder forms of the disease. An uncommon complication of prolonged hemolysis, which is not limited to HS, is chronic leg ulceration.

### Clinical Laboratory Findings

**Evidence of Hemolytic Process.** The laboratory features of extravascular hemolysis outlined earlier are usually apparent. Hyperbilirubinemia is found in about half the patients, and haptoglobins are variably reduced. Classic features of intravascular hemolysis such as hemoglobinemia, hemoglobinuria, or hemosiderinuria do not occur. The reticulocyte production index is elevated above 2.5 in most cases (presplenectomy).

**Red Cell Indices.** Anemia is usually mild. The mean level of hemoglobin in several series is about 12 to 13 g/dl, but individual cases may vary widely depending on the severity of hemolysis and the degree of compensation. The mean corpuscular volume (MCV) is usually within the normal range both before and after splenectomy but can be low, normal, or high. The MCH tends to parallel the MCV. Although the MCV is usually normal, because of the red cell's spheroidal shape, the diameter of some cells is substantially decreased and these appear as dark, rounded microspherocytes on the peripheral smear (see further on). The mean corpuscular hemoglobin concentration (MCHC) is elevated (>36 percent) in about 50 percent of cases and probably reflects mild cellular dehydration, particularly of cells that have undergone splenic conditioning and that have low levels of cell water and potassium (see section on etiology and pathophysiology).

**Morphology of Peripheral Smear.** The morphologic hallmark of HS is the spherocyte **(see Color Figure 87).** Although in many instances the detection of these cells may present no difficulty, in some patients their detection may provoke argument even among experienced hematologists. It is particularly important to examine well-prepared smears free of any artifact. In typical cases prior to splenectomy there may be varying degrees of polychromasia, poikilocytosis, and anisocytosis with many normal discoid cells, but the overriding impression is one of increased numbers of uniformly round cells (Fig. 7-5). Some of the cells appear as microspherocytes and are dark and round and lack a pale center.

**Special Laboratory Tests.** *Osmotic Fragility Test.* This test is essentially a measure of the surface-to-volume ratio of the red cell. If the test is done on fresh red cells it is then also a measure of the proportion of cells that have undergone splenic conditioning. When red cells are placed in a series of graded hypotonic salt solutions, water rapidly enters the cells and osmotic equilibrium is achieved. The cells swell and become spherical, and eventually a critical volume is reached at which point the cellular contents (hemoglobin) leak out and ultimately the cell may burst. Red cells of patients with HS, because of their decreased surface area–to-volume ratio can tolerate less swelling than normal cells and lyse at higher concentrations of salt than do normal cells. It is important to note that about 25 percent of HS patients have normal osmotic fragility of fresh red cells, particularly in the very group that is mildly affected and is difficult to diagnose on morphologic grounds. Patients in the latter group as well as patients with more typical cases with vary rare exception have abnormal osmotic fragility of red cells that have been stressed by prior sterile incubation for 24 hours. During the 24-hour incubation, because of relative membrane instability, HS cells have greater loss of membrane surface. A corollary of the use of the incubated osmotic fragility test is that if the test result is normal,

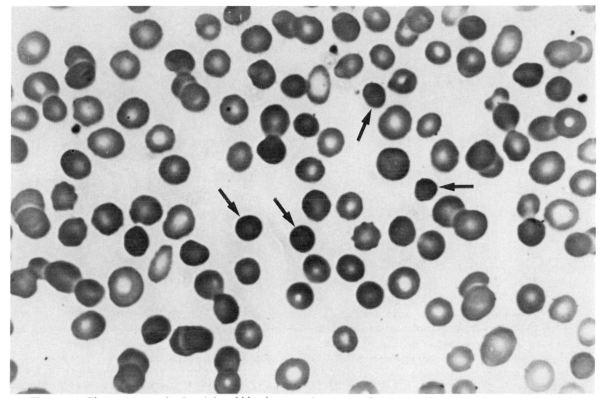

**Figure 7-5.** Photomicrograph of peripheral blood smear of patient with HS. Note the microspherocytes (arrows).

it is highly unlikely that one is dealing with a patient with HS. Representative osmotic fragility curves for fresh and incubated normal and HS red cells are shown in Figure 7 – 6. It is important to note that increased osmotic fragility is independent of the cause of spheroidal cells (e.g., it may be found in autoimmune hemolytic anemia, burns, and so on) (see Chapter 31).

*Autohemolysis Test.* This relatively sensitive test in the diagnosis of HS measures the structural and metabolic integrity of the HS red cell membrane under conditions of erythrostasis and relative glucose lack, i.e., sterile incubation of red cells in their own plasma for 48 hours at 37°C. The HS red cell is leaky to sodium. To "keep its head above water" the cell utilizes ATP and glucose to drive the cation pump to a greater extent than normal. Associated with the increased activity of the pump, there is a greater turnover of membrane phospholipids and associated membrane fragmentation with a decrease in surface-to-volume ratio until the critical hemolytic volume is reached and autohemolysis occurs. The usual range of autohemolysis in HS cells is variable and is about 10 to 50 percent, compared with control values of 0.2 to 3.0 percent. However, a minority of patients show only minimally elevated autohemolysis or may even be within the normal range. In most HS patients, addition of glucose markedly diminishes autohemolysis but not usually to within the normal range of samples incubated with glucose (0 to 1.0 percent). A minority of patients show no correction of autohemolysis with glucose, a finding also obtained with many patients with spherocytosis associated with autoimmune hemolytic anemia. It should be noted that many laboratories do not use this test routinely (see Chapter 31 for the procedure).

## Treatment

From the foregoing discussion of the pathophysiology of the HS red cell and the central role of the spleen in "conditioning" such cells and ultimately leading to their destruction, it should not be surprising that splenectomy is functionally curative in this disease. Although spherocytosis persists, "conditioned" microspherocytes are no longer seen and red cell lifespan is normal or very near normal. At one time, many authorities recommended splenectomy uniformly in all patients with HS because of the risks of biliary tract disease and the development of aplastic crises, but this view has been considerably tempered in recent years. Patients with mild, compensated cases of HS are usually not offered splenectomy unless the previously mentioned complications intervene. An important consideration in infants and young children is the risk of postsplenectomy sepsis, particularly with Streptococcus pneumoniae, so that most authorities recommend deferment of splenectomy until about 6 years of age. In severe cases, however, splenectomy

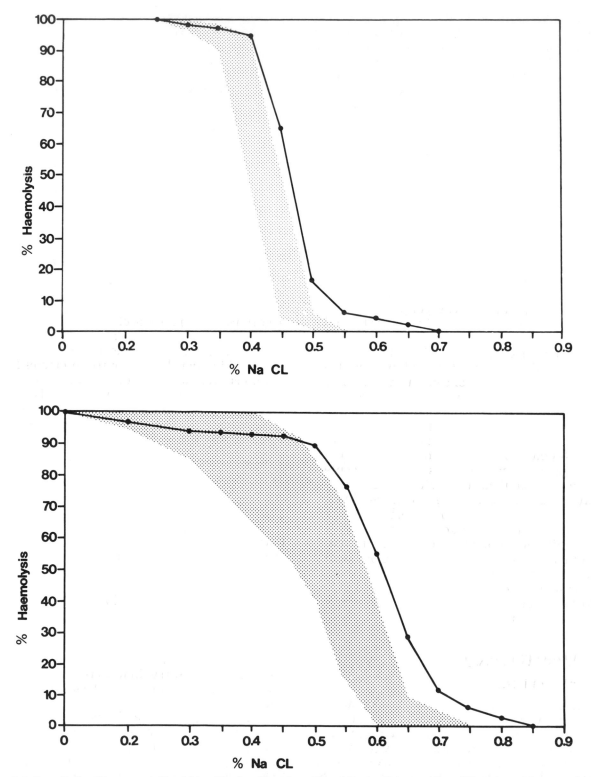

**Figure 7-6.** Osmotic fragility curves of fresh blood *(top)* and incubated blood *(bottom)* obtained from HS subjects. The normal range is shown by *dotted areas.* Note the increased fragility of HS red cells to osmotic lysis.

may have to be performed earlier; but in either event, treatment with pneumococcal vaccine is recommended, preferably starting before splenectomy. Younger children may also require prophylactic penicillin or other antibiotics postsplenectomy, but the latter course is controversial. Failure of splenectomy is almost always associated with an accessory spleen not removed at surgery.

## Case History

Mrs. T.P., aged 40 years, presented to her physician with an attack of acute cholecystitis. Physical examination revealed a palpable spleen in addition to the signs of acute cholecystitis. On investigation she was found to have numerous gallstones, and a routine blood count showed a mild, compensated hemolytic state: Hb 13.8 g/dl, HCT 38 percent, MCV 80 fl, MCHC 36 percent, reticulocyte count 7 percent, "shift" cells present, RPI 3.9. The peripheral smear showed moderate numbers of spherocytes and a few microspherocytes. The Coombs test was negative. Unconjugated bilirubin was 2.5 mg/dl, and conjugated bilirubin was 0.5 mg/dl. Haptoglobin concentration was less than 10 mg/dl (normal range: 25 to 180 mg/dl). Further investigation revealed that osmotic fragility of both fresh and incubated venous blood was increased. Autohemolysis was 25 percent after 48 hours' incubation, corrected to 3 percent in the presence of glucose. After the acute episode had settled, an elective cholecystectomy was performed. A diagnosis of hereditary spherocytosis was made and confirmed in a subsequent study of her family when two of her three children were found to have mild, compensated hemolytic states associated with spherocytosis. In view of the risk of recurrence of common bile duct calculi, an elective splenectomy was performed six months later, curing the hemolytic state.

## Hereditary Elliptocytosis

### Mode of Inheritance

Hereditary elliptocytosis is a disorder characterized by the presence of large numbers of elliptical red cells in the peripheral blood (see Color Figure 88). It has become clear over the past few years that this relatively common disorder (incidence about 1:4000), which shows variable linkage to the Rh gene, is genetically, biochemically, and clinically heterogeneous. All the variants are inherited in autosomal dominant fashion, except for a morphologically and clinically distinct syndrome found almost exclusively in Melanesian populations. In addition, there is a biochemical and genetic relationship to hereditary pyropoikilocytosis (HPP), which will be considered in a separate section.

### Clinical Phenotypes

Three major clinical and morphologic syndromes have been delineated by Palek and Lux in an extensive recent review.[4] The most frequently occurring group is designated "common HE," in which five subgroups have been categorized, the most common being mild HE in which there is minimal or no hemolysis and in which one parent has mild HE. Some of these kindreds have members who exhibit mild to moderate hemolysis (HE with sporadic hemolysis). Rarely, both parents have mild HE and the homozygote proband presents with a severe hemolytic state that resembles HPP (see further on). Another subgroup is HE with poikilocytosis in infancy, in which there is a transient neonatal state resembling HPP with gradual development of mild HE during the first two years of life. A rare variety of HE linked to families of Italian origin has associated ineffective erythropoiesis and erythroblast dysplasia.

The second major clinical category of HE is spherocytic HE, a phenotypic hybrid of mild HE and HS, in which the clinical course resembles HS and responds well to splenectomy. Stomatocytic HE constitutes the last major category. It is common only in Melanesian populations in whom it may have a selective protective effect against malaria and is probably inherited in a recessive fashion.

### Etiology and Pathogenesis of Membrane Disorder

It is now well established that a defect in the red cell membrane skeleton exists in HE. A fundamental observation is that both red cell ghosts and membrane skeletons of HE subjects retain their elliptical shape and also show marked instability when subjected to mechanical stress. A puzzling feature of the pathogenesis of HE is that in recent years several different molecular defects have been described in HE that affect the quantitative expression of skeletal proteins or their functional interaction with each other, yet have the same morphologic expression. To date, the most tenable hypothesis put forward to explain these findings is that of Palek and Lux,[4] who suggest that mild defects lead to a weakened skeleton and to an alteration in the material properties of the HE membrane. This results in a greater tendency for the membrane to develop permanent plastic deformation (i.e., remain in an elongated elliptical form) when subjected to the repeated shear stresses in the microcirculation. This is in contrast to normal cells, which develop only transient elliptical deformation in traversing the microcirculation. More severe defects, such as may occur in homozygous HE states (or in double heterozygous states as in HPP), lead to greater membrane instability and actual fragmentation and poikilocytosis. A summary of this hypothesis is shown diagrammatically in Figure 7–7 and contrasts the pathogenesis of HE with that of HS.

Several molecular lesions have been detected in the various phenotypic expressions of HE. The most common functional defect leading to a weakened membrane skeleton in mild HE is defective spectrin dimer association to form tetramers and occurs in about 20 percent of white patients and 40 percent of black patients who have this HE variant. This defect has been shown to be due to an abnormality of the functional domain ($\alpha$I domain) at the N-terminus of the alpha chain of spectrin, which is necessary for dimer association. This domain can be isolated after limited tryptic digestion of spectrin and has a molecular weight of 80,000.[3] Limited tryptic proteolysis of spectrin in this group of HE subjects reveals a decrease in the 80,000 dalton $\alpha$I domain, with recip-

rocal increases in either a 74,000 dalton peptide in some kindreds or a 50,000 dalton peptide in other kindreds. These defects are designated HE [SpD$\alpha$ $^{1/74}$-SpD] and HE [SpD$\alpha$ $^{1/50}$-SpD], the superscripts $^{1/74}$ and $^{1/50}$ referring to the abnormality in the $\alpha$I domain manifesting an abnormal tryptic peptide of molecular weight 74,000 or 50,000. Identical functional (i.e., altered spectrin tetramer assembly) and structural defects of spectrin have been described in patients with HPP, in whom there is thought to be greater membrane instability. The functional defect of tetramer assembly is, however, greater in patients with HPP than in patients with HE, which is consistent with the hypothesis outlined in Figure 7–7. Other much rarer molecular and functional variants associated with HE are defective spectrin dimer-dimer interaction due to a beta chain variant – HE [SpD$\beta$-SpD]; deficiency of protein 4.1

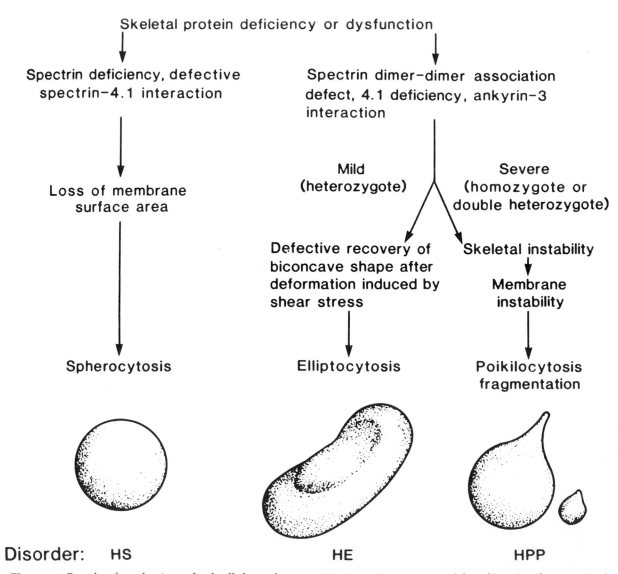

Figure 7-7. Postulated mechanisms of red cell shape change in HS, HE, and HPP. (From Palek and Lux,[4] with permission.)

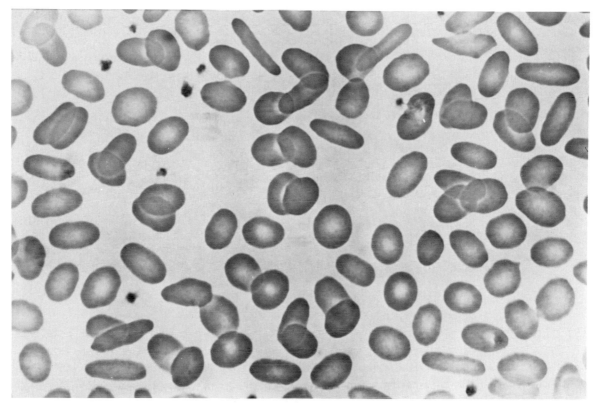

**Figure 7-8.** Photomicrograph of peripheral blood smear of a patient with mild HE (compensated hemolysis).

associated with a spherocytic form of He-[HE 4.1$^+$] and HE [4.1°]; a reduction in the number of high affinity binding sites (i.e., protein 3) for ankyrin −[HE Ank-3], and defective binding of spectrin to ankyrin in a kindred with atypical HE.

## Clinical Laboratory Findings

**Evidence of Hemolytic Process.** The usual picture in the most common variant (mild HE) is that of a very mild, compensated hemolytic anemia in which the only features may be a slight reticulocytosis and decreased haptoglobin levels. Many patients show no biochemical evidence of a hemolytic process. In the more severe cases, such as in spherocytic HE or in HE with infantile poikilocytosis, the usual features of extravascular hemolysis outlined earlier are found.

**Morphology of Peripheral Smear.** The morphology of the peripheral smear obviously varies with the clinical phenotypes of HE. In the usual variant of mild HE with no hemolysis or a compensated hemolytic state, the red cells show prominent uniform elliptocytosis, the cells being elliptic rather than oval or egg-shaped (Fig. 7-8). Usually greater than 30 percent of the red cells are elliptocytic, but many patients have a higher proportion of elliptocytes, e.g., greater than 75 percent. Very elongated or rodshaped cells are characteristic and often constitute more than 10 percent of the red cells. In patients with uncompensated hemolysis (mild HE with sporadic hemolysis) the red cells show more prominent poikilocytosis and a small proportion of elliptocytes may have bud-like projections. The rare patient with homozygous HE presents with a picture resembling HPP, as does the infant with mild HE and poikilocytosis of infancy. In such infants, there is prominent poikilocytosis, microspherocytosis, fragmentation, budding of red cells, and a variable degree of elliptocytosis (Fig. 7-9). By the time the infant reaches the age of 1 to 2 years, the morphology has changed to that characteristic of mild HE. In the neonatal period, the red cells show increased thermal sensitivity (which is also a characteristic of HPP), but the diagnosis is suggested by finding evidence of mild HE in one parent.

Red cell morphology in spherocytic HE is very variable, but the hallmarks are less prominent elliptocytosis with spherocytes and microspherocytes. The proportion of spherocytes and elliptocytes varies in different kindreds and even within the same kindred. Patients with stomatocytic HE have a characteristic red cell morphology. The elliptocytes are more rounded and have one or two transverse bars giving them the appearance of double stomatocytes.

**Red Cell Indices.** In the common variants of mild HE with compensated and uncompensated hemoly-

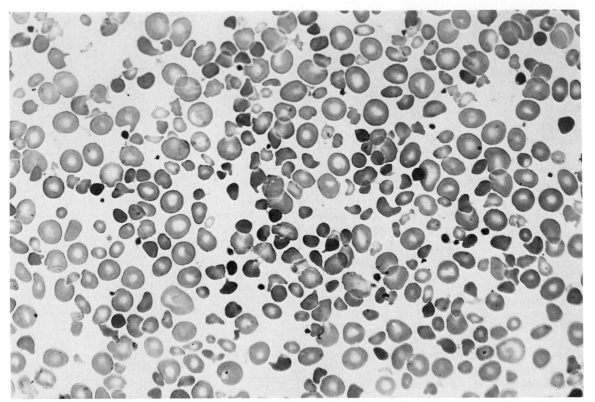

**Figure 7-9.** Photomicrograph of peripheral blood smear of a patient with mild HE and poikilocytosis of infancy. Note the bizarre poikilocytosis and fragmentation.

sis, the MCV is usually normal or slightly elevated, the latter finding probably reflecting an associated reticulocytosis. MCH and MCHC are also usually within the normal range. In infants with HE and poikilocytosis who have morphology representing that seen in HPP, the MCV may be decreased and the MCHC is either normal or slightly elevated.

**Special Laboratory Tests.** The osmotic fragility and autohemolysis tests are useful additional tests in delineating some of the HE phenotypes. In patients with mild HE (compensated and uncompensated) both the preincubation and the postincubation osmotic fragility and autohemolysis test results are normal. Rarely patients with mild HE and uncompensated hemolysis may have increased autohemolysis corrected by glucose. Preincubation and postincubation osmotic fragility is uniformly increased in spherocytic HE and autohemolysis is characteristically increased but corrected by glucose. Children with HE and infantile poikilocytosis have increased osmotic fragility and autohemolysis in the early neonatal period that reverts to normal with the development of more prominent elliptocytosis.

In laboratories with a specialized interest in HS and HE, further studies can be undertaken to define some of the structural and functional abnormalities of the membrane skeleton proteins, particularly of spectrin, outlined earlier. In brief, these involve one- and two-dimensional SDS-PAGE of membrane proteins as a screen for quantitating putative deficiencies of the skeletal proteins. Studies of the functional interactions of spectrin, actin, protein 4.1, ankyrin, and band 3 can be determined either in solution or in some cases with appropriately treated membrane vesicles. Structural studies of isolated skeletal proteins using techniques such as limited tryptic proteolysis and separation of tryptic peptides by one- and two-dimensional SDS-PAGE are powerful tools in delineating such defects (see Fig. 7-11).

## Treatment

Patients with mild HE (compensated) have a benign disorder with no splenomegaly and require no therapeutic intervention. Those with HE and uncompensated hemolysis usually benefit from splenectomy, which is also uniformly beneficial to patients with spherocytic HE. Patients with HE and infantile poikilocytosis should be recognized and treated symptomatically, as they will improve spontaneously with the development of a picture indistinguishable from mild HE.

## Case History

Mrs. R.L., aged 45 years, presented to her physician complaining of malaise and tiredness on mild exertion. On physical examination, she was found to have slight scleral icterus and a two-finger splenomegaly. A blood count revealed the following: Hb 11.0 g/dl, HCT 32 percent, MCHC 34.3 percent, MCV 100 fl, reticulocyte count 12.0 percent, shift cells on peripheral smear, and RPI 5.7. The peripheral smear showed about 80 percent elliptocytes with some poikilocytosis consisting of a few fragmented cells and budding elliptocytes. Unconjugated bilirubin was 3.5 mg/dl, conjugated bilirubin 0.6 mg/dl, and haptoglobin 15 mg/dl (normal range 25 to 180 mg/dl). Preincubation and postincubation osmotic fragility and autohemolysis were within the normal range. Examination of her family showed striking elliptocytes with normal hemoglobin and reticulocyte count in her father and in one of her three children. A diagnosis of mild HE with sporadic hemolysis was made, and a good response to splenectomy was obtained.

## Hereditary Pyropoikilocytosis (HPP)

HPP is a relatively rare severe hemolytic state first recognized in 1975 as a distinct clinical entity, which has subsequently been found to have a close genetic and biochemical relationship to mild HE. The hallmarks of the condition are (1) striking bizarre micropoikilocytosis in which red cell budding, fragments, microspherocytes, and elliptocytes are prominent (Fig. 7-10) **(see Color Figure 89)**; (2)

thermal instability of red cells in which heparinized venous blood heated to 45° or 46°C in vitro for 15 minutes leads to striking fragmentation of the red cells in contrast to normal red cells which fragment only at 49°C; and (3) autosomal recessive inheritance.

The MCV is characteristically very low (55 to 70 fl), preincubation and postincubation osmotic fragility is markedly increased, and autohemolysis is increased and unaffected by glucose.

The thermal instability of the red cells in HPP reflects thermal instability of the spectrin of the membrane skeleton and accounts for the in vitro fragmentation on heating to 45°C. However, the bizarre red cell picture found in vivo is thought to be a manifestation of a functional defect in spectrin dimer-dimer association more severe than that found in HE, leading to an unstable membrane skeleton that undergoes fragmentation on exposure to shear stresses in the circulation, with attendant decrease in surface-to-volume ratio and decreased cellular deformability (see Fig. 7-7). It should be noted that both normal and functionally abnormal populations of spectrin can be detected in probands with HPP. More recently, two types of structural abnormalities have been described in different kindreds with HPP, both affecting the 80,000 molecular weight αI domain of spectrin, which is involved in the dimer-dimer interaction. These are identical to that described in some HE kindreds and are designated HPP [SpDα $^{1/74}$-SpD] and HPP [SpDα

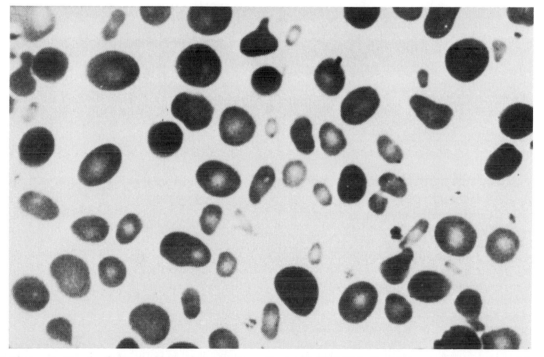

**Figure 7-10.** Photomicrograph of peripheral blood smear of a patient with HPP. Note the bizarre poikilocytosis and fragmentation similar to that seen in Figure 7-9. (From Palek and Lux,[4] with permission.)

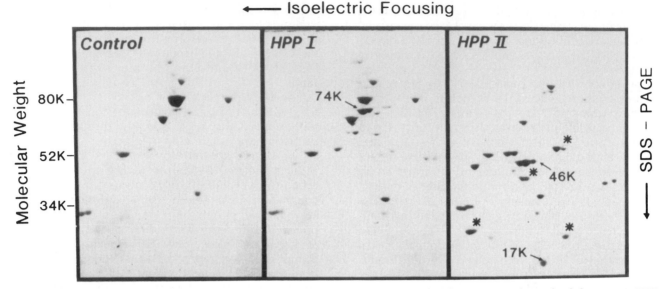

**Figure 7-11.** Two-dimensional SDS-PAGE of tryptic peptides of spectrin from patients with HPP. HPP I shows the defect seen in HPP [SpDα $^{1/74}$-SpD], and HPP II represents the defect in HPP [SpDα $^{1/46}$-SpD]. The positions of the 74K peptide characteristic of HPP I and the 46K and 17K peptides characteristic of HPP II are *arrowed*. Peptides that are variable both in patients and controls are denoted by *asterisks*. (From Palek and Lux,[4] with permission.)

$^{1/50}$-SpD]. The latter variant is probably identical to HPP [SpDα $^{1/46}$-SpD] described also by Palek and Lux[4] and reflects minor differences in technique in identifying the abnormal tryptic peptide on limited tryptic digestion of spectrin. Figure 7–11 shows the tryptic peptides of spectrin obtained in two representative HPP kindreds.

The parents of HPP probands are usually clinically normal and have normal red cell morphology. In a few families, one carrier parent has mild HE. In all families, one of the carrier parents has a functional defect of spectrin dimer-dimer interaction but not as severe as in the proband. The most feasible explanation for these findings is that patients with HPP are double heterozygotes for a spectrin dimer association defect due to alpha chain abnormality and another as yet undefined abnormality of spectrin that compounds the defect in tetramer assembly.

## Disorders of Membrane Cation Permeability: Hereditary Hydrocytosis (Stomatocytosis) and Hereditary Xerocytosis

This is a heterogeneous group of rare disorders characterized by alterations in the permeability of the red cell membrane to cations. Two main clinical and morphologic syndromes have been described and consist on the one hand of hereditary stomatocytosis (hydrocytosis) in which the red cells are swollen **(see Color Figure 90)** and on the other hand of hereditary xerocytosis in which the red cells are markedly dehydrated **(see Color Figure 91)**. A num-

ber of intermediate syndromes have been described, but these will not be considered here.

### Modes of Inheritance

Most reported cases of hereditary hydrocytosis are inherited in autosomal dominant fashion, but some patients who have a more severe degree of hemolysis show autosomal recessive inheritance. Hereditary xerocytosis is inherited by autosomal dominant transmission.

### Etiology and Pathophysiology

An important determinant of the water content of red cells is their total content of sodium and potassium. To maintain osmotic equilibrium water enters cells in which the total cation content is increased leading to swelling and hydrocyte formation. In contrast, a net loss of cations results in a movement of water out of the cell with formation of dehydrated cells or xerocytes.

The basic abnormality of hydrocytic red cells is a marked increase in the passive permeability of sodium into the cell and of potassium out of the cell. The defect in sodium permeability is greater than that for potassium. Although the sodium-potassium pump is stimulated by the influx of sodium, it cannot cope with the influx, and the total cation content of the cell increases with resultant water influx and formation of hydrocytes. There is some evidence for functional defects in the membrane skeleton of red cells with hydrocytosis (e.g., diminished phosphorylation of spectrin), but how these relate to the permeability defect is unknown. Recently a deficiency of one component of band 7 has been reported in red cell membranes of such patients, which may be important in determining the permeability lesion. Because of the influx of water, hydrocytes have an increased volume with a decreased surface-to-volume ratio and its attendant consequences of decreased red cell deformability and susceptibility to splenic sequestration. While splenectomy is predictably of benefit in the majority of patients with hereditary hydrocytosis, paradoxically some patients with severe permeability defects do not have significant hemolysis, suggesting that other as yet unknown factors may be of importance in the destruction of these cells.

Red cells from patients with hereditary xerocytosis have an increased efflux of potassium that is greater than the sodium influx. Although the influx of sodium leads to stimulation of the sodium-potassium pump, it is insufficient to correct the loss of potassium. Irreversible potassium and total cation loss occurs with resultant dehydration and formation of xerocytes that have an *increased* surface-to-volume ratio. These dehydrated cells, however, have an increased MCHC and presumably increased cell viscosity, which makes them less deformable and liable to sequestration in the reticuloendothelial system. The red cells are not specifically sequestered in the spleen, so that splenectomy does not have a beneficial effect.

## Clinical Laboratory Findings

**Morphology of Peripheral Smear.** The characteristic morphologic features of hereditary hydrocytosis are a tendency to macrocytosis and the presence of increased numbers of stomatocytes on the peripheral smear. These are red cells with a central slit or stoma **(see Color Figure 90)**. On phase contrast or scanning electron microscopy the cells have a bowl-like appearance. In hereditary xerocytosis there is an increase in the number of target cells (reflecting the greater surface-to-volume ratio of these cells). Small spiculated red cells and cells with

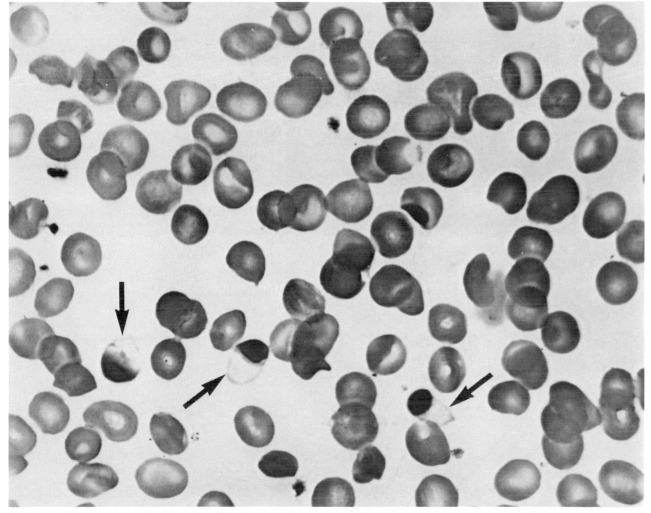

**Figure 7-12.** Photomicrograph of peripheral blood smear of a patient with hereditary xerocytosis. Note the characteristic target cells and cells with "puddled" hemoglobin (*arrows*).

hemoglobin concentrated in one part of the cell are also features of hereditary xerocytosis (Fig. 7-12).

**Red Cell Indices.** The MCV in both hereditary hydrocytosis and hereditary xerocytosis is elevated, notwithstanding the cellular dehydration in the latter condition. The MCHC is decreased in hereditary hydrocytosis and increased in hereditary xerocytosis.

**Special Laboratory Tests.** Osmotic fragility is increased in hereditary hydrocytosis and reflects the decreased surface-to-volume ratio. Red cell sodium concentration is elevated and potassium concentration is decreased. Total monovalent cation content is increased. In contrast, red cells in hereditary xerocytosis have strikingly decreased osmotic fragility, reflecting the increased surface-to-volume ratio. Red cell potassium concentration is markedly decreased, sodium concentration may be normal or slightly increased, and total cation concentration is decreased.

## Treatment

Most patients with hemolysis due to hereditary stomatocytosis show a good response to splenectomy. However, patients with hereditary xerocytosis, as stated earlier, do not benefit from splenectomy, presumably because of more generalized sequestration of these cells.

## Case History

T.R., a 6-year-old boy, was noted to have slight scleral icterus by his mother and was referred for further investigation. He complained of some tiredness on exertion but was otherwise symptom free. Physical examination showed only a one-finger splenomegaly. A blood count showed the following: Hb 10.8 g/dl, HCT 29 percent, MCHC 37 percent, MCV 100 fl, reticulocyte count 10 percent. Numerous target cells, some spiculated cells, and a few cells showing eccentric concentration of hemoglobin at one pole of the red cell were seen on the peripheral smear. The unconjugated bilirubin level was mildly elevated, and serum haptoglobins were decreased. There was no hemoglobinemia or hemosiderinuria. The osmotic fragility curve was strikingly decreased. Determination of red cell cation concentrations revealed a markedly decreased red cell postassium level of 65 mEq/l RBC (normal 90 to 104 mEq/1 RBC) and a slightly elevated red cell sodium level of 15 mEq/1 RBC (normal 5 to 12 mEq/1 RBC). Similar findings were obtained in the child's father, who had previously been diagnosed at another center as having an "unusual" form of anemia. A diagnosis of hereditary xerocytosis was made. Splenectomy was not advised and the child has remained with a hemoglobin level varying between 9.5 and 11.0 g/dl over the past two years.

## References

1. Hillman, RS and Finch, CA: Red Cell Manual, ed 4. FA Davis, Philadelphia, 1974, p 60.
2. Lux, SE and Glader, BE: Disorders of the red cell membrane. In Nathan, DG and Oski, FA (eds): Hematology of Infancy and Childhood, ed 2. WB Saunders, Philadelphia, 1981, p 456.
3. Marchesi, VT: The red cell membrane skeleton: recent progress. Blood 61:1, 1983.
4. Palek, J and Lux, SE: Red cell membrane skeletal defects in hereditary and acquired hemolytic anemias. Semin Hematol 20:184, 1983.

# CHAPTER 8

JEANNINE R. MELOON, M.S., M.T.(ASCP)

# Hemolytic Anemias: Intracorpuscular Defects

## II. Hereditary Enzyme Deficiencies

Since anemia is not in itself a disease but rather the result of a disease process, treatment of an anemic condition depends on the accurate assessment of the underlying cause. In 1953 Dacie and his associates[1] reported on an apparently heterogeneous group of congenital hemolytic anemias that had several common characteristics. There was no detectable abnormal hemoglobin, the antiglobulin test was negative, and the osmotic fragility was normal. The term "nonspherocytic" was used to describe this group of anemias. Investigators have since that time been able to pinpoint specific chemical explanations for many of these anemias.

The most commonly encountered anemia in this group is caused by deficiency of glucose-6-phosphate dehydrogenase, an enzyme in the pentose phosphate pathway. The second most frequently encountered enzyme deficiency is that of pyruvate kinase, an essential enzyme in the Embden-Meyerhof pathway. Many other enzyme deficiencies have also been identified, and laboratory testing is directed toward identification of the specific enzyme deficiency.

## GLUCOSE-6-PHOSPHATE DEHYDROGENASE DEFICIENCY

**Historic Aspects.** In the early 1950s it was known that certain antimalarial drugs caused hemolysis in certain susceptible individuals. The use of primaquine as an antimalarial treatment for soldiers in the Korean War enabled investigators to study the effects of the drug in controlled situations. In 1954, by using a new technique of radiolabeling erythrocytes, it was reported that the susceptibility to hemolysis induced by primaquine was due to an intrinsic abnormality of the erythrocyte.[2] The intrinsic defect was shown to be an inborn error in erythrocyte glucose metabolism and specifically identified as a deficiency of the enzyme glucose-6-phosphate dehydrogenase (G-6-PD).[3] Since that time, many different varieties of G-6-PD deficiency have been identified.

**Mode of Inheritance.** G-6-PD deficiency is transmitted by a mutant gene, located on the x-chromosome.[4] The disorder is fully expressed in the male (hemizygote) who inherits the mutant gene. Full expression of the disorder occurs only in females who inherit two mutant genes (homozygous). The heterozygous female may exhibit partial expression of the disorder, depending on random gene inactivation.

Distribution of the mutant gene for G-6-PD deficiency is worldwide; however, the highest incidence occurs in the darkly pigmented racial and ethnic groups. Normally active G-6-PD is designated type Gd B. It is the most common form of the enzyme in all populations. Gd B is present in 99 percent of Caucasians in the United States. There is another variety of the G-6-PD enzyme which is commonly found in Africans that also has normal activity but differs from Gd B by a single amino acid substitution that alters its electrophoretic mobility. This variant is designated as Gd A. The Gd A variant is found in about 16 percent of American black males. Among the American blacks who possess the Gd A variant mutant gene, the type designated A— ([ − ] because of reduced activity) is the most common, occurring in approximately 10 to 15 percent of the males. Approximately 20 percent of the females are heterozygous for the Gd A− gene. Among Caucasians, G-6-PD Mediterranean is the most common variant although the overall prevalence is low. However, among Kurdish Jews, the incidence of this enzyme may be as high as 50 to 60 percent. Gd Canton is a variant that is commonly found in the Chinese and in people of Southeast Asia. Table 8 – 1 lists the type of G-6-PD variant found in certain populations. More than 150 variants of G-6-PD have been identified. These variants are generally named according to geographic locations.

**Pathogenesis.** G-6-PD catalyzes the first step in the pentose phosphate pathway (aerobic pathway).

Oxidative catabolism of glucose is accompanied by reduction of NADP to NADPH (Fig. 8-1), which is required to reduce glutathione. Reduced glutathione (GSH) is an important source of reducing potential, that protects hemoglobin from oxidative denaturation.

G-6-PD activity is highest in young erythrocytes and decreases as aging of the cell occurs. Under normal conditions, the individual with G-6-PD deficiency compensates for the shortened lifespan of the erythrocytes. Oxidative stress, however, can lead to a mild to severe hemolytic episode. GSH deficiency results in oxidative destruction of certain erythrocyte components, including sulfhydryl groups of globin chains and the cell membrane.[5] More than 50 chemical agents may induce hemolysis in G-6-PD–deficient erythrocytes. Table 8–2 lists the drugs commonly leading to hemolysis in G-6-PD deficiency. The drug-induced hemolytic episode results when G-6-PD–deficient erythrocytes fail to produce sufficient NADPH and subsequently fail to maintain adequate levels of GSH.[6] The resulting oxidation of hemoglobin leads to progressive precipitation of irreversibly denatured hemoglobin (Heinz bodies). The cells lack normal deformability when sulfhydryl groups are oxidized and consequently encounter difficulties navigating in the microcirculation. Premature destruction of the cells results when they undergo intravascular lysis or when they are sequestered and destroyed in the liver or spleen. This early destruction may sometimes be detected in the peripheral smear with the formation of small condensed "bite"- or "helmet"-shaped red cells **(see Color Figure 93).**

Certain G-6-PD–deficient individuals also exhibit a sensitivity to the fava bean (favism) **(see Color Figure 95).** These individuals develop severe hemolysis after ingesting the fava bean or even after inhaling the plant's pollen. Favism is found in some individuals with G-6-PD deficiency of the Mediterranean and Canton types.

**Clinical Manifestations.** Stress, which may occur with exposure to certain drugs, following infections, or during the newborn period, challenges the G-6-PD–deficient erythrocytes, resulting in varying degrees of hemolysis. Consequently, symptoms of the disorder are related to the severity of the hemolytic episode. Two to three days following the administration of the offending drug, the erythrocyte count decreases, along with the hemoglobin content. The anemia will appear normochromic and normocytic with an increase in reticulocytes. The patient may or may not experience back pain. Hemoglobinuria and jaundice may also be evidence of the hemolytic process. Table 8–3 compares the clinical features of the two most common variants.

The hemolytic episode is generally self-limiting. Young cells that are produced in response to the anemia have G-6-PD levels that are nearly normal.[7]

**Table 8 – 1. DISTRIBUTION OF SOME COMMON G-6-PD VARIANTS**

| Enzyme Type | Population Affected |
| --- | --- |
| Gd B+ (normal) | All |
| Gd A+ | Africans |
| Gd A− | Blacks |
| Gd Med | Caucasians (Mediterranean area) |
| Gd Canton | Orientals |

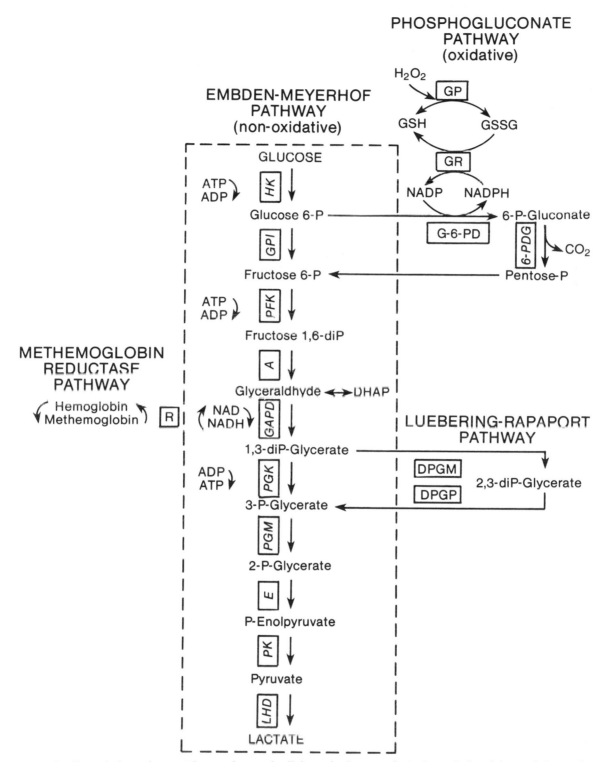

**Figure 8-1.** Red cell metabolic pathways. The anucleate red cell depends almost exclusively on the breakdown of glucose for energy requirements. The Embden-Meyerhof (nonoxidative or anaerobic) pathway is responsible for most of the glucose utilization and generation of ATP. In addition, this pathway plays an essential role in maintaining pyridine nucleotides in a reduced state to support methemoglobin reduction (the methemoglobin reductase pathway) and 2,3-diphosphoglycerate synthesis (the Leubering-Rapaport pathway). The phosphogluconate pathway couples oxidative metabolism with pyridine nucleotide and glutathione reduction. It serves to protect red cells from environmental oxidants. (From Hillman, RS and Finch, CA: Red Cell Manual, ed. 5. FA Davis, Philadelphia, 1985, p. 14, with permission.)

## Table 8–2. DRUGS COMMONLY LEADING TO HEMOLYSIS IN G-6-PD DEFICIENCY

| Antimalarials | Analgesics |
|---|---|
| Primaquine | Acetanilid |
| Quinacrine (Atabrine) | Acetylsalicylic acid* |
| | Acetophenetidin (Phenacetin)* |
| **Sulfonamides** | **Sulfones** |
| Sulfanilamide | Diaminodiphenyl |
| Salicylazosulfapyridine (Azulfidine) | sulfone (Dapsone) |
| Sulfisoxazole (Gantrisin) | |
| **Other Antibacterials** | **Miscellaneous** |
| Nitrofurantoin (Furadantin) | Dimercaprol (BAL) |
| Nitrofurazone (Furacin) | Napthalene (moth balls) |
| Chloramphenicol* | Methylene blue* |
| Para-aminosalicylic acid | Vitamin K (water-soluble analogues)* |
| Nalidixic acid | Ascorbic acid* |

*Hemolysis is infrequent and generally requires high concentrations of the drug. Probably a risk in Gd Med but not in Gd A– or Gd Canton.

From Hyun, Ashton, and Dolan: Practical Hematology: A Laboratory Guide With Accompanying Filmstrip. WB Saunders, Philadelphia 1975, p 69.

**Laboratory Tests.** Laboratory investigation of a hemolytic anemia when there is evidence (family history or drug sensitivity or both) of G-6-PD deficiency may include several screening procedures. It has already been noted that oxidative denaturation of hemoglobin results in formation of Heinz bodies. These small particles of precipitated hemoglobin can be visualized by supravital staining using certain basic dyes such as crystal violet **(see Color Figure 94)**. Heinz bodies will appear as small (1 to 4 $\mu$m), purple inclusions, usually seen on the cell periphery. Heinz bodies will not be seen with Romanowsky stains such as Wright's stain. Although Heinz bodies may be seen in other enzyme deficiencies, they are not seen in pyruvate kinase deficiency. Some of the unstable hemoglobins will also form

## Table 8–3. COMPARISON OF CLINICAL FEATURES OF Gd A– AND Gd MED

| Clinical Feature | Gd A– | Gd Med |
|---|---|---|
| Cells affected by defect | Aging erythrocytes | All erythrocytes |
| Hemolysis with drugs | Unusual | Common |
| Hemolysis with infection | Common | Common |
| Favism | No | Occasionally |
| Degree of hemolysis | Moderate | Severe |
| Transfusions required | No | Occasionally |
| Chronic hemolysis | No | No |
| Hemolytic disease of newborn | Rare | Occasionally |

Heinz bodies when the erythrocytes have been incubated at 37°C for 48 hours.

Other test procedures that may be used to screen for G-6-PD deficiency include the methemoglobin reduction test[8] and the ascorbate-cyanide test.[9] The methemoglobin reduction test is a simple and sensitive screening procedure in which G-6-PD–deficient erythrocytes fail to reduce methemoglobin in the presence of methylene blue. The ascorbate-cyanide test measures perioxidative denaturation of hemoglobin. This test is not specific for G-6-PD deficiency, as it will be moderately positive for pyruvate kinase deficiency and in the presence of certain unstable hemoglobins.

The fluorescent spot test and the G-6-PD assay will be positive only with G-6-PD deficiency. When a mixture of glucose-6-phosphate, NADP, saponin, and buffer is mixed with blood and placed on filter paper, G-6-PD acts to convert NADP to NADPH. The filter paper is observed under fluorescent light. G-6-PD–deficient erythrocytes fail to convert NADP to NADPH and will lack fluorescence. The quantitative assay of G-6-PD[10] is based on the measurement of the rate of reduction of NADP to NADPH measured at 340 nm.

It should be noted that diagnosis of G-6-PD deficiency during an acute hemolytic episode may be difficult. The deficiency may be obscured by a younger erythrocyte population as the older G-6-PD–deficient erythrocytes are destroyed.

## PYRUVATE KINASE DEFICIENCY

**Historic Aspects.** Investigations of the "nonspherocytic" anemias pointed to a possible defect in erythrocyte glucose utilization. In 1961 Valentine, Tanaka, and Miwa[11] reported that three patients with congenital nonspherocytic anemia had a severe deficiency of pyruvate kinase (PK). This enzyme catalyzes one of the steps in the Embden-Meyerhof pathway of glycolysis.

**Mode of Inheritance.** The deficiency of erythrocyte PK is inherited as an autosomal recessive trait[12] affecting both sexes equally. Individuals who are homozygous for the trait develop a hemolytic anemia, while those who are heterozygous are clinically normal. Although studies have shown that the defect is distributed worldwide, there appears to be a predominance of the trait in individuals whose ancestors originated from northern Europe.

**Pathogenesis.** PK catalyzes the formation of pyruvate from phosphoenolpyruvate (PEP) with the generation of ATP from ADP (see Fig. 8-1). Erythrocytes generate about 90 percent of their energy requirements through the anaerobic Embden-Meyerhof pathway of glycolysis. The PK-deficient erythrocyte fails to generate sufficient quantities of ATP to maintain normal erythrocyte membrane function. The cells exhibit cell membrane changes and are prematurely destroyed. The exact sequence of events resulting in the premature destruction of erythrocytes that are deficient in PK is not known.

**Clinical Manifestations.** The severity of the hemolytic disease associated with PK deficiency varies widely. Since clinical features are related to the effects of the hemolysis and the severity of the anemia, there are also variations in the clinical manifestations. Onset may be during infancy or early childhood; however, some mild cases may not be detected until adulthood.

The peripheral blood film will show varying degrees of polychromasia and poikilocytosis. Nucleated red blood cells may be seen. No significant leukocyte or platelet abnormalities are seen. Physical findings commonly include splenomegaly, and radiologic evaluation may demonstrate cholelithiasis.

**Laboratory Tests.** Several screening tests may be used to distinguish the nonspherocytic anemia of PK deficiency from the anemias of hereditary spherocytosis and the unstable hemoglobinopathies. These tests are nonspecific and serve only as a mechanism for classifying the type of anemia. Diagnosis is made on the basis of specific testing for the PK enzyme.

Screening tests may include the osmotic fragility test and the autohemolysis test, (see Chapter 31), as well as the antiglobulin and red blood cell survival tests. PK-deficient erythrocytes will show osmotic fragility that is near normal when the test is performed on freshly drawn blood. If the blood is incubated, some patients with nonspherocytic anemia will show an increase in osmotic fragility.[5] Sterile defibrinated blood is used to perform the test for autohemolysis. When normal erythrocytes are incubated in their own serum at 37°C they will gradually lyse, showing up to 3.5 percent lysis after 48 hours.[13] Erythrocytes from patients with nonspherocytic anemias, as well as those with hereditary spherocytosis, show an increased amount of autohemolysis. When glucose is added prior to incubation, erythrocytes from the patient with hereditary spherocytosis will show a normal amount of hemolysis. The addition of glucose does not correct the increased autohemolysis of PK-deficient erythrocytes (Fig. 8-2). The antiglobulin test in PK deficiency is negative and the red blood cell survival is decreased.

Differential diagnosis of PK deficiency is dependent on qualitative and quantitative assays for the specific enzyme. The fluorescent spot test[10] detects the decrease in fluorescence when PK catalyzes the reaction of PEP to pyruvate, and NADH is subsequently reduced to NAD by the pyruvate with the formation of lactate. Erythrocytes that are PK deficient fail to produce this reaction, and the fluorescence of NADH persists even after 60 minutes. It should be noted that leukocytes contain a PK isoen-

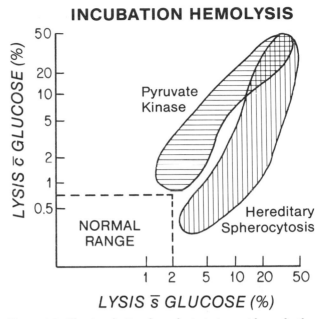

**Figure 8-2.** The incubation hemolysis test provides a further measure of cell resistance to hemolysis. Pyruvate kinase–deficient blood demonstrates an abnormal rate of hemolysis that is independent of the presence or absence of glucose in the incubation media. In contrast, the blood from a patient with hereditary spherocytosis shows more marked hemolysis when glucose is absent. (From Hillman, RS and Finch, CE: Red Cell Manual, ed. 5. FA Davis, Philadelphia, 1985, p. 97, with permission.)

zyme that will also catalyze the same reaction. Therefore, blood must be centrifuged and plasma and buffy coat removed prior to testing the erythrocytes. In addition, patients who have recently been transfused may have enough donor cells remaining in circulation to give erroneous test results. A quantitative assay for PK is also available. The principle is the same as the fluorescent spot test, and the change in absorbance at 340 nm is measured to quantify PK activity.

In the orthocresol red test, the formation of lactic acid in the normal Embden-Meyerhof pathway is detected by the change of the indicator from red to yellow at an acid pH. Although the test has been proposed as a specific test for PK deficiency, it is probable that any enzyme deficiency in the Embden-Meyerhof pathway will result in decreased production of lactic acid. Therefore, the test may be useful as a nonspecific screening test for these enzyme deficiencies.[14]

## METHEMOGLOBIN REDUCTASE DEFICIENCY

Hemoglobin that is oxidized from the ferrous to the ferric state is called "methemoglobin." Normally, about 1 percent of the circulating hemoglobin is in the form of methemoglobin. A balance is maintained between methemoglobin formation and reduction by the NADH-methemoglobin reductase (also called "diaphorase") pathway. Methemoglobinemia may occur either when there is decreased enzyme activity or when production of methemoglobin exceeds the reducing capacity of the enzyme system. Hereditary deficiency of NADH-methemoglobin reductase results in increased levels of methemoglobin. This congenital deficiency is inherited as an autosomal recessive trait.[15] The heterozygote does not usually show signs of methemoglobinemia unless challenged with certain drugs.

The major clinical feature of methemoglobinemia is cyanosis. Since methemoglobin cannot carry oxygen, some patients exhibit symptoms similar to those of anemia. Some patients develop a mild polycythemia (see Chapter 15). The course of this disorder is generally benign, and patients are treated only for cosmetic reasons. In cases of severe cyanosis, methylene blue is administered intravenously to activate the NADPH-methemoglobin reductase system.

In addition to the hereditary deficiency of NADH-methemoglobin reductase, methemoglobinemia may be due to the hemoglobin M diseases or to acute reaction to various drugs or toxic substances. The abnormality in the globin structure of hemoglobin that results in the hemoglobin M diseases is discussed further in Chapter 9. Hemoglobin may be oxidized by various substances such as nitrites, sulfonamides, and aniline derivatives. Toxic methemoglobinemia results when the methemoglobin-reducing system is unable to reduce the excess being formed.

The laboratory differentiation of the types of methemoglobinemia is shown in Table 8-4. Methemoglobin has a maximum absorbance band at 630 nm. The addition of cyanide causes the band to disappear and the change in absorbance is directly proportional to the concentration of methemoglobin.[16] While the concentration of methemoglobin is increased to varying degrees in all three disorders, enzyme activity is decreased only in hereditary NADH-methemoglobin reductase deficiency. Hemoglobin electrophoresis is normal except in the hemoglobin M diseases.

## Table 8-4. LABORATORY DIFFERENTIATION OF METHEMOGLOBINEMIA

| Methemoglobinemia resulting from | Methemoglobin level | Enzyme Activity | Hemoglobin Electrophoresis |
|---|---|---|---|
| Hereditary enzyme deficiency | Increased | Decreased | Normal |
| Toxic substance exposure | Increased | Normal | Normal |
| Hemoglobin M disease | Increased | Normal | Abnormal |

## OTHER ENZYME DEFICIENCIES

Except for the deficiencies of G-6-PD and PK, reports of hereditary enzyme deficiencies have been limited to a few rare cases. In a study of 350 cases of suspected enzyme-deficient hemolytic anemia, Beutler[17] reported 13.9 percent G-6-PD deficiencies and 9.9 percent PK deficiencies. Glucose phosphate isomerase was the third most commonly identified enzyme deficiency (1.7 percent). Although there have been reports of other enzyme deficiencies (glycolytic and nonglycolytic), not all such deficiencies have been associated with hemolytic anemia. There is considerable controversy in the literature regarding the role of certain enzyme deficiencies in hemolytic anemia.

Laboratory tests are available to assay many of the specific enzymes. Some of these tests may be available only through reference laboratories. Most laboratories, however, will be able to screen patients with a suspected hemolytic anemia due to enzyme deficiency. The antiglobulin, erythrocyte survival, autohemolysis, osmotic fragility, and Heinz body tests can all be effectively used to distinguish the enzyme deficiencies from hereditary spherocytosis and the unstable hemoglobinopathies.

## CASE HISTORY

A 26-year-old black male patient was referred to the clinical laboratory for investigation of reported hemoglobinuria. The patient had recently been diagnosed as having infectious mononucleosis. The following laboratory data were obtained.

| | |
|---|---|
| RBC | $3.7 \times 10^{12}$/l |
| Hb | 11.0 g/dl |
| HCT | 0.32 |
| MCV | 86.0 fl |
| MCHC | 34.0 g/dl |
| WBC | $9.5 \times 10^9$/l |
| Differential | |
|   Segs | 40% |
|   Bands | 3% |
|   Lymphs | 48% (many atypical) |
|   Monos | 7% |
|   Eos | 2% |
| Platelets | Adequate |
| Reticulocytes | 14.5% (uncorrected) |

The red blood cell morphology was normochromic and normocytic. Polychromasia was noted owing to the increase in reticulocytes. A slight poikilocytosis was noted with some red cells showing irregular protrusions. Further testing showed that the anti–human globulin test was negative. The hemolytic process was not due to an immune reaction. A previously negative history would tend to rule out any of the hemoglobinopathies. This was confirmed by a normal hemoglobin electrophoresis.

The hematologist suggested that the patient return in 30 days for testing for erythrocyte enzyme deficiency. At that time, the patient was found to have erythrocyte G-6-PD activity 15 percent of normal.

Hemolysis can be induced in G-6-PD–deficient individuals by infection with certain viral agents. Testing to confirm erythrocyte G-6-PD activity should be done after the patient has had sufficient time to recover from the hemolytic episode.

## References

1. Dacie, JR, Mollison, PL, Richardson, N, et al: Atypical congenital haemolytic anemia. QJ Med 22:79, 1953.
2. Dern, RJ, Weinstein, IM, LeRoy, GV, et al: The hemolytic effect of primaquine. I. The localization of the drug-induced hemolytic defect in primaquine-sensitive individuals. J Lab Clin Med 43:303, 1954.
3. Carson, PE, Flanagan, CL, Ickes, CE, et al: Enzymatic deficiency in primaquine-sensitive erythrocytes. Science 124:484, 1956.
4. Desforges, JF: Genetic implications of G-6-PD deficiency. N Engl J Med 294:1438, 1976.
5. Beutler, E: Glucose-6-phosphate dehydrogenase deficiency. In Williams, WJ, Beutler, E, Erslev, AJ, et al (eds): Hematology, ed 2. McGraw-Hill, New York, 1977, p 466
6. Beutler, E: GLucose-6-phosphate dehydrogenase deficiency. In Stanbury, JB, et al: (eds): The Metabolic Basis of Inherited Disease. McGraw-Hill, New York, 1978, p 1430.
7. Beutler, E, Dern, RJ, and Alving, AS: The hemolytic effect of primaquine. IV. The relationship of cell age to hemolysis. J Lab Clin Med 44:439, 1954.
8. Brewer, GJ, et al: The methemoglobin reduction test for primaquine-type sensitivity of erythrocytes: a simplified procedure for detecting a specific hypersusceptibility to drug hemolysis. JAMA 180:386, 1962.
9. Jacob, HS, and Jandl, JH: A simple visual screening test for glucose-6-phosphate dehydrogenase deficiency employing ascorbate and cyanide. N Engl J Med 274:1162, 1966.
10. Beutler, E: Red Cell Metabolism. A Manual of Biochemical Methods, ed 2. Grune & Stratton, New York, 1975.
11. Valentine, WN, Tanaka, KR, and Miwa, S: A specific glycolytic enzyme defect (pyruvate kinase) in three subjects with congenital non-spherocytic hemolytic anemia. Trans Assoc Am Phys 74:100, 1961.
12. Valentine, WN and Tanaka, KR: Pyruvate kinase deficiency hemolytic anemia. In Stanbury, JB, Wyngaarden, JR, and Frederickson, DS (eds): The Metabolic Basis of Inherited Disease, ed 2. McGraw-Hill, New York, 1966, p 1051.
13. Beutler, E: Autohemolysis. In Williams, WJ, Beutler, E, Erslev, AJ, et al (eds): Hematology, ed 2. McGraw-Hill, New York, 1977, p 1610.
14. Miale, JB: Laboratory Medicine Hematology, ed 6. CV Mosby, St Louis, 1982, p 588.
15. Jaffe, ER: Hereditary methemoglobinemias associated with abnormalities in the metabolism of erythrocytes. Am J Med 41:786, 1966.
16. Evelyn, KA and Malloy, HT: Micro determination of oxyhemoglobin, methemoglobin and sulfhemoglobin in a single sample of blood. J Biol Chem 126:655, 1938.
17. Beutler, E: Red cell enzyme defects as nondiseases and as diseases. Blood 54:1, 1979.

# CHAPTER 9

H. ZERINGER, M.T.(ASCP), S.H., AND
D. HARMENING PITTIGLIO, Ph.D., M.T.(ASCP)

# Hemolytic Anemias: Intracorpuscular Defects
## III. The Hemoglobinopathies

Hemoglobinopathies are disorders or aberrations of hemoglobin synthesis leading to production of an abnormal hemoglobin.

The pathophysiologic basis for the anemia is increased red cell destruction, which classifies these disorders as hemolytic anemias. They are all inherited or genetic mutations, the ultimate result being interference with structural integrity or function of or upset of the hemoglobin molecule.

## STRUCTURE AND FUNCTION OF NORMAL HEMOGLOBIN

Hemoglobin is a conjugated protein that is linked to both a metal atom, ferrous iron (divalent), and a complex organic group, a porphyrin, specifically protoporphyrin IX type III. The combination of the iron and the porphyrin is referred to as the heme moiety. The ferrous iron is set into four pyrrole rings of the porphyrin. The globin portion is composed of four chains of amino acids that in normal adult hemoglobin consist of two alpha and two beta chains. The hemoglobin molecule consists therefore of four polypeptide chains with an attached heme molecule (see Chapter 2).

The heme moiety is positioned such that it is suspended in the center of the globin chains. The environment is created so that the ferrous ion can exist in the reduced state, a feature that is critical for oxygen transport.

## Structure

There are six known polypeptide chains that make up the globin portion of the hemoglobin molecule. These chains are alpha ($\alpha$), beta ($\beta$), gamma ($\gamma$), delta ($\delta$), epsilon ($\epsilon$), and zeta ($\zeta$). The two latter are embryonic chains. The structure of the chains and the resulting hemoglobin molecule can be described in four steps:

1. The primary structure is the number and sequence of amino acids comprising the chain. Alpha chains have 141 amino acids; the other chains have 146 amino acids.
2. The secondary structure occurs with the twisting of the amino acid chain around an axis in a helical conformation.
3. The tertiary structure consists of bending the twisted amino acid chain into a three-dimensional shape resembling an irregular pretzel.[2] The polar groups are oriented outward, and the nonpolar groups are interior. The heme molecule is nestled in a nonpolar pocket and attached to a proximal histidine residue of the chain ($\alpha^{87}$ or $\beta^{92}$).
4. The quaternary structure is the assembling of the four three-dimensional chains with their attached heme groups into a completed, functional molecule.[2,3]

## Function

The function of the hemoglobin molecule is to carry oxygen to the tissues and carbon dioxide from the tissues to be expelled by the lungs. To quote Tietz, "Hemoglobin is uniquely adapted to take up and discharge oxygen within a relatively narrow range of oxygen pressure ($pO_2$). This is a function of a chain-to-chain interaction whereby an alteration in spatial relationships of portions of the molecule to another facilitates the uptake or release of $O_2$."[1] The shape of the oxygen dissociation curve indicates that with only a slight increase or decrease of oxygen tension the hemoglobin molecule can be made to take up or release oxygen. Also, as one heme group is oxygenated, the oxygen affinity of the remaining groups is increased. The increased partial pressure of $O_2$ and pH of the lungs allows oxygen loading, whereas the decreased pressure and pH of the tissues facilitates release. The molecule in effect "breathes" (Fig. 9-1).[1,3]

## Normal Hemoglobins[2–5]

**Hemoglobin A: $\alpha_2 \beta_2$.** HbA is the major hemoglobin fraction in adults and constitutes of total hemoglobin 92 to 96 percent. It consists of two alpha chains and two beta chains.

**Hemoglobin $A_2$: $\alpha_2 \delta_2$.** $HbA_2$ is present in a small amount in adult blood (1.5 to 3.5 percent) and con-

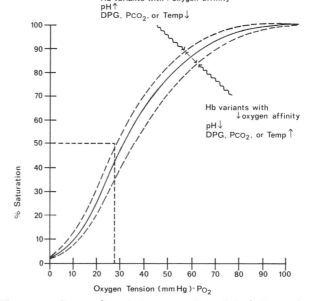

**Figure 9–1.** Oxygen dissociation curve. (From Spivak, JL: Fundamentals of Hematology. Harper & Row, Philadelphia, 1984, p. 50, with permission.)

sists of two alpha chains, as in HbA, plus two delta chains. The delta chains are similar to beta chains, differing by only eight amino acids.

**Hemoglobin F: $\alpha_2 \gamma_2$.** HbF is the major hemoglobin fraction of the fetus and newborn (50 to 85 percent) and consists of two alpha chains and two gamma chains. By the age of 2 years, it comprises less than 1 percent of the total hemoglobin. The gamma chain has two configurations: position 136 is either glycine ($^G\gamma$) or alanine ($^A\gamma$). The ratio of $^G\gamma$ to $^A\gamma$ is 3:1 at birth but 2:3 by age 1 year.

**Embryonic Hemoglobins.** Two other chains, epsilon ($\epsilon$) and zeta ($\zeta$) chains, along with the alpha and gamma chains, are constituents of embryonic hemoglobins. These hemoglobins are present only in fetal life. Three embryonic hemoglobins are described—Hb Gower 1 ($\epsilon_4$ or $\epsilon_2 \zeta_2$), Hb Gower 2 ($\alpha_2 \epsilon_2$), and Hb Portland 1 ($\zeta_2 \gamma_2$).

Figure 9-2 shows the relative percentages of the various chains and the time during fetal development that they are present. The epsilon and zeta chains are present only through the third month of fetal life. The alpha chain is present always. Gamma chain production is active from the third fetal month until one year postnatally. Beta chain production rises gradually during prenatal life and reaches adult percentages between three and six months after birth.[2–5]

## ABNORMAL HEMOGLOBINS (HEMOGLOBINOPATHIES)

By far, the majority of abnormal hemoglobins are clinically insignificant, as they do not demonstrate

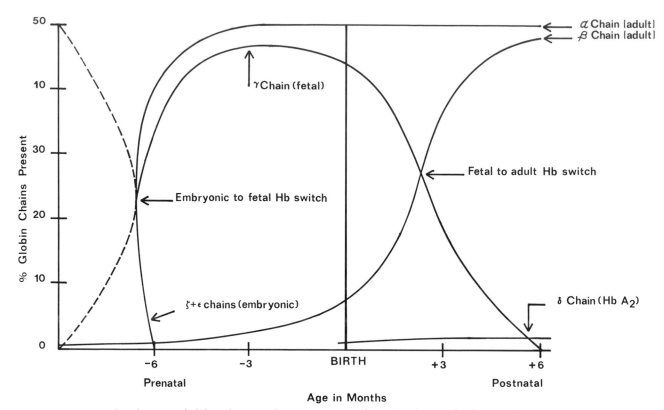

**Figure 9–2.** Prenatal and postnatal globin chain synthesis. (From Spivak, JL: Fundamentals of Hematology. Harper & Row, Philadelphia, 1984, p. 53, with permission.)

any physiologic consequence. Most abnormalities occur in the beta chain, and a greater number of patients with these beta chain abnormalities present with abnormal physical properties resulting in clinical disease than do patients with alpha chain abnormalities.

Most variants arise from a single substitution in the coding for a specific amino acid. For example, in the bases on DNA coding for glutamic acid in the sixth position of the beta chain, there is a single substitution that changes the coding to valine in that position. The result is hemoglobin S instead of hemoglobin A. A different base substitution coding for that same position produces lysine instead of glutamic acid in production of hemoglobin C. These disorders truly represent a "molecular disease," a feature that was initially appreciated by Pauling in the late 1940s. There are more than 350 known hemoglobin variants. Other such replacements can cause unstable molecules, deformation of the three-dimensional structure, oxidation of the ferrous ion, or alteration in residues that interact with heme, with 2,3-DPG, or at subunit contact points.[3]

A single base substitution is only one cause of abnormal hemoglobins. There are also cases of (1) multiple base substitutions, (2) abnormally long or short subunits, (3) frame shift mutations, (4) crossover in phase, and (5) fusion subunits. These are

beyond the scope of this chapter, and the reader is referred to the appropriate references for a more indepth discussion.[4]

## Genetics

There are nine different loci or positions on two chromosomes that code for the polypeptide chains. The alpha ($\alpha$) and zeta ($\zeta$) coding is on chromosome 16, with two loci for each chain. As a result, a total of four genes are inherited: two from each parent. This may explain why alpha variants are less severe than beta variants. The inheritance of two genes from each parent is also important in the expression of alpha thalassemias. The beta ($\beta$), delta ($\delta$), gamma ($\gamma$), and epsilon ($\epsilon$) coding is on chromosome 11. There are two loci for gamma chains — $^G\gamma$ and $^A\gamma$, and one each for the other chains.

Inheritance of abnormal hemoglobins is shown in Figure 9-3. This chart uses as examples hemoglobins S and C but is applicable to any hemoglobin variant.

## Nomenclature

Investigators began by naming the abnormal hemoglobins with capital letters but, with the end of the alphabet rapidly approaching, changed to the use of

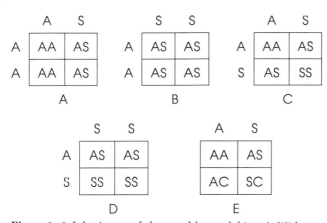

**Figure 9–3.** Inheritance of abnormal hemoglobins. *A*, With one parent heterozygous for an abnormal hemoglobin, the offspring have a 1-in-2 chance of carrying the trait. *B*, With one parent homozygous for an abnormal hemoglobin, all offspring will carry the trait, as that parent can contribute *only* an abnormal gene. *C*, With both parents heterozygous for the abnormality, the chances are 1-in-4 normal, 2-in-4 heterozygous, and 1-in-4 homozygous. *D*, With both parents carrying the same abnormal hemoglobin—one homozygous and one heterozygous—the offspring have a fifty-fifty chance of being either homozygous or heterozygous. *E*, With parents carrying two different abnormal hemoglobins, offspring have a 25 percent chance of not inheriting an abnormality, a 50 percent chance of carrying the trait for one or the other abnormality, and a 25 percent chance of carrying both abnormalities in codominance.

place names. A letter plus a place name indicates identical mobility on electrophoresis but different substitutions. The description of the variant can also involve naming the chains and the substitution. For example, homozygous hemoglobin S is $\alpha_2 \beta_2^S$ or $\alpha_2 \beta_2^{6\ val}$ or $\alpha_2 \beta_2^{6\ glu \rightarrow val}$. Hemoglobin G Philadelphia is written $\alpha_2^{G\ Phil} \beta_2^A$ or $\alpha_2^{68\ lys} \beta_2$ or $\alpha_2^{68\ asn \rightarrow lys} \beta_2$. Additionally, the exact helix of the secondary structure and the position in that helix can be indicated. Using these examples, the designations would be $\alpha_2 \beta_2^{6\ (A3)}$ for HbS and $\alpha_2^{68\ (E17)} \beta_2$ for HbG Philadelphia. The reader is referred to other texts for complete lists of the abnormal hemoglobins[2,5,6] (see Table 9–1 for a limited list).

## HEMOGLOBINOPATHY SYNDROMES

The term "hemoglobinopathy" refers to production of an *abnormal* hemoglobin of which there are many variants. Only the more common variants will be discussed here.

### Sickle Cell Disease

The structural formula for the S hemoglobin is $\alpha_2 \beta_2^{6\ glu \rightarrow val}$. The sixth position on the beta chain has valine substituted for glutamic acid.

The abnormality occurs with greatest frequency in tropical Africa, particularly Central Africa. Many social and historic factors, such as slavery and con-

quest, are responsible for the appearance of hemoglobin S in the North American and Middle Eastern populations.

The frequency of the carrier state in Africa is between 20 and 40 percent.[6] In the United States, the frequency of the carrier state is approximately 8 percent, with the incidence of the homozygous state at birth being 0.16 percent.[3]

Although the distribution of the gene through slavery or conquest is easily understood, the relationship between the incidence of the malarial parasite and the frequency of the abnormal hemoglobin requires explanation. Malaria, caused by a parasite of the Plasmodium species, is still a serious disease in tropical areas, with Plasmodium falciparum responsible for the most life-threatening situations. Cells carrying the abnormal S hemoglobin, when parasitized by P. falciparum, will sickle more quickly than will nonparasitized cells. The sickling affects the cycle of the parasite in two ways: directly, by killing the parasite; or indirectly, by causing the parasitized sickle cells to be sequestered in the spleen.[7] The fact that persons homozygous for the S hemoglobin often lack spleens by the time they reach adulthood (autosplenectomy or functional asplenia) may be one reason why malaria is exceptionally severe, often fatal, in these cases.

### Pathophysiology

The abnormal Hb S is soluble and gives no problem when oxygenated. When the oxygen tension decreases, the S hemoglobin polymerizes, forming "tactoids" or "fluid crystals" **(see Color Figure 97).**[5] The hemoglobin realigns and distorts the red cell into the characteristic sickle shape. The sickling process works in a vicious cycle: once triggered, the cycle builds on itself. The sickle cells in circulation increase the viscosity of the blood, which slows circulation, thereby increasing the time of exposure to an hypoxic environment. This promotes further sickling. The formation of rigid sickle cells is likely to plug small circulation, further lowering the pH and oxygen tension and increasing the number of sickled cells (Table 9–2). All of this leads to hypoxia, painful crises and infarction of organs.[8-11]

There are two types of sickle cells: reversible and irreversible (ISC). The sickling of the cell is reversible up to a point. However, repeated sickling eventually damages the cell permanently. For a more detailed discussion, the reader is referred to an article by Nagel and colleagues,[10] in which the possible relationship between these irreversibly sickled cells and painful sickle crises is discussed.

### Clinical Features

Sickle cell disease (HbSS) is usually diagnosed early in life, as the level of HbF declines. The homozygous form of the disease is usually fatal by middle age. It is a chronic hemolytic anemia with many compli-

## Table 9-1. FUNCTIONAL CLASSIFICATION OF HEMOGLOBIN VARIANTS

I. Homozygous: Hemoglobin polymorphisms; the variants that are most common.

| | | |
|---|---|---|
| HbS | $\alpha_2\beta_2^{6Val}$ | Severe hemolytic anemia; sickling |
| HbC | $\alpha_2\beta_2^{6Lys}$ | Mild hemolytic anemia |
| HbD Punjab | $\alpha_2\beta_2^{121Gln}$ | No anemia |
| HbE | $\alpha_2\beta_2^{26Lys}$ | Mild microcytic anemia |

II. Heterozygous: Hemoglobin variants causing functional aberrations or hemolytic anemia in the heterozygous state.
  A. Hemoglobins associated with methemoglobinemia and cyanosis.

| | | | | |
|---|---|---|---|---|
| 1. HbM Boston | $\alpha_2^{58Tyr}\beta_2$ | 3. HbM Saskatoon | $\alpha_2\beta_2^{63Tyr}$ | |
| 2. HbM Iwate | $\alpha_2^{87Tyr}\beta_2$ | 4. HbM Milwaukee | $\alpha_2\beta_2^{67Glu}$ | |
| | | 5. HbM Hyde Park | $\alpha_2\beta_2^{92Tyr}$ | |

  B. Hemoglobins associated with altered oxygen affinity.
    1. Increased affinity and polycythemia.

| | |
|---|---|
| a. Hb Chesapeake | $\alpha_2^{92Leu}\beta_2$ |
| b. HbJ Cape Town | $\alpha_2^{92Gln}\beta_2$ |
| c. Hb Malmö | $\alpha_2\beta_2^{97Gln}$ |
| d. Hb Yakima | $\alpha_2\beta_2^{99His}$ |
| e. Hb Kemp | $\alpha_2\beta_2^{99Asn}$ |
| f. Hb Ypsi (Ypsilanti) | $\alpha_2\beta_2^{99Tyr}$ |
| g. Hb Hiroshima | $\alpha_2\beta_2^{146Asp}$ |
| h. Hb Rainier | $\alpha_2\beta_2^{145Cys}$ |
| i. Hb Bethesda | $\alpha_2\beta_2^{145His}$ |

    2. Decreased affinity—may have mild anemia or cyanosis.

| | |
|---|---|
| a. Hb Kansas | $\alpha_2^{102Thr}\beta_2$ |
| b. Hb Titusville | $\alpha_2^{94Asn}\beta_2$ |
| c. Hb Providence | $\alpha_2\beta_2^{82Asn,Asp}$ |
| d. Hb Agenogi | $\alpha_2\beta_2^{90Lys}$ |
| e. Hb Beth Israel | $\alpha_2\beta_2^{102Ser}$ |
| f. Hb Yoshizuka | $\alpha_2\beta_2^{108Asp}$ |

  C. Unstable hemoglobins
    1. Hemoglobins which may precipitate as Heinz bodies after splenectomy: "congenital Heinz body hemolytic anemia."

| a. α-chain abnormalities | | b. β-chain abnormalities | | |
|---|---|---|---|---|
| Hb Torino | $\alpha_2^{42Val}\beta_2$ | Hb Leiden | $\alpha_2\beta_2^{6or7}$ | (Glu deleted) |
| Hb L-Ferrara | $\alpha_2^{47His}\beta_2$ | Hb Sogn | $\alpha_2\beta_2^{14Arg}$ | |
| Hb Hasharon | $\alpha_2^{47His}\beta_2$ | Hb Freiburg | $\alpha_2\beta_2^{23}$ | (Val deleted) |
| Hb Ann Arbor | $\alpha_2^{80Arg}\beta_2$ | Hb Riverdale Bronx | $\alpha_2\beta_2^{24Arg}$ | |
| Hb Etobicoke | $\alpha_2^{84Arg}\beta_2$ | Hb Genova | $\alpha_2\beta_2^{28Pro}$ | |
| Hb Dakar | $\alpha_2^{112Glu}\beta_2$ | Hb Tacoma | $\alpha_2\beta_2^{30Ser}$ | |
| Hb Bibba | $\alpha_2^{136Pro}\beta_2$ | Hb Philly | $\alpha_2\beta_2^{35Phe}$ | |
| | | Hb Louisville | $\alpha_2\beta_2^{42Leu}$ | |
| 2. Tetramers of normal chains; appear in thalassemias. | | Hb Hammersmith | $\alpha_2\beta_2^{42Ser}$ | |
| Hb Bart's | $\gamma_4$ | Hb Zurich | $\alpha_2\beta_2^{63Arg}$ | |
| HbH | $\beta_4$ | Hb Toulouse | $\alpha_2\beta_2^{66Glu}$ | |
| Hbα4A | $\alpha_4$ | Hb Bristol | $\alpha_2\beta_2^{67Asp}$ | |
| | | Hb Sydney | $\alpha_2\beta_2^{67Ala}$ | |
| | | Hb Shepherd's Bush | $\alpha_2\beta_2^{74Asp}$ | |
| | | Hb Seattle | $\alpha_2\beta_2^{76Glu}$ | |
| | | Hb Böras | $\alpha_2\beta_2^{88Arg}$ | |
| | | Hb Santa Ana | $\alpha_2\beta_2^{88Pro}$ | |
| | | Hb Gun Hill | $\alpha_2\beta_2^{91-97}$ | (5 a.a. deleted) |
| | | Hb Sabine | $\alpha_2\beta_2^{91Pro}$ | |
| | | Hb Köln | $\alpha_2\beta_2^{98Met}$ | |
| | | Hb Kansas | $\alpha_2\beta_2^{102Thr}$ | |
| | | Hb Wein | $\alpha_2\beta_2^{130Asp}$ | |
| | | Hb Olmsted | $\alpha_2\beta_2^{141Arg}$ | |

(From Henry,[5] with permission.)

## Table 9-2. FACTORS AFFECTING THE SEVERITY OF HbS

| | | | |
|---|---|---|---|
| 1. | Amount of HbS | 6. | Vascular stasis |
| 2. | Other hemoglobins | 7. | Temperature |
| 3. | Thalessemia | 8. | pH |
| 4. | G-6-PD deficiency | 9. | Viscosity |
| 5. | Deoxygenation | 10. | MCHC |

Adapted from Williams et al.[6]

cations, both hematologic and nonhematologic. The major hematologic manifestations are called "crises" and there are three types: aplastic, hemolytic, and vaso-occlusive or "painful."

The aplastic crisis is usually associated with infections and results in a temporary marrow aplasia. The marrow is simply overworked as a result of the stress related to the continuous stimulus for production of new red cells. With an already shortened red cell lifespan, even a temporary decrease or arrest in red cell production causes a drastic anemia.[6]

The hemolytic crisis is an acute exacerbation of an anemia with a falling hemoglobin and hematocrit, increased reticulocyte count, and jaundice. It is difficult to diagnose, as other complications of the disease could be responsible for the jaundice (for example, gallstones, which are a feature of most chronic hemolytic anemias).[6]

The vaso-occlusive or "painful" crisis is the hallmark of sickle cell anemia. This crisis is an episode of severe pain caused by plugs of rigid sickle cells in the small circulation, resulting in tissue damage and necrosis. Infarcts can occur anywhere—bones, joints, lungs, liver, spleen, kidney, eye, central nervous system. Repeated splenic infarcts result in autosplenectomy by the adult years.[6] These patients are thereby more prone to serious infections with capsulated organisms (for example, pneumococcus and Haemophilus influenzae).

Nonhematologic manifestations of sickle cell anemia are many and varied. For the most part, they are sequelae of repeated infarctive crises. They include bone abnormalities due to marrow proliferation, arthritis, renal papillary necrosis, autosplenectomy, liver dysfunction, enlarged heart, retinal hemorrhage, and leg ulcers (Table 9–3).

## Laboratory Diagnosis

The anemia of sickle cell disease is quite severe, with a hemoglobin ranging between 6 and 8 grams. It is a chronic hemolytic anemia classified as normochromic and normocytic. The peripheral blood picture is striking. If the patient is in crisis, there is a marked amount of anisocytosis and poikilocytosis, which includes numerous target cells, fragmented red cells, nucleated red cells, and, of course, sickled cells **(see Color Figure 96)**. Howell-Jolly bodies may present as red cell inclusions, indicating functional asplenia, as well as siderocytes which may be present due to the increased chronic hemolysis which results in relative iron overloading. There is a moderate to marked amount of polychromasia reflecting the hemolytic state and marrow response, with an average reticulocyte count between 10 and 20 percent.[6] Even when not in active crisis, the patient presents with an elevated reticulocyte count, approximately 10 percent. The reticulocyte count will of course be decreased during an aplastic crisis, and indeed a falling reticulocyte count may herald the onset of an aplastic crisis. The peripheral blood smear also shows a neutrophilic leukocytosis with a "left shift" and a thrombocytosis. The bone marrow shows a marked erythroid hyperplasia (except during an aplastic crisis) and sickled cells may be noted in the marrow. In general, there is panmyelosis reflecting increased production of all cell lines.

Though a diagnosis may seem possible from the smear, it is necessary to confirm the presence of HbS. There are several easy screening methods available such as Sicklequik (General Diagnostics), a tube test that isolates the abnormal sickling hemoglobin at an interface; or Sickledex (Ortho) or Sickle Sol (Dade), a tube test that precipitates the abnormal hemoglobin, causing a turbid solution. It is important to remember that some hemoglobins other than HbS can sickle (for example, HbC Harlem, HbC Ziguinchor, HbS Memphis, HbS Travis, Hb Alexandra, and Hb Porto-Alegre).[7] Another common screening method used is the Sodium Metabisulfite Preparation **(see Color Figure 99)**.

The definitive test for any hemoglobinopathy is a hemoglobin electrophoresis, first at an alkaline pH and then, if necessary for further separation, at an acid pH. The patient with sickle cell disease is producing no normal beta chains; therefore, there will be no HbA on alkaline electrophoresis (unless the patient has been recently transfused). HbS will be 80 to 95 percent. HbF will be 1 to 20 percent. Values of HbF greater than 20 percent show evidence of mediating the severity of the disease (for example, in newborns and in a combination of HbS with hereditary persistence of fetal hemoglobin [HPFN]).[12] HgA$_2$ shows a slight increase, 2 to 4.5 percent. Higher values of HbA$_2$ may suggest the possibility of an S/B thalassemia. On alkaline electrophoresis, HbS, HbD, and HbG Philadelphia all migrate at the same position; therefore, further differentiation is necessary. They will differentially separate at an acid pH; but even easier is the fact that only HbS will have a positive solubility test.

## Treatment

There are a variety of drugs being tested for their potential in ameliorating sickle cell disease. At present, no single drug is effective, and there is controversy about most. Ideally, the best drug or drug combination is one that would inhibit polymeriza-

### Table 9–3. CLINICAL FEATURES OF SICKLE CELL ANEMIA

| | |
|---|---|
| I. Hematologic | 4. Spleen and liver |
|   1. Aplastic crisis |   a. Autosplenectomy |
|   2. Hemolytic crisis |   b. Hepatomegaly |
|   3. Vaso-occlusive crisis |   c. Jaundice |
| II. Nonhematologic | 5. Cardiopulmonary |
|   1. Growth |   a. Enlarged heart |
|   2. Bone and joint |   b. Heart murmurs |
|     abnormalities |   c. Pulmonary infarction |
|     a. Pain | 6. Eye |
|     b. Salmonella |   a. Retinal hemorrhage |
|       infection | 7. CNS |
|     c. Hand-foot | 8. Leg ulcers |
|       dactylitis | 9. Risky pregnancy |
|   3. Genitourinary | |
|     a. Renal papillary | |
|       necrosis | |
|     b. Priapism | |

tion of the abnormal hemoglobin while having little effect on the oxygen affinity of the hemoglobin molecule. Most drugs seem to increase the oxygen affinity, which increases the hemoglobin and hematocrit and, thus, the viscosity of the blood. This effect should be avoided, as the lower hemoglobin and hematocrit is protective in sickle cell disease. A recent study by Chang and coworkers,[13] evaluating several antisickling agents, found butylurea and the bifunctional dibromosalicylates to be strong inhibitors of gelation in vitro. Several drugs, including nitrogen mustard and cyanate, work well but are toxic to the body.[14] They can perhaps best be used in extracorporeal treatment of the blood.[13] Drugs such as S-azacytidine and hydroxyurea have been used to facilitate methylation of DNA to enhance HbF synthesis. These results, although initially interesting, are experimental, and clinical effects are very hazardous. The use of amniocentesis and recombinant DNA technology is becoming more feasible for prenatal detection.

Because there is as yet no "cure" for sickle cell disease, efforts are concentrated on keeping the patient healthy and easing crises if and when they occur. Exchange transfusions have been proven beneficial in certain situations. A good diet, prevention and early treatment of infection, and avoidance of situations that could precipitate a crisis are the best medicine. Also, the prophylactic administration of folic acid to supplement the greater need of this vitamin owing to the panmyelosis will reduce the frequency of aplastic crises.

## Sickle Cell Trait

In discussing hemoglobinopathies, the term "trait" refers to the heterozygous state. Sickle cell trait is a combination of HbA and HbS. The structural formula is $\alpha_2 \beta_1, \beta_1^{6\ glu \rightarrow val}$, indicating one normal beta chain and one abnormal beta chain. In the United States, this trait is common, appearing in 8 percent of blacks. The patient is normally asymptomatic. The potential for sickling exists, however, and drastic lowering of pH or reduction in oxygen tension can precipitate a crisis. The usual causes are severe respiratory infection, air travel in unpressurized aircraft, anesthesia, and congestive heart failure.

The peripheral blood smear is usually normal, with the exception of a few target cells (see Color Figure 98). Solubility screening tests are positive. Hemoglobin electrophoresis at an alkaline pH shows 50 to 70 percent HbA and 30 to 45 percent HbS, normal HbF, and normal $HbA_2$. All traits show an electrophoretic pattern with approximately a 60:40 ratio of normal to abnormal hemoglobin, regardless of whether the abnormal hemoglobin is type S, D, C, or E. It should be noted that HbE, however, more often exhibits a 70:30 pattern.

## Hemoglobin C Disease and Trait

The structural formula for hemoglobin C is $\alpha_2 \beta_2^{6\ glu \rightarrow lys}$. The same amino acid on the beta chain that is replaced with valine to give HbS results in an entirely different hemoglobinopathy when replaced by lysine. The gene occurs with great frequency in West Africa, particularly Northern Ghana, at a rate of 17 to 28 percent.[6] In the United States, it shows up in 2 to 3 percent of blacks. The clinical manifestation in the homozygous state is a mild chronic hemolytic anemia with *splenomegaly* and abdominal discomfort. Patients with the trait are clinically asymptomatic.[5]

The peripheral blood picture of HbC disease is much more striking than the clinical picture (see Color Figure 100). The morphology is normochromic, normocytic to occasionally hypochromic, microcytic. There is marked poikilocytosis with numerous target cells (50 to 90 percent),[5] occasional microspherocytes and fragmented red cells, plus the abnormal rod-shaped crystallization of HbC which resembles a "bar of gold" (HbC crystals) (see Color Figures 101 and 102). The reticulocyte count is slightly increased. The heterozygous state (HbC trait) presents with only a moderate number of target cells on the peripheral smear. The alkaline electrophoretic pattern of HbC disease shows 95 to 100 percent HbC, less than 7 percent HbF, and no HbA. The trait shows 50 to 70 percent HbA and 30 to 40 percent HbC. Several other hemoglobins migrate with HbC at an alkaline pH, including $HbA_2$, HbE, and HbO Arab. They will separate at an acid pH or by quantitating $HbA_2$ by the column method. The crystals of HbC can be demonstrated in a wet prep by washing the red cells, then suspending them in a sodium citrate solution.[15]

## Hemoglobin D Disease and Trait

Hemoglobin D (HbD Punjab $\alpha_2 \beta_2^{121\ glu \rightarrow gln}$) is a rare abnormality. It shows up with slight frequency in northwest India, approximately 3 percent.[6] It is not a cause of a serious disease in either the homozygous or the heterozygous state. The peripheral blood smear is unremarkable; it does not even have many target cells. The importance of this abnormal hemoglobin arises from its electrophoretic pattern at an alkaline pH. In this situation, it migrates in the same position as HbS (HbG Philadelphia also migrates here). The red cells with HbD do not sickle; therefore, the solubility test will be negative. Electrophoresis at an acid pH demonstrates the absence of HbS, as HbD migrates with HbA.

## Hemoglobin E Disease and Trait

Hemoglobin E ($\alpha_2 \beta_2^{26\ glu \rightarrow lys}$) occurs with greatest frequency in Southeast Asia, including Thailand, Cambodia, and Burma. The incidence of the gene is as much as 30 percent in some places.[6] It has become more important in the United States with the influx of refugees from that area. The trait is asymptomatic with 30 to 40 percent HbE on electrophoresis. The homozygous state shows a mild anemia that is usually microcytic with target cells (which may well be because of a coexistent alpha thalassemia). It may also resemble a severe iron deficiency. Electrophoresis shows 95 to 97 percent HbE. This abnormal hemoglobin also occurs frequently in combination with beta thalassemia. The clinical severity of this combination is very similar to beta thalassemia major.[18] Electrophoresis will show 70 to 90 percent HbE. HbE is slow moving on alkaline electrophoresis and migrates with $HbA_2$, HbC, and HbO Arab. They can be separated on acid electrophoresis, in which HbE migrates with HbA, and HbC and HbO Arab separate out.

As with HbS, there is some question of HbE being protective against malaria. Areas of Thailand that are highly endemic for malaria show the highest incidence of the HbE gene.[19] Some authors also indicate that the parasite (P. falciparum) multiplies more slowly in red cells homozygous for HbE than in HbAE or HbAA red cells.[20]

## Sickle Cell Syndromes

### Hemoglobin SC Disease

Hemoglobin SC disease $\alpha_2 \beta^{6\,val}, \beta^{6\,lys}$ occurs with the inheritance of a different abnormal hemoglobin from each parent. The frequency of the disease in western Africa is up to 25 percent of the population. The incidence in the United States is approximately 1 in 833 blacks.[6] Both beta chains are abnormal but are substituted with two different amino acids. The presence of HbC moderates the severity of the disease somewhat, as the lysine substitution makes the hemoglobin more water soluble and less likely to sickle.[16] A recent study by Ballas and associates,[17] comparing the severity of hemoglobin SC disease to sickle cell disease, found a wide range of severity in SC disease but overall a generally milder course than in sickle cell disease. The hemolytic process is milder and there are fewer painful crises as the cells are much less likely to sickle. The patients are less anemic, but perhaps because of this and the resulting increased blood viscosity, there is a greater instance of retinal hemorrhage and renal papillary necrosis as well as aseptic necrosis of the femoral head.

Peripheral blood findings in SC disease include many target cells, folded red cells, and attempts at crystal formation that may resemble the "Washington Monument" (see Color Figure 103). The abnormal hemoglobin condenses in a "glove" shape (see Color Figure 104). Only occasionally will a typical sickle cell be seen. Screening tests for HbS are positive. Hemoglobin electrophoresis shows HbS and HbC in equal amounts, with a slight bias toward HbC (see Color Figure 107).[17] HbF is usually less than 2 percent in hemoglobin SC disease, compared with sickle cell disease, in which HbF averages about 6 percent.[17] Electrophoresis at an acid pH will confirm HbC, since it separates HbC from HbE and HbO Arab.

### Hemoglobin SD Disease

The combination of the S and D abnormal hemoglobins, although rare, presents an interesting diagnostic problem. Because they migrate in the same position, the electrophoretic pattern will be that of sickle cell disease. However, the clinical severity of this disease is much less than that of sickle cell anemia and falls between sickle cell disease and sickle cell trait. Any solubility tests will be positive, as abnormal HbS is present; but acid electrophoresis will separate the two hemoglobins. HbS migrates by itself at an acid pH, and HbD moves with HbA.

### Hemoglobin S/B Thalassemia Combination

The severity of HbS combined with beta thalassemia depends on how much the beta chain synthesis is suppressed. S/B° thalassemia is a severe disease similar to sickle cell disease (see Color Figure 105). S/B+ thalassemia more resembles sickle cell trait. The peripheral blood shows hypochromic, microcytic red cells characteristic of thalassemia. Sickle cells are rarely seen in either case. The electrophoretic pattern in S/B° thalassemia shows no HbA, 75 to 90 percent HbS, increased HbF, and increased $HbA_2$. The pattern in S/B+ thalassemia shows 15 to 30 percent HbA, more than 50 percent HbS, increased HbF, and increased $HbA_2$.[5]

## HEREDITARY PERSISTENCE OF FETAL HEMOGLOBIN

Hereditary persistence of fetal hemoglobin (HPFH) is a benign condition associated with mild decreased beta chain production with gamma chain synthesis persisting into adult life. There is 15 to 35 percent fetal hemoglobin on electrophoresis. However, HPFH can occur in combination with HbS and HbC. This excess of fetal hemoglobin is a definite modifier of the abnormal S hemoglobin. If it were necessary to determine whether the increased HbF came from HPFH or from simply a compensatory increase in HbF, the Kleinhauer-Betke stain for fetal hemoglobin could be used. HPFH shows a homogenous distribution of fetal hemoglobin (present uniformly in all cells), as opposed to a heterogenous distribution in a high HbF/HbS state.

## HEMOGLOBIN M AND METHEMOGLOBINEMIA

### Physiologic Mechanisms

Methemoglobin contains the oxidized ferric form of iron ($Fe^{+++}$) rather than the usual ferrous form ($Fe^{++}$). In this state, the molecule is unable to bind oxygen, which results in hypoxia and cyanosis. The blood is chocolate-brown.

### Causes of Methemoglobinemia

The causes of methemoglobinemia are basically three: (1) hemoglobin M variants (autosomal dominant); (2) congenital deficiency of NADH-diaphorase, which converts naturally occurring ferric iron back to ferrous iron (autosomal recessive); and (3) acquired from the toxic effect of various drugs, especially aniline dyes and derivatives, nitrates, and nitrites.

Hemoglobin M presents in five variants. They are the result of a single substitution on either the alpha or the beta chain, which stabilizes the hemoglobin molecule in the ferric form instead of the ferrous form.

Clinically, the patient is cyanotic with no significant hemolytic disease, although HbM Saskatoon and HbM Hyde Park are slightly unstable and may cause a mild hemolytic anemia. Variants affecting the alpha chain are manifested as cyanosis in the patient at birth. The beta chain variants show up as cyanosis in the patient by 6 months of age, with the switch from gamma to beta chain production. Laboratory diagnosis consists of electrophoresis at a pH of 7.1 to separate HbM from HbA, as they migrate in the same position at an alkaline or acid pH. HbM methemoglobinemia also shows different spectral absorption patterns from the other forms of methemoglobinemia. There is no therapy for HbM, although the enzyme deficiency and drug effects are reversed with methylene blue or ascorbic acid[2,3,6,23]

## UNSTABLE HEMOGLOBINS

The unstable hemoglobins are those hemoglobins that denature and precipitate within the red cells as Heinz bodies. The disease is known as congenital Heinz body hemolytic anemia; or, more recently, as unstable hemoglobin hemolytic anemia such as hemoglobin Zurich (see Color Figure 106). The precipitated Heinz bodies attach to the red cell membrane, affecting permeability and decreasing deformability. The cells are not able to traverse the spleen, and, while the spleen can pit out the Heinz bodies, the red cell is damaged, hypochromic, and prematurely destroyed.[24] The instability of the hemoglobin molecule can be caused by (1) substitutions of amino acids around the heme pocket, (2)

substitutions at contact points between the alpha and beta chains (particularly at the $\alpha_1 \beta_1$ bridge), (3) substitution of polar for nonpolar amino acids in the interior of the molecule, (4) deletions or elongations in the primary structure, and (5) substitution with proline.[6]

The disease is inherited as an autosomal dominant, and all patients are heterozygous. The homozygous state is probably not compatible with survival. Most instabilities affect the beta chain. Clinically, the patient has a compensated chronic hemolytic anemia with jaundice, splenomegaly, and perhaps dark urine from excretion of dipyrroles. The severity of the anemia depends on the degree of instability of the hemoglobin molecule.

The peripheral smear is not helpful in diagnosis, because Heinz bodies are not visible on a Wright's stain. They must be demonstrated with a supravital stain, such as brilliant cresyl blue (see Color Figure 94). The specific tests for unstable hemoglobins are the heat and isopropanol precipitations. Positive test results differentiate an unstable hemoglobin from an enzyme deficiency or a drug-induced hemolytic anemia. Hemoglobin electrophoresis is only moderately helpful. Most hemoglobins migrate with HbA, although there may be increased HbF and increased HbA.[3,6,24,25]

## HEMOGLOBINS WITH ALTERED OXYGEN AFFINITY

Hemoglobins with increased oxygen affinity bind oxygen more readily and release it less easily to the tissues. The result is tissue anoxia and increased hemoglobin concentration to compensate, resulting therefore in polycythemia. An example is hemoglobin Chesapeake. The patient has high hemoglobin and hematocrit levels but a normal white count, platelet count, and spleen. Erythropoietin production is usually normal once a balance is established between tissue anoxia and an increased hemoglobin concentration.

Hemoglobins with decreased oxygen affinity release oxygen quite readily to the tissues. With more oxygen released per gram of hemoglobin, the result is a normal to decreased hemoglobin concentration and slight anemia. There may be mild cyanosis due to decreased oxygen saturation.[3,6,23] Table 9–4 lists some of the hemoglobins with increased or decreased oxygen affinity.

## CASE HISTORY

### History

H.M., a 13-year-old black female, was admitted to the hospital appearing acutely ill with fever and abdominal pain. On physical exami-

**Table 9–4. VARIOUS HEMOGLOBINS WITH ALTERED OXYGEN AFFINITY**

| Hb with increased $O_2$ affinity | Hb with decreased $O_2$ affinity |
|---|---|
| Chesapeake | Torino |
| Rainer | Seattle |
| Hiroshima | Kansas |
| Tacoma | Hammersmith |
| Zurich | Beth Israel |
| Gun Hill | Bristol |
| Freiberg | |
| Koln | |
| Yakima | |
| Bethesda | |
| Ypsi | |
| Kempsey | |
| J Capetown | |

nation, splenomegaly was quite evident. Laboratory examination revealed the following:

Hb: 5.0 g/dl
HCT: 15%
RBC count: 1.4 million/mm³
WBC count: 22,000/mm³
Reticulocyte count: 1%
Differential count:
    Segmented neutrophils: 62%
    Bands: 12%
    Lymphocytes: 19%
    Monocytes: 4%
    Eosinophils: 2%
    Basophils: 1%
Red cell indices: Normal
Platelet count: 400,000
Peripheral smear **(see Color Figure 103)**
Hemoglobin electrophoresis **(see Color Figure 107, patient 4)**
Normal electrophoretic controls **(see Color Figure 107, patients 3 and 6)**

## Questions

1. Describe the morphologic features of this peripheral smear and *interpret the laboratory results.*

2. What possible explanation could be given for the hematologic results? Comment on the clinical condition exhibited by this patient. Is it consistent with this disease?

3. Comment on crystal formation in this disease.

4. Do you notice any red cell inclusions in the peripheral smear? If so, identify the inclusion and name other inclusions that are possible in this patient's condition.

5. Comment on the pathophysiology in-

volved in the formation of this inclusion, and its significance.

6. What stain could be used to confirm the nature of this inclusion?

## Answers

1. On the peripheral smear (br.see Color Figure 103) numerous target cells are present with several sickle-shaped cells appearing to have shadows of precipitating intra-erythrocytic crystals. On examination of the electrophoretic pattern **(see Color Figure 107,** patient 4) in comparison with a normal pattern **see Color Figure 107,** patient 6), there appears to be no $HbA_1$ present with HbS and HbC comprising practically all the patient's hemoglobin, with C type being the major portion.

2. Generally hemoglobin SC disease is milder than SS sicle cell anemia, but as exemplified by this patient severe attacks called "crisis" may occur. The clinical picture indicates that this patient is proba bly experiencing a severe episode of an SC crisis indicated by her acute illness and abdominal pain and drop in hemoglobin and hematocrit without an increase in reticulocyte count.

    Usually the spleen is considerably enlarged, as this case demonstrates, in comparison to that in sickle cell disease. As indicated by the normal red cell indices, the anemia is classified morphologically as normocytic normochromic, which is generally the case with all hemolytic anemias.

    Precipitation of HbC is *independent* of the oxygen tension present, but sickling of red cells with HbS depends on the oxygenation of the hemoglobin, with enhanced HbS polymerization (sickling) in the deoxygenated state.

3. HbC crystal formation in HbSC disease is distinct from crystal formation in HbCC disease. In CC disease, the shape of the intraerythrocytic crystals appear as a "bar of gold," whereas crystals seen in HbSC disease are shaped similarly to the "Washington Monument," i.e., the crystals always seem to protrude through the red cell membrane.

4. One red cell exhibits the presence of a Howell-Jolly body. In episodes of acute

hemolysis, siderotic granules and basophilic stippling may be observed.

5. Howell-Jolly bodies are DNA in nuclear composition. They are 1 to 2 $\mu$ in size and may appear singly or doubly in an eccentric position on the periphery of the cell membrane. They are thought to develop in periods of accelerated or abnormal erythropoiesis and are most commonly seen in hemolytic anemias, megaloblastic anemias, and following splenectomy.

In normal conditions, Howell-Jolly bodies are thought to result from nuclear fragmentation or incomplete nuclear expulsion from the red cell. In pathologic states, they are believed to represent a chromosome detached from the spindle apparatus during abnormal mitosis. Under ordinary circumstances, the spleen effectively "pits" these nondeformable bodies from the cell, but in periods of erythroid stress the pitting mechanism cannot keep pace with inclusion formation.

6. Howell-Jolly bodies gave a positive Feulgen reaction for DNA when stained.

# References

1. Tietz, NW: Fundamentals of Clinical Chemistry, ed 2. WB Saunders, Philadelphia, 1976, pp 401–454.
2. Miale, JB: Laboratory Medicine Hematology, ed 6. CV Mosby, St. Louis, 1982.
3. Spivak, JL: Fundamentals of Clinical Hematology, ed 2. Harper & Row, Philadelphia, 1984, pp 47–74.
4. Bunn, HF, Forget, BG, and Ranney, HM: Human Hemoglobins. WB Saunders, Philadelphia, 1977.
5. Henry, JB: Clinical Diagnosis and Management by Laboratory Methods, ed 16. WB Saunders, Philadelphia, 1979.
6. Williams, WJ, Beutler, E, Erslev, AJ, et al: Hematology, ed 2. McGraw-Hill, New York, 1977.
7. Luzzatto, L: Genetics of Red Cells and Susceptibility to Malaria. Blood 54(5):961, 1979.
8. May, A and Huehns, ER: The mechanism and prevention of sickling. Br Med Bull 32(3):223, 1976.
9. Noguchi, CT and Schechter, AN: The intracellular polymerization of sickle hemoglobin and its relevance to sickle cell disease. Blood 58(6):1057, 1981.
10. Nagel, RL, Fabry, ME, and Paul, DK: New insights on sickle cell anemia. Diagn Med 7:26, 1984.
11. Fabry, ME and Nagel, RL: The effect of deoxygenation on red cell density: Significance for the pathophysiology of sickle cell anemia. Blood 60(6):1370, 1980.
12. Powars, DR, Weiss, JN, Chan, LS, et al: Is there a threshold level of fetal hemoglobin that ameliorates morbidity in sickle cell anemia? Blood 63(4):921, 1984.
13. Chang, H, Ewert, SM, Bookthin, RM, et al: Comparative evaluation of fifteen anti-sickling agents. Blood 61(4):693, 1983.
14. Benjamin, LJ, Kokkini, G, and Peterson, CM: Cetiedil: its potential usefulness in sickle cell disease. Blood 55(2):265, 1980.
15. Hyun, BH, Ashton, JK, and Dolan, K: Practical Hematology. WB Saunders, Philadelphia, 1975.
16. Richardson, MA: Hemoglobin SC Disease. ASCP Check Sample. (H-134) 1983 (H 83-3).
17. Ballas, SK, Lewis, CN, Noone, AM, et al: Clinical, hematological, and biochemical features of hg SC disease. Am J Hematol 13(1):37, 1982.
18. Fairbanks, VF and Pierre, RV: Hemoglobin E/Alpha Thalassemia. ASCP Check Sample. (H-122) 1982 (H 82-3).
19. Cunningham, TM: Hemoglobin E in Indochinese refugees. West J Med 137:186, 1982.
20. Nagel, RL, Raventos-Suarez, C, Fabry, ME, et al: Impairment of the growth of P. falciparum in hgb EE erythrocytes. J Clin Invest 68(1):303, 1981.
21. Ward, PCJ, Freier, E, Schellekens, A, et al: Hgb Lepore: Diagnosis by Differential Electrophoresis and Isoelectric Focusing. ASCP Check Sample. (H-93) 1978.
22. Hoffman, GC: Thalassemia Minor—Hg Lepore Trait. ASCP Check Sample. (H-75) 1975.
23. Liebhaber, SA and Manno, CS: Update on hemoglobinopathies. Disease-a-Month 29(10):1, 1983.
24. Vichinsky, EP and Lubin, BH: Unstable hemoglobins, hemoglobins with altered oxygen affinity, and M hemoglobin. Pediatr Clin North Am 27(2):421, 1980.
25. White, JM: The Unstable Hemoglobins. Br Med Bull 32(3):219, 1976.
26. Simmons, A: Technical Hematology, ed 2. JB Lippincott, Philadelphia. 1976.
27. Basset, P, Beuzard, Y, Garel, MC, et al: Isoelectric focusing of human hemoglobins: its application to screening, to the characterization of 70 variants, and to the study of modified fractions of normal hemoglobins. Blood 51(5):971, May 1978.
28. Eaton, JW, Jacob, HS, and White, JG: Membrane abnormalities of irreversibly sickled cells. Semin Hematol 16(1):52, 1979.
29. Fairbanks, VF, Gilchrist, GS, Brimhall, B, et al: Hemoglobin E trait reexamined: a cause of microcytosis and erythrocytosis. Blood 53(1):109, 1979.
30. Inchausti, BC, Levin, B, and DiBella, J: Hemoglobin C Disease (Hgb CC). ASCP Check Sample. (H-139) 1983 (H 83-8).
31. International Committee for Standardization in Hematology: Simple electrophoretic system for presumptive identification of abnormal hemoglobins. Blood 52(5):1058, 1978.
32. International Committee for Standardization in Hematology: Recommendations of a system for identifying abnormal hemoglobins. Blood 52(5):1065, 1978.
33. Mears, JG, Lachman, HM, Labie, D, et al: Alpha thalassemia is related to prolonged survival in sickle cell anemia. Blood 62(2):286, 1983.
34. Sunshine, HR: Effects of other hemoglobins on gelation of sickle cell hemoglobin. Tex Rep Biol Med 40:233, 1981.
35. Steinberg, MH and Hibbel, RP: Clinical diversity of sickle cell anemia: genetic and cellular modulation of disease severity. Am J Hematol 14(4):405, 1983.

# CHAPTER 10

CHANTAL RICAUD HARRISON, M.D.

# Hemolytic Anemias: Intracorpuscular Defects
## IV. Thalassemia

The thalassemia syndromes consist of a diverse group of inherited disorders, which clinically manifest themselves as anemia of varying degrees. These disorders are the result of a defective production of the globin portion of the hemoglobin.

In 1925 Thomas B. Cooley and Pearl Lee described the first case of severe thalassemia in several North American children of Mediterranean origin. "Cooley's anemia" is still a commonly used term for this form of severe thalassemia, which is also termed "thalassemia major." The name of "thalassemia" was actually applied to these clinical syndromes a few years later. The term is derived from the Greek word "thalassa," which means "sea," since at that time, all of the cases described were from Mediterranean coastal origin. It is now well known that the distribution of thalassemia is worldwide and not restricted to the Mediterranean Sea area. It was later realized that the original severe clinical disease described by Cooley was the result of a homozygous defect in hemoglobin production, whereas many milder cases described as "thalassemia minima" or "thalassemia minor" were manifestations of a heterozygous defect.

The thalassemia syndromes are often considered part of a larger category of hematologic disorders called hemoglobinopathies (disorders in hemoglobin synthesis or production). Hemoglobinopathies are further divided into two main categories. One group is the result of an inherited structural defect in one of the globin chains resulting in an abnormal hemoglobin (true hemoglobinopathies), which may have abnormal physical or physiologic properties. Examples of these structural abnormalities are hemoglobin S, hemoglobin C, hemoglobin E, and so on. The second group consists of the thalassemia syndromes, which are caused by an abnormality in the rate of synthesis of the globin chains. With a few minor exceptions, the globin chains produced are structurally normal, but there is an imbalance in production of the two different types of chain resulting in an absolute decrease in the amount of normal hemoglobin formed, as well as an excess production of one type of chain that may precipitate and induce hemolysis. Therefore, these disorders are also considered "inherited" hemolytic anemias, which represent a form of intracorpuscular defect.

The globin portion of hemoglobin is formed by four polypeptide chains consisting of two identical dimers. Ninety-seven percent of adult hemoglobin consists of hemoglobin A, which contains two alpha chains and two beta chains (Fig. 10-1). There are two major types of thalassemia: alpha thalassemia, which is caused by a defect in the rate of synthesis of alpha chains; and beta thalassemia, caused by a defect in the rate of synthesis of beta chains. The original cases described by Cooley were cases of homozygous beta thalassemia. In the "Old World," thalassemia was present in a wide tropical geographic band originating in Portugal, Spain, and North Africa, surrounding the Mediterranean Sea, including southern Italy, Greece, Bulgaria, Turkey, and the Middle East, continuing through Afghanistan, Pakistan, India, Southeast Asia, China, Malaysia, and the Philippines, and extending as far as New Guinea. Another pocket of beta thalassemia is

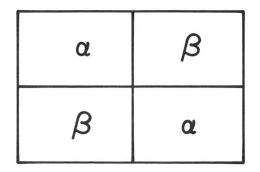

**Figure 10-1.** Diagram of the structure of hemoglobin A. Tetrameric structure consisting of two identical dimers linked to each other by weak noncovalent bonds in such a way as to minimize contact between like subunits.

found in West Africa. While beta thalassemia appears to have its highest frequency in the Mediterranean area, alpha thalassemia has its highest frequency in Southeast Asia, particularly in Thailand. Alpha thalassemia is also common throughout Africa. In the new world thalassemia has been imported and is present in immigrant populations originating mostly from Italy, Greece, West Africa, and Southeast Asia. For all practical purposes thalassemia is absent from American Indian populations. The world distribution of thalassemia is summarized in Figure 10-2. The marked similarity in worldwide distribution of thalassemia with malignant malaria caused by Plasmodium falciparum has given rise to the hypothesis that persons who are heterozygous for the thalassemia gene are resistant to Plasmodium falciparum infections and that the high frequencies of thalassemia can be explained by the process of gene selection by malaria.

Because the hemoglobin structural variants (such as hemoglobin S and hemoglobin C in West African and North American blacks or hemoglobin E in Southeast Asians) occur in the same population where alpha or beta thalassemia is frequent, the two types of genetic defects may be found in the same person resulting in variability of clinical expression of the two defects.

## GENETICS OF HEMOGLOBIN SYNTHESIS

All normal human hemoglobins have a general tetrameric structure consisting of two alpha-like (alpha or zeta, respectively abbreviated as $\alpha$ or $\zeta$) and two beta-like (beta, delta, G-gamma, A-gamma, or epsilon, respectively abbreviated as $\beta$, $\delta$, $^{G}\gamma$, $^{A}\gamma$, and $\epsilon$) chains. During embryonic and fetal development there is a progression in activation of the globin genes from the zeta to the alpha gene and from the epsilon to G-gamma to A-gamma to delta and beta genes, so that the majority of the hemoglobin found in the embryo are $\zeta_2 \epsilon_2$ (hemoglobin Gower 1), $\zeta_2 \gamma_2$ (hemoglobin Portland), and $\alpha_2 \epsilon_2$ (hemoglobin Gower 2). In the fetus until birth the major hemoglobin is $\alpha_2 \gamma_2$ (hemoglobin F). The gamma chains occur as a mixture of two types of chain differing only by one amino acid at position 136. G-gamma contains glycine, whereas A-gamma has alanine at that position. In the normal adult, the majority (97 percent) of the hemoglobin is $\alpha_2 \beta_2$ (hemoglobin A) and a minor fraction (about 2.5 percent) is $\alpha_2 \delta_2$ (hemoglobin $A_2$). A small amount of hemoglobin F (always less than 2 percent) may also be found. Figure 10-3 demonstrates the relative amount of the different globin chains produced from embryonic stage to early childhood. Table 10–1 lists the different normal hemoglobins found throughout human development, as well as the abnormal hemoglobins found in patients with thalassemia. Figure 10-4 is a diagram of the location of the different globin genes on

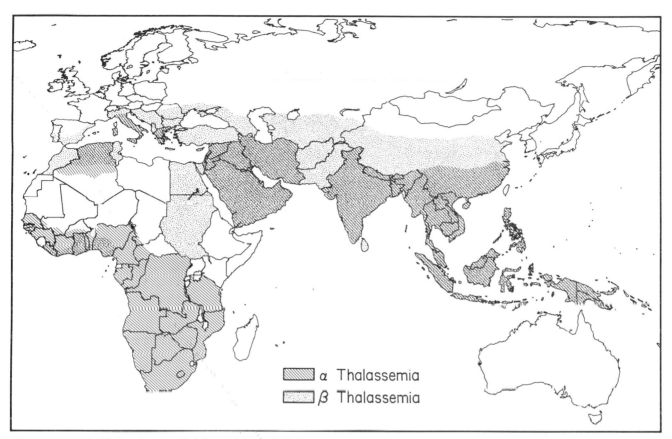

**Figure 10-2.** World distribution of alpha and beta thalassemia. Although alpha thalassemia is probably present in Pakistan and Afghanistan, no data on population screens are available yet.

the human chromosomes. The zeta and alpha genes are found on chromosome 16. There are two closely linked alpha genes, both active and coding for identical alpha globin chains in the normal adult. On chromosome 11 are found the genes for the epsilon, G-gamma, A-gamma, delta, and beta globins. Detailed mapping of the DNA by restriction endonucleases shows great similarity between the two alpha genes, as well as the two gamma genes, the delta gene, and the beta gene. (For an explanation of the DNA analysis method, see the section on gene analysis.) It is tempting to speculate that multiple occurrences of these similar genes on the same chromosome were caused by duplication of an ancestral gene during evolution. Figure 10-5 illustrates the formation of the normal human hemoglobin from two identical globin chains coded by chromosome 11 and two identical globin chains coded by chromosome 16.

Figure 10-6 is a diagram of the biochemical progression from the original chromosomal deoxyribonucleic acid (DNA) to the final globin chain polypeptide. The gene is represented by a length of chromosomal DNA, which consists of alternating coding and noncoding (or intervening) sequences. Only the coding sequences contain the information that will be finally translated into the polypeptide

chain. The exact role of the intervening sequences is not clear at present, although it is thought that they may be involved in the initiation and the rate of progression of the synthetic process. The DNA is transcribed into a large ribonucleic acid (RNA) called heterogenous nuclear RNA (HnRNA), which contains all the coding and noncoding sequences of the genes. This HnRNA is then processed into the messenger RNA (mRNA), which contains only the coding sequences and which diffuses into the cytoplasm to be translated by the ribosomes into the final globin chain.

## PATHOPHYSIOLOGY OF THALASSEMIA

The genetic defect in thalassemia is the result of one of two processes: (1) a mutation in one of the noncoding intervening sequences of the original globin chain gene, producing inefficient splicing from HnRNA to mRNA, thereby decreasing the amount of mRNA produced; or (2) the partial or total deletion of a globin gene, probably resulting from an unequal crossover. In both cases the final result is a decreased or absent production of one globin chain. There ensues a decrease in the amount of normal physiologic hemoglobin produced, resulting in a microcytic, hypochromic anemia. There will also

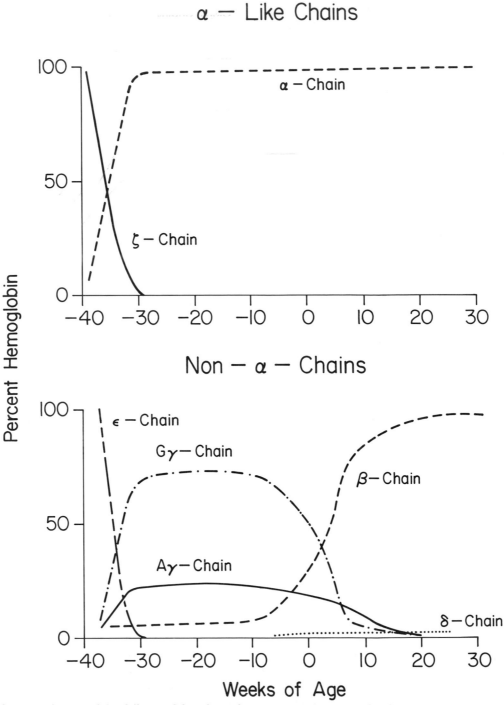

**Figure 10-3.** Relative production of the different globin chains from conception to 30 weeks after birth. *Top,* zeta embryonic chain production has been almost totally replaced by alpha chain production around 12 weeks after conception. *Bottom,* epsilon chain production runs in parallel with zeta chain production. The beta chain production stays at very low levels from 6 weeks after conception until it increases suddenly a few weeks before birth, while the gamma chain production suddenly decreases. The delta chain production starts a few weeks before birth and stays low. The $^G\gamma$ chain to $^A\gamma$ chain production ratio is 3:1 before birth and gradually reverses to 2:3 during the first few months of life.

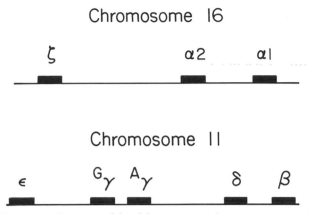

**Figure 10-4.** Location of the globin genes on chromosomes 16 and 11.

Table 10-1. COMPOSITION OF HEMOGLOBINS FOUND IN NORMAL HUMAN DEVELOPMENT AND ABNORMAL HEMOGLOBINS FOUND IN THALASSEMIA

| Globin Chains | Hemoglobin | State |
|---|---|---|
| $\alpha_2\beta_2$ | A $\}$ | |
| $\alpha_2\delta_2$ | $A_2$ $\}$ | Adult |
| $\alpha_2{}^A\gamma_2$ | F $\}$ | |
| $\alpha_2{}^G\gamma_2$ | F $\}$ | Fetus |
| $\alpha_2\epsilon_2$ | Gower 2 $\}$ | |
| $\zeta_2\epsilon_2$ | Gower 1 $\}$ | Embryo |
| $\zeta_2\gamma_2$ | Portland $\}$ | |
| $\beta_4$ | H $\}$ | $\alpha$ Thalassemia |
| $\gamma_4$ | Bart's $\}$ | |
| $\alpha_2$ precipitate | — | $\beta$ Thalassemia |

be an excess of globin chains produced by the unaffected genes. In the case of alpha thalassemia, the excess gamma chains and beta chains can form stable tetramers: hemoglobin Bart's ($\gamma_4$) and hemoglobin H ($\beta_4$), respectively. However, these hemoglobins are physiologically useless and will precipitate in older red cells, causing a shortened red cell lifespan. In the case of beta thalassemia, the excess alpha chains will form $\alpha_2$ precipitates, which will cause hemolysis of the red cell precursors in the bone marrow, resulting in ineffective erythropoiesis.

## Beta Thalassemia

In beta thalassemia the disease will not manifest itself until the switch from gamma chain to beta

chain synthesis has been completed. This usually occurs several months after birth. Thus, the clinical presentation of a patient with this disease usually occurs during the first year of life. There often is a compensatory absolute or relative increase in production in gamma chains and delta chains, resulting in an increased level of hemoglobin F and hemoglobin $A_2$. The genetic background for beta thalassemia is very heterogeneous but may be broadly subdivided into $\beta^\circ$ and $\beta^+$ thalassemia.

### $\beta^\circ$ Thalassemia

This gene results in complete absence of production of beta chains. This particular gene is commonly found in the Mediterranean area, particularly in northern Italy, Greece, Algeria, and Saudi Arabia. It is also common in Southeast Asia. At the molecular

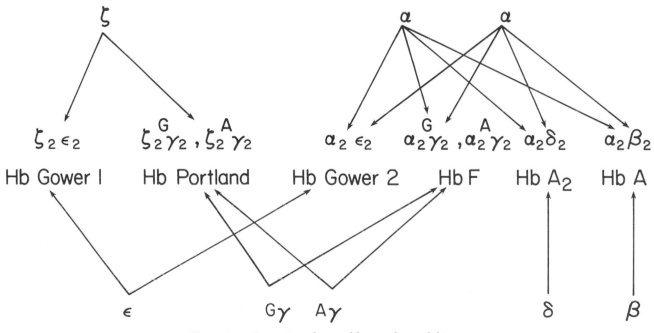

**Figure 10-5.** Formation of normal human hemoglobins.

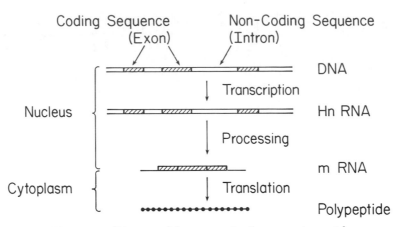

**Figure 10-6.** Diagram of the progression from gene to peptide.

level, there is heterogeneity in the basis for the genetic abnormality with at least eight genetic backgrounds described, each found in a specific geographic area.

## $\beta^+$ Thalassemia

The $\beta^+$ thalassemia gene produces a reduced amount of beta chains. There is heterogeneity again in $\beta^+$ thalassemia, and at least three different genes have been described. The type 1 $\beta^+$ thalassemia gene produces the least amount of beta chains (about 10 percent of normal production) and is found throughout the Mediterranean region, the Middle East, the Indian subcontinent, and Southeast Asia. The type 2 $\beta^+$ thalassemia gene produces a greater amount of beta chains (about 50 percent of normal production) and is characteristically found in the blacks of West Africa and North America. The type 3 $\beta^+$ thalassemia gene produces an even greater amount of beta chains and causes a much milder form of beta thalassemia. It is found sporadically in Italy, Greece, and the Middle East.

## Clinical Expression of the Different Gene Combinations

Homozygosity for the $\beta^\circ$ or $\beta^+$ thalassemia gene, or compound heterozygosity for the $\beta^\circ$ and $\beta^+$ genes, causes a severe form of thalassemia called "thalassemia major." The only exception is perhaps the homozygous type 2 or type 3 $\beta^+$ thalassemia, which causes a milder form of thalassemia that has sometimes been called "thalassemia intermedia." In thalassemia major a severe hypochromic, microcytic anemia develops during the first year of life. The hemoglobin level is usually below 7 g/dl and consists mostly of hemoglobin F and hemoglobin $A_2$. This severe chronic anemia starting so early in life is a strong stimulus for erythropoiesis. This causes marked expansion of the marrow space and characteristic skeletal changes of the skull, long bones, and

hand bones. The skull roentgenograms show widening of the diploic space and demonstrate characteristic radiating striations giving typical "hair on end" appearance (Fig. 10-7). The marrow expansion of the facial bones produces a characteristic facial appearance with hypertrophy of the maxilla causing forward protrusion of the upper teeth and overbite, a relatively sunken nose, widely spaced eyes, and prominent cheek bones resulting in a Mongoloid facies (Fig. 10-8). The long small bones of the hands and feet have cortical thinning with porosity of the medullary space. These changes are not a specific feature of thalassemia and are found in other severe chronic congenital anemias, but it may be in beta thalassemia major that these changes are most prominent. Without careful medical supervision and a therapeutic program including blood transfusions, iron chelation, and early treatment of infection, these children will have numerous complications such as massive hepatosplenomegaly, recurrent infections, spontaneous fractures, leg ulcers, dental and orthodontic problems, and compression syndromes due to tumor masses from extramedullary hematopoiesis. If the condition is left untreated, these children will usually die in early childhood.

Heterozygosity for the $\beta^\circ$ or $\beta^+$ thalassemia gene causes a mild form of chronic hypochromic, microcytic anemia that has been called "thalassemia minor." While the degree of anemia is variable with hemoglobin levels from 10.5 to 13.9 g/dl, it is impossible to determine whether the patient has the $\beta^\circ$ or $\beta^+$ gene on clinical grounds alone. In general the levels of hemoglobin F and hemoglobin $A_2$ are mildly elevated. The patients are usually completely asymptomatic, although symptoms may occur under stressful situations, such as pregnancy. The patient with heterozygous $\beta^+$ type 3 thalassemia usually shows no clinical or laboratory evidence of anemia and has been called the silent carrier.

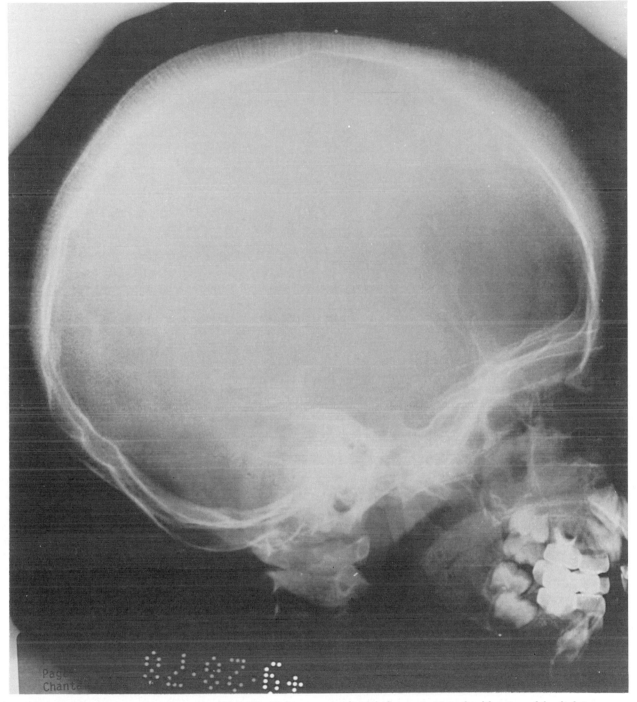

**Figure 10-7.** Skull roentgenogram of a 5-year-old child with homozygous beta thalassemia. Note the dilatation of the diploic space and the typical "hair on end" appearance due to subperiostial bone growth in radiating striations.

## Alpha Thalassemia

In contrast to beta thalassemia, alpha thalassemia is usually manifested immediately at birth and even in utero, as the alpha genes are activated early in fetal life. Another characteristic of alpha thalassemia is that, because each chromosome 16 carries two alpha genes, the total normal complement of alpha genes is four. Thus, there will be a greater variety in severity of disease, as there may be one, two, three, or four alpha genes affected in a patient.

Owing to the wide variety of genetic backgrounds and the difficulty in defining the heterozygous carrier state, there has been much confusion in the

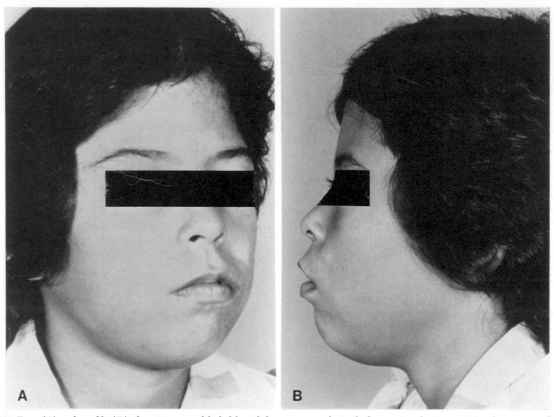

**Figure 10-8.** Face (A) and profile (B) of an 11-year-old child with homozygous beta thalassemia who is receiving hypertransfusion. The characteristic facial changes are not as prominent as in an untransfused child but are still present. Note bossing of the skull, hypertrophy of the maxilla, with prominent malar eminences, depression of the bridge of the nose, and mongoloid slant of the eyes.

classification and nomenclature of alpha thalassemias. Much of this confusion is the result of the indiscriminate use of a phenotypic or a genotypic classification without clear definition. We will use a genotypic classification that parallels the classification used for beta thalassemia.

Another characteristic of alpha thalassemia is the fact that the decreased or absent alpha chain production will result in excess gamma chains during fetal life and at birth and in excess beta chains later on. This will cause the formation of stable tetramers, such as $\gamma_4$ or hemoglobin Bart's and $\beta_4$ or hemoglobin H, that can be detected by hemoglobin electrophoresis. These stable, nonfunctional tetramers precipitate in older red cells, forming inclusion bodies, which results in decreased red cell survival and which may, thereby, induce a hemolytic crisis during infectious episodes.

### $\alpha°$ Thalassemia (Alpha Thalassemia 1)

"$\alpha°$ Thalassemia" and "alpha thalassemia 1" have been used equally in the past to describe a genetic determinant. However, because "alpha thalassemia 1" has been used also to describe the phenotypic or clinical expression of a disease, "$\alpha°$ thalassemia" is the preferred term for the description of the genetic determinant. This gene results in complete absence

of production of alpha chains. This means that both alpha genes on chromosome 16 are nonfunctional. Studies by DNA hybridization techniques have shown that the $\alpha°$ determinant is the result of alpha gene deletions. In addition, they also demonstrated that there are at least five major haplotypes resulting in $\alpha°$ thalassemia, depending on the amount of DNA that has been deleted from the chromosome. Each haplotype appears to be characteristic of a certain population in the world. $\alpha°$ Thalassemia genes are found frequently in Southeast Asia and less frequently in the Mediterranean area. They also occur sporadically in other parts of the world. Recent studies published in early 1986 seem to indicate that this gene can be recognized in adults through the detection of small amounts of zeta globin chain by radioimmunoassay.

### $\alpha^+$ Thalassemia (Alpha Thalassemia 2)

Again, "$\alpha^+$ thalassemia" is the better term to describe the genetic determinant, as "alpha thalassemia 2" has been used to describe both the genetic determinant and a phenotypic expression. The $\alpha^+$ thalassemia gene is characterized by a reduction in the output of alpha chains. This may be due to a deletion of a single alpha gene on chromosome 16, which leaves the other alpha gene intact and able to function. Other types of $\alpha^+$ thalassemia genes are due to nondeletion mutants which affect the regulation of the alpha chain synthesis. This is similar to the situation in the beta thalassemias. A third type of $\alpha^+$ thalassemia genetic background is associated with alpha globin structural mutants, which may be a termination mutant such as hemoglobin Constant Spring (CS), hemoglobin Koya Dora (KD), hemoglobin Seal Rock (SR), or hemoglobin Icaria (Ic) or a single amino acid change such as hemoglobin Quong Sze (QS) or hemoglobin Swan Dok (SW). These structural mutants result in a decreased output of alpha chains due either to an instability of the corresponding mRNA or to a direct degradation of the abnormal alpha chain produced. Overall, a minimum of 12 major genetic defects resulting in the $\alpha^1$ thalassemia gene have been defined using DNA hybridization techniques, sequencing analysis of the alpha genes as well as population studies. These different $\alpha^+$ thalassemia genes result in different levels of alpha chain output. For example, the nondeletion regulatory type of defect, also called $\alpha\alpha^T$ and found in Saudi Arabia, is more severe than the single gene deletion type of defect, also called $-\alpha$ and commonly found throughout the Mediterranean area, Middle East area, Indian subcontinent, Southeast Asia, Africa, and Malaysia.

## Clinical Expression of the Different Gene Combinations

Alpha thalassemia can be divided into four clinical categories depending on the severity of the disease. The most severe expression of alpha thalassemia is the hemoglobin Bart's hydrops fetalis syndrome, which is caused by homozygosity of the $\alpha^°$ thalassemia gene. This is a lethal disease, and infants with hemoglobin Bart's hydrops fetalis die either in utero or soon after birth. They produce no alpha chain, and the only hemoglobins found are hemoglobin Bart's ($\gamma_4$) and hemoglobin Portland ($\zeta_2\gamma_2$). Because hemoglobin Bart's is useless as an oxygen carrier, survival of these fetuses into the third trimester or until birth is entirely due to the presence of hemoglobin Portland. At birth, these infants are severely anemic and edematous, and demonstrate ascites, marked hepatomegaly, and splenomegaly. Significant morbidity and mortality can occur in the mothers owing to obstetric complications. This condition is quite common in Southeast Asia and is found sporadically in the Mediterranean area.

The second most severe clinical expression of alpha thalassemia is hemoglobin H disease. In this entity only one alpha gene out of four is functioning. This is usually the result of a double heterozygosity of an $\alpha^°$ thalassemia gene with an $\alpha^+$ thalassemia gene but is also found in Saudi Arabia as the result of homozygosity of the more severe form of the $\alpha^+$ thalassemia gene — the nondeleted $\alpha\alpha^T$ gene. Clinically, hemoglobin H disease is characterized by a variable degree of microcytic, hypochromic anemia, which is somewhat intermediate between the clinical pictures of thalassemia minor and thalassemia major and which has often been called "thalassemia intermedia." The patients will have a mild to moderate degree of anemia and may develop the physical and bony characteristics of thalassemia major, as well as splenomegaly and hepatomegaly. They will, however, survive into adulthood without blood transfusion and do not usually suffer from severe iron overload. The anemia usually becomes worse with infections, pregnancy, and folic acid deficiency states. Hemolytic crises may occur with infections. Adults with hemoglobin H disease will have from 5 to 40 percent hemoglobin H, with the remainder being mostly hemoglobin A with a small amount of hemoglobin $A_2$ and hemoglobin Bart's. Infants who will later develop hemoglobin H disease usually have between 19 and 27 percent hemoglobin Bart's at birth, with the remainder composed of hemoglobin F and hemoglobin A. Hemoglobin H and hemoglobin Bart's can easily be identified by hemoglobin electrophoresis, because they migrate anodally at pH 6.5 to 7.0. In addition, hemoglobin H shows a characteristic appearance of multiple ragged inclusions in many red cells after incubation with brilliant cresyl blue, the so-called golf-ball appearance.

The $\alpha^°$ thalassemia trait, also called "alpha thalassemia 1 trait," is caused by the defect of two of the four alpha genes. This is usually the result of heterozygosity for the $\alpha^°$ thalassemia gene but could also be the result of homozygosity for the $\alpha^+$ thalassemia gene. The condition is characterized by the presence at birth of 5 to 15 percent hemoglobin Bart's, which disappears with development and is not replaced by hemoglobin H. There is a minimal amount of anemia with slight hypochromia and microcytosis present. After hemoglobin Bart's disappears, the hemoglobin electrophoretic pattern becomes normal.

The last category of alpha thalassemia is the $\alpha^+$ thalassemia trait, also called "alpha thalassemia 2 trait." This is the result of a defect in one of the four alpha globin genes and is characterized by the presence of a very small amount (up to 2 percent) of hemoglobin Bart's at birth; after the disappearance of hemoglobin Bart's during development, no recognizable hematologic abnormality will be present.

Table 10–2 summarizes the different genetic backgrounds associated with the four different clinical expressions of alpha thalassemia.

## Delta-Beta Thalassemias and Hemoglobin Lepore Syndrome

Delta-beta thalassemias are a diverse group of thalassemias characterized by a combined defect in delta and beta chain synthesis. They can be de-

Table 10-2. GENETIC BACKGROUND OF ALPHA THALASSEMIA CLINICAL SYNDROMES (MATING COMBINATIONS)

| Chromosome → | Normal | $\alpha^+$ | | | | $\alpha^\circ$ |
|---|---|---|---|---|---|---|
| Genes ↓ | $\alpha\alpha$ | $-\alpha$ | $\alpha^{cs}\alpha$ | $\alpha\alpha^T$ | | $--$ |
| $\alpha\alpha$ | N | $\alpha$thal 2 | $\alpha$thal 2 | $\alpha$thal 2 | | $\alpha$thal 1 |
| $-\alpha$ | $\alpha$thal 2 | $\alpha$thal 1 | $\alpha$thal 1 | $\alpha$thal 1 | | H |
| $\alpha^{cs}\alpha$ | $\alpha$thal 2 | $\alpha$thal 1 | $\alpha$thal 1 | $\alpha$thal 1 | | H |
| $\alpha\alpha^T$ | $\alpha$thal 2 | $\alpha$thal 1 | $\alpha$thal 1 | H | | H |
| $--$ | $\alpha$thal 1 | $\alpha$thal 1 | H | H | | Bart's |

$\alpha\alpha \pm$ normal haplotype; $-\alpha =$ deletion of one alpha gene: $\alpha^{cs}\alpha =$ Hb Constant Spring: $\alpha\alpha^T =$ nondeletion alpha thalassemia gene; $-- =$ deletion of both alpha genes. (The clinical phenotype resulting from the combination of these haplotypes is found at the intersection of the corresponding column and row.) N = normal clinical phenotype; $\alpha$thal 1 = $\alpha^\circ$ trait, 5–15% Hb Bart's at birth, mild anemia; $\alpha$thal 2 = $\alpha^+$ trait, 0–2% Hb Bart's at birth, minimal hematologic changes; H = hemoglobin H disease; Bart's = hemoglobin Bart's hydrops fetalis.

scribed as demonstrating a normal level of hemoglobin $A_2$ and an unusually high level of hemoglobin F in the heterozygote, and absent hemoglobin A and $A_2$ in the homozygote. The delta-beta thalassemias can be subdivided into two groups according to the type of hemoglobin F produced. If both $^G\gamma$ and $^A\gamma$ chains are produced—that is, if both gamma genes are active—this variety is then called $^G\gamma^A\gamma\,\delta\beta$ thalassemia. If only $^G\gamma$ chains are produced, which means that the A-gamma gene as well as the delta and the beta genes are inactive, this variety is then called $^G\gamma\delta\beta$ thalassemia. Another syndrome of delta-beta chains involves the production of an abnormal hemoglobin. This abnormal hemoglobin, called hemoglobin Lepore after the name of the family in which it was first found, has been shown to be a fusion of the delta and beta chains, which is the product of a fusion gene formed by an unequal crossing over.

Figure 10-9 indicates diagrammatically the production of hemoglobin Lepore by this unequal crossing over. At least three different hemoglobin Lepores have been described, varying in the exact location of the unequal crossing over.

All delta-beta thalassemias studied thus far have been shown to be the result of a deletion. They can be described at the genetic level as three different entities, depending on the amount of DNA lost: hemoglobin Lepore syndrome results from a partial deletion of the delta and beta genes, $^G\gamma^A\gamma\delta\beta$ thalassemia from a complete deletion of the delta and beta genes, and $^G\gamma\delta\beta$ thalassemia from a deletion of the A-gamma gene in addition to the deletion of the delta and beta genes.

Delta-beta thalassemias are less common than beta thalassemias and have been found sporadically in Greeks, American blacks, Italians, and Arabs.

The gamma chain synthesis in delta-beta thalassemia is usually more efficient than that in beta thalassemia, and in general the former results in a milder clinical disease than the latter. Patients with homozygous delta-beta thalassemia will have a mild to moderate degree of anemia and rarely require blood transfusion, except occasionally during times of stress such as infection or pregnancy. The clinical course is usually described as "thalassemia intermedia." This is also true of the double heterozygous delta-beta and beta thalassemias. However, the homozygous state for hemoglobin Lepore appears to be somewhat more severe and closer to the clinical state of homozygous beta thalassemia. The majority of patients with homozygous hemoglobin

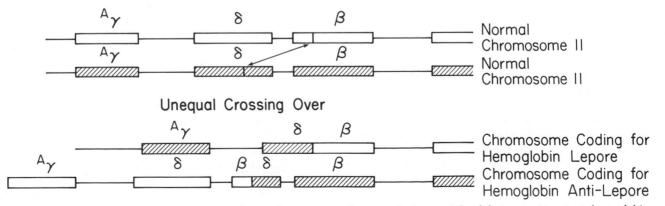

**Figure 10-9.** Hemoglobin Lepore formation. An abnormal crossing over between the beta and the alpha genes gives rise to hemoglobin Lepore and to hemoglobin anti-Lepore.

Lepore are transfusion dependent. Double heterozygosity for beta thalassemia and hemoglobin Lepore also causes a clinical disorder similar to homozygous beta thalassemia.

Heterozygosity for delta-beta thalassemia and hemoglobin Lepore results in a mild form of anemia that is clinically described as "thalassemia minor" and is similar to the condition of patients with heterozygous beta thalassemia.

## Hereditary Persistence of Fetal Hemoglobin (HPFH)

Hereditary persistence of fetal hemoglobin consists of a group of conditions characterized by the persistence of fetal hemoglobin synthesis into adult life. These conditions can be classified into two different categories according to the distribution of hemoglobin F among the red cells. Fetal hemoglobin is more resistant than adult hemoglobin to elution at acid pH and can be demonstrated on a peripheral smear by the acid elution test of Kleihauer and Betke **(see Color Figure 245)**. Using this stain, the hereditary persistence of fetal hemoglobin conditions can be divided into a pancellular form, in which hemoglobin F is uniformly distributed among the red cells, and a heterocellular form, in which hemoglobin F is found in a small percentage of the cells only. In the normal adult, cells containing hemoglobin F can occasionally be found, but the amount is always less than 2 percent and is usually less than 1 percent. These cells are called F cells.

Heterocellular HPFH appears to be an inherited condition in which the number of F cells is increased without concurrent abnormalities in delta and beta chain production. Its most common form is the Swiss type, in which individuals have up to 3 percent hemoglobin F but are otherwise hematologically normal. At the DNA level, there appears to be no gross abnormalities of the delta and beta genes.

On the other hand, pancellular HPFH appears to be a form of delta-beta thalassemia in which the gamma genes were not switched off and are able to compensate fully for the lack of delta and beta chain production. The most common form of pancellular HPFH is the Negro type, in which there is a deletion of the beta and delta globin genes that is associated with synthesis of $^G\gamma$ and $^A\gamma$ chains, which almost compensates for the lack of production of delta and beta chains. Hemoglobin F constitutes 100 percent of the hemoglobin in the homozygous state and 15 to 30 percent of the hemoglobin in the heterozygous state. The hemoglobin F is homogeneously distributed among the red cells and consists of a mixture of $^G\gamma$ and $^A\gamma$ chains. Clinically, the homozygotes will demonstrate features of thalassemia minor and the heterozygotes will be hematologically normal.

Another form of pancellular HPFH is the Greek type, in which about 15 percent hemoglobin F is present in the heterozygous state. This hemoglobin F is also found uniformly distributed among the red cells but is only of the A-gamma type. The homozygous state for this type of pancellular HPFH has not been described. In general, heterozygous or homozygous HPFH causes no significant clinical abnormalities.

## Thalassemia Associated with Hemoglobin Variants

The molecular basis of the hemoglobinopathies can be broadly divided into two groups. In the first group the genetic defect involves the synthesis of the beta chain; this group includes beta thalassemia, hemoglobin S, hemoglobin C, and hemoglobin E. In the second group the genetic defect involves the alpha chain synthesis; the alpha thalassemias compose this group. Homozygosity or double heterozygosity for defective genes within the same group usually results in severe disease that is often lethal. Double heterozygosity with one gene from one group and a second gene from the other group usually shows no interaction, and a defective gene in one group may even result in a clinical improvement of the condition of a patient who is homozygous for a defective gene in the other group. Although thalassemia has been described in association with a large number of hemoglobin structural variants, we will only consider the interactions with the more common hemoglobin variants (that is, beta thalassemia with hemoglobin S, hemoglobin C, and hemoglobin E, and alpha thalassemia with hemoglobin S).

### Beta Thalassemia/Hemoglobin S

This condition was first recognized in individuals who had inherited a single hemoglobin S gene and who demonstrated about 65 percent hemoglobin S and 35 percent hemoglobin A, which is the reverse of the proportions found in patients with sickle cell trait. It was discovered that this condition was the result of the inheritance of a hemoglobin S gene from one parent and the beta thalassemia gene from the other. Beta thalassemia/hemoglobin S (also called the beta thalassemia sickle cell syndrome) has been widely seen in Africa, the Mediterranean area, the Middle East, and the West Indies, as well as in North American blacks. There is great variety in the clinical severity of this syndrome, depending mostly on the type of beta thalassemia gene inherited. If the beta thalassemia gene is the $\beta°$ type, no hemoglobin A will be produced and the clinical condition will be indistinguishable from classic sickle cell anemia, characterized by severe anemia presenting in early childhood and recurrent sickling crises. If the beta thalassemia gene is $\beta^+$ type 1, a small amount of hemoglobin A will be produced, possibly representing up to 15 percent of the total hemoglobin. Patients in this group will have severe anemia with a hemoglobin level in the 7 to 8 g/dl range and will experience less frequent and less severe sickling crises than will those in the $\beta°$ group. If the beta thalassemia gene is $\beta^+$ type 2, as found in most American blacks, a greater amount of hemoglobin A will be produced, representing up to 30 percent of the total hemoglobin. Patients in this group have a very mild refractory anemia with hemoglobin in the 11 g/dl range and are usually asymptomatic, the condition being diagnosed later in life or during the course of a family study. These patients, as a rule, will not experience any sickling crisis except under the most severe hypoxic conditions.

## Beta Thalassemia/Hemoglobin C

The beta thalassemia/hemoglobin C syndrome demonstrates great variability in clinical and hematologic manifestations, which is directly related to the type of beta thalassemia gene that interacts with the hemoglobin C gene; however, the great majority of patients with this syndrome are West African and North American blacks. In this racial group the more common beta thalassemia gene is $\beta^+$ type 2. In this case the beta thalassemia/hemoglobin C syndrome will be characterized by a mild degree of usually asymptomatic anemia in which the clinical and hematologic findings are very similar to those found in heterozygous beta thalassemia.

## Beta Thalassemia/Hemoglobin E

Double heterozygosity for beta thalassemia and hemoglobin E is unusual in that it results in a severe clinical disorder that is much more severe than homozygous hemoglobin E disease. Patients with this syndrome are distributed widely throughout the Far East. The condition follows a clinical course very similar to that of homozygous beta thalassemia, with a very severe anemia occurring in early childhood and the development of the characteristic features of thalassemia major if the patient is not started on a regular blood transfusion program.

## Alpha Thalassemia with Sickle Cell Anemia

The occurrence of alpha thalassemia in conjunction with sickle cell anemia has a positive influence on the clinical expression of the disease. Patients with such a genetic background have an increased percentage of hemoglobin F, which is thought to result in a decreased severity of the sickling process. Of interest is the fact that the amount of hemoglobin F present is roughly proportional to the number of alpha genes affected. Patients with the $\alpha°$ thalassemia trait will have an average of 16 percent hemoglobin F, and those with the $\alpha^+$ thalassemia trait will have an average of 8 percent hemoglobin F.

## CLINICAL COURSE AND THERAPY

The clinical course and therapy of patients with thalassemia can be broadly subdivided into three categories: thalassemia major, thalassemia intermedia, and thalassemia minor. Table 10–3 summarizes the different genetic backgrounds that result in each of these clinical outcomes.

By itself, as a single entity, stands hemoglobin Bart's hydrops fetalis, in which the affected infants are either stillborn or die within a few days after birth. For this condition, no therapy is available. The clinical significance of this entity is related more to the obstetric problems that may arise in the affected infants' mothers. Pregnancy is often complicated by toxemia, obstructed labor, and postpartum hemorrhage, which may result in severe morbidity and mortality. Clinical emphasis for this entity is in the prevention of the disease through early antenatal diagnosis, which should result in termination of pregnancy for the protection of the mother's health.

Thalassemia major is the most severe clinical expression of thalassemia and characteristically occurs in patients with homozygous $\beta°$ or $\beta^+$ thalassemia or with double heterozygous $\beta°$ and $\beta^+$ thalassemia, as well as in patients with homozygous hemoglobin Lepore, double heterozygous beta thalassemia/hemoglobin Lepore, and double heterozygous beta thalassemia/hemoglobin E.

Untreated thalassemia major is lethal, resulting in death within the first few years of life, secondary to one of the complications described earlier. Appropriate therapy for thalassemia major is based on a regular blood transfusion program, splenectomy, and iron chelation, along with close medical supervision, good nutrition, and early treatment of infections.

Infants with thalassemia major will usually present within the first year of life with failure to thrive, pallor, a variable degree of jaundice, and abdominal enlargement, with hemoglobin levels from 4 to 8 g/dl. All diagnostic work necessary to define exactly the type of thalassemia should be done at this time before blood transfusions are started.

It is now clear that a high transfusion program (hypertransfusion) that maintains the hemoglobin level at 11.5 g/dl on the average is better than an intermittent program that allows the hemoglobin level to drop to a point when the child is severely symptomatic. Hypertransfusion allows for better development, depresses ineffective erythropoiesis (thus preventing the serious bony deformities), and provides for an overall better quality of life. This, however, draws on considerable blood resources and may not be available in the very countries where thalassemia major is a main public health concern.

Table 10-3. GENETIC BACKGROUND OF THE DIFFERENT CLINICAL COURSES OF THALASSEMIA

| Major | Intermedia | Minor | Minima* |
|---|---|---|---|
| Homozygous $\beta°$ thal | Homozygous $\beta°$ or $\beta^+$ thal or double heterozygous | Heterozygous $\beta°$ thal | Heterozygous $\beta^+$ thal (type 3) |
| Homozygous $\beta^+$ thal (type 1) | $\beta°$/$\beta^+$ thal in association with $\alpha$ thal | Heterozygous $\beta^+$ thal (type 1 or type 2) | |
| Double heterozygous $\beta°$/$\beta^+$ thal | Homozygous $\beta^+$ thal (type 2 or type 3) | Heterozygous $\delta\beta$ thal | |
| Homozygous Hb Lepore (some) | Homozygous Hb Lepore (some) | Heterozygous Hb Lepore | |
| Double heterozygous Hb Lepore/$\beta°$ or $\beta^+$ thal | Double heterozygous $\delta\beta$ thal/$\beta$ thal | Double heterozygous $\beta$ thal/HPFH | Homozygous HPFH |
| Double heterozygous HbE/$\beta°$ or $\beta^+$ thal | Double heterozygous Hb Lepore/$\delta\beta$ thal | | Heterozygous HPFH |
| | Hemoglobin H disease | $\alpha$ thalassemia 1 | $\alpha$ thalassemia 2 |

*Thalassemia minima is a term used for thalassemia carriers with no clinical symptoms and minimal to no hematologic abnormalities.

In the presence of splenomegaly, splenectomy plays a clear role in decreasing the blood transfusion requirement. However, it should preferably not be performed until the child has reached at least 5 years of age, to decrease the risk of overwhelming infection — particularly of pneumococcal origin.

With regular blood transfusion, these children will survive but will develop severe iron overload owing to increased iron absorption and to the loading of iron from the blood transfusions. This iron overload results in hemochromatosis, and these patients will die in their second or third decade, usually of cardiac failure. In the meantime, these patients will have developed multiple organ damage, with lack of pubertal development probably due to iron toxicity to the pituitary gland, cirrhosis of the liver (which may be the result of either hemochromatosis or post-transfusion hepatitis), and diabetes due to iron toxicity to the pancreas. This iron overload may be improved with the early introduction of iron chelation therapy. Recent assessment of iron chelation therapy with desferrioxamine seems to indicate that an adequate iron balance can be achieved and that longer survival will be attained.

Alternate modes of therapy for thalassemia major in the future may be found in the areas of bone marrow transplantation, genetic engineering, and pharmacologic manipulations that may induce the "switching back on" of the gamma globin gene. The current optimal therapy for thalassemia major relies on intensive use of a fairly sophisticated level of health care that cannot be achieved in most of the countries where thalassemia major is a serious problem without shunting the major thrust of the health resources in that direction.

Another approach to this problem at the health planning level is to decrease the number of births of infants with thalassemia major. This has been successful in certain countries, particularly Cyprus, with the implementation of mass population screening for the detection of heterozygous carriers, genetic counseling, and antenatal diagnosis for couples at risk. Recent developments in antenatal diagnosis, using DNA hybridization techniques in association with chronic villi sampling, enable physicians to make a diagnosis during the first trimester of pregnancy, thus making early termination of pregnancy much more widely available and acceptable.

Thalassemia intermedia covers a broad spectrum of clinical expression of thalassemia, bridging the gap between the severe, lethal form of thalassemia major and the mild, often asymptomatic anemic state of thalassemia minor. The definition of thalassemia intermedia is relative, since the clinical state of patients in this group varies from a mild disability to severe incapacitation without transfusion. Thalassemia intermedia could be defined as a form of thalassemia in which patients have variable degrees of symptomatic anemia, jaundice, splenomegaly, and many of the complications of thalassemia major, but will survive into adulthood without a large blood transfusion requirement.

The genetic background of thalassemia intermedia is also extremely varied. It includes patients with homozygosity for the less severe forms of the beta thalassemia gene (such as $\beta^+$ type 2 and $\beta^+$ 3 thalassemia), homozygous delta-beta thalassemia, double heterozygous delta-beta thalassemia/beta thalassemia, hemoglobin H disease, and patients who are homozygous for beta thalassemia but who have also inherited a gene for alpha thalassemia or who have the ability to synthesize the gamma chains more efficiently. The exact definition of the genetic background of a patient with thalassemia intermedia requires a careful and extensive family study.

Patients with thalassemia intermedia will usually present at a somewhat older age — usually after the age of 2 — and with a slightly higher level of hemoglobin (between 6 and 10 g/dl) than patients with thalassemia major. There is great overlap between the two conditions at presentation; however, it is very important to differentiate between them, as the only therapy for thalassemia major is regular blood transfusion in conjunction with iron chelation, whereas the management of thalassemia intermedia involves mostly supportive therapy with only occasional blood transfusion under special circumstances.

The serum bilirubin level is significantly more elevated in patients with thalassemia intermedia than in those with thalassemia major. Patients with thalassemia intermedia may develop the severe bony deformities and compression syndromes due to marrow hyperplasia and extramedullary erythropoiesis characteristic of thalassemia major. They are susceptible to frequent, sometimes severe, infections, and gallbladder problems due to the formation of gallstones. These children will usually have an acceptable level of growth and development (although puberty may be delayed by a few years), and they will reach adulthood if infections are controlled and if they enjoy good nutrition with particular emphasis on prevention of folic acid deficiency. They will usually develop splenomegaly and may become transfusion dependent if severe hypersplenism occurs. This will usually require splenectomy. Children with thalassemia intermedia may develop iron overload due to increase gastrointestinal absorption, but this is a much slower process than that experienced in patients with thalassemia major, and the complications due to iron overload will occur much later in life. Women with thalassemia intermedia may get pregnant and will require blood transfusions as well as folic acid supplementation throughout the pregnancy.

Thalassemia minor is a clinical entity in which the genetic defects of thalassemia are expressed as a mild microcytic, hypochromic anemia, usually in the 9 to 11 g/dl range, and is asymptomatic except during periods of stress such as pregnancy, infection, or folic acid deficiency. Most patients with thalassemia minor are heterozygous for the $\beta^+$ thalassemia gene, the $\beta^\circ$ thalassemia gene, or the $\alpha^\circ$ thalassemia gene. The genetic background of thalassemia minor also includes heterozygosity for hemoglobin Lepore and for delta-beta thalassemia. Patients with thalassemia minor are usually diagnosed incidental to a family study of an index case with thalassemia major or by population screening. They usually require no therapy if they maintain good nutrition.

## BLOOD TRANSFUSION IN THALASSEMIA

The three main concerns that need to be addressed regarding patients with thalassemia major who will be on a regular blood transfusion program are (1) the development of iron overload, (2) the development of alloimmunization, and (3) the risk of transfusion-transmitted diseases. The problem of iron overload can be approached from two directions — by increasing the iron excretion or by decreasing the amount of iron transfused. This latter option can be performed by increasing the length of survival time of the transfused red cells, which requires selection of the younger red cells (also called neocytes) for transfusion. Young red cells and reticulocytes have a lower specific gravity than old red cells, and by using a differential centrifugation technique the blood unit can be separated so that the upper layer of cells is collected. These red cells will have a much longer life expectancy and can decrease the transfusion requirement of a patient by lengthening the interval of the blood transfusion schedule.

Alloimmunization is a recurrent problem of all chronically transfused patients. These patients often develop antibodies to white cell as well as to red cell antigens. Antibodies to white cell antigens cause febrile nonhemolytic transfusion reactions that are unpleasant. These reactions can be avoided by routinely transfusing leukocyte-poor red cells. Alloimmunization to red cell antigens is a more serious problem, since this can cause acute or delayed hemolytic transfusion reactions and may seriously affect the availability of compatible blood. It is a good idea to obtain a complete phenotype of the patient's red cell before embarking on a regular transfusion program.

Transfusion-transmitted diseases are a common complication in multitransfused patients. Patients with thalassemia major will often develop hepatitis, which is usually non-A, non-B hepatitis in countries where blood is routinely screened for the presence of the hepatitis B surface antigen (HBsAg). Hepatitis B as well as delta hepatitis can also be transmitted through blood transfusions and are the most common threat in certain parts of the world. Some patients may develop a chronic form of hepatitis that, in conjunction with the iron toxicity of iron overload, may damage the liver severely and result in cirrhosis of the liver.

## LABORATORY DIAGNOSIS OF THALASSEMIA

The hallmark of thalassemia is the finding of a microcytic, hypochromic anemia. Although more sophisticated laboratory procedures are needed to define exactly the type of thalassemia, the original diagnosis of thalassemia can be made or strongly suspected on the basis of the result of routine hematology procedures.

### Routine Hematology Procedures

#### Automated Blood Cell Analyzer

Modern electronic cell analyzers now routinely give the following parameters: red cell count (RBC), hemoglobin level (Hb), hematocrit (HCT), mean corpuscular volume (MCV), mean cell hemoglobin (MCH), mean corpuscular hemoglobin concentration (MCHC), and red cell volume distribution width (RDW). The thalassemias in general are characterized by a decrease in Hb, HCT, MCV, and MCH in conjunction with a normal-to-increased RBC, a normal to mildly decreased MCHC, and a normal RDW. The only exception is thalassemia major, in which the degree of anisocytosis is such that the RDW will be increased. The decrease in MCV is usually striking and disproportionate to the decrease in hemoglobin and hematocrit. This fact, in conjunction with the relatively high RBC and the normal RDW, offers a reliable discrimination index between heterozygous alpha or beta thalassemia and iron deficiency. In iron deficiency, the RDW will be increased and the decrease in MCV will be less striking and only observed when the anemia is more severe. In heterozygous thalassemia, the MCH will usually be below 22 pg and the MCV below 70 fl, whereas the hemoglobin level will be in the 9 to 11 g/dl range.

### Peripheral Smear Examination

The careful examination of a well-prepared peripheral smear is essential to the diagnosis of thalassemia.

**Wright's Stain.** In homozygous beta and double heterozygous non-alpha thalassemia, the peripheral smear demonstrates extreme anisocytosis and poikilocytosis with bizarre shapes, target cells, ovalocytes, and a large number of nucleated red cells **(see Color Figure 108)**. There is marked hypochromia and microcytosis. In heterozygous beta thalassemia, the cells are hypochromic and microcytic with a mild to moderate degree of anisocytosis and poikilocytosis. Target cells are frequent, and basophilic stipling is often present **(see Color Figure 109)**. The peripheral smear of a patient with the sickle cell thalassemia syndrome can be differentiated from that of a patient with pure sickle cell anemia by the presence of hypochromia, microcytosis, and numerous target cells, and by the somewhat less frequent finding of sickled cells, in sickle cell thalassemia.

In hemoglobin H disease, the peripheral smear will demonstrate hypochromia with microcytosis, target cells, and mild to moderate anisopoikilocytosis. Patients with heterozygous $\alpha°$ thalassemia usually demonstrate a mild hypochromia and microcytosis, whereas those with heterozygous $\alpha^+$ thalassemia usually have a perfectly normal peripheral smear.

**Supravital Stains.** The reticulocyte count is usually elevated up to 10 percent in hemoglobin H disease and up to 5 percent in homozygous beta thalassemia but is disproportionately low in relation to the degree of anemia in the latter condition.

In hemoglobin H disease, incubation of the red cells with brilliant cresyl blue stain will cause in vitro precipitation of hemoglobin H owing to the redox action of the dye. This will result in a characteristic appearance of the majority of the red cells, in which they contain multiple discrete inclusions, the appearance of which has often been compared to that of a golf-ball **(see Color Figure 110)**. Occasionally, and after extensive searching, such cells containing hemoglobin H inclusions can be found in the $\alpha°$ thalassemia carrier.

Incubation of the blood with methyl violet stain can demonstrate Heinz body–like inclusions, which represent in vivo precipitation of the abnormal hemoglobin in splenectomized patients with homozygous beta thalassemia or hemoglobin H disease.

**Acid Elution Stain.** The acid elution technique originally described by Kleihauer and Betke is based on the fact that at an acid pH of about 3.3, hemoglobin A is eluted from an air-dried, alcohol-fixed blood smear, whereas hemoglobin F is resistant to elution. After such treatment and subsequent staining with eosin or erythrosin, normal adult red cells will appear as very faint ghosts. Red cells containing hemoglobin F will demonstrate a variable amount of stain, depending on the amount of hemoglobin F present. A controlled preparation containing a mixture of adult and cord cells must also be stained and examined in parallel to check the quality of the technique, as this technique is very sensitive to many variables.

This stain is very useful in demonstrating the distribution of hemoglobin F and can be used to differentiate between pancellular and heterocellular HPFH. It is also useful in differentiating heterozygous delta-beta thalassemia from heterozygous pancellular HPFH, since the former usually has a heterocellular distribution of hemoglobin F.

### Osmotic Fragility

The red cells of patients with homozygous or heterozygous beta thalassemia, hemoglobin H disease, and $\alpha°$ thalassemia trait have a decreased osmotic fragility. This fact is not very useful for diagnostic purposes in a specific patient, but it is the basis of a simple, inexpensive method of screening for the thalassemia carrier state in large populations.

## Hemoglobin Electrophoresis

Hemoglobin electrophoresis plays an important role in the diagnosis of thalassemias by allowing the detection of increased levels of hemoglobin $A_2$ and hemoglobin F as well as the presence of abnormal hemoglobins, such as hemoglobin H, hemoglobin Bart's, hemoglobin Lepore, hemoglobin Constant Spring, or other structurally abnormal hemoglobins that can be found in association with thalassemia (hemoglobin S, hemoglobin C, hemoglobin E). Table 10–4 contains a summary of the different patterns

Table 10-4. HEMOGLOBINS A, A₂, AND F LEVELS IN THE DIFFERENT NON-ALPHA THALASSEMIAS

|  | HbA % | HbA₂ % | HbF % |
|---|---|---|---|
| Homozygous $\beta°$ thal | 0 | 2–5 | 95–98 |
| Homozygous $\beta^+$ or double heterozygous $\beta^+/\beta°$ thal | 5–35 | 2–5 | 60–95 |
| Homozygous $\delta\beta$ thal | 0 | 0 | 100 |
| Homozygous Hb Lepore | 0 | 0 | 75 (25% Hb Lepore) |
| Heterozygous $\beta$ thal | 90–95 | 3.5–7 | 2–5 |
| Heterozygous $\delta\beta$ thal | 80–92 | 1–2.5 | 5–20 |
| Heterozygous Hb Lepore | 75–85 | 2 | 1–6 (7–15% Hb Lepore) |
| Homozygous HPFH | 0 | 0 | 100 |
| Heterozygous HPFH (Negro type) | 65–85 | 1–2.5 | 15–35 |
| Heterozygous HPFH (Greek type) | 75–85 | 1.5–2.5 | 15–25 |
| Normal | 97.5 | 2.5 | 0.2–1 |

of the hemoglobins present in the different thalassemia syndromes.

Routine hemoglobin electrophoresis to confirm the diagnosis of thalassemia is done at an alkaline pH around 8.4 on cellulose acetate or starch gel. At that pH the hemoglobins will migrate from the most cathodal to the most anodal in the following order: first hemoglobin Constant Spring, then hemoglobins A₂, C, and E migrate in the same band; next hemoglobins S and Lepore, again in the same band; next hemoglobin F, followed by hemoglobin A, then hemoglobin Bart's, and last hemoglobin H. The different patterns of migration of the different hemoglobins is illustrated in Figure 10-10. Cellulose acetate or starch gel electrophoresis can be done at low to neutral pH to detect easily hemoglobin H and hemoglobin Bart's, as they migrate anodally (that is, in opposite direction of other hemoglobins) at this pH.

## Cellulose Acetate

Cellulose acetate electrophoresis is becoming more popular and has replaced starch gel electrophoresis in many laboratories, owing to its simple, rapid method. It uses a smaller sample than starch gel electrophoresis, and minor components such as hemoglobin Constant Spring and small amounts of hemoglobin A₂ may be overlooked. Small amounts of hemoglobin A in the presence of mostly hemoglobin F also can be difficult to detect. Figure 10-11 demonstrates a strip of a cellulose acetate after electrophoresis of several hemoglobins.

## Starch Gel

Starch gel electrophoresis is a little more cumbersome than cellulose acetate electrophoresis, because the starch gel must be prepared and poured and is more difficult to handle. The staining procedure is also more time consuming, and long-term storage is more difficult. However, the result of the starch gel electrophoresis is similar to that of the cellulose acetate procedure. Electrophoresis with starch gel is better at defining the presence of hemoglobin Constant Spring and should always be used if such a variant is suspected.

## Citrate Agar Gel

Citrate agar gel electrophoresis, which is performed at an acid pH between 5.9 and 6.2, has a minor role

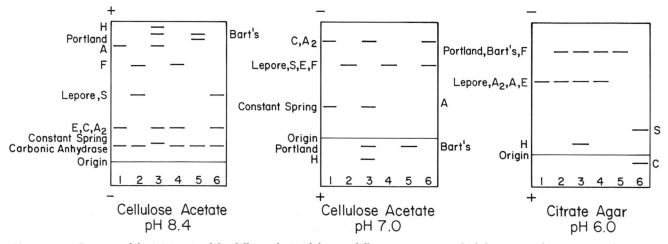

**Figure 10-10.** Diagram of the migration of the different hemoglobins at different pH. *1*, Normal adult (A, A₂); *2*, homozygous Hb Lepore (F, Lepore); *3*, HbH/Constant Spring disease $\alpha^{CS}\alpha/$—— (Constant Spring, A₂, A, Bart's, H); *4*, double heterozygous HbE/beta thalassemia (E, F); *5*, Hb Bart's hydrops fetalis syndrome (Portland, Bart's); *6*, HbS/C disease (S, C).

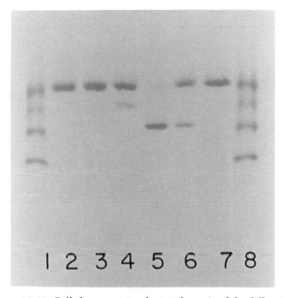

**Figure 10-11.** Cellulose acetate electrophoresis of the following samples: *1,* AFSC control; *2 and 3,* beta thalassemia carriers (increased $A_2$ and F); *4,* normal newborn; *5,* HbS/beta thalassemia (more hemoglobin S than A); *6,* HbS heterozygote; *7,* normal adult; *8,* AFSC control.

In the diagnosis of the thalassemias. It is mostly useful in defining structurally abnormal hemoglobins that are interacting with thalassemia, since it allows the distinction between hemoglobin C and hemoglobin E and between hemoglobin S and hemoglobin Lepore.

## Hemoglobin Quantitation

Although an increased level in hemoglobin $A_2$ or hemoglobin F can be detected by an experienced observer on cellulose acetate or starch gel electrophoresis, actual quantitation is necessary to further define the diagnosis of thalassemia.

### Hemoglobin $A_2$ Quantitation

The elevation of hemoglobin $A_2$ is an excellent tool for the detection of a heterozygote carrier of beta thalassemia. It is characteristic of heterozygous beta thalassemia and specific with no overlap values between heterozygous carriers and normal individuals. The level of hemoglobin $A_2$ ranges between 3.5 and 7 percent in heterozygous beta thalassemia, whereas normal values are always below 3.5 percent. A few rare variants of beta thalassemia with normal $A_2$ do exist, which are called normal $A_2$ beta thalassemia, and can only be distinguished in the carrier state from heterozygous alpha thalassemia by globin chain synthesis. The percent hemoglobin $A_2$ can be quantified either by elution following cellulose acetate electrophoresis or by microcolumn chromatography.

## Hemoglobin F Quantitation

The hemoglobin F levels are useful in the definition of the type of thalassemia involved, and a summary of the levels of hemoglobin F corresponding to the different types of thalassemia can be found in Table 10–4. The hemoglobin F level is normally below 2 percent. Approximately half of the beta thalassemia carriers will have a mildly elevated level of hemoglobin F — usually below 5 percent. Quantitation of hemoglobin F can be done by an alkali denaturation method, in which hemoglobin A is denatured in the presence of an alkali solution while hemoglobin F is unaffected. Immunologic techniques using a specific antibody to hemoglobin F have been developed and are more accurate and practical. Preprepared radioimmunodiffusion plates containing agarose with antihemoglobin F antisera are now available.

## Routine Chemistry

The indirect bilirubin level is elevated in thalassemia major and intermedia, ranging from 1 to 6 mg/dl. It is characteristically more elevated in thalassemia intermedia than in thalassemia major.

The assessment of the iron status of the patient by the determination of the serum iron level, total iron-binding capacity (TIBC), and serum ferritin level is useful in the differentiation of a thalassemia carrier from a patient with iron-deficiency anemia, as well as in the assessment of the iron load in a patient with thalassemia major or intermedia. The serum iron and the serum ferritin will be low and the TIBC increased in patients with iron deficiency. These values are normal in patients with thalassemia minor, unless they have concurrent iron deficiency. Patients with thalassemia major who have been transfused have increased levels of serum iron that will approach 100 percent saturation of the TIBC. The serum ferritin level will be elevated and will indicate the amount of iron deposited in the tissues.

## Miscellaneous

### Alpha/Beta Globin Chain Synthesis

The rate of synthesis of the globin chains can be measured in vitro by culturing reticulocytes from peripheral blood or nucleated red cells from the bone marrow in the presence of radioactively labeled leucine. The radioactive leucine is incorporated into the globin chains that are being synthesized. After the incubation is stopped, the red cells are lysed and the globin is precipitated and washed. The different globin chains are then separated by fractionation using CM-cellulose chromatography, and the radioactivity of each fraction is counted. In this way, a ratio of synthesis of alpha/beta globin

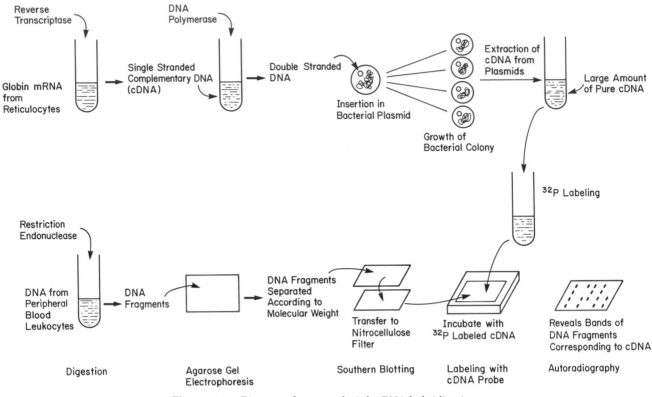

**Figure 10-12.** Diagram of gene analysis by DNA hybridization.

chains can be determined. This is a very sophisticated technique that can be used on special occasions when it is vitally important to differentiate an alpha thalassemia carrier from a normal $A_2$ beta thalassemia carrier, to identify a silent carrier of the alpha thalassemia gene, or to unravel a complicated inheritance pattern of multiple types of thalassemia within a family.

## Gene Analysis

This even more sophisticated technique using restriction endonucleases and hybridization with complementary DNA probes can study the genetic defects at the DNA level. The DNA is extracted from the nuclei of peripheral blood leukocytes and fragmented by enzymes called "restriction endonucleases." These enzymes recognize specific sequences in the DNA and will cleave the DNA at that particular point. Agarose gel electrophoresis is then performed on this fragmented DNA, which will separate the fragments according to their molecular weight. The separated DNA fragments are then transferred on a nitrocellulose filter and fixed to this filter by baking. Specific complementary DNA probes (cDNA) that will recognize the globin genes can be synthesized, using an enzyme called "reverse transcriptase" that can synthesize cDNA from globin mRNA that has been isolated from reticulocytes. These cDNA can be labeled with radioactive

nucleotides and then incubated with the DNA fragments on the nitrocellulose filter. They will bind or hybridize to any DNA fragment whose sequence is complementary to theirs. In this way, one can locate the specific globin genes that the cDNA probe recognizes. This technique can detect complete deletion of a globin gene, partial deletion of a globin gene, and some minute mutations that may abolish a normal cleavage site or create a new cleavage site that will be recognized by the specific restriction endonuclease used. These minute mutations that occur around the globin genes are inherited and have been found to be in linkage disequilibrium with specific defects of the globin gene complex. This type of analysis, called restriction fragment length polymorphism (RFLP), is now used in the antenatal diagnosis of thalassemia major. This method is illustrated in Figure 10-12.

## DIFFERENTIAL DIAGNOSIS OF MICROCYTIC HYPOCHROMIC ANEMIA

The differential diagnosis of microcytic hypochromic anemia includes iron deficiency, alpha thalassemia, beta thalassemia, anemia of chronic disease, hemoglobin E disease, sideroblastic anemia, and lead poisoning. The evaluation of the clinical history, the hemoglobin level, and the red cell indices (in particular MCV and MCH) usually narrow down

Table 10–5. DIFFERENTIAL DIAGNOSIS OF MICROCYTIC HYPOCHROMIC ANEMIA

| | RDW | Serum Iron | TIBC | Serum Ferritin | FEP | A₂ Level |
|---|---|---|---|---|---|---|
| Iron deficiency | ↑ | ↓ | ↑ | ↓ | ↑ | nl |
| Alpha thalassemia | nl | nl | nl | nl | nl | nl |
| Beta thalassemia | nl | nl | nl | nl | nl | ↑ |
| Hemoglobin E disease | nl | nl | nl | nl | nl | nl |
| Anemia of chronic disease | nl | ↓ | ↓ | ↑ | ↑ | nl |
| Sideroblastic anemia | ↑ | ↑ | nl | ↑ | ↓ | nl |
| Lead poisoning | nl | nl | nl | nl | ↑ | nl |

RDW = red cell volume distribution width; TIBC = total iron-binding capacity; FEP = free erythrocyte protoporphyrin; nl = normal.

the diagnosis. The difficult differential between the thalassemia carrier and iron deficiency can be done by evaluating the serum iron and ferritin levels and the TIBC. A markedly elevated free erythrocyte protoporphyrin (FEP) will identify a child with lead poisoning. Cellulose acetate electrophoresis will usually allow differentiation between a beta thalassemia carrier, an alpha thalassemia carrier, or the presence of hemoglobin E. The differentiation between these diseases is summarized in Table 10–5.

## CASE HISTORY

A 25-year-old man of Chinese extraction is being evaluated because when he attempted to donate blood he was found to be anemic. He otherwise has no complaints; he is active in sports and feels healthy. A complete blood count gives the following results: The RBC is 5.76 million, the Hb is 10.4 g/dl, the HCT is 35.9 percent, the MCV is 62 fl, the MCH is 18.1 pg, the MCHC is 29 pg, and the RDW is 13.5. The peripheral blood smear shows hypochromic, microcytic erythrocytes with a mild anisocytosis; occasional target cells but no basophilic stippling can be found.

The serum iron is 95 mg/dl (normal 60 to 150 mg/dl), the TIBC 305 mg/dl (normal 260 to 360 mg/dl), and the ferritin level 175 μg (normal 30 to 300 μg/dl). Cellulose acetate electrophoresis show an increased amount of hemoglobins F and A₂, which are quantitated to 4.5 percent and 5 percent, respectively.

### Questions

1. What are the diagnoses that you entertain at this time?
2. What laboratory tests do you think are most useful to diagnose the cause of his anemia?
3. What is your diagnosis now, and what is the significance of this diagnosis for this patient?

### Answers

1. On clinical history alone, the possibilities of anemia of chronic disease and lead poisoning can be ruled out in a healthy young man. We are left with the possibility of iron deficiency, a beta thalassemia carrier, an alpha thalassemia carrier, sideroblastic anemia, and hemoglobin E disease (which should be considered in a person of Chinese extraction).
2. A serum iron level, TIBC, serum ferritin level, and cellulose acetate electrophoresis are appropriate tests that may differentiate among these conditions.
3. Sideroblastic anemia and iron deficiency can be ruled out by the normal iron level, TIBC, and ferritin level. Although hemoglobin E migrates in the same area as hemoglobin A₂ on cellulose acetate electrophoresis, a patient with heterozygous or homozygous hemoglobin E would have a much larger amount of hemoglobin in that band; thus, hemoglobin E disease is ruled out. An alpha thalassemia carrier would have a normal hemoglobin electrophoresis pattern; therefore, the diagnosis in this patient is heterozygous beta thalassemia.

   Making the diagnosis of beta thalassemia heterozygosity in this patient is important for two reasons. First, the patient must be reassured that this level of hemoglobin and hematocrit is normal for him, and he should not be placed on iron therapy which could be harmful. Second, the patient needs to be educated regarding the possibility of his having a child with a severe congenital anemia and its therapeutic implications, if he marries someone who is a carrier of beta thalassemia, hemoglobin E, or hemoglobin S. His spouse should be screened for the presence of these genes and genetic counseling such as antenatal diagnosis offered if she in fact is a carrier.

## Bibliography

Bank, A: Genetic defects in the thalassemias. Curr Topics Hematol 5:1, 1985.

Bunn, HF, Forget, BG, and Ranney, HM: Human hemoglobins. WB Saunders, Philadelphia, 1977.

Higgs, DR and Weatherall, DS: Alpha thalassemia. Curr Topics Hematol 4:37, 1983.

Lehman, H and Huntsman, RG: Man's hemoglobin. JB Lippincott, Philadelphia, 1974.

Liebhaber, SA and Manno, CS: Update on hemoglobinopathies. Diagn Med 29:1, 1983.

Lin-Fu, JS: Cooley's anemia, a medical review. US Department of Health and Human Services, Washington, DC, 1981.

Modell, B and Berdoukas, V: The clinical approach to thalassemia. Grune & Stratton, New York, 1984.

Weatherall, DJ (ed): The Thalassemias. Methods in Hematology. Churchill-Livingstone, New York, 1983.

Weatherall, DJ and Clegg, JB: The thalassemia syndromes. Blackwell Scientific Publications, Boston, 1981.

WHO Working Group: Community control of hereditary anemias: Memorandum from a WHO meeting. Bull WHO 61:63, 1983.

WHO Working Group: Hereditary anemias: Genetic basis, clinical features, diagnosis and treatment. Bull WHO 60:643, 1982.

## CHAPTER 11

KATHRYN GRENIER-HUGHES, M.T.(ASCP), C.L.S.(NCA)

# Hemolytic Anemias: Intracorpuscular Defects
## V. Paroxysmal Nocturnal Hemoglobinuria

## DEFINITION

Paroxysmal nocturnal hemoglobinuria (PNH) is an acquired hemolytic anemia with an insidious onset, resulting in a chronic hemolytic state. In this disorder, the red cell membrane is abnormal, causing the red cells to be highly sensitive to the hemolytic action of complement. This defect also affects leukocytes and platelets.[1] The membrane defect present in the blood cells is the result of an abnormal clone of hematopoietic stem cells. Frequently associated with the chronic hemolysis is leukopenia, thrombocytopenia, hemosiderinuria, and hemoglobinuria.

## HISTORY

In 1866, William Gull published the first case of PNH.[2] He described an anemic patient with "hematinuria," which varied throughout the day but was worse in the morning. He recognized that the urinary pigment was due to some breakdown product of the red cells. The second case of PNH was published in 1882 by Paul Strübing, a German physician.[3] He reported a case of "paroxysmal hemoglobinuria," and, as Gull had, he too noted that this finding was most pronounced in the morning. Strübing related the hemolysis and hemoglobinuria to exercise and to the consumption of beer and hypothesized that the abnormality was a defect in the red cells and that hemolysis occurred when the abnormal red cells circulated through the kidney.

Furthermore, he believed that an accumulation of carbon dioxide and lactic acid from the previous day's exertion caused the hemolysis. Subsequent to Strübing's report, several other descriptions of PNH appeared. In addition to the hemoglobinuria, Marchiafava[4] and Micheli[5] separately observed and described the presence of "perpetual hemosiderinuria." In 1911, Hijmas van den Bergh,[6] a Dutch physician, made the next significant observation by demonstrating that PNH red cells underwent lysis when the serum and cells were exposed to carbonic acid. This was the first acidified serum lysis test.

In 1930, Thomas H. Ham described in detail the acidified serum lysis test (Ham Test).[7,8] He acidified serum to a pH of 6.4 and noted that when mixed with red cells from a patient with PNH, the cells lysed. Ham observed that these cells had an increased sensitivity to some serum hemolytic protein (complement) that caused the cells to lyse when acidified. Ham also demonstrated that some patients with PNH, presenting with chronic hemolysis, had positive acidified serum lysis test results but did not have hemoglobinuria.

Although paroxysmal nocturnal hemoglobinuria is fairly rare, much progress and research have increased our understanding of the mechanism of hemolysis, the role of complement, and possible causes of the defect.

## ETIOLOGY AND PATHOPHYSIOLOGY

PNH is an acquired intracorpuscular defect due to an abnormality in hematopoietic cell membranes.

This abnormality causes the cells, especially the erythrocytes, to be more sensitive than normal to the lytic action of complement (Fig. 11-1). This defect is probably associated with an abnormal clone of hematopoietic stem cells, resulting from a mutagenic event occurring during the course of bone marrow hypoplasia or recovery from an aplastic episode,[9] although it has also occurred without evidence of marrow hypoplasia.

Although the exact membrane defect is unknown, there has been much speculation about its possible mechanisms. Studies on the affected erythrocytes have shown the following abnormalities: altered membrane lipids,[10] increased sensitivity to peroxidation,[12] decreased membrane acetycholinesterase activity,[13] and craters and pits on the erythrocyte membrane as demonstrated by electron microscopy.[11] Unfortunately, there is no conclusive evidence as to the actual membrane defect.

Complement has a major role in the pathogenesis of PNH and will be discussed in detail at the end of this chapter. The PNH erythrocytes have been classified into three categories based on their interaction with complement. In PNH, the erythrocytes react abnormally with complement components C3 and C5-C9. PNH I erythrocytes react normally with complement and are thought to be residual normal cells because they are similar to normal erythrocytes in all respects.[14] PNH II erythrocytes have moderate sensitivity to complement component C3 and are three to five times more sensitive to lysis by complement than are normal erythrocytes.[15] PNH

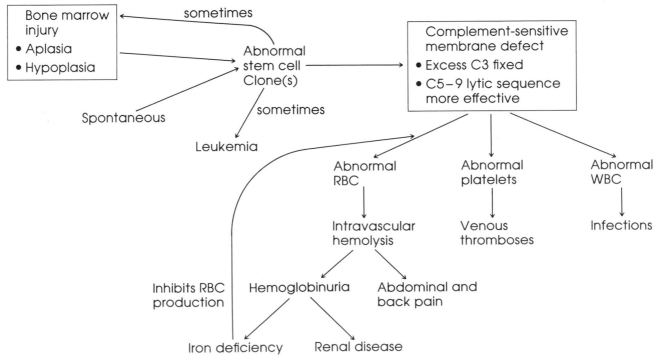

**Figure 11-1.** Pathophysiology of PNH. (From Beck, WS: Hematology, ed 3. MIT Press, Cambridge, 1982, with permission.)

III erythrocytes are the cells most sensitive to complement, being 15 to 25 times more sensitive to complement component C3 than normal erythrocytes; in addition to binding increased amounts of C3, they also have increased sensitivity to the terminal complement component, C5-C9.[16]

Patients with PNH usually have variable combinations of the three different types of PNH erythrocytes. Eighty percent of all patients with PNH have the combination of PNH I and PNH III cells, whereas the other 20 percent have variable combinations of PNH I, PNH II, and PNH III cells.[16] The degree of hemolysis depends on the proportion of abnormal cells and the severity of the defect. The proportion of abnormal cells varies from patient to patient, and the intensity of the clinical symptoms is related to the percentage of PNH III cells present.

## CLINICAL FEATURES

Diverse clinical presentations of PNH are common. The disease most often occurs in middle-aged adults, but occasionally occurs in children and the elderly as well. Both genders are equally affected. Most patients with PNH present with symptoms of anemia, which may be mild to severe and are due to the chronic hemolysis.

The classic presentation of hemoglobinuria, due to significant intravascular hemolysis, is most noticeable in the patients' first morning urine specimen. Twenty-five percent or less of patients present with this classic symptom;[16] however, irregular episodes of intravascular hemolysis with hemoglobinuria may be triggered by infections (most commonly viruses), surgical operations, menstruation, administration of iron, and a variety of drugs.

In contrast to hemoglobinuria, hemosiderinuria is present in most patients. Recurrent hemolysis results in loss of body iron into the urine. This iron is derived from plasma hemoglobin that is absorbed and catabolized in the renal tubules. Iron-laden tubular cells appear in the urine and can be stained for hemosiderin. Prolonged loss of iron can lead to iron-deficiency anemia, which may mask the diagnosis of PNH.

Patients commonly present with abdominal pain, headaches, and back pain—symptoms thought to be caused by intravascular thrombi. One of the major complications of PNH is the formation of venous thromboses of the portal, mesenteric, or hepatic veins. Formation of these thrombi may be attributed to the activation of complement sensitive platelets by the complement component C3.[9,17] Also, during the thrombotic episodes, features of disseminated intravascular coagulation (DIC) may appear (see Chapter 29).

Aplastic anemia may precede or coexist with PNH. In such cases, pancytopenia and marrow hypoplasia are present. Complement sensitive erythrocytes will occur transiently and in small numbers in certain patients of aplastic anemia, and in a few patients complement-sensitive erythrocytes are increased in number and persist, making these rare cases indistinguishable from PNH.

## DIAGNOSIS OF PNH

The diagnosis of PNH depends on the detection of complement-sensitive erythrocytes in the peripheral blood.[9] The diagnosis is difficult if based solely on clinical features and evaluation of the bone marrow and peripheral blood smears. PNH should be included in the differential diagnosis of patients with the following disorders: (1) hemolytic anemia of unknown etiology, (2) pancytopenia associated with a hypoplastic or aplastic bone marrow, (3) iron deficiency of unknown etiology, and (4) unexplained episodic hemoglobinuria.[18] PNH must also be differentiated from other causes of chronic hemolytic anemia (both inherited and acquired), congenital dyserythropoiesis type II, or hereditary erythroblast multinuclearity with positive acidified serum test (HEMPAS), and paroxysmal cold hemoglobinuria.[1]

### Laboratory Evaluation

Characteristic laboratory findings in PNH are anemia, leukopenia, and thrombocytopenia.[19] The anemia may be mild to severe, depending on the number and type of PNH erythrocytes present. Hemoglobin levels may vary from normal to less than 6 g/dl. No characteristic red blood cell morphologic abnormalities are observed in the peripheral blood; in fact, patients most commonly present with a normocytic, normochromic anemia. Slight macrocytosis and polychromasia, due to increased numbers of reticulocytes in the peripheral blood, may be seen. This reticulocytosis is a compensatory mechanism for the hemolytic process, and, although the reticulocyte count is usually elevated (5.0 percent to 10.0 percent), the absolute reticulocyte count may be low with respect to the degree of anemia present. This discrepancy is attributed to the presence of iron deficiency or to the bone marrow stem cell defect itself.[20] With associated iron deficiency, the erythrocytes appear microcytic and hypochromic. During an exacerbation of hemolysis, nucleated red blood cells may be seen in the peripheral blood smear. Spherocytes, although present in other types of hemolytic anemias, are generally not seen. Schistocytes or fragmented red blood cells are occasionally seen with acute hemolysis and may suggest intravascular thrombosis.[16]

Also commonly present in PNH erythrocytes is decreased membrane acetylcholinesterase, a finding that is most apparent in the reticulocytes.[9] The severity of the decrease in acetylcholinesterase activity parallels the severity of the disease.

Granulocytes, like the red cells, have a membrane defect that renders them more sensitive to the lytic action of complement and to antibodies.[21] When observed by light microscopy and with routine staining, however, they appear to have no characteristic morphologic abnormality. Leukopenia, primarily due to a decrease in granulocytes, is often observed, and the granulocytes have decreased leukocyte alkaline phosphatase (LAP) activity ranging from zero to low normal. The LAP score can aid in distinguishing PNH from aplastic anemia because in the latter the LAP score is normal to elevated.

Platelet counts vary in PNH. Moderate thrombocytopenia is present, with counts ranging from 50,000/mm³ to 100,000/mm³. The platelets have the same membrane defect as the erythrocytes and granulocytes. Although decreased in number, the platelets have a normal function and lifespan.

Because almost all patients have hemosiderin in their urine, testing for urinary hemosiderin will aid in confirming the diagnosis of PNH. A random urine sample is centrifuged and the sediment stained with potassium ferrocyanide (Prussian blue) for hemosiderin, turning the iron granules blue.

Hemoglobinuria, when present, must be differentiated from hematuria. This may be accomplished by performing a routine urinalysis with microscopic examination looking for the absence of intact red cells. The hemoglobinuria can lead to formation of hemoglobin casts in the renal tubules and eventually cause renal failure.

Other laboratory procedures that aid in diagnosing PNH are nonspecific test for intravascular and extravascular hemolysis, including indirect bilirubin (increased), plasma hemoglobin (increased), haptoglobin (decreased, but not very reliable), and Coombs test (negative).

As expected, the bone marrow shows erythroid hyperplasia. This is the result of increased erythropoiesis subsequent to chronic hemolysis. The increased erythropoiesis is usually normoblastic, although some megaloblastic changes may be noted. Occasionally, a hypoplastic or even aplastic marrow is seen. The bone marrow usually reveals adequate numbers of myeloid and platelet precursors, except after an aplastic episode when the myeloid and platelet precursors are decreased. Bone marrow iron stains often reveal decreased iron stores.

## Diagnostic Tests

### Sugar Water Test (Sucrose Hemolysis Test)

The sugar water test is used as a screening procedure when the diagnosis of PNH is considered. The sucrose provides a medium of low ionic strength that promotes the binding of complement, especially C3, to the red cell membrane. The low ionic strength solution used in the sugar water test activates complement via the classic or alternate pathway. The complement sensitive PNH red cells are lysed, whereas normal cells will be unaffected.

To perform the sugar water test, the patient's cells are first washed and then mixed with ABO/Rh-compatible serum and "sugar water." The tubes are incubated at room temperature for 30 minutes, after which time they are centrifuged. The percent hemolysis is then determined. Ten to 80 percent lysis is seen in PNH (see Color Figure 111). Less than 5 percent hemolysis is usually considered negative for PNH. A small amount of lysis (less than 5 percent) has been observed in patients with megaloblastic anemia, autoimmune hemolytic anemia, and leukemia. False-negative results occasionally occur if the serum lacks complement or if an unbuffered sucrose solution is used.

However, a definitive diagnosis of PNH depends on the results obtained with the Ham's test.

### Ham's Test (Acidified Serum Lysis Test)

The Ham's test, or acidified serum lysis test, is used to confirm the diagnosis of PNH. Serum is acidified, which activates complement via the alternate pathway and enhances the binding of C3 to the cell membrane. The PNH erythrocytes lyse because of their increased sensitivity to complement, whereas normal erythrocytes will be unaffected. In order to confirm a positive Ham's test result, the following characteristics must be demonstrated: (1) hemolysis occurs with the patient's cells and not with control cells, and (2) hemolysis is enhanced by acidified serum and does not occur with the heat-inactivated serum[20] (heating serum to 56°C for 30 minutes destroys complement activity) (Table 11–1; see Color Figure 112). This test is specific for PNH when it is shown that the patient's own serum is capable of lysing his or her own cells.[22]

A positive Ham's test result will be seen in the rare disorder congenital dyserythropoiesis type II, or HEMPAS. In this disorder, lysis does not occur with the patient's own serum; lysis in this case is due to an unusual red cell antigen that reacts with IgM, a complement-activating antibody, present in many normal sera.[19] The sugar water test for this disorder will also have negative results. Spherocytes also lyse in acidified serum because of the decreased pH, and they lyse in the tube containing the inactivated serum.[19]

Table 11–2 gives a summary of the laboratory tests that are most useful in confirming the diagnosis of PNH.

## THERAPY

No specific therapeutic regimen is employed in the treatment of PNH. There is also no known therapeu-

Table 11–1. ACIDIFIED SERUM TEST

|  | 1 | 2 | 3 | 4 | 5 | 6 | 7 |
|---|---|---|---|---|---|---|---|
| Fresh normal serum | 0.5 | 0.5 |  |  | 0.5 | 0.5 |  |
| Patient's serum |  |  | 0.5 |  |  |  |  |
| Heat-inactivated normal serum |  |  |  | 0.5 |  |  | 0.5 |
| 0.2 N HCL |  | 0.05 | 0.05 | 0.05 |  | 0.05 | 0.05 |
| 50% patient's red cells | 0.05 | 0.05 | 0.05 | 0.05 |  |  |  |
| 50% normal red cells |  |  |  |  | 0.05 | 0.05 | 0.05 |
| Pattern of lysis in positive test | Trace | +++ | + | − | − | − | − |

Modified from Dacie, JV and Lewis, SM: Practical Haematology, ed 4. Grune & Stratton, New York, 1968; by Nelson, D: Clinical Diagnosis and Management by Laboratory Methods, ed 17. WB Saunders, Philadelphia, 1984, p. 673.

tic agent for the erythrocyte membrane abnormality. Treatment is usually directed toward the complications that arise from infections, anemia, and thromboses. In uncomplicated mild cases, therapy is not needed.

In patients with severe iron-deficiency anemia, iron therapy is usually given, either orally or parenterally. However, patients may experience hemolytic episodes after iron therapy. Iron therapy causes an increase in the production of normal as well as abnormal erythrocytes. Oral administration of iron produces less hemolysis, but the iron loss as hemosiderin may be so great that the oral doses cannot compensate for the iron deficiency present.[23]

In the severely anemic patient, blood transfusions are required; however, stored whole blood or packed red cells may cause an exacerbation of hemolysis. This hemolysis is thought to be due to infusion of activated complement components; therefore, it is best to use washed or frozen deglycerolized red blood cells. Transfusions cause an increase in the hemoglobin level, and at the same time cause a temporary decrease in the production of the abnormal erythrocytes.

Hemolytic episodes associated with PNH may be controlled with the use of adrenocorticosteroids. Patients with any degree of bone marrow hypoplasia respond best to therapy with androgens. The androgens have a stimulatory effect on erythropoiesis and are thought to inhibit complement activation. Although androgens may be helpful, one must consider the possible side effects. Prednisone, a corticosteroid, has been used with success in suppression of hemolytic episodes. High doses have proven the most beneficial but may be associated with various side effects. However, moderate to high doses given on alternate days significantly decrease the side effects that may occur.[23]

Table 11–2. USEFUL LABORATORY METHODS FOR PNH

Complete blood cell count (CBC)
Leukocyte alkaline phosphatase (LAP)
Urinary hemosiderin
Sugar water test
Ham's test

Anticoagulant therapy is indicated in patients who are prone to the formation of venous thromboses or in whom a known life-threatening thrombosis exists. Heparin is the anticoagulant of choice in treating thromboses, but it can precipitate a hemolytic crisis. Administered in low doses, heparin can activate complement and thereby increase the probability of a hemolytic crisis.[24] Administered in high doses, however, it has been effective in the treatment of thromboses and has been shown to inactivate complement, thereby diminishing the chance of a hemolytic crisis.[24]

Certain patients with PNH have such severe bone marrow hypoplasia that a bone marrow transplant may be indicated. Transplants have been reported successful in severe cases. After the transplant the abnormal clone of cells may be eliminated and replaced by a normal cell population.

## CLINICAL COURSE AND PROGNOSIS

PNH is a chronic disease. Patients have survived 20 to 43 years after diagnosis, although the average survival is 10 years.[19] The most common cause of death is thromboembolism. Patients with bone marrow hypoplasia often die from infections or hemorrhage.[16] In a minority of patients, the disease may decrease in severity or completely disappear with time. Some patients have complete clinical remissions with persisting laboratory abnormalities. Rarely, acute myelogenous leukemia develops in patients with PNH.[25,26] When PNH in these patients transforms to acute leukemia, the abnormal complement-sensitive population of erythrocytes disappears.[19] PNH has also been classified as a preleukemic or myelodysplastic syndrome.[27]

## ROLE OF COMPLEMENT

Complement is a group of serum proteins that interact with each other to bring about, among other events, complement-dependent cell-mediated lysis. Complement can be activated by two different routes, the classic or the alternate (properdin) pathway.

## Classic Pathway

Activation of the classic pathway is initiated by immune complexes containing IgG ($IgG_1$, $IgG_2$, $IgG_3$) or IgM. The first complement component, C1, consists of three subunits, C1q, C1r, and C1s, as well as calcium (recognition unit). C1q initiates the complement cascade by interacting with the Fc (antibody fragment) portion of the immunoglobulin. C1q then causes the activation of $\overline{C1r}$, which then activates $\overline{C1s}$. (A bar across the top of a complement component denotes its active form.) C4 is the second complement protein to be activated. This occurs when C1s cleaves C4 into its activated components, $\overline{C4a}$, which remains in the plasma, and $\overline{C4b}$, a small portion of which attaches to the cell membrane with the rest remaining in the plasma, inactivated. C2 attaches to $\overline{C4b}$ in the presence of magnesium and is then cleaved by $\overline{C1s}$ into a and b subunits. $\overline{C2a}$ remains attached to $\overline{C4b}$ and forms the enzyme C3 convertase ($\overline{C4b2a}$), and $\overline{C2b}$ is released into the plasma.

Amplification of complement activity occurs now with the action of C3 convertase on C3. This enzyme ($\overline{C4b2a}$) cleaves C3 into its active components, $\overline{C3a}$ and $\overline{C3b}$, and is able to cleave hundreds of C3 molecules. $\overline{C3a}$ is released into the plasma and acts as an anaphylatoxin. $\overline{C3b}$ binds to the cell membrane and combines with $\overline{C4b2a}$ to form another enzyme, C5 convertase ($\overline{C4b2a3b}$). Some of the C3b molecules attach to other sites on the cell, are inactivated (C3bi), or are cleaved by C3 inactivator to C3c, which is released into the plasma, and to C3d, an inactive subunit that remains attached to the cell. The components C4, C3, and C2 are referred to as the "enzyme activation unit."

C5 convertase ($\overline{C4b2a3b}$) cleaves C5 into the components $\overline{C5a}$, which is released into the plasma and acts as an anaphylatoxin and a chemotactic agent, and $\overline{C5b}$, which binds C6 and C7 to the cell membrane. Membrane-bound $\overline{C5b67}$ causes binding of C8, resulting in immediate ion flux into the cell. The $\overline{C5b678}$ complex can bind up to six C9 molecules, together forming the membrane attack unit,

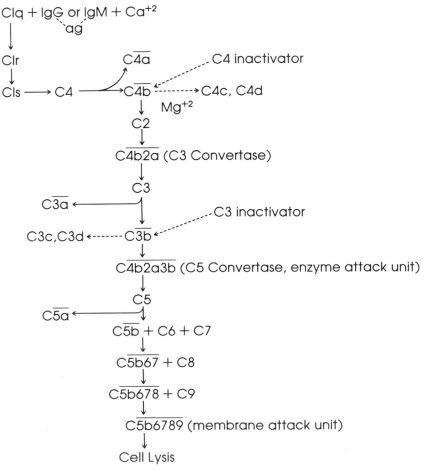

**Figure 11–2.** Classic pathway of complement activation.

C5b6789, which causes cell lysis and accelerated movement of ions into the cell. With binding of C9, cell lysis results (Fig. 11-2).

Complement activity is regulated by certain inhibitors (C1s inhibitor, C3b inactivator, C4 inactivator) and by the instability of certain components ($C\overline{4b2a}$, $C\overline{4b2a3b}$).[28]

## Alternate (Properdin) Pathway

The alternate, or properdin, pathway of complement activation also results in cell lysis but by a different mechanism and group of proteins. The alternate pathway bypasses the complement components C1, C2, and C4 and enters at C3. This pathway consists of a distinct group of proteins: factor A (complement component C3); factor B (C3 proactivator), which is enzymatically cleaved into fragments Bb (biologically active) and Ba; factor D (C3 proactivator convertase), which cleaves factor B; properdin (P), a serum protein that stabilizes the $C\overline{3bBb}$ complex; and beta-1H (C3b inactivator accelerator), which aids in controlling activation of the alternate pathway.[29]

The alternate pathway may be triggered by certain microorganisms, polysaccharides, liposaccharides, aggregates of IgA, and cells or particles even in the absence of specific antibody. Present in the plasma are small amounts of a "priming" C3 convertase ($C\overline{3Bb}$). The "priming" C3 convertase is produced continuously owing to spontaneous interaction of intact C3, factor B, factor D, and properdin, an event not requiring activating substances. This results in the formation of small amounts of $C\overline{3b}$. $C\overline{3b}$ binds to the cell surface and under appropriate conditions and in the presence of magnesium causes the attachment of factor B. The bound factor B is cleaved by factor D, releasing the Ba fragment and uncovering the C3 cleaving site on the Bb fragment. The $C\overline{3bBb}$ complex can rapidly lose activity or dissociate unless properdin is present. Properdin binds to the $C\overline{3b}$ part of the complex and stabilizes it. The $C\overline{3bBb}$ fragment (C3 convertase) then cleaves more C3, resulting in $C\overline{3a}$ and $C\overline{3b}$ fragments. A complex of $C\overline{3bBbPC3b}$ (C5 convertase) forms and cleaves C5 into its fragments, $C\overline{5a}$ and $C\overline{5b}$. C5b along with C6, C7, C8, and C9 forms the membrane attack unit, the same way as in the classic pathway, which causes cell lysis (Fig. 11-3).

Control mechanisms also exist in the alternate pathway, just as they do in the classic pathway. Spontaneous dissolution of $C\overline{3bBb}$ may occur, beta-1H protein may compete with factor B, as may Bb for the C3b fragment, then blocking the formation of C3 convertase ($C\overline{3bBb}$). Beta-1H may increase the susceptibility of $C\overline{3b}$ to be destroyed by C3b inactivator.[29]

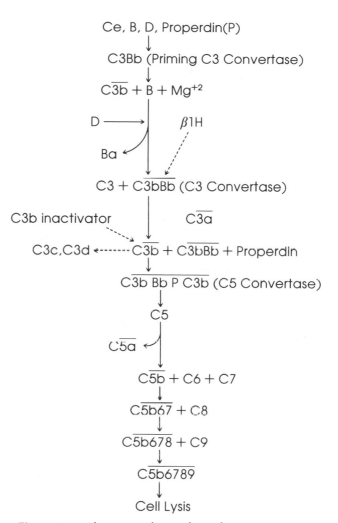

**Figure 11–3.** Alternate pathway of complement activation.

## CASE HISTORY

A 43-year-old male presented to his physician with complaints of lower back pain, fatigue, easy bruising, and a sudden onset of dark urine upon arising in the morning. Laboratory studies and a bone marrow aspirate were then ordered by his physician, which disclosed the following:

A. CBC:

| | |
|---|---|
| HCT | 28% |
| WBC | 3300/mm³ |
| Platelet Count | 76,000/mm³ |
| Retic | 5.1% |
| Corrected Retic | 3.2% |

Differential:

| | |
|---|---|
| Segmented neutrophils | 34% |
| Lymphocytes | 64% |
| Monocytes | 2% |
| 1   Nucleated red cell (NRBC) | |

Red Cell Morphology:
1+ Poikilocytosis
2+ Anisocytosis
1+ Polychromasia

**Color Figure 113** shows the peripheral blood smear from this patient.

 B. Chemistries were normal except for an increased lactic dehydrogenase (LDH) (780 IU/l) and bilirubin (total 2.9 mg/dl, direct 0.4 mg/dl).

 C. A urinalysis was performed and was positive for hemoglobin.

 D. The bone marrow aspirate revealed a hypocellular marrow with relative erythroid hyperplasia. There were adequate numbers of myeloid and platelet precursors **(see Color Figure 114)**.

Further studies were then performed after initial tests were finished.

 E. Urinary hemosiderin: Positive

 F. Sugar water test: Positive (12%)

 G. Ham's test: Positive

Diagnosis: Paroxysmal nocturnal hemoglobinuria

## References

1. Williams, WJ, Buetler, E, Erslev, AJ, et al: Hematology, ed 2. McGraw-Hill, 1977, p 560.
2. Gull, WP: A case of intermittent hematuria, with remarks. Guys Hospital Reports 12;381, 1866.
3. Strübing, P: Paroxysmale Hämoglobinurie. Dtsch Med Wschr 8:1, 1882.
4. Marchiafava, E: Anemia emolitica con emosiderinuria perpitua. Policlinico (sez med) 18:241, 1931.
5. Micheli, F: Anemia (splenomegalia) emolitica con emoglobinuria-emosiderinuria tipo Marchiafava. Hematologica 12:101-123, 1931.
6. Hijmas van den Bergh AA: Ictère hémolytique avec crises hemoglubinuriques. Fragilité globulaire Rev Med 31:63, 1911.
7. Ham, TH and Dingle, JH: Studies on destruction of red blood cells-II. Chronic hemolytic anemia with paroxysmal nocturnal hemoglobinuria — Certain immunological aspects of the hemolytic mechanism with special reference to serum complement. J Clin Invest 18:657, 1939.
8. Ham, TH: Chronic hemolytic anemia with paroxysmal nocturnal hemoglobinuria — A study of the mechanism of hemolysis in relation to acid base equilibrium. N Engl J Med 217:915, 1937.
9. Beck, WS: Hematology, ed 3. Massachusetts Institute of Technology Press, Cambridge, MA, 1982, p 211.
10. Mengal, CE, Kann HE, Meriwether WD, et al: Studies of Paroxysmal Nocturnal Hemoglobinuria erythrocytes: increased lysis and lipid peroxide formation by hydrogen peroxide. J Clin Invest 46:1715, 1967.
11. Lewis, SM, Lambertenghi G, Ferrone S, et al: Electron microscope study of PNH red cells and AET-treated normal cells (PNH-like cells). J Clin Pathol 24:677, 1971.
12. Mengal, CE, Ebbert L, Stickney D, et al: Biochemistry of PNH cells; nature of the membrane defect. Ser Haematol 5:88, 1972.
13. Metz, J, Bradow BA, Lewis SM, et al: Acetylcholinesterase activity of the erythrocytes in paroxysmal nocturnal hemoglobinuria in relation to the severity of the disease. Br J Haematol 6;372, 1960.
14. Rosse, WF and Adams, JP: The membrane abnormalities in paroxysmal nocturnal hemoglobinuria. Prog Clin Biol Res 30;457, 1979.
15. Dacie, JV: Paroxysmal nocturnal hemoglobinuria. Sangre 25:890, 1980.
16. Wintrobe, ME, Lee GR, Boggs DR, et al: Clinical Hematology, ed 8. Lea & Febiger, Philadelphia, 1981, 312, 978.
17. Rosse, WF: Paroxysmal nocturnal hemoglobinuria in aplastic anemia. Clin Haematol 7;3:541, 1978.
18. Sun, NC: Hematology — An Atlas and Diagnostic Guide, ed 1. WB Saunders, Philadelphia, 1983, p 90.
19. Dacie, JV and Lewis, SM: Paroxysmal nocturnal hemoglobinuria, clinical manifestations, hematology and nature of the disease. Ser Haematol 5:3, 1972.
20. Maslow, WC, Buetler, E, Bell, C, et al: Hematologic Diseaase, Practical Diagnosis, ed 1. Houghton-Mifflin, Boston, 1980, p 154.
21. Aster, RH and Enright, SE: A platelet and granulocyte membrane defect in paroxysmal nocturnal hemoglobinuria, usefulness for the detection of platelet antibodies. J Clin Invest 48:1199, 1969.
22. Hoffbrand, AV and Lewis, SM: Post Graduate Hematology, ed 2. Appleton-Century-Crofts, New York, 1981, p 232.
23. Rosse, WF: Treatment of paroxysmal nocturnal hemoglobinuria. Blood 60(1):20, 1982.
24. Logue, GL: Effects of heparin on complement activation and lysis of paroxysmal nocturnal hemoglobinuria red cells. Blood 50(20):239, 1977.
25. Cowell, DE, Pasquale, DN, and Dekker, P: Paroxysmal nocturnal hemoglobinuria terminating as acute leukemia. Cancer 43:1914, 1979.
26. Krause, JR: Paroxysmal nocturnal hemoglobinuria and acute non-lymphoblastic leukemia. Cancer 51:2078, 1983.
27. Rosse, WF: Paroxysmal nocturnal hemoglobinuria — present status and future prospects. West J Med 132(3):219, 1980.
28. Muller-Eberhard, HJ: Complement. Ann Rev Biochem 44:697, 1975.
29. Fearson, DT and Austen, KF: The alternate pathway of complement — a system of host resistance to microbial infections. N Engl J Med 303:259, 1980.

## Bibliography

Dacie, JV and Lewis, SM: Paroxysmal nocturnal hemoglobinuria, clinical manifestations, hematology and nature of the disease. Ser Haematol 5:3, 1972.

Forman, K, Sokol, RJ, Hewitt, et al: Paroxysmal nocturnal hemoglobinuria — a clinicopathological study of 26 cases. Acta Haematol 71:217, 1984.

Goetz, O and Muller-Eberhardt, HJ: The alternate pathway of complement activation Adv Immunol 24:1, 1976.

Hartman, RC and Jenkins, DE, Jr: The "sugar water" test for paroxysmal nocturnal hemoglobinuria. N Engl J Med 275:155, 1966.

Hartman, RC, Jenkins, DE, Jr, and Arnold, AB: Diagnostic specificity of sucrose hemolysis test for paroxysmal nocturnal hemoglobinuria. Blood 35:462, 1970.

Muller-Eberhard, HJ: Complement. Ann Rev Biochem 44:697, 1975.

Rosse, WF: Paroxysmal nocturnal hemoglobinuria — present status and future prospects. West J Med 132(3):219, 1980.

# CHAPTER 12

D. HARMENING PITTIGLIO, Ph.D., M.T.(ASCP) AND
RALPH L.B. GREEN, B.App.Sci. (MLS), F.A.I.M.L.S.

# Hemolytic Anemias: Extracorpuscular Defects

## I. Immune Hemolytic Anemia

ALLOIMMUNE HEMOLYTIC ANEMIA
Transfusion Reactions
Hemolytic Disease of the Newborn (HDN)
    ABO HDN
    Rh HDN
Treatment
Prophylaxis
AUTOIMMUNE HEMOLYTIC ANEMIA (AIHA)
Warm Auto Immune Hemolytic Anemia (WAIHA)
    RED CELL HEMOLYSIS
    SEROLOGIC EVALUATION
    AUTOANTIBODY SPECIFICITY
    TREATMENT
        Corticosteroid Administration
        Splenectomy
        Immunosuppressive Drugs
Cold Autoimmune Hemolytic Anemia (Cold AIHA)
    NORMAL COLD AUTOANTIBODIES
    PATHOLOGIC COLD AUTOANTIBODIES
        Cold Agglutinin Syndrome (Idiopathic Cold
            AIHA)
        Secondary Cold AIHA (Cold Autoantibodies
            Related to Infection)
        Paroxysmal Cold Hemoglobinuria (PCH)
DRUG-INDUCED IMMUNE HEMOLYTIC ANEMIA
    IMMUNE COMPLEX MECHANISM
    DRUG ADSORPTION (HAPTEN) MECHANISM
    MEMBRANE MODIFICATION MECHANISM
        (NONIMMUNOLOGIC PROTEIN ADSORPTION)
    METHYLDOPA-INDUCED MECHANISM (UNKNOWN
        MECHANISM)
Treatment

Immune hemolytic anemia is defined as a shortened red cell survival mediated through the immune response, specifically by humoral antibody.

Immune-mediated hemolysis represents the results of an acquired extracorpuscular abnormality associated with demonstrable antibodies, as opposed to the inherited intracorpuscular defects described in Chapters 7 through 11, which represent intrinsic abnormalities of the patient's red cells.

Numerous classifications of immune hemolytic anemias have been proposed; however, three broad categories are generally used:

1. Alloimmune
2. Autoimmune
3. Drug-Induced

In an alloimmune response, patients produce alloantibodies to foreign red cell antigens introduced into their circulation either through transfusion or pregnancy. An autoimmune response occurs when patients produce autoantibodies directed against their own red cell antigens. A drug-induced immune hemolytic anemia is the result of a patient's production of antibodies to a particular drug or drug complex, with subsequent damage to the patient's red cells.

## ALLOIMMUNE HEMOLYTIC ANEMIA

Alloimmunization is the process in which the immune system of an individual is stimulated by a foreign antigen with production of the corresponding antibody. The antibody produced by this immune response is termed an "alloantibody." The antibody coats the foreign red cells introduced into the circulation, resulting in hemolysis. Alloantibody, or alloimmune, hemolytic anemia, is produced through two processes: (1) transfusion reactions (exposure to foreign donor red cell antigens) or (2) pregnancy (foreign antigens on fetal cells released into the mother's circulation).

## Transfusion Reactions

Hemolytic transfusion reactions may be classified as immediate (acute) or delayed.

**Immediate hemolytic transfusion reactions** are characterized by acute intravascular hemolysis and are most commonly associated with ABO IgM isoantibodies, which activate complement.

Clinical features of an immediate transfusion reaction may be associated with a variety of signs and symptoms. Typical symptoms are fever, shaking, chills, pain at the infusion site, nausea, vomiting, lower back pain, hypotension, and chest pain (Table 12–1). In an anesthetized patient, the reaction may manifest itself as disseminated intravascular coagulation (DIC) with generalized bleeding and shock. This type of transfusion reaction is termed "immediate" or "acute," because its manifestations occur within minutes to hours.

The process of hemolysis is initiated by the binding of the patient's alloantibody to the donor's (foreign) corresponding red cell antigen, which activates the complement cascade to completion, causing intravascular lysis of the transfused erythrocytes. (For a review of the process of intravascular hemolysis and the complement cascade, see Chapters 2 and 11.) The immediate type of transfusion reaction is most commonly associated with ABO incompatibilities. These reactions are severe because potent naturally occurring IgM anti-A or anti-B are circulating in the patient's plasma at the time of transfusion.

The majority of other circulating blood group antibodies destroy foreign red cell antigens through extravascular hemolysis, since complement activation is only partial or is absent. However, in rare circumstances, some IgG antibodies can bind complement and induce intravascular hemolysis. The most common offender is anti-Jk[a] (Kidd blood group system).

**Table 12–1. CLINICAL FEATURES OF ACUTE HEMOLYTIC TRANSFUSION REACTION**

| | |
|---|---|
| Fever | Hemoglobinuria |
| Chills | Shock |
| Chest pains | Generalized bleeding |
| Hypotension | Oliguria |
| Nausea | Anuria |
| Flushing | Back pain |
| Dyspnea | Pain at infusion site |

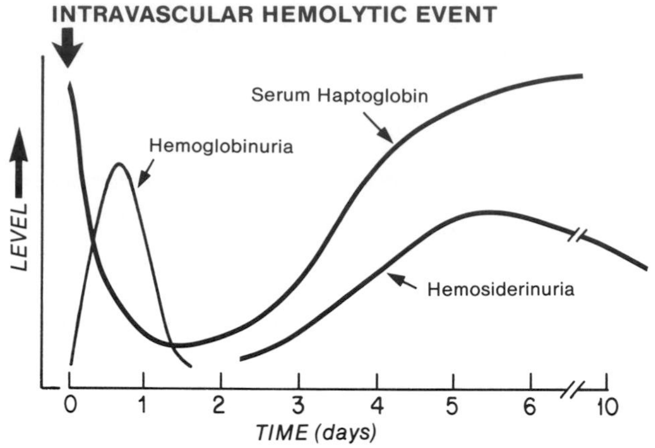

**INTRAVASCULAR HEMOLYTIC EVENT**

**Figure 12-1.** Indicators of acute intravascular hemolysis. Within a few hours of an acute hemolytic event, free hemoglobin is cleared from plasma and the serum haptoglobin falls to undetectable levels. Hemoglobinuria ceases soon after this. If no further hemolysis occurs, the serum haptoglobin level recovers, and methemalbumin disappears within several days. The urinary hemosiderin can provide more lasting evidence of the hemolytic event.

Laboratory findings include signs of a hemolytic process. Figure 12–1 charts the sequence of events that occur as a result of an intravascular hemolytic episode. Within hours plasma haptoglobin is depleted, since as little as 5 ml of lysed red cells can bind all the haptoglobin available. It is important to have a pretransfusion baseline level of haptoglobin available for comparison to the post-transfusion level, since many factors affect the synthesis of haptoglobin and could result in misinterpretation of results. Within 24 hours, the liver will synthesize new haptoglobin, replenishing the levels.

Other laboratory findings include the presence of free plasma hemoglobin resulting in hemoglobinemia. The free hemoglobin is filtered through the kidneys, resulting in hemoglobinuria and hemosiderinuria. Hemoglobinuria may be confused with hematuria, especially when the urine is bright red. The urine in hemoglobinuria is clear, whereas in hematuria it is smokey. The urinary sediment will usually distinguish the two quite readily, since intact red cells will be found in hematuria, provided that the osmolality is not too low. Hemoglobinuria is always accompanied by hemoglobinemia.

Other abnormal laboratory findings include elevated bilirubin (primarily indirect). Table 12–2 summarizes the laboratory findings of an acute, or immediate, hemolytic transfusion reaction. (For a review of the process of intravascular hemolysis and the laboratory parameters used to monitor the severity of the hemolysis, see Chapter 2.)

Treatment of an immediate hemolytic transfusion reaction focuses on prompt termination of the transfusion. Therapy is then directed toward maintaining diuresis, management of coagulopathy, promoting adequate renal blood flow, and treatment of hypotension.

Table 12–2. LABORATORY FINDINGS IN AN
IMMEDIATE (ACUTE) HEMOLYTIC TRANSFUSION
REACTION

1. Decrease in haptoglobin
2. Hemoglobinemia
3. Increase in lactic dehydrogenase (LDH)
4. Hemoglobinuria
5. Bilirubinemia (primarily indirect)
6. Methemalbuminemia (dependent on the severity of
   hemolysis)
7. Hemosiderinuria

The most common type of **delayed hemolytic transfusion reaction (DHTR)** results from an anamnestic or secondary response to transfused red cell antigens. This occurs in previously sensitized patients whose alloantibody level has dropped to the point of being undetectable, after initial stimulation. As a result, the initial antibody screen performed on the patient's pretransfusion serum sample is negative. In most cases of DHTR, the antibodies implicated in the reactions are IgG immunoglobulins and are usually demonstrable in the patient's serum as early as 48 hours after transfusion, reaching a peak level within six days. This type of reaction is termed "delayed," because it takes time for the patient to produce increasing levels of IgG antibodies that attack and destroy the transfused red cells.

As with most hemolytic anemias, the erythrocyte destruction is primarily extravascular, occurring within the cells of the reticuloendothelial system. As a result, spherocytes may be characteristically seen on the peripheral smear. (For a review of the process of extravascular hemolysis, see Chapter 2.)

Hemoglobinemia and hemoglobinuria are not present as described in immediate hemolytic transfusion reactions. However, there are increases both in serum bilirubin (primarily indirect) and in urobilinogen in the urine and stools. Usually, antibodies can be found in the patient's serum (positive antibody screen) and coating the circulatory transfused cells (positive direct antiglobulin test).

Symptoms of a DHTR include fever, an unexpected fall in hemoglobin, mild jaundice, and anemia.

Treatment is rarely necessary, and investigation focuses on accurately identifying the antibody to ensure that blood in future transfusions will be antigen negative for the patient's corresponding antibody. Table 12–3 lists the antibodies most commonly implicated in DHTR.

## Hemolytic Disease of the Newborn (HDN)

HDN is a immune hemolytic disorder in which red cells of the fetus and newborn are destroyed by maternal IgG antibody. Generally, maternal antibodies provide the fetus with immune protection, since the fetus is incapable of adequate immunoglobulin synthesis. This transport mechanism is selective in that only IgG antibodies can cross the placenta. When a mother is sensitized, either through a previous pregnancy or through transfusion, all maternal IgG antibodies (including the IgG blood group–specific antibodies) cross the placenta. If this antibody is specific for any antigen on the fetal red cells, destruction of these fetal red cells occurs, resulting in anemia. The term "erythroblastosis fetalis" is a synonym for HDN and describes the marked erythroblastic response to the immune hemolytic anemia present in the fetus.

The mother usually becomes immunized to foreign fetal red cell antigens during larger fetal-maternal bleeds that occur at the time of delivery. During the last half of pregnancy, small amounts of fetal red cells regularly enter maternal circulation. However, this is rarely sufficient to induce sensitization. Even though the average bleed at the time of delivery is less than 1 ml of whole blood, it is estimated that at least 0.5 ml of fetal blood is necessary to promote alloimmunization.

Fetal red cells coated with maternal antibody are removed from circulation by extravascular hemolysis. Responding to this increased red cell destruction, fetal hematopoietic tissue increases erythrocyte production, which results in liver and splenic enlargement. However, the fetus may not be able to compensate, and an anemia characterized by increased numbers of erythroblasts present during fetal development will then result. Hence, "erythroblastosis fetalis" has been traditionally used to describe HDN. The spectrum of clinical features ranges from mild anemia, jaundice, and hepatosplenomegaly to severe congestive cardiac failure with edema ("hydrops fetalis").

The characteristic jaundice is a result of high levels of unconjugated bilirubin that have accumulated owing to increased red cell destruction. In utero, increased bilirubin crosses the placenta where the maternal liver conjugates and excretes it, since the fetal liver is not developed enough to handle this process. After birth, however, this maternal

Table 12–3. ANTIBODIES MOST COMMONLY
IMPLICATED IN DHTR

| Antibody | Blood Group System |
|---|---|
| Anti-Jk$^a$ | Kidd |
| Anti-K | Kell |
| Anti-c̄ | Rh |
| Anti-E | Rh |
| Anti-Fy$^a$ | Duffy |
| Anti-Jk$^b$ | Kidd |
| Anti-C | Rh |
| Anti-e | Rh |

mechanism is no longer available and there is a buildup of the unconjugated bilirubin in the newborn. Since unconjugated bilirubin has a predilection for lipid tissue, a major potential consequence is the deposition of this bilirubin in the brain of the newborn with the development of a condition known as "kernicterus." This disorder occurs only in the newborn infant, since the enzyme, glucuronyl transferase, which is necessary to conjugate bilirubin, is poorly developed at that time.

Table 12-4 summarizes the clinical features characteristic of HDN.

By far, the majority of the cases of HDN are caused by ABO and Rh incompatibility. HDN due to ABO incompatibility is the more common form and is also generally much milder in severity than Rh hemolytic disease. The once-common Rh HDN is now a "dying disease," because the routine prophylactic use of Rh immune globulin (RhIg) has markedly decreased its incidence. However, cases are still reported occasionally even today, and these represent relatively severe forms of the disease. Table 12-5 lists the frequency of the various types of HDN.

Laboratory findings in patients with HDN include anemia, may be mild (Hb = 13 g%) to severe (Hb = 8 g%) (normal hemoglobin for newborns is 14 to 20 g%); reticulocytosis; leukocytosis; numerous spherocytes (in ABO HDN); and nucleated red cells on the peripheral smear.

As mentioned previously, bilirubinemia is present, and the direct antiglobulin test result is usually positive.

## ABO HDN

ABO incompatibility, the most common form of HDN, rarely produces a clinical disease. The major clinical manifestation that occurs in approximately 10 to 20 percent of ABO-incompatible pregnancies is jaundice. This usually appears in the first 24 hours of life and is much milder than Rh HDN. Anemia is uncommon, and ABO HDN rarely causes stillbirths. Spherocytosis, however, is usually present on the peripheral smear. A group O mother delivering a group A or B infant is usually responsible for the disorder, since O blood groups contain a significant amount of "naturally occurring" IgG isoantibodies as well as IgM. Therefore, ABO HDN characteristically can occur in the first-born child, as well as in subsequent pregnancies. Antenatal examination of the maternal serum is, however, un-

**Table 12-5. FREQUENCY OF TYPES OF HDN**

| | |
|---|---|
| ABO HDN | 65% |
| Rh HDN | 33% |
| Other | 2% |

necessary in almost all cases, since the serologic findings do not accurately predict or correlate with the incidence of ABO HDN. The direct Coombs test on cord blood is generally weakly positive, but the results can vary from negative to moderately positive, because they reflect whether antibody-coated cells have been lysed and destroyed or are still circulating. The offending maternal anti-A,B IgG is easily identified in the infant's serum and in eluates of the infant's red cells by indirect antiglobulin testing. Table 12-6 summarizes the main differences between ABO and Rh HDN.

## Rh HDN

This disease occurs from primary sensitization of an Rh-negative mother with Rh-positive blood either by a previous pregnancy, blood transfusion, or abortion. The subsequent pregnancy of the Rh-negative mother carrying an Rh-positive fetus after initial sensitization results in HDN due to Rh incompatibility. Clinical manifestations include jaundice (appearing within four or five hours of birth), anemia, and hepatosplenomegaly. Hematologic laboratory results reflect the severity of the disease demonstrating decreased hemoglobin, increased reticulocyte count, and increased numbers of nucleated red cells in the peripheral smear. The previous discussion of "erythroblastosis fetalis" is characteristic of Rh HDN. Serologic findings include a positive antibody screen and the identification of anti-D or other Rh antibodies in the serum of an Rh-negative mother, and a positive direct Coombs test result on the Rh-positive cells of the infant. Antenatal diagnosis is very important in Rh HDN and should be performed. Additionally, hemoglobin levels should be followed in a successfully delivered infant during the first month because of the risk of severe anemia developing during this time. Stillbirths and hydrops fetalis (previously described) are still major problems in Rh HDN. It is interesting to note that ABO incompatibility between mother and infant is protective for Rh HDN, because the fetal cells entering the mother's circulation will be destroyed by naturally occurring isoagglutinins preventing Rh sensitization. (For comparison of Rh and ABO HDN, see Table 12-6.)

## Treatment

Treatment of HDN depends on the severity of the hemolysis and usually involves one of the following forms of therapy:

**Table 12-4. MAJOR CLINICAL FEATURES OF HDN**

1. Anemia (erythroblastosis fetalis)
2. Jaundice (icterus gravis)
3. Severe edema (hydrops fetalis)
4. Hepatosplenomegaly

## Table 12-6. COMPARISON OF ABO AND Rh HDN

|  | ABO | Rh |
|---|---|---|
| Severity | Mild | Severe |
| Child affected | First-born (40–50% of cases) | Usually second or subsequent births (first-born: 5% of cases) |
| Blood groups | Mother: O<br>Child: A or B | Mother: Rh negative<br>Child: Rh positive |
| Anemia | Uncommon/mild | Severe |
| Stillbirths/hydrops fetalis | Rare | Frequent |
| Jaundice | Mild | Severe |
| Spherocytes on peripheral smear | Usually present | None |
| Direct Coombs test result | Negative or weakly positive | Positive |
| Maternal antibodies | Inconsistent/inconclusive | Always present |
| Antenatal diagnosis | Unnecessary | Necessary |
| Treatment (dependent on severity) | Phototherapy (common)<br>Exchange transfusion (rare) | Exchange transfusion (common newborn treatment)<br>Intrauterine (common antenatal treatment) |
| Types of antibody | IgG (immune) | IgG (immune) |
| Prophylaxis | None | RhIG<br>Antenatal RhIG |

1. Intrauterine transfusion ⎫ Antenatal
2. Maternal plasmapheresis ⎭ treatment
3. Exchange transfusion ⎫ Treatment of
4. Phototherapy ⎭ newborn

An intrauterine transfusion may be performed when there is a threat of stillbirth or hydrops fetalis, before the baby is mature enough for inducing labor. The antenatal antibody screening of the mother's serum will help determine the severity of the disease, the need for aggressive monitoring, and a management strategy for the clinician. If Rh anti-D antibodies are demonstrated in an Rh-negative mother, then Rh HDN will occur if the fetus is Rh positive. The degree of alloimmunization should be determined by an antibody titer in the presence of a positive antibody screen.

Using serial dilutions of the mother's serum, the strength of the antibody (titer) can be determined with corresponding D-positive cells. The value of the titer represents the lowest dilution with which the serum will react with the positive cells used. A titer of 1:2 reactivity represents very mild sensitization, whereas a titer of 1:512 reactivity represents severe immunization. It is important to note that following a secondary immune response, as a result of a subsequent pregnancy and continued transplacental hemorrhage immunizing the mother, the titer may be initially low and then increase to higher levels with a significant risk of fetal death. Therefore, repeated serial titers (every two to three weeks) are particularly helpful in terms of the management of Rh HDN in the immunized Rh-negative mothers.

If the titer remains below a determined critical level, then delivery can be performed at 38 weeks' gestation with a neonatal team present and blood available for an exchange transfusion. The critical titer is determined by each institution and represents the maximum value at which there have been no stillbirths or severely affected infants. If the antibody titer reaches or exceeds the critical level, then amniocentesis and amniotic fluid analyses are performed to determine fetal condition. The practical spectrophotometric method of measuring amniotic fluid bilirubin developed by Liley provides a useful severity grading based on the gestational age and the relationship of amniotic fluid bilirubin levels. If intervention treatment is necessary and the fetus is too premature to deliver, then intrauterine transfusion remains the current therapy of choice. This procedure involves localization of the fetal peritoneal cavity with ultrasound waves and the injection of group O Rh-negative irradiated packed red cells into the fetal peritoneal cavity. The volumes used are determined according to the gestational age, and approximately 80 percent of the transfused red cells are eventually absorbed via lymphatic channels into fetal circulation. Once the transfusions are started, they should be repeated every 10 to 21 days until the infant is viable. The blood is routinely irradiated in this procedure to prevent the possible complication of graft-versus-host disease (GVHD).

Experimental maternal plasma exchange has been used in conjunction with this procedure. The objective of plasmapheresis in Rh HDN is the removal of the large quantities of circulating anti-D antibody in an attempt to reduce the amount of fetal red cell destruction. Plasma exchange is usually automated involving the use of cell-separating instruments and the routine removal of 2 to 3 liters of plasma, which is replaced with an albumin or plasma solution. The efficiency of this procedure has not yet been proven with any degree of certainty, and the reported clinical trials have not been controlled. Furthermore, the procedure does not reduce the level of anti-D in the majority of cases, its overall value in preventing severe Rh HDN and fetal death has not been proven, and it is very expensive.

Exchange transfusion is the treatment of choice in affected infants requiring more than a single transfusion for correction of the anemia that is usually characteristic of Rh HDN. Serum bilirubin levels are generally used as the criteria for determining whether an exchange transfusion is necessary. Values vary, but bilirubin levels of greater than 12 to 15 mg% suggest the need for an exchange transfusion. However, the infant's entire clinical status must be considered before such a decision is made. An exchange transfusion attempts to accomplish four main objectives:

1. Remove antibody-coated fetal cells, reducing hemolysis
2. Lower bilirubin levels
3. Correct anemia by providing compatible red cells with adequate oxygen-carrying capacity
4. Decrease amount of circulating incompatible antibody

One major goal of exchange transfusion in Rh HDN is removal of bilirubin, not only in the initial exchange but also in subsequent exchanges. In Rh HDN, the blood selected for exchange transfusion should be Rh negative, ABO group–specific if the ABO group of the infant and mother are the same. If different ABO groups exist between the mother and infant, then group O blood should be used. For the first exchange transfusion, the selected blood is crossmatched against the mother's serum. Blood selected for subsequent exchange transfusions should be crossmatched with the mother's and infant's post–exchange transfusion serum.

Treatment of patients with ABO HDN with phototherapy is usually sufficient, because the anemia in these patients is usually mild. If there is a need for exchange transfusion, which is rare, group O blood of the same Rh type as the infant's blood should be used, and this should be crossmatched with the mother's serum prior to transfusion.

## Prophylaxis

Prevention of Rh HDN may be accomplished through the use of Rh immune globulin (RhIg), which is a passive form of anti-D given within 72 hours of delivery to all Rh-negative mothers delivering a Rh-positive fetus. Postpartum testing to detect fetal-maternal hemorrhage (FMH) should be performed in all Rh-negative women at risk to determine if more than a single dose of RhIg is necessary. The Kleihauer-Betke acid elution procedure (Table 12–7) is the most commonly used method for quantitating FMH. Using this stain, HbF is resistant to acid elution and stains red with eosin dyes, whereas HbA is eluted with acid and the red cells appear as colorless ghosts with the Kleihauer-Betke staining procedure **(see Color Figure 244)**. If the FMH is greater than 30 ml of whole blood, then one dose of RhIg will not be sufficient to prevent alloimmunization.

Antenatal prophylactic administration of RhIg is currently being routinely administered at 28 weeks' gestation (300 $\mu$g) to Rh-negative nonimmunized women to protect against FMH occurring during the third trimester. This type of prophylaxis eliminates the low failure rate of alloimmunization prevention that occurs when RhIg is administered only post-delivery. Serologically, at the time of delivery, the mother receiving this antenatal prophylactic dose of RhIg may demonstrate a positive antibody screen, owing to detectable levels of the passive anti-D in her serum. The weakly reacting passive anti-D may also cause a microscopically positive direct Coombs test result in a Rh-positive newborn. Accurate records from the obstetrician and laboratory facilitates the blood bank's role in ascertaining whether the antibody was passively acquired or represents active alloimmunization. This confusion must be resolved, as postpartum RhIg must also be given to these women following delivery. If the cause of the maternal anti-D is still in doubt in an Rh-negative mother who has received antenatal doses, it must be

---

**Table 12–7. KLEIHAUER-BETKE PROCEDURE**

1. Peripheral blood slides are made from a 1:1 dilution with saline of EDTA blood.
2. After 10 sec of air drying, slides are fixed with 80% ethyl alcohol.
3. Citric acid buffer for 10 sec.
4. Counterstain with erythrocin for 3 sec, rinse, and dry.
5. $\dfrac{\text{Stained cells}}{\text{Unstained cells}} \times$ Adjusted maternal red cell volume (2400) = FMH.

assumed that it is a result of passive transfer, and the woman is still considered a candidate for RhIg at the time of delivery.

## AUTOIMMUNE HEMOLYTIC ANEMIA (AIHA)

AIHA represents an abnormality within the immune system whereby the ability for self-recognition of an individual's own red cell antigens is lost. As a result, patients destroy their own red cells by producing autoantibodies, which bind to the patients' erythrocytes, inducing hemolysis. The majority of cases of AIHA can be divided into warm and cold types. The warm type (WAIHA) is the most common, representing approximately 70 percent of the cases of autoimmune hemolytic anemia. The term "warm" is used to define autoantibodies whose serologic reactivity is optimal at 37°C. "Cold" AIHA defines autoantibodies whose optimal serologic reactivity occurs at 4°C but which also react at between 25 and 31°C. Two types of cold AIHA have been described: (1) cold agglutinin syndrome and (2) paroxysmal cold hemoglobinuria (PCH).

Drug-induced immune hemolytic anemia, which is sometimes difficult to distinguish from other cases of WAIHA, is the third type of AIHA, representing approximately 12 percent of the cases of AIHA in various studies.

Table 12–8 lists the frequency of the various types of AIHA.

## Warm Autoimmune Hemolytic Anemia (WAIHA)

Patients with WAIHA present a special problem to the blood bank. A significant percentage of cases suffer from an anemia of sufficient severity to suggest the need for a possible transfusion. The degree of anemia is variable; however, hemoglobins less than 7 g/dl are frequently manifested. The onset of WAIHA is usually insidious and may be precipitated by a variety of factors such as infection, trauma, surgery, pregnancy, or psychologic stress. In other patients the onset is sudden.

WAIHA may be idiopathic, with no underlying disease process, or it may be secondary to a pathologic disorder. Table 12–9 lists the disorders reported to be associated with WAIHA.

### Table 12–8. PERCENTAGE OF REPORTED CASES OF AIHA

| | |
|---|---|
| Warm AIHA | 70% |
| Cold agglutinin syndrome | 16% |
| Paroxysmal cold hemoglobinuria (PCH) | 1–2% |
| Drug-induced | 12% |

Signs and symptoms appear when a significant anemia has developed. Pallor, weakness, dizziness, dyspnea, jaundice, and unexplained fever occasionally are presenting complaints. Hemolysis is usually acute at onset and may stabilize or continue to accelerate at a variable rate.

The blood smear usually displays polychromasia, reflecting reticulocytosis, which is characteristic of a hemolytic anemia **(see Color Figure 115)**. Spherocytosis and occasionally red cell fragmentation, indicating extravascular hemolysis, can be demonstrated along with nucleated red blood cells. An uncommon manifestation of WAIHA is reticulocytopenia. It is usually seen in the presence of a hyperplastic marrow, although it may also be associated with a hypoplastic marrow that is secondary to another underlying disease state. Since antigenic determinants on erythrocyte precursors can also react with the patient's red cell autoantibodies, reticulocytes can be destroyed as they are released from the bone marrow. Reticulocytopenia at the time of intense hemolysis, therefore, is associated with a high mortality rate. Products of hemolysis such as bilirubin (particularly the unconjugated/indirect fraction) and urinary urobilingen are increased. In severe cases, depleted serum haptoglobin, hemoglobinemia, hemoglobinuria, and increases in lactic dehydrogenase (LDH) may be demonstrated.

### Red Cell Hemolysis

In 80 percent of cases of WAIHA, the antibody causing the hemolysis is an IgG immunoglobulin, with IgG subclasses 1 and 3 being associated with patients demonstrating clinical signs of a hemolytic anemia.

The subclasses or isotypes of IgG are distinguished by the number of disulfide bonds present in the hinge region of the molecule. This accounts for their differences in electrophoretic mobility and biologic properties. Table 12–10 summarizes the biologic properties of the IgG subclasses. IgG antibodies in the serum of healthy individuals show a spread of all four isotypes. In some instances, such as in an immune response, antibodies tend to be predominantly or exclusively of one class. (For example, anti-Rh antibodies are usually IgG1 or IgG3; anti-Duffy and anti-Kell antibodies are usually IgG1; and anti-Jk$^a$ are usually IgG3.) In terms of biologic half-life, IgG3 is the shortest, 7 to 8 days, whereas all the other subclasses possess a half-life of 21 days. All IgG subclasses except IgG4 possess the ability to bind complement via the classic pathway of activation, with IgG3 being more efficient than IgG1, which in turn is more efficient than IgG2. Macrophages possess receptors for the Fc fragment of IgG1 and IgG3.

Immune red cell destruction is primarily extra-

**Table 12-9. DISORDERS REPORTED TO BE FREQUENTLY ASSOCIATED WITH WAIHA**

1. Reticuloendothelial neoplasms such as chronic lymphocytic leukemia, Hodgkin's disease, non-Hodgkin's lymphomas, thymomas
2. Collagen disease such as systemic lupus erythematosus, scleroderma, and rheumatoid arthritis.
3. Infectious diseases such as viral syndromes in childhood
4. Immunologic diseases such as hypogammaglobulinemia, dysglobulinemia, and other immune-deficiency syndromes
5. Gastrointestinal diseases such as ulcerative colitis
6. Benign tumors such as ovarian dermoid cysts

Modified from Petz and Garratty, 1980, p 32.

vascular, taking place in the fixed reticuloendothelial system (RES) cells primarily of the liver and spleen. However, the spleen has been demonstrated to be 100 times more efficient in removal of (Rh) IgG–sensitized red cells. The macrophages are equipped with two important biologic receptors on their membranes: (1) a receptor for the Fc fragments of IgG1 and IgG3 immunoglobulins, and (2) a receptor for the C3b fragment of complement. Sensitized red cells are phagocytized by interaction with RES mononuclear phagocytes, depending on what is coating the erythrocytes. If only IgG is coating the red cells, phagocytosis of erythrocytes occurs. If both C3b and IgG are coating the red cells, then there is a rapid phagocytosis, as the C3b fragment augments the action of IgG, enhancing sequestration and phagocytosis of the coated erythrocytes. If only C3b is coating the red cells, then transient immune adherence primarily occurs. It has been estimated that greater than 100,000 molecules of the complement fragment would be required to induce phagocytosis. Therefore, the activity of the macrophages and the severity of hemolysis via phagocytosis of sensitized red cells are dependent on various factors, summarized in Table 12-11.

## Serologic Evaluation

Laboratory evaluation reveals a positive direct antiglobulin test (DAT) result. The autoantibody can present several different problems in serologic testing. The serologic problems of WAIHA are twofold:

1. The patient's red cell antigens are strongly coated with autoantibody, which interferes with phenotyping
2. Autoantibody present in the serum may mask any underlying alloantibody

A typical serologic pattern from a patient with WAIHA can be found in Table 12-12.

## Autoantibody Specificity

The autoantibodies producing WAIHA usually display broad specificity, reacting with all cells tested. Sometimes the autoantibody will demonstrate a narrow specificity, the most common being anti-e. On rare occasion, other specificities have also been reported.

## Treatment

Therapy is generally aimed at treating the underlying disease first, if one is present. General measures to support cardiovascular function are important in patients who are severely anemic. Transfusion is generally avoided if possible, as this may only accelerate the hemolysis instead of ameliorating the anemia. However, transfusion is used in life-threatening situations.

Three forms of treatment are generally used, depending on the severity of the disorder.

**Corticosteroid Administration.** This form of therapy involves the use of corticosteroids, such as prednisone. Initially, high doses of 100 to 200 mg of prednisone are maintained until the patient's hematocrit stabilizes. Patients who are not transfused respond to steroid therapy more rapidly than those who are transfused. Several mechanisms have been proposed for the action of prednisone, including (1) reduction of antibody synthesis, (2) altered antibody avidity, and (3) alteration of macrophage receptors for IgG and C3, which reduces the clearance of antibody-coated red cells.

The dosage of prednisone should be reduced when the hematocrit begins to rise and the reticulocyte count drops. Finally, the steroids are withdrawn slowly over a period of two to four months. A beneficial response to the administration of prednisone is demonstrated in 50 to 65 percent of all cases of WAIHA. Recent reports on the use of the andro-

**Table 12-10. BIOLOGIC PROPERTIES OF IgG ISOTYPES**

| Characteristic | IgG1 | IgG2 | IgG3 | IgG4 |
|---|---|---|---|---|
| % Total serum IgG | 65–70 | 23–28 | 4–7 | 3–4 |
| Complement fixation (classic pathway) | Yes | Yes | Yes | No |
| Binding to macrophage Fc receptors | Yes | No | Yes | No |
| Placental transfer | Yes | Yes | Yes | Yes |
| Biologic half-life (days) | 21 | 21 | 7–8 | 21 |

From Pittiglio, Baldwin, and Sohmer, p 66, with permission.

**Table 12–11. FACTORS AFFECTING ACTIVITY OF MACROPHAGES**

1. Subclass of IgG
2. Presence of complement
3. Quantity of immunoglobulin of complement
4. Number and activity of helper T cells ($T_4$)
5. Number and activity of suppressor T cells ($T_8$)

genic steroid Dana 20 have also indicated some benefit in predisone-resistant cases.

**Splenectomy.** If steroid treatment fails, or if a patient requires large steroid doses to control hemolysis, then splenectomy is usually recommended. The decision to perform a splenectomy requires clinical evaluation and judgment. However, there are three reasons for performing a splenectomy: (1) failure of steroid therapy, (2) need for continuous high steroid maintenance doses, and (3) complications of steroid therapy. Splenectomy accomplishes two functions: (a) it decreases the production of antibody and (b) it removes a potent site of red cell damage and destruction. Patients who had a good initial response to steroids respond better with splenectomy than do those who failed steroid therapy initially.

It has been reported that as many as 60 percent of the patients with WAIHA benefit from splenectomy if steroid dosages greater than 15 mg/day are also used to maintain remission.

**Immunosuppressive Drugs.** This is usually the last approach used in the management of WAIHA. Azathioprine (Imuran) and cyclophosphamide are examples of cytotoxic immunosuppressive drugs that interfere with antibody synthesis by destroying dividing cells.

Experience in using this therapy is limited. The most detrimental side effect that threatens the common use of these drugs is the potential for neoplastic growth, as immunosuppressed patients have defective immune surveillance.

## Cold Autoimmune Hemolytic Anemia (Cold AIHA)

### Normal Cold Autoantibodies

Cold autoagglutinins are present in all human sera to a greater or lesser degree. Cold autoantibodies found in the serum of normal, healthy individuals include anti-I, anti-H, and anti-IH even though practically all adult red cells have the I and H antigens present on their red cells. Generally, most examples of anti-I, anti-H, and anti-IH have no clinical significance, and most of these autoantibodies are often too weak to be detected by routine serologic testing. This is primarily due to their low concentration in serum, failure to react at body temperature (37°C), and the fact that their optimal reactivity is at lower temperatures. Table 12–13 compares the characteristics of a normal cold autoagglutinin found in healthy adults with that of a pathologic cold autoantibody. These autoantibodies termed "autoagglutinins" differ in many ways from the "pathologic" cold autoagglutinins that produce cold AIHA.

### Pathologic Cold Autoantibodies

Pathologic cold autoantibodies can be divided into the following types: (1) cold agglutinin syndrome (idiopathic cold AIHA); (2) secondary cold AIHA (cold autoantibodies related to infection); and (3) paroxysmal cold hemoglobinuria (PCH).

**Cold Agglutinin Syndrome (Idiopathic Cold AIIIA).** Cold agglutinin syndrome, also called cold hemagglutinin disease (CHD) or idiopathic cold AIHA, represents approximately 16 percent of the cases of AIHA. A moderate chronic hemolytic anemia is produced by a cold autoantibody which optimally reacts at 4°C and also reacts between 25 to 31°C. The antibody is usually an IgM immunoglobulin, which quite efficiently activates complement.

CHD occurs predominantly in older individuals with a peak incidence beyond 50 years of age. Antibody specificity in this disorder is almost always anti-I, less commonly anti-i, and rarely anti-Pr.

Cold hemagglutinin disease is rarely severe and usually seasonal, since the winter cold months often precipitate the signs and symptoms of a chronic hemolytic anemia. Acrocyanosis of the hands, feet, ears, and nose is frequently the patient's main complaint, along with a sense of numbness in the extremities. Changes take place when the person is exposed to the cold, since the cold autoantibody will precipitate autoagglutination of the individual's red cells in the skin capillaries causing local

**Table 12–12. PRELIMINARY TESTING: SEROLOGIC PATTERN FROM A PATIENT WITH WAIHA**

| Anti-A | Anti-B | Anti-A,B | $A_1$ cells | B cells | Anti-D | Rh control |
|---|---|---|---|---|---|---|
| 4+ | neg | 4+ | neg | 4+ | 3+ | 1+ |

Antibody Screen

| | I.S. | 37°C | AHG |
|---|---|---|---|
| I | neg | neg | 2+ |
| II | neg | neg | 2+ |

PANEL RESULTS: 2+ reaction (AHG phase only) with all cells tested.

Table 12-13. COMPARISON OF CHARACTERISTICS OF NORMAL COLD AUTOANTIBODY AND PATHOLOGIC COLD AUTOAGGLUTININ

| Characteristic | Healthy | Pathologic |
|---|---|---|
| Thermal amplitude | <22°C | Broad: up to 32°C |
| Visible agglutination (in anticoagulated tube of blood) | None | Huge mass of agglutinated cells (disperses after incubation at 37°C) |
| Titer (concentration) | <64 (seldom >16 at 4°C) | >1000 |
| Albumin enhancement | Usually none | Enhances reactivity |
| Clonal production | Polyclonal | Monoclonal |
| Clinical significance | None | Produces cold AIHA |
| Common antibody specificity | Anti-I | Anti-I |
| DAT | Neg/+ or wk (polyspecific) Coombs sera | 2 to 3+ (polyspecific) Coombs sera |

blood stasis. During winter cold weather, the temperature of an individual's blood falls to as low as 28°C, activating the cold autoantibody in these patients. This activated cold antibody agglutinates red cells and fixes complement as the erythrocytes flow through the capillaries of the skin, causing autoagglutination and signs of acrocyanosis. In addition, these patient's may also experience hemoglobinuria, as complement fixation may result in intravascular hemolysis after cold exposure. However, this intravascular hemolytic episode is not associated with fever, chills, or acute renal insufficiency, which is characteristic of patients with PCH or severe WAIHA.

Patients usually display weakness, pallor, and weight loss, which are characteristic symptoms of a chronic anemia. Cold hemagglutinin syndrome usually remains quite stable, and if it does progress in severity, it is insidious in intensity. Physical findings such as hepatosplenomegaly are infrequent owing to the mechanism of hemolysis. Other clinical features of cold agglutinin disease include jaundice and Raynaud's phenomenon (symptoms of cold intolerance, such as pain and a bluish tinge in the fingertips and toes, owing to vasospasm).

Laboratory findings in cold agglutinin syndrome include reticulocytosis and a positive DAT result (owing to complement coating only). It is suggested and recommended that a simple serum screening procedure be performed initially to test the ability of the patient's serum to agglutinate normal saline–suspended red cells at 20°C after a room temperature incubation. If this test result is positive, further steps must be taken to determine the titer and thermal amplitude of the patient's cold autoantibody; if negative, the diagnosis of cold agglutinin syndrome is unlikely. The peripheral smear in patients with cold agglutinin syndrome may show rouleaux or autoagglutination, polychromasia, and a mild to moderate anisocytosis, and poikilocytosis (see Color Figure 116). Autoagglutination of anticoagulated whole blood samples is characteristic of cold agglutinin syndrome and occurs quickly as blood cools to room temperature, causing the binding of cold autoantibodies to the patient's red cells. As a result of this autoagglutination, performance of blood counts and preparation of blood smears are extremely difficult in these patient samples. Leukocyte and platelet counts are usually normal.

Table 12-14 summarizes the clinical criteria for diagnosis of cold agglutinin syndrome.

**Secondary Cold AIHA (Cold Autoantibodies Related to Infection).** Cold hemagglutinin disease can also occur as a transient disorder that is secondary to infections. Episodes of cold autoimmune hemolytic anemia often occur following upper respiratory infections. Approximately 50 percent of patients suffering from pneumonia due to Mycoplasma pneumoniae have elevated titers of cold autoagglutinins of greater than 64. In the second or third week of the patient's illness, cold hemagglutinin disease may occur in association with the infection, and a rapid onset of hemolysis is observed. Pallor and jaundice are characteristically present, and splenomegaly is generally found. Uncharacteristically, acrocyanosis and hemoglobinuria are un-

Table 12-14. CLINICAL CRITERIA FOR THE DIAGNOSIS OF COLD AGGLUTININ SYNDROME

1. Clinical signs of an acquired hemolytic anemia, with a history (which may or may not be present) of acrocyanosis and hemoglobinuria upon exposure to cold
2. A positive direct antiglobulin test (DAT) result using polyspecific antisera
3. A positive DAT result using monospecific C3 antisera
4. A negative DAT result using monospecific IgG antisera
5. The presence of reactivity in the patient's serum owing to a cold autoantibody
6. A cold agglutinin titer of 1000 or greater in saline at 4°C with visible autoagglutination of anticoagulated blood at room temperature.

usual and are not consistently present. Usually, resolution of the episode occurs in two to three weeks, as the hemolysis is self-limiting. The offending cold autoantibody is an IgM immunoglobulin with characteristic anti-I specificity. Very high titers of the cold autoagglutinin are seen almost exclusively in patients with Mycoplasma pneumonia. It has been reported that the cold agglutinin produced in this infection is an immunologic response to the mycoplasmal antigens and this antibody cross-reacts with the red cell I antigen.

The antibodies produced in cold agglutinin syndrome and in this disorder secondary to Mycoplasma pneumonia both have anti-I specificity. Red cells are again sensitized with complement components owing to the cold autoantibody produced, which is related to the particular infection. If the complement cascade does not proceed to C9 (cell death by lysis), the macrophages of the RES system can still clear the sensitized red cells through their receptors for C3b fragments, thereby causing hemolysis.

Infectious mononucleosis may also be associated with a hemolytic anemia due to a cold autoagglutinin. Although rather infrequent, it has been well documented that a high titered IgM cold agglutinin with a wide thermal range anti-i specificity plays a major role in the hemolytic anemia associated with this viral infection. Acute illness with sore throat and high fever, followed by weakness, anemia, and jaundice are characteristic features of infectious mononucleosis.

Lymphadenopathy and hepatosplenomegaly are common findings. A larger percentage of patients with infectious mononucleosis have been reported to develop anti-i, but only a small number of these patients develop the antibody of sufficient titer and thermal amplitude to induce in vivo hemolysis. (For a review of infectious mononucleosis, see Chapter 18.) Table 12–15 lists the cold autoantibody specificity most commonly found in the various infections that cause secondary cold hemagglutinin disease.

***Treatment.*** Therapy for cold agglutinin syndrome is generally unsatisfactory. Most patients require no treatment and are instructed to avoid the cold, keep warm, or move to a milder climate. Patients with moderate anemia are given the same

instructions, urging them to tolerate the symptoms rather than to use drugs on a therapeutic trial basis. There is some advantage to the use of plasma exchange in more severe cases, as IgM antibodies have a predominantly intravascular distribution. However, response to plasma exchange is still variable in this patient population. Corticosteroids have also been used but generally have a poor effect. In some patients whose red cells are strongly sensitized with C3, successful results have been reported with corticosteroids. Some favorable responses have also been reported with the alkylating drug chlorambucil. Splenectomy is generally considered ineffective.

**Paroxysmal Cold Hemoglobinuria (PCH).** PCH is the least common type of AIHA, with an incidence of only 1 to 2 percent. It is, however, more common in children in association with viral disorders such as measles, mumps, chicken pox, infectious mononucleosis, and the ill-defined "flu syndrome."

Originally, PCH was described in association with syphilis, in which an autoantibody was formed in response to the Treponema pallidum infection, the causative agent of the disease. However, with the discovery and use of antibiotics to treat syphilis, PCH is no longer a commonly reported disorder related to syphilis.

Red cell destruction is due to a cold autoantibody termed an "autohemolysin," which binds to the patient's red cells at low temperatures and fixes complement. Hemolysis occurs when the body temperature rises to 37°C and the sensitized cells undergo complement-mediated intravascular lysis. *Uncharacteristically*, this cold autoagglutinin is an IgG antibody with "biphasic" activity; therefore, it is termed a "biphasic hemolysin." The classic antibody produced in PCH is called the Donath-Landsteiner antibody, which characteristically is an IgG biphasic hemolysin with anti-P specificity.

During the Donath-Landsteiner laboratory test, two blood samples are drawn from the patient and maintained at different temperatures. One specimen is used as the control and kept at 37°C for 60 minutes. The other sample is cooled at 4°C for 30 minutes and then incubated at 37°C for an additional 30 minutes. Both samples are then centrifuged and observed for hemolysis. In a positive Donath-Landsteiner test result, hemolysis will be demonstrated in the sample placed at 4°C and then at 37°C, while no hemolysis is observed in the control sample. Table 12–16 summarizes the Donath-Landsteiner test. Determination of the specificity of the autoantibody is indicated in all positive Donath-Landsteiner test results.

As the name of PCH implies, paroxysmal or intermittent episodes of hemoglobinuria occur upon exposure to the cold. These acute attacks are characterized by a sudden onset of fever, shaking chills, malaise, abdominal cramps, and back pains. All the

**Table 12–15. SECONDARY COLD AIHA**

| Type of Infection | Cold Autoantibody Specificity |
|---|---|
| Mycoplasma pneumonia | Anti-I |
| Infectious mononucleosis | Anti-i |
| Lymphoproliferative disorder | Anti-i |

**Table 12–16. DONATH-LANDSTEINER TEST**

| | Whole Blood Sample 1 (Control) | Whole Blood Sample 2 |
|---|---|---|
| **Procedure** | | |
| 1. 30 min | 37°C | 4°C |
| 2. 30 min | 37°C | 37°C |
| 3. Centrifuge and observe | | |
| **Results** | | |
| Positive | No hemolysis | Hemolysis |
| Negative | No hemolysis | No hemolysis |
| Inconclusive | Hemolysis | Hemolysis |

signs of intravascular hemolysis are evident, along with hemoglobinemia, hemoglobinuria, and bilirubinemia depending on the severity and frequency of the attack (see Fig. 12-1). This results in a severe and rapidly progressive anemia with hemoglobin values frequently around 4 to 5 g%. Polychromasia, nucleated red blood cells, and poikilocytosis are demonstrated in the peripheral smear; these are consistent findings associated with a hemolytic anemia.

These signs and symptoms, as well as hemoglobinuria, may resolve in a few hours or persist for days. Splenomegaly, hyperbilirubinemia, and renal insufficiency may also develop.

PCH is an acute hemolytic anemia occurring almost exclusively in children and young adults and almost always representing a transient disorder. Table 12–17 compares and contrasts PCH versus cold agglutinin syndrome.

***Treatment.*** For chronic forms of PCH, protection from cold exposure is the only useful therapy. Acute postinfection forms of PCH usually terminate spontaneously following resolution of the infectious process. Steroids and transfusions may be required, depending on the severity of the attacks.

Table 12–18 reviews and compares characteristics of warm and cold autoimmune hemolytic anemias.

## DRUG-INDUCED IMMUNE HEMOLYTIC ANEMIA

The administration of drugs may lead to the development of a wide variety of hematologic abnormalities, including immune hemolytic anemia. Drug-induced immune hemolytic anemia, which is sometimes difficult to distinguish from other cases of WAIHA, represents approximately 12 percent of cases in various studies. However, drug-related immune hemolytic processes do not involve any known abnormality intrinsic to the red cell.

Four recognizable mechanisms lead to the development of drug-related antibodies and drug-induced immune hemolytic anemia.

### Immune Complex Mechanism (Fig. 12-2)

The most common drugs involved in this response include quinidine and phenacetin. Table 12–19 lists other drugs involved in the immune complex mechanism. The patient responds to these drugs by producing an antidrug antibody, which forms an

**Table 12–17. COMPARISON OF PCH AND COLD AGGLUTININ SYNDROME**

| | PCH | Cold Agglutinin Syndrome |
|---|---|---|
| Patient population | Children or young adults | Elderly or middle-aged |
| Pathogenesis | Following viral infection | Idiopathic/lymphoproliferative disorder/ following Mycoplasma pneumoniae infection |
| Clinical features | Hemoglobinuria: acute attacks upon exposure to cold (symptoms resolve in hours or days) | Acrocyanosis/autoagglutination of blood at room temperature |
| Severity of hemolysis | Acute and rapid | Chronic and rarely severe |
| Hemolysis | Intravascular | Extravascular/Intravascular |
| Autoantibody | IgG (anti-P specificity) (biphasic hemolysin) | IgM (anit-I/i) (monophasic) |
| DAT | 3+ (polyspecific Coombs sera)/neg IgG/ 3–4+ C3 monospecific Coombs sera | 3+ (polyspecific Coombs sera)/neg IgG/ 3–4+ C3 monospecific Coombs sera |
| Thermal range | Moderate (<20°C) | High (up to 30–31°C) |
| Titer (4°C) | Moderate (<64) | High (>1000) |
| Donath-Landsteiner test | Positive | Negative |
| Treatment | Supportive (disorder terminates when underlying illness resolves) | Avoid the cold |

**Table 12-18. COMPARISON OF WARM AND COLD AUTOIMMUNE HEMOLYTIC ANEMIAS**

|  | WAIHA | Cold AIHA |
| --- | --- | --- |
| Optimal reactivity | >32°C | <30°C |
| Immunoglobulin class | IgG | IgM (exception: PCH-IgG) |
| Complement activation | May bind complement | Binds complement |
| Hemolysis | Usually extravascular (no cell lysis) | Usually intravascular (cell lysis) |
| Frequency | 70–75% of cases | 16% of cases (PCH: 1–2%) |
| Specificity | Frequently Rh | Ii system (PCH: anti-P) |

immune complex. The antibody drug complex then adsorbs onto the patient's red cells, which become "innocent bystanders."

Clinical laboratory findings include signs of intravascular hemolysis, with hemoglobinemia and hemoglobinuria being most notable. The antibody, which is usually either IgM or IgG, is capable of activating complement. Only a small amount of the drug is necessary to produce an antibody response in a particular patient. The DAT result is positive, often only because of the presence of complement components on the red cell surface, since the immune complex has dissociated. In vitro agglutination reactions are generally observed during serologic testing only when the patient's serum, drug, and red cells are *all* incubated together. In addition, elution procedures often demonstrate nonreactive eluates.

Treatment is aimed at stopping the use of the drug. Although hemolysis by this mechanism is rare, onset is sudden and characterized by intravascular hemolysis and frequent renal failure. Therefore, immediate cessation of the drug is essential. Steroid treatment may also be given.

## Drug Adsorption (Hapten) Mechanism (Fig. 12-3)

The drugs implicated in this response include the penicillins (which produce the second most common drug-induced hemolytic anemia) and rarely the cephalosporins and streptomycins. In this response, the drug is nonspecifically bound to the pa-

**Table 12-19. DRUGS IMPLICATED IN IMMUNE COMPLEX, OR "INNOCENT BYSTANDER," MECHANISM**

| | |
| --- | --- |
| Quinidine | Insecticides |
| Quinine | Dipyrone |
| Phenacetin | Anhistine |
| Stibophen | Antazoline |
| P-Aminosalicylic acid | Chlorpromazine |
| Sulfonamides | Aminopyrine |
| Thiazide | Isoniazid |

tient's red cells. It remains firmly adsorbed to the cells regardless of whether the patient develops an antibody to the drug. "Hapten mechanism" is also used to describe this response, because the drug's immunogenicity is determined by its ability to chemically react with serum proteins to form several haptenic groups. If the patient develops an anti-drug antibody, it will react with the red cell–bound drug protein.

Clinical laboratory findings include signs of extravascular hemolysis. Large doses of intravenous penicillin (10 million units daily) are needed to produce a response. The onset is much less acute than that of the immune complex mechanism; the disorder develops over a period of 7 to 10 days. The DAT result is strongly positive owing to IgG sensitization, and a high titer of IgG antibody is present in the serum. Red blood cell eluates react only with antibiotic-coated red cells. Treatment focuses on the discontinuation of the drug in the presence of an overt hemolytic anemia.

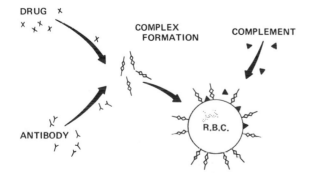

**Figure 12-2.** Immune complex mechanism. (From Petz, LD and Garraty, G (eds): Acquired Immune Hemolytic Anemias. Churchill Livingstone, New York, 1980, with permission.)

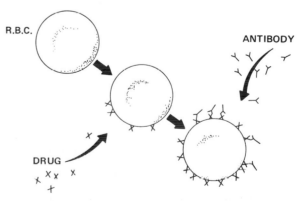

**Figure 12-3.** Drug absorption mechanism. (From Petz, LD and Garraty, G (eds): Acquired Immune Hemolytic Anemias. Churchill Livingstone, New York, 1980, with permission.)

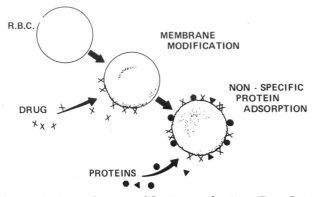

**Figure 12-4.** Membrane modification mechanism. (From Petz, LD and Garraty, G (eds): Acquired Immune Hemolytic Anemias. Churchill Livingstone, New York, 1980, with permission.)

## Membrane Modification Mechanism (Nonimmunologic Protein Adsorption) (Fig. 12-4)

As the name implies, the drug modifies the red cell membrane so that normal plasma proteins are adsorbed nonimmunologically. Cephalosporins are the drugs implicated in this response. Cephalothin-sensitized cells become coated with numerous plasma proteins such as albumin, fibrinogen, and globulins. Approximately 3 percent of the patients receiving the drug develop a positive DAT result from the nonspecific protein adsorption onto the red cells. However, hemolytic anemia has not been reported in association with this mechanism of drug-induced positive DAT results. Elution procedures result in nonreactive eluates. There is no treatment approach, as hemolytic anemia associated with ingestion of these drugs has not been described in relation to membrane modification.

## Methyldopa-Induced Mechanism (Unknown Mechanism)

This represents the most common drug-induced immune hemolytic anemia, with an incidence of 0.8 percent. The drugs implicated in this response include methyldopa and related drugs (i.e., Aldomet, L-dopa), which are commonly prescribed for the treatment of hypertension. Drug-induced AIHA by this mechanism is difficult to diagnose, because it mimics WAIHA. A positive DAT result develops in approximately 12 to 15 percent of the patients receiving Aldomet (alphamethyldopa), but AIHA develops only rarely in these patients (1 to 3 percent). Patients may continue to have a positive DAT result for up to two years after discontinuation of the drug. If anemia develops, it will do so gradually in this type of drug-induced hemolytic anemia, and its development depends on the dose of the drug. The antibodies produced by the patients suffering from this disorder are of the IgG immunoglobulin class with specificities similar to those found in WAIHA. Hemolysis is extravascular, and the DAT result is strongly positive owing to IgG sensitization.

Atypically, the eluate is positive, unlike all the other drug-induced positive DAT mechanisms in which the eluates are negative.

There are several hypotheses suggested for this drug-related hematologic problem; however, the exact mechanism is still unknown. Table 12–20 presents the four different theories proposed for the methyldopa-induced mechanism of immune hemolytic anemia.

## Treatment

Discontinuation of the drug is the treatment of choice for patients with a drug-induced hemolytic anemia. The presence of a positive DAT result does not necessarily imply that the drug must be discontinued, if the effects of the drug are of therapeutic benefit. In general, however, other drugs should be substituted and the patient observed for resolution of the anemia to confirm a drug-induced hemolytic process. If the patient has a positive DAT result *without* hemolysis, continued administration of the drug is optional.

Generally, the prognosis for patients with drug-induced hemolytic anemia is excellent. In Table 12–21, the four recognized mechanisms leading to the development of drug-related antibodies are compared. Table 12–22 contrasts the antibody characteristics of the various types of autoimmune hemolytic anemias.

This chapter has focused on acquired red cell problems associated with demonstrable antibodies, known as immune hemolytic anemias. These represent only one type of hemolytic anemia due to extracorpuscular defects. (See Chapter 13 on nonim-

## Table 12–20. PROPOSED THEORIES FOR METHYLDOPA-INDUCED MECHANISM OF IMMUNE HEMOLYTIC ANEMIA

1. Normal red cell antigens are altered by the drug and are no longer recognized as "self," resulting in production of autoantibodies to these red blood cell antigens.
2. The drug acts as a hapten, resulting in the production of antibodies, which cross-react with normal red cell antigens.
3. The drug produces aberrations in the proliferation of normal lymphocytes, producing clones of abnormal immunologically competent cells, which produce antibodies against normal red blood cell antigens.
4. The drug affects the synthesis of IgG, exerting a direct effect on T lymphocytes, which results in a loss of suppressor function and subsequent proliferation of autoantibodies by B lymphocytes.

Table 12-21. MECHANISMS LEADING TO DEVELOPMENT OF DRUG-RELATED ANTIBODIES

| Mechanism | Prototype Drugs | Immunoglobulin Class | DAT | Biologic Results | Frequency of Hemolysis |
|---|---|---|---|---|---|
| Immune complex formation (innocent bystander) | Quinidine<br>Phenacetin | IgM or IgG | Positive (often to complement fragments only; however, IgG may be present) | Eluate often negative | Small doses of drug may cause acute intravascular hemolysis with hemoglobinemia and hemoglobinuria; renal failure is common |
| Drug adsorption (Hapten) | Penicillins<br>Cephalosporins<br>Streptomycin | IgG | Positive (strongly) due to IgG sensitization | Eluate often negative | 3–4% of patients on large doses (10 million units) daily of penicillin, which is one of the most common causes of drug induced immune hemolysis, usually extravascular in nature |
| Membrane modification (nonimmunologic protein adsorption) | Cephalosporins | Numerous plasma proteins (nonimmunological sensitization) | Positive due to a variety of serum proteins | Eluate negative | No hemolysis; however, 3% of patients receiving the drug develop a +DAT |
| Methyldopa-induced (unknown) | Methyldopa (Aldomet) | IgG | Strongly positive (due to IgG sensitization) | Eluate positive (warm autoantibody identical to antibody found in WAIHA) | 0.8% develop a hemolytic anemia that mimics a WAIHA (depends on the dose of the drug); 15% of patients receiving Aldomet develop a +DAT |

Table 12–22. SUMMARY OF ANTIBODY CHARACTERISTICS IN AIHA

| | Warm Reactive Autoantibody | Cold Reactive Autoantibody | Paroxysmal Cold Hemoglobinuria | Drug Related Autoantibody |
|---|---|---|---|---|
| Immunoglobulin Characteristics | Polyclonal IgG, IgM, and IgA may also be present. Rarely IgA alone | Polyclonal IgM–infection Monoclonal kappa chain IgM in cold agglutinin disease | Polyclonal IgG | Polyclonal IgG |
| Complement activation | Variable | Always | Always | Depends on mechanism of drug, antibody, and red cell interaction |
| Thermal reactivity | 20°C–37°C Optimum 37°C | 4°C–32°C occasionally to 37°C. Optimum 4°C | 4°C–20°C Biphasic hemolysin | 20°C–37°C Optimum 37°C |
| Titer of free antibody | Low (<32) May only be detectable using enzyme treated cells | High (>512 at 4°C) | Moderate to low (<64) | Depends on mechanism of drug, antibody and red cell interaction |
| Reactivity of eluate with antibody screening cells | Usually pan-reactive | Nonreactive | Nonreactive | Panreactive with Aldomet type antibody. Nonreactive in all other circumstances |
| Most common specificity | Anti-Rh precursor -common Rh -LW -Enª/Wrᵇ -U | -I -i -Pr | Anti–P | Anti-'e' like–Aldomet, antidrug |
| Site of red cell destruction | Predominantly spleen with some liver involvement | Predominantly liver, rarely intravascular | Intravascular | Intravascular and spleen |

160

mune mechanisms to complete the category of hemolytic anemias due to extracorpuscular defects.)

## Bibliography

Bowman, JM: Rh erythroblastosis fetalis. Semin Hematol 12:189, 1975.

Bowman, JM, Chown, B, Lewis, M, et al: Rh iso-immunization during pregnancy: Antenatal prophylaxis. Canad Med Assoc J 118:623, 1978.

Calvo, R, Stein, W, Kochwa, S, et al: Acute hemolytic anemia due to anti-i; frequent cold agglutinins in infectious mononucleosis. J Clin Invest 44:1033, 1965.

Candle, MR, Scott, JR: The potential role of immunosuppression, plasmapheresis and desensitization as treatment modalites for Rh immunization. Clin Obstet Gynecol 25:313, 1982.

Carter, P, Koval, JJ, and Hobbs, JR: The relation of clinical and laboratory findings to the survival of patients with macroglobinaemia. Clin Exp Immunol 28:241, 1977.

Chaplin, H and Avioli, LV: Autoimmune hemolytic anemia. Arch Intern Med 137:346, 1977.

Czuba, TL: Special problems in the mother and newborn. In Approaches to Serological Problems in the Hospital Transfusion Service. American Association of Blood Banks. Arlington, VA, pp 73–99, 1985.

Dacie, JV: Autoimmune hemolytic anemia. Arch Intern Med 135:1293, 1975.

Dike, AE: The role of plasma exchange in the management of hemolytic disease of the newborn: The Oxford Experience. Plasma Ther Transfus Technol 5:23, 1984.

Evans, RS, Baxter, E, and Gilliland, BC: Chronic hemolytic anemia due to cold agglutinins: A 20-year history of benign gammopathy with response to chlorambucil. Blood 42:463, 1973.

Frank, MM, Atkinson, JP, and Cadok, J: Cold agglutinins and cold agglutinin disease. Ann Rev Med 28:291, 1977.

Golbus, MS, Stevens, JD, Cairn, HM, et al: Rh isoimmunization following genetic amniocentesis. Prenat Diagn 2:49, 1982.

Hemolytic Disease of the Newborn. American Association of Blood Banks, 1984.

Hensleigh, PA: Preventing rhesus iso-immunization: Antepartum Rh immune globulin prophylaxis versus a sensitive test for risk identification. Am J Obstet Gynecol 146:749, 1983.

Leddy, JP and Swisher, SN: Acquired immune hemolytic disorders (including drug-induced immune hemolytic anemia). In Samter, M (ed): Immunological Diseases. Ed 3. Vol I. 1978, p 1187.

Marchand, A: Charting a course for hemolytic anemia. Diagn Med 19, 1981.

Marchand, A: Immune hemolytic anemia. Part I: Classification, manifestations and mechanism of destruction. Diagn Med 51, 1982.

Marchand, A: Immune hemolytic anemia. Part II: Test procedures and strategy. Diagn Med 25, 1983.

Mollison, PL: Blood Transfusion in Clinical Medicine, ed 6. Blackwell Scientific Publications, Oxford, 1979, pp 693–709.

Petz, LD and Garraty, G: Acquired Immune Hemolytic Anemias. Churchill Livingstone, New York, 1980.

Pittiglio, DH, Baldwin, AJ, and Sohmer, PR: Modern Blood Banking and Transfusion Practices. FA Davis, Philadelphia, 1983.

Queenan, JT: Current management of the Rh sensitized patient. Clin Obstet Gynecol 25:293, 1982.

Rosenfield, RE, Schmidt, PJ, Calvo, RC, et al: Anti-i, a frequent cold agglutinin in infectious mononucleosis. Vox Sang 10:631, 1965.

Rote, NS: Pathophysiology of Rh iso-immunization. Clin Obstet Gynecol 25:243, 1982.

Sacher, RA and Lenes, BA: Exchange transfusion. Clin Lab Med 1:265, 1981.

Scott, JR, Warenski, JC: Tests to detect and quantitate feto-maternal bleeding. Clin Obstet Gynecol 25:277, 1982.

Tanowitz, HB, Robbins, N, and Leidich, N: Hemolytic anemia: Associated with severe mycoplasma pneumoniae pneumonia. NY State J Med 78:2231, 1978.

Taswell, HF, Pineda, AA, and Moore, SB: Hemolytic transfusion reactions: Frequency and clinical laboratory aspects. American Association of Blood Banks 4:71, 1981.

Whitfield, CR: An obstetric overview of trends in the management of Rh hemolytic disease. Plasma Ther Transfus Technol 5:47, 1984.

# CHAPTER 13

ERROL A. HOLLAND, M.B., B.Ch., F.C.P.(SA), AND
RONALD A. SACHER, M.D., F.R.C.P.(C)

# Hemolytic Anemias: Extracorpuscular Defects
## II. Nonimmune Hemolytic Anemias

Table 13–1. MECHANISMS OF RED CELL DAMAGE

| Mechanism | Pathogenesis |
|---|---|
| **Mechanical Pressure** | |
| In heart and great vessels | Artificial valves |
| In microcirculation | Hemolytic uremic syndrome (HUS) |
| | Thrombotic thrombocytopenic purpura (TTP) |
| | Disseminated intravascular coagulation (DIC) |
| **Membrane Disorders** | |
| Loss of membrane | Hypersplenism |
| Lipid peroxidation | Oxidant drugs |
| Lipid dissolution | Clostridium perfringens (Welchii) |
| Thermal damage | Burns |
| **Intracellular Pressure** | |
| Parasites | Malaria |
| Water (Osmotic) | Drowning |
| **Altered Energy Production** | Lead poisoning |

Normal red cells may have shortened intravascular survival if subjected to the harmful effects of abnormal or unusual physical or chemical stress. Cells may be damaged by mechanical forces within the circulation. The lipids and proteins of the cell membrane may be damaged by heat, radiation, chemicals, enzymes, and toxins. Pressure from within the red cell exerted by osmotic forces or intracellular parasites may cause cell rupture. These processes are acquired hemolytic anemias that represent usually non–immune-mediated extracorpuscular damage to red cells. This contrasts with the inherited causes of hemolysis discussed in previous chapters, which illustrate intracorpuscular defects of the erythrocyte. Table 13–1 lists the mechanisms of red cell damage with typical examples. It should be noted that in many instances an agent will cause damage by multiple mechanisms, including immunologic and nonimmunologic means.

## INFECTIONS

### Malaria

Malaria is the most prevalent infectious hematologic condition in the world. Red cell hemolysis due to intracellular asexual multiplication of the parasite is the cardinal process producing hemolysis. Immunologic mechanisms as manifested by a positive Coombs test result may also contribute to the red cell sequestration.

Malaria is a protozoan with a complex life cycle (Fig. 13–1). The bite from an infected mosquito injects into the blood sporozoites that travel to the liver, where they invade hepatic parenchymal cells. Within these cells asexual reproduction takes place, to form merozoites. After an incubation period of about 10 days, the hepatic cells rupture, releasing thousands of merozoites into the circulation. These are the parasitic forms that invade the circulating red cells. Apparently, the attachment of the para-

sites to red cells and their subsequent ability to enter depend on normal cell-surface structures. The most intensively investigated of these normal structures are the blood group antigens known as the Duffy system. When red cells that are missing the Duffy antigens are incubated with Plasmodium knowlesi, invasion does not occur. Thus, this antigen may constitute one of the attachment sites of the parasite.

Once the merozoite enters the red cell, it divides asexually to form 16 to 32 merozoites per cell. Red cells packed with merozoites are called schizonts. At regular intervals, these schizonts rupture, releasing the merozoites, which in turn attack other red cells. The rupture of the schizonts is often synchronized and occurs at regular intervals. Clinically, the rupture causes severe fever, chills, and prostration.

There are four species of Plasmodium that infect humans. Three of these have their own "preference" for subpopulations of red cells that they attack. For example, P. vivax invades reticulocytes, whereas P. malariae prefers older, mature cells. P. falciparum, however, can infect red cells at any stage, and it is not surprising that this organism causes the greatest amount of parasitemia and is clinically the most severe of the malarial infections **(see Color Figure 117)**.

### Laboratory Findings

Anemia is usually normocytic, normochromic. Hematocrits of less then 35 percent develop in approximately 20 percent of cases. The causes are multifactorial and include the hemolysis of parasitized red cells, marrow depression, and shortened red cell survival due to altered energy production. Immune hemolysis due to the development of autoantibodies may also occur. Generally, the degree of anemia is proportional to the parasitization of the cells. Therefore, the most severe anemia is usually seen in the P. falciparum infestation.

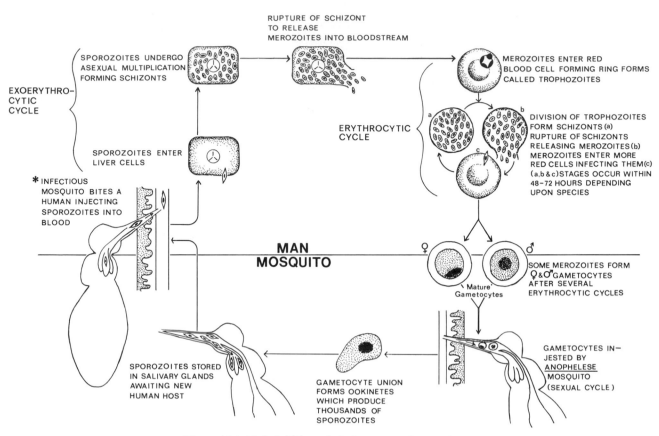

**Figure 13-1.** Malarial life cycle in humans and mosquitoes.
*Beginning of cycle.

**Leukopenia.** The white count may be normal but is frequently reduced.

**Thrombocytopenia.** This is a frequent finding. This is possibly due to a marked increase in macrophage proliferation and phagocytosis within the spleen, which is palpable in 70 to 80 percent of patients.

**Hemolytic Studies.** Evidence of intravascular hemolysis, as discussed in the introduction to hemolytic diseases, is found. Occasionally a severe hemolytic state with hemoglobinuria occurs, called "blackwater fever." This descriptive term was used to describe the severe hemoglobinuria that followed quinine therapy. The mechanism is thought to be a Coombs-positive hemolytic anemia due to quinine sensitivity. This contrasts with the Coombs-negative findings in the inherited hemolytic anemia G-6-PD deficiency, which also demonstrates intravascular hemolytic episodes.

**Smear Identification.** This establishes the definitive diagnosis. Blood smears stained with Wright's or Giemsa's stain demonstrates the Plasmodium parasite. Schizonts with about 15 merozoites in the shape of a rosette, ring forms, or occasionally the banana-shaped gametocyte may be seen. P. vivax produces a stippled appearance in red cells called Schüffner's dots **(see Color Figure 118).**

## Babesiosis

Hemolysis as a result of infection by the protozoan Babesia may produce features clinically similar to those of a malarial infestation. The organism is usually transmitted by ticks, and this zoonotic disease has a natural animal reservoir in certain species of wild and domestic animals. Cases of the disorder have been reported from Nantucket Island, off the New England coast of the United States.

Clinically, patients present with flu-like illness, night sweats, and fever. Like malaria, the organism can be identified on peripheral smears within red blood cells with Giemsa staining **(see Color Figure 119).** The disease is often self-limited, but patients who have previously undergone a splenectomy seem to be at greater risk of a more severe illness. Treatment involves chemotherapy with clindamycin and quinine.

## Bartonella Bacilliformis (Oroya Fever, Carrión's Disease, Bartonellosis)

Oroya fever is a fatal disease found in Peru, Ecuador, and Columbia. People visiting these areas may develop a verrucous skin lesion and a severe hemolytic disease with fever after a bite from a Phlebotomus verrucarum sand fly infected with Bartonella bacilliformis. Hepatosplenomegaly and lymphadenopathy may occur. The parasite is demonstrated on the *surface* of the red cells in the Giemsa-stained blood smear. Patients respond well to penicillin, streptomycin, chloramphenicol, or tetracycline. Untreated, the infection carries a high mortality rate.

## Clostridium perfringens (Welchii)

Clostridia are spore-forming gram-positive bacilli that grow in anaerobic conditions. Because they also produce gas, the term "gas-gangrene" is given to the clinical infection. Tissues damaged by trauma, surgical incisions, or septic abortions, create the anaerobic conditions within which the organisms thrive.

The organisms produce a variety of toxins that serve to break down healthy tissues. The alpha toxin is a lecithinase, which, together with proteases, attacks the lipoprotein membrane of the red cell to produce severe hemolysis.

### Laboratory Diagnosis

**Blood Counts.** Normocytic, normochromic anemia, leukocytosis with a high percentage of early forms, and thrombocytopenia are characteristic features.

**Smear.** Microspherocytes represent cells with partially destroyed membranes.

**Hemolytic Studies.** Hemoglobinemia sufficient to cause the serum to appear a brilliant red and hemoglobinuria are found. The prognosis is poor since concomitant renal and hepatic failure exist.

## Other Bacterial Infections

A few bacterial species are known to cause hemolysis or agglutination of red cells in vitro but to have little if any effect in vivo. The types of hemolysins produced in blood agar plates by the Streptococcus species are used for subtype identification. Similarly, Haemophilus influenzae, Escherichia coli, and Salmonella organisms produce questionable hemolytic effects in vivo.

Bacterial infections (particularly gram-negative organism) may also precipitate microangiopathic hemolytic anemia, which will be discussed subsequently.

## Viral Infections

Hemolytic reactions associated with viral infections are chiefly due to immune mechanisms. Autoantibody production has been observed after viral hepatitis, cytomegalovirus infections, Epstein-Barr virus, rubella, and other viral infections. Cold agglutinin production with subsequent clinical hemolysis is found with Mycoplasma pneumoniae infection and in some cases of infectious mononucleosis (see Chapter 12).

## CHEMICALS, TOXINS, AND PHYSICAL AGENTS

### Oxidative Hemolysis

The mechanisms of oxidative damage to red cells are discussed in Chapter 8.

Certain individuals are susceptible to the oxidant stress of drugs. Their susceptibility relates to a decreased production of NADPH (glucose-6-phosphate dehydrogenase deficiency), glucolytic enzyme deficiency, methemoglobin reductase enzyme deficiency, or structurally abnormal hemoglobin. These clinical entities and the drugs to which they are susceptible are discussed in Chapters 8 and 9 dealing with intracorpuscular defects.

Some of the drugs listed in Table 8–2 are powerful enough to overcome the defense mechanisms of normal cells. Others produce hemolysis if given in very high dosages or in normal dosages in the presence of renal failure.

### Nonoxidative Hemolysis

#### Arsenic

Arsine gas inhalation encountered during industrial exposure may cause a severe anemia, jaundice, and hemoglobinuria. The morphology of the red cells remains normochromic and normocytic, despite severe hemolysis. Patients present after 2 to 24 hours with nausea, vomiting, and abdominal pain. Treatment is directed at chelation with dimercaprol and exchange transfusion to remove arsenic compounds bound to the red cell membrane.

#### Lead

Intoxication is usually found in children ingesting flaking lead-containing paint or in adults inhaling fumes from burning batteries. Hemolysis is due to the interference with energy production of the cell, but the principal effect of lead is the interference in heme production. Several enzymes are inhibited, including $\delta$-aminolevulinic acid synthetase, $\delta$-aminolevulinic acid dehydrase, heme synthetase, porphyrinogen deaminase, uroporphyrinogen decarboxylase, and coproporphyrinogen oxidase.

**Laboratory Features**

**Blood Examination.** Microcytic, hypochromic cells with basophilic stippling may be seen **(see Color Figure 120)**. Shortened red cell survival may be demonstrated with radiolabeled chromium studies.

***Marrow Examination.*** Ringed sideroblasts are frequently found. This represents iron accumulation within the mitochondria owing to inhibited heme production (protoporphyrin IX + $Fe^{++}$ → heme).

## Copper

The toxic effects relate to the inhibition of reducing enzyme systems of the cell membrane, as well as enzymes of the glycolytic pathway. High levels of copper are found in persons attempting suicide by ingestion of large amounts of this substance, and in those with Wilson's disease.

## Osmotic Damage (Water)

Accidental intravenous injections of large amounts of distilled water will cause hemodilution, with water entry into cells leading to red cell rupture. This is also the mechanism of hemolysis associated with drowning.

## Venoms

Poisoning by a variety of insects (e.g., bees, wasps, spiders, and scorpions) is associated with hemolysis.

Occasionally, snake bites are associated with hemolysis. Certain snake venoms are known to contain lecithinase, which is able to dissolve the lecithin within the red cell membrane. Snakes belonging to the Elapidae group (cobras and other hooded snakes) are more likely to be associated with hemolysis. In general, hemolysis is uncommon following snake bites.

## Burns

Red cells damaged by heat are osmotically and mechanically fragile and are rapidly removed from the circulation. Blood smears from burn patients reveal microspherocytes and red cell fragments **(see Color Figure 124)**. Hemoglobinemia and hemoglobinuria may be found within the first 24 hours after a severe burn. Hemolysis occurring one or more days after the burn occurs may be associated with infused AB isohemagglutinins present in the transfused fresh frozen plasma.

## MICROANGIOPATHIC AND MACROANGIOPATHIC HEMOLYTIC ANEMIAS

Any impedence to the flow of blood propelled through the large and small blood vessels by the pumping action of the heart will create turbulence, producing sufficient shear stress to cause the rupture of red cells. The site of impedence may be within the heart and great vessels or in the microcirculation containing fibrin strands.

The pathogenesis is one of red blood cell contact with damaged blood vessels, valves, or artificial surfaces. Red cells contact vessels partially occluded with fibrin strands or with roughened or necrotic endothelium may produce the characteristic features. The clinical syndromes produced depend on the etiology of the disease process, the extent and degree of anemia and renal failure, the lumen size and extent of the vascular lesion of the involved blood vessels, and whether disseminated intravascular coagulation coexists (Table 13–2).

Fragments of red cells are typically seen in the peripheral smears, and laboratory evidence of intravascular hemolysis is found **(see Color Figure 122)**. Therefore, the macroangiopathic and microangiopathic hemolytic anemias are syndromes characterized by shortened red cell survival (hemolysis) and a typical red cell morphology (schistocytes). Active marrow compensation for the hemolytic process is revealed by the presence of reticulocytosis or earlier red cell precursors within the peripheral blood (normoblasts). Varying degrees of consumptive coagulopathy are encountered, from a mildly decreased platelet count and increased fibrinogen turnover to decreased levels of clotting factors and increased levels of fibrin and fibrinogen degradation products.

### Thrombotic Thrombocytopenic Purpura (TTP)

TTP is a rare disorder that can occur at any age, with a peak incidence between the ages of 30 and 40 years. The majority of cases develop spontaneously but may be associated with a variety of etiologic agents: for example, drugs, including oral contraceptives; pregnancy; connective tissue disorders; and viral infections. TTP is discussed in more detail in Chapter 27.

**Pathogenesis.** Although the initiating stimulus is unknown in most cases, precapillary arterioles and capillaries of the brain, kidney, heart, adrenals, and pancreas become occluded by platelet aggregates and fibrin, leading to hyaline thrombi.

The critical event is thought to be intravascular platelet aggregation and adhesion at the endothelial surface of the involved arteriole or capillary. The plasma in patients with TTP has been demonstrated to contain a platelet-aggregating factor, and the endothelium in some cases has been shown to be depleted of the natural platelet antiaggregant prosta-

**Table 13–2. FACTORS INFLUENCING THE CLINICAL SYNDROMES OF ANGIOPATHIC HEMOLYTIC ANEMIA**

1. Etiology of disease process
2. Extent and degree of anemia/renal failure
3. Luminal size of involved vessels
4. Distribution of involved vessels: localized/generalized
5. Disseminated intravascular coagulation (DIC)

cyclin. Once platelets are activated, platelet adhesion and aggregation followed by release of platelet products and fibrin strand formation occur, thus partially occluding the microvasculature. Hemolytic anemia then occurs, as the red cells flowing through these vessels are frankly "chopped."

Thrombotic thrombocytopenic purpura is a syndrome with a pentad of clinical and laboratory features: thrombocytopenia, microangiopathic hemolytic anemia, renal dysfunction, neurologic abnormalities, and fever. Varying degrees of severity of each of these features are found in every patient. Bleeding into skin, retina, gastrointestinal tract, and genitourinary tract is common. Some patients have hepatosplenomegaly, although this is uncommon.

**Laboratory Features.** Microangiopathic hemolytic anemia and thrombocytopenia are the principal hematologic findings **(see Color Figure 121)**. The reticulocyte count is elevated and nucleated red blood cells may be seen. The reticulocyte count is above 10 percent in 66 percent of cases. Leukocytosis exists in 70 percent of cases, often with a significant shift to the left. Coagulation factor consumption generally does not occur. Proteinuria, hematuria, urinary casts, or azotemia occur in most patients but are not the predominant feature, as in the hemolytic uremic syndrome. The serum lactic dehydrogenase is usually markedly increased, and patients may be clinically jaundiced.

**Therapy.** Plasma exchange with fresh frozen plasma replacement has been successful in some cases. Occasionally, simple plasma infusion appears to improve the patient's disorder, and this modality should be tried first. Most patients are also treated with high-dose corticosteroids and antiplatelet drugs.

Once the process is controlled, patients are given maintenance therapy with antiplatelet agents such as aspirin and dipyridamole for a few months (see Chapter 27).

## Hemolytic Uremic Syndrome (HUS)

This disorder usually affects young children. Although it resembles thrombotic thrombocytopenic purpura (TTP), it has a much lower mortality rate. As with TTP, intravascular thrombi with an associated microangiopathic blood picture occur, but in this syndrome the kidneys are usually the only organs affected. The endothelium of the glomeruli and renal arterioles are damaged with localized deposition of platelets and fibrin located predominantly subendothelially.

**Clinical Features.** A prodromal acute febrile illness with nausea and vomiting is followed by renal dysfunction, leading to renal failure and significant hypertension. The syndrome may be seasonal, occurring in the autumn months.

**Laboratory Features.** The presence of schistocytes on the peripheral smear is the predominant hematologic finding. The platelet count may or may not be decreased. Reticulocytosis is often present, and nucleated red blood cells are often found in the peripheral blood (normoblastemia). The white cell count is usually also elevated.

Impairment in renal function is reflected by increased blood urea nitrogen and creatinine levels. Urinalysis shows red blood cells and granular and hyaline casts. Deteriorating renal function is the rule, as evidenced by decompensated fluid and electrolyte balance.

**Management.** Supportive therapy, antihypertensive therapy, blood transfusion, and hemodialysis during the acute phase of HUS produces favorable results. Only a small number of patients have residual (renal) damage; however, 25 percent of patients may have persisting hypertension.

## Postpartum Hemolytic Uremic Syndrome

A disorder that is analogous to HUS that occurs in children may rarely complicate pregnancy. The disorder may be a focal (renal) expression of the TTP syndrome. The etiology is unknown; pathologically, the vessels show subendothelial deposition of periodic acid–Schiff (PAS)–positive material, a feature that is seen in both HUS and TTP.

## Disseminated Intravascular Coagulation (DIC)

This condition is discussed more completely in Chapter 30. The principal event is the activation of the coagulation system, leading to intravascular generation of thrombin. The clinical and laboratory features are manifestations of various pathogenetic events, producing a DIC syndrome with differing clinical manifestations.

Fragmentation in the peripheral blood smear, together with the hemoglobinemia and hemoglobinuria that result, is a characteristic feature of DIC.

Low levels of platelets and the clotting factors fibrinogen, prothrombin, factor V, and factor VIII result from constant activation and consumption. This is an important cause of the bleeding disorder that is seen in this syndrome and accounts for the term "consumptive coagulopathy."

Disseminated intravascular coagulopathy may also manifest a varied clinical spectrum, depending on whether the thrombo-occlusive events or the coagulopathy is most prominent. Often both may coexist, making therapeutic management difficult (see Chapter 29).

## Disseminated Carcinoma

Microangiopathic hemolytic anemia is seen in epithelial malignancies, particularly gastric carcinoma. When present, it is associated with severe anemia and a poor prognosis **(see Color Figure 125)**. The hemolytic anemia improves only with effective therapy of the primary lesion, chemotherapy for gastric carcinoma, or hormonal therapy (breast or prostate carcinoma).

The chemotherapeutic drug mitomycin C has been reported to be associated with a TTP/HUS-like syndrome, occasionally occurring in patients who are apparently in remission from their primary tumor. The drug is a commonly used agent in the treatment of bowel cancer. The actual mechanism is uncertain but is felt to be mediated through immune complexes.

### Miscellaneous

**Malignant Hypertension.** The cardinal feature of this disease is appearance of fibrin-like material in the walls of small arteries and arterioles, called fibrinoid necrosis. The high blood pressure and impedence to flow causes red cell fragmentation **(see Color Figure 126)**.

**Pre-eclampsia and Eclampsia.** The uterine spiral and basal arteries are partially or completely blocked by internal aggregates of fibrin, thrombi, and large lipid-laden cells. In the advanced form, the disease may progress to DIC. Hemolysis is manifested by a sudden drop in hemoglobin, an increased reticulocyte count, and red cell fragmentation (schistocytes).

**Vasculitis.** Immune-related vascular injury, with an inflammatory infiltrate on biopsy of involved vessels, may occur in systemic lupus erythematosus, rheumatoid arthritis, polyarteritis, and Sjögren's syndrome. Red cell fragmentation may be seen owing to microvascular inflammation with partial vascular occlusion.

**Renal Allograft Rejection.** Acute rejection causes intravascular thrombosis, endothelial swelling and proliferation, and fibrinoid necrosis. In chronic rejection these vascular changes progress to extensive intimal fibrosis with obliteration of the vessel lumen, and glomerular fibrosis and ischemia. All these vascular changes may cause mechanical impairment of blood flow producing red cell fragmentation.

All the aforementioned conditions may or may not have an associated DIC syndrome. In most cases when erythrocyte fragmentation is seen, DIC is coexistent.

### Macroangiopathic Hemolytic Anemia

Abnormalities within the heart and large vessels may cause hemolysis of red cells, with or without surgical correction of the abnormality. Impedence to flow or prosthetic material within the heart or great vessels can lead to erythrocyte fragmentation. Stenosed aortic valves, particularly if severe, with a high pressure gradient across the valve, generate great shear stresses on the red cells. Prosthetic valves with inadequate apertures cause hemolysis in a similar way. The material of the prosthetic valves or patches used to repair intracardiac defects may create roughened surfaces; the red cells are caused to rupture when propelled against these surfaces by the pumping action of the heart. Faulty fixation of prosthetic valves and patches may create abnormal channels through which red cells are forced, causing hemolysis. Large pressure gradients across cardiac valves — especially the aortic valve in conditions such as idiopathic subaortic stenosis — may also lead to the erythrocyte fragmentation and chronic intravascular hemolysis.

Anemia caused by the fragmentation hemolysis leads to compensatory tachycardia and greater forces of cardiac contraction, thus aggravating the increased stresses the red cells are subjected to. Exercise will aggravate hemolysis similarly.

### March Hemoglobinuria

A mild hemolytic disorder, usually manifested only by hematuria, may occur with repetitive traumatic stress exerted upon intradermal vascular channels, as occurs in strenuous marching. Similar stresses are produced during running, karate exercises, and bongo drumming.

The degree of march hemolysis can be lessened by advising athletes to pad the insoles of their shoes.

## HYPERSPLENISM

Red cell survival is shortened in the presence of an enlarged spleen. The degree of anemia produced depends on the capacity of the marrow to compensate for the excessive red cell loss. Reticulocytosis and occasionally earlier red cell precursors may appear in the peripheral circulation as a manifestation of marrow stress. The number of conditions associated with splenic enlargement is great. Those associated with hypersplenism, as listed in Table 13–3.

**Mechanisms of Anemia.** The hemoconcentration within the spleen presents an unfavorable microenvironment for the red cell. Prolonged transit of red cells through an enlarged spleen leads to the loss of membrane surface area. The resultant decreased red cell survival, together with the pooling of a significant fraction of red cells within the enlarged spleen, is the principal cause of the anemia.

## GENERAL SYSTEMIC DISORDERS ASSOCIATED WITH NONIMMUNE HEMOLYTIC ANEMIA

Nonimmune hemolytic phenomena may be a contributing factor producing anemia in patients with

**Table 13-3. CAUSES OF SPLENOMEGALY ASSOCIATED WITH HYPERSPLENISM**

Congestive
  Intrahepatic obstructive portal hypertension
  Extrahepatic obstructive portal hypertension
    Portal vein
    Splenic vein
  Chronic passive congestion of cardiac origin
Reactive
  Acute infections
    Bacterial
    Viral
  Chronic infections
    Tuberculosis
    Brucellosis
    Malaria
    Kala-azar
  Inflammatory conditions
    Felty's syndrome
    Systemic lupus erythematosus
    Sarcoidosis
  Chronic hemolytic disorders
Infiltrative
  Storage disorders
  Malignant disorders
    Leukemias
    Lymphomas
    Secondary carcinoma
Idiopathic

general systemic disorders; such anemia is multifactorial in most cases. In addition, as in renal disease, more than one cause of shortened red cell survival is found. For instance, red cells from patients with renal disease have inherently shortened survival in addition to the microangiopathy associated with many renal disorders. General systemic disorders associated with microangiopathy and hypersplenism will not be mentioned here.

## Anemia of Chronic Disorders

Chronic infections (such as osteomyelitis), chronic inflammatory disorders (such as collagen diseases), and various malignancies are associated with an anemia of "chronic disorders." Shortened red cell survival is one of four established mechanisms producing anemia. Other mechanisms include a reticuloendothelial iron blockade, decreased serum levels of essential compounds, and marrow depression. (For a more complete description, see Chapter 14.)

## Lipid Disorders

Changes in blood lipid concentrations cause abnormalities in the red cell membrane lipid composition. Resultant alterations in red cell deformability lead to decreased red cell survival. The condition of spur cell anemia **(see Color Figure 129)**, in which abundant sharp, spiculated red cells occur in associ-

ation with hyperlipidemia and liver disease, has been called Zieve's syndrome. Patients with this condition have a hemolytic anemia.

## Liver Disease

Two types of nonimmune hemolytic anemia are found in patients with liver disease. In the first type, decreased red cell survival with anemia and acanthocytosis is associated with markedly distorted red cell shapes called spur cells, or acanthocytes **(see Color Figure 130)**. This type of anemia may occur in patients with advanced alcoholic cirrhosis and portal hypertension. Acanthocytes are also seen in the rare disorder abetalipoproteinemia. The red cell abnormality is due to its excessive cholesterol content, which decreases its deformability. As the membrane becomes more rigid, it can no longer negotiate small vascular channels and it is damaged every time it passes through the microvasculature of the spleen, where it is eventually destroyed.

The second type of nonimmune hemolytic anemia found in patients with liver disease appears more acutely and is associated with abdominal pain and hyperlipidemia. These episodes usually coincide with alcoholic binges, producing acute fatty necrosis of the liver of patients with chronic alcoholic cirrhosis. This acute form has been termed Zieve's syndrome, mentioned earlier.

## Renal Disease

Retained excretory products found in patients with renal disease create unfavorable conditions for red cells. Red cell survival is shortened, but excessive plasma volumes (dilutional anemia), a direct suppressive effect on the bone marrow (hypoproliferative anemia), blood loss, and iron and folate deficiency all contribute to the anemia universally found in such patients.

The cells are normochromic and normocytic; a few cells appear distorted by multiple blunted projections and are called burr cells, or echinocytes **(see Color Figure 123)**. These cells are round or crenated cells with multiple tiny, round-ended spicules covering the entire surface. Burr cells are occasionally seen in patients with pyruvate kinase deficiency or with conditions associated with gastrointestinal bleeding such as peptic ulcers. They may be seen also in patients in dehydration states and are thought to occur from changes in tonicity of the intravascular fluid.

Fibrin deposition in the capillary loops of the glomeruli is found in many renal diseases. Thus, red cell fragmentation is thought to be the principal cause of the shortened red cell survival. Metabolically stressed cells are particularly vulnerable. A dialyzable factor is believed to impair the sodium-potassium pumps of the red cell membrane, rendering the red cell rigid. The rigid cells pass through the fibrin strands with difficulty, and portions of the membrane are sliced off to appear as fragments in the peripheral blood smear.

Hemodialysis may improve the anemia as well as the red cell survival. However, hemodialysis may produce additional problems. Blood is lost within the disposable membrane filter, and folic acid is dialyzable and supplementation is essential. Hemolysis may occur also. The tap water used in the dialysis machine creates a hypotonic medium, causing the cells to imbibe water, swell, and rupture. A cold reacting anti-N red cell antibody may cause hemolysis. These antibodies are associated with the use of ethylene oxide used to sterilize the disposable dialysis membrane.

The anemia of renal disease is discussed further in Chapter 14.

## Vitamin E Deficiency

Premature infants fed on polyunsaturated fatty acids in artificial foods may develop hemolysis in four to six weeks, owing to vitamin E (alpha-tocopherol) deficiency. This fat-soluble vitamin serves as an antioxidant to maintain red cell membrane integrity. These patients respond to vitamin E supplementation with brisk reticulocytosis.

## CASE HISTORIES
### Case 1

A 34-year old patient presented to the medical service with a two-day history of episodic chills and rigors. He had been completely well before, having just returned from a safari tour in Central Africa. On closer questioning, he admitted that he had neglected taking regular prophylaxis against malaria.

Examination revealed a fit, anxious man, with severe rigors, who had mild pallor and appeared jaundiced. Abdominal examination revealed a normal-sized liver, but the patient's spleen was enlarged to 2 cm below the left costal margin. Blood studies revealed a normochromic, normocytic anemia, with a hematocrit of 25 percent, and a reticulocyte count of 20 percent (corrected to 5 percent); LDH levels were raised to 1250 IU/l and bilirubin levels to 6 mg/dl, mostly unconjugated. Urine examination was positive for hemoglobin on dipstick testing, but no red cells were observed on microscopic examination. A fingerprick was performed and thin and thick slides were made and stained with Wright's stain. Typical ring forms of Plasmodium falciparum were observed. The patient was started on chloroquine therapy, to which he had a prompt response.

**Comment.** Splenomegaly is a frequent finding in malarial infection and an important aid in the clinical diagnosis. Red cells contain the enzyme lactic dehydrogenase (LDH), and high levels of this enzyme together with increase amounts of unconjugated bilirubin are important indicators of red cell hemolysis. With severe hemolysis, free hemoglobin appears in the urine. The dipstick urine testing will appear positive for blood, but no red cells are visible on microscopy.

### Case 2

A 40-year-old man presented to the emergency room, complaining of severe shortness of breath and cough. Two years earlier, he had undergone aortic valve replacement for tight aortic valve stenosis. He remained well for a year after surgery, but then noted dyspnea on exertion. The soft ejection murmur noted earlier had increased in intensity, and a paravalvular leak due to loosening of a small section of anchoring sutures of the valve prosthesis was suspected. Since then, his hematocrit fell gradually, associated with mild reticulocytosis, mildly raised LDH, and normal serum bilirubin levels. His urine test for hemoglobin was positive, and red cells were not present on microscopic examination, which indicated hemoglobinuria. Two weeks before his present illness, the patient developed a cough productive of purulent sputum. He became pyrexial two days before presentation.

On examination, the patient appeared ill and pale, with a temperature of 39°C, a rapid pulse rate of 100 beats/min, and a blood pressure of 150/50 mm Hg. Chest examination revealed signs of a right lower-lobe consolidation. His jugular venous pressure was raised to 4 cm above the clavicle, with a liver enlarged to 4 cm below the costal margin, and pedal edema. Heart examination revealed a harsh systolic murmur at the aortic region radiating to the neck, with a soft early diastolic component.

His hematocrit was measured at 26 percent, MCV 72 fl, MCH 20 pg ($\mu\mu$g), with a reticulocyte count of 12 percent (corrected to 3 percent). The platelet count was 350,000/mm³. The blood smear showed anisocytosis and anisochromia with microspherocytes and fragmented forms **(see Color Figure 122)**. The urine tested positive for both hemoglobin and hemosiderin, indicating longstanding hemolysis. Serum bilirubin levels were raised to 4 mg/dl, LDH was raised to 430 IU/l, and haptoglobin levels were decreased to 0 mg/dl. The serum iron was 21 $\mu$g/dl and total iron-binding capacity (TIBC) 380 $\mu$g/dl.

The patient was treated for cardiac failure, transfused slowly with packed cells, and treated with antibiotics. Following resolution of his infection, he was subjected to cardiac catheterization and angiography and was found to have a significant leak alongside the prosthetic valve. At surgery the defective valve was removed and replaced. The patient had good recovery and is well one year after surgery.

**Comment.** Initially the mild hemolysis was well tolerated, but the increasing anemia, causing a raised heart rate, accentuated the degree of hemolysis. The lung infection caused fever and even greater cardiac stress, leading to increased hemolysis of red cells across the defective cardiac valve.

A macroangiopathic hemolytic anemia is suggested by the patient's history (cardiac valve prosthesis), the red cell morphology (schistocytes), and the normal platelet count.

Iron deficiency is not uncommon in patients with chronic intravascular hemolysis, as the ongoing hemolytic state depletes haptoglobin, allowing for hemosiderin loss in the urine. Over time this can amount to a substantial iron loss as reflected in the patient's red cell morphology and serum iron levels. Many patients with cardiac valve prostheses are given prophylactic iron supplementation for this reason.

## Bibliography

Amorosi, EL and Ultmann, JE: Thrombotic thrombocytopenic purpura: Report of 16 cases and review of the literature. Medicine 45:139, 1966.

Antman, KH, Skarin, AT, Mayer, RJ, et al: Microangiopathic hemolytic anemia and cancer: A review. Medicine 58:377, 1979.

Bowdler, AJ: Splenomegaly and hypersplenism. Clin Haematol 12(2):467, 1983.

Brain, MC: The hemolytic-uremic syndrome. Semin Hematol 6:162, 1969.

Brain, MC, Sacie, JV, and Hourihane DO'B: Microangiopathic haemolytic anaemia:The possible role of vascular lesions in pathogenesis. Br J Haematol 8:355, 1962.

Bull, BS, Rubenberg, ML, Dacie, JV, et al: Microangiopathic hemolytic anemia: Mechanism of red cell fragmentation; in vitro studies. Br J Haematol 14;643, 1968.

Goldstein, E; Bartonellosis. In Hoeprich, PD (ed): Infectious Disease, ed 2. Harper & Row, Hagerstown, MD, 1977, p 1072.

Gordon-Smith, EC: Drug-induced oxidative haemolysis. Clin Haematol 9:557, 1980.

Harlan, JM: Thrombocytopenia due to non-immune platelet destruction. Clin Haematol 12(1):39, 1983.

Healy, GR: Babesia infections in man. Hosp Pract 14:107, 1979.

Miller, LH, Mason, SJ, Dvorak, JA, et al: Erythrocyte receptors for (Plasmodium Knowlesi) malaria: Duffy blood group determinants. Science 189:561, 1975.

Perrin, LH, Mackey, LJ, and Miescher, PA: The hematology of malaria in man. Semin Hematol 19:70, 1982.

Remuzzi, G, Marchesi, D, Mecca, G, et al: Hemolytic-uremic syndrome: Deficiency of plasma factors regulating prostacycline activity. Lancet 2:871, 1978.

Rosner, F, Zarrabi, MH, Benach, JL, et al: Babesiosis in splenectomized adults: Review of 22 reported cases. Am J Med 76:696, 1984.

Wu, EC-Y, Harkness, DR, Byrnes, JJ, et al: Presence of a platelet aggregating factor in the plasma of patients with thrombotic thrombocytopenic purpura and its inhibition by normal plasma. Blood 53:333, 1979.

CHAPTER **14**

HARVEY LUKSENBURG, M.D.

# Anemia Associated With Other Disorders: Infection, Renal Disease, Liver Disease, Endocrine Disease, Connective Tissue Disease, and Malignancies

A clinician usually encounters anemia in one of three ways: (1) as a concurrent finding in a patient with an already diagnosed illness or illnesses; (2) as a finding in the investigation of new or undiagnosed complaints in a previously stable patient; and (3) as an unexpected laboratory finding in an asymptomatic patient (e.g., in the course of a routine physical examination). Anemia is a common laboratory finding in many systemic illnesses and is often mild and asymptomatic. It is not always clear whether anemia is due to a single cause (e.g., a known pre-existing illness) or to more than one cause (e.g., a pre-existing illness plus a new undiagnosed neoplasm). Elucidating the causes of anemia is often difficult and may require a hematologist's assistance.

It is helpful to know some of the characteristic types of anemia in various systemic illness, what laboratory findings to expect, and when to become suspicious that more than one process may be occurring. If a patient with chronic rheumatoid arthritis with a previously stable hematocrit (HCT) of 32 percent and a normal mean corpuscular volume (MCV) (these values are typical for this disease) returns for re-evaluation a few months later with a hematocrit of 22 percent and MCV of 69 fl, then suspicions should be raised that something new is occurring. Rheumatoid arthritis is not associated with a low MCV. A workup may reveal chronic gastrointestinal blood loss, which could possibly be due to a coexisting malignancy or to gastritis from aspirin the patient is taking for the arthritis.

It is also important to know that some diseases, if uncomplicated, are *not* associated with anemia. The "anemia of chronic disease" is a potentially misleading term, for it seems to imply that any chronic disease may be associated with anemia. This is not true. Diabetes mellitus is not associated with anemia, unless the diabetes is complicated by renal failure, a chronic infection, or a previously undiagnosed disease. Atherosclerotic coronary artery disease, certainly a "chronic disease," does not cause anemia. "Old age" also is not a cause of anemia. By neglecting to note the appearance of a mild abnormality such as anemia, a clinician may miss the first signs of a potentially serious disease.

This chapter discusses the major categories of systemic illness — infections, renal and hepatic disease, endocrine disease, connective tissue disease, and malignancies — with some of the characteristic features of the anemias associated with each type of illness.

## INFECTION: ITS EFFECT ON RED BLOOD CELLS

Infections tend to affect the production or destruction of red blood cells in one of four ways: (1) through the effects of chronic inflammation on the bone marrow (the so-called anemia of chronic disease), (2) through direct parasitization of the red cell, leading to hemolysis (malaria, babesiosis), (3) via the production of infection-associated cold agglutinins, and (4) through direct infection of the red cell precursors of the bone marrow (human parvovirus) (Table 14–1).

## Anemia of Chronic Disease

The persistence of any infection for a period of more than two or three weeks sets in motion a complex, multisystem series of events, called the "acute-

phase response." Many of the effects of this response seem to be mediated by interleukin-1, a polypeptide that is produced by the monocyte/macrophage system, and by several other specialized cells scattered throughout the body. Interleukin-1 has numerous effects on many different tissues, the most important being the production of fever, the increased synthesis of the so-called acute-phase reactants (fibrinogen, C-reactive protein, haptoglobin) by the liver, the neutrophilic leukocytosis commonly seen in infections, and the lowering of the serum iron that is the hallmark of the anemia of chronic disease.[1]

The striking characteristic of the anemia of chronic disease is a low serum iron and low total iron-binding capacity in the face of increased tissue stores of iron. The iron is trapped in the macrophages of the spleen, liver, and bone marrow, and the normal plasma transport system that shuttles the iron from these storage sites to the bone marrow seems to be operating at a reduced level.[2] A mild to moderate anemia ensues. Characteristically, the anemia develops over the first weeks of a chronic infection and persists at the same level. The hematocrit settles at a value between 30 and 40 percent and is either normocytic and normochromic or slightly hypochromic and microcytic (**see Color Figure 00**). The reticulocyte count is decreased. Usually, other commonly measured markers of the acute-phase response are present, such as elevations in the white blood cell count, erythrocyte sedimentation rate, haptoglobin, and fibrinogen.

In some patients it may be difficult to differentiate between the anemia of chronic of disease and iron-deficiency anemia. These patients may have a low MCV (usually 78 to 80 fl) and a transferrin saturation of 10 to 15 percent. The easiest way to make this distinction is to perform a bone marrow aspiration for the purpose of examining iron stores. A patient with iron-deficiency anemia will have no stainable iron, while the patient with anemia of chronic disease will have increased iron, most of which is "locked up" in the bone marrow macrophages.[3] Alternatively, serum ferritin can be measured, and it correlates well with bone marrow iron stores, except in acute inflammatory conditions (see Chapter 4).

The anemia of chronic disease can be found in any patients with persistent infection. Common causes seen in contemporary medical practice are subacute bacterial endocarditis, pulmonary tuberculosis, lung abscesses, and chronically infected decubitus ulcers or diabetic foot ulcers. Since the anemia of chronic disease seems to be an adaptive response of the body to chronic infection, only the treatment of the infection can reverse it. As mentioned earlier, the iron stores are adequate or increased, and treatment with oral or parenteral iron is of no value.

**Table 14–1.** EFFECT OF INFECTIONS ON RED BLOOD CELLS

1. Suppressive effects
   "Anemia of Chronic Disease" — Anemia of Inflammation
2. Direct parasitization of the red cell
   Malaria
   Babesiosis
   Bartonella bacilliformis
3. Immune hemolysis through cold agglutinins
   Infectious mononucleosis (anti-i)
   Mycoplasma pneumoniae (anti-I)
   Syphillis (anti-P)
   Rubella, rubeola, mumps (anti-P)
4. Direct infection of red cell precursors
   Parvovirus
   Hepatitis B

## Organisms that Parasitize the Erythrocyte

By far the most important organism in this category is the malarial parasite. Malaria is a protozoan that has a complex life cycle involving both mosquitoes and humans (see Chapter 13). The bite of an infected mosquito injects plasmodial sporozoites into the blood. These develop into merozoites, which invade the circulating erythrocytes **(see Color Figures 117 and 118)**. Following intraerythrocytic development, the merozoites cause the cell to rupture. The rupture of the schizonts is often synchronized and occurs at regular intervals. Clinically, the rupture causes severe fever, chills, and prostration.

Anemia is an important manifestation of all malarial infections. The hemolysis caused by the mechanical disruption of red cells from the bursting of schizonts is an important component of this anemia, but recent studies seem to indicate that it is not the only component. The bone marrow production of red cells is depressed, and examination of marrows in infected patients has shown abnormalities in the appearance of red cell precursors (dyserythropoiesis). These abnormalities disappear with resolution of the infection. In addition, an immune-mediated destruction of red cells occurs during active malarial infection. This immunologic hemolysis results in the destruction of both parasitized and nonparasitized erythrocytes in the spleen. This process may be due to the binding of immune complexes to red cell surfaces, leading to the activation of components of the complement system (see also Chapter 12).[4]

Babesiosis produces a hemolytic anemia through intraerythrocyte parasitization by Babesia protozoan species (see Chapter 13 and **Color Figure 119)**.

Bartonella bacilliformis is a gram-negative bacterium transmitted to humans through the bite of infected sand flies. This results in destruction of the red cells by the liver and spleen, with a severe hemolytic anemia and severe systemic symptoms.

## Infection-Associated Cold Agglutinin Hemolytic Anemias

The organisms discussed immediately above directly attack red cells. There are two relatively common organisms that by contrast produce antibodies that may adhere to red cells and thereby indirectly cause their destruction. These organisms are Mycoplasma pneumoniae and the Epstein-Barr virus (the causative agent of infectious mononucleosis).[5-7]

## Infections of Red Cell Precursors

In patients with chronic congenital hemolytic anemias (sickle cell disease, hereditary spherocytosis,

and so on), occasionally there are periods during which the bone marrow stops manufacturing red cells, resulting in a precipitous drop in the hematocrit ("aplastic crisis"). This phenomenon usually occurs in children and is often associated with a clinical syndrome consistent with a viral illness. Bone marrow samples obtained during aplastic crises show a dramatic depletion of red cell precursors.

The etiology of aplastic crisis had been obscure, but recently convincing evidence has accumulated that the causative agent is a DNA virus, human parvovirus. Experiments in which human parvovirus has been cultured with bone marrow elements have demonstrated this agent's cytotoxicity toward erythroid precursors.[8]

## ANEMIA OF CHRONIC RENAL DISEASE

Normocytic, normochromic anemia frequently accompanies chronic renal disease. Morphologically, the red cells often show burr cell formation, most likely a result of osmotic changes in the intravascular fluid **(see Color Figure 127)**. The etiology of this anemia is multifactorial (Table 14–2).

## Decrease in Erythropoietin Production

The kidneys are the site of most of the production of erythropoietin, the hormone that mediates the control of red blood cells. Thus, in chronic renal disease, when the kidneys often become atrophied or sclerosed, a concurrent decrease in erythropoietin production is seen. Many patients with chronic renal disease maintain hemotocrit levels in the range of 20 to 25 percent. Patients who have had both kidneys removed tend to have even lower hematocrit values. The liver is thought to produce some erythropoietin in compensation. The trans-

**Table 14–2. MECHANISMS INVOLVED IN ANEMIA OF RENAL DISEASE**

1. Hypoproliferative Anemia
   ↓ Erythropoietin — ↓ Erythroid committed precursors
   Suppressive effects of uremic toxins on erythroid precursors
   Folate deficiency (hemodialysis)
2. Hemolytic Anemia
   Unfavorable chemical environment
   Uremic toxins
3. Dilutional Anemia
   Abnormal fluid retention
4. Blood Loss Anemia
   Gastrointestinal bleeding
   Blood drawn for laboratory tests
   Hemodialysis
   Chronic iron deficiency
5. Hypersplenism
   Chronic renal dialysis associated splenomegaly

plantation of a viable kidney into a patient with chronic renal disease can restore the hematocrit level to normal.

## Uremia

The milieu created by the accumulation of "uremic toxins" (substances that are normally excreted by the kidneys but that build up in the plasma owing to impaired renal function) affects the synthesis of red blood cells at the site of their production in the bone marrow and the length of their survival in the peripheral circulation. In vitro experiments in which bone marrow cultures have been incubated with uremic plasma have demonstrated impaired production of late red cell precursors. Red blood cell survival studies (carried out with radiochromium-labeled red cells) demonstrate a decline in the average cell lifespan.[9]

In addition, a platelet dysfunction that results in a bleeding disorder is associated with the buildup of uremic toxins.

## Hemodialysis

A certain amount of red blood cells are hemolyzed after each dialysis session as a result of mechanical injury associated with instrumentation. This form of chronic blood loss may result in iron-deficiency anemia if the iron is not replaced. In addition some patients on hemodialysis may develop a folate deficiency, as folate is a dialyzable substance. Development of iron-deficiency anemia or folate deficiency would change the morphologic classification of the anemia from normocytic, normochromic to microcytic, hypochromic and macrocytic anemia, respectively.

Thus, the entire apparatus of red cell production, regulation, and peripheral survival is impaired during chronic renal failure. Despite a frequent reduction of the hematocrit to half its normal value, many patients can tolerate this anemia quite well. Other patients, however, require tranfusions to alleviate symptoms due to anemia. Dialysis alone brings about only a minor improvement in the hematocrit level. Androgenic steroids, particularly if given subcutaneously, may be of some benefit, but the improvement in hematocrit, which may be slight, is often outweighed by the drugs' side effects.[10]

Critical evaluation of the status, progression, and severity of the disease state will determine which patients are candidates for renal transplant. **Color Figure 128** shows the peripheral blood of a patient after renal transplant and splenectomy.

## ANEMIA ASSOCIATED WITH LIVER DISEASE

The anemia of chronic liver disease, like that of renal failure, is often complicated by other factors, such as iron deficiency (owing to blood loss) or folate deficiency (a vitamin often lacking in the diet of alcoholics) (Table 14–3).

The most common form of anemia associated with chronic liver disease is the "anemia of chronic disease," which is often a normocytic, normochromic anemia. However, in many cases a macrocytosis may be seen (MCV 100 to 115) that is not associated with folate or vitamin $B_{12}$ deficiency. In contradistinction to the macrocytosis of megaloblastic anemia, in which there are *oval* macrocytes, the macrocytic cells of liver disease morphologically are *round*. The macrocytosis of liver disease is often associated with the morphologic finding of *target cells* on the peripheral smear **(see Color Figure 129)**. Target cells (so called because of the "bull's eye" appearance they present on peripheral smears) are thin red cells with an increased diameter. An increased proportion of cholesterol from the plasma to the red cell membrane exists, which is thought to be due to a transfer of cholesterol from the plasma to the red cell membrane. Target cells do not have an increased propensity to be destroyed in the spleen.[11]

Patients with severe liver disease often develop the red cell morphologic finding of *acanthocytosis*, or "spur cell anemia" **(see Color Figure 130)**. These cells show five to 10 irregular sharp spicules, and are destroyed by the reticuloendothelial system, resulting in a hemolytic anemia. The presence of spur cells on the peripheral smear of a patient with cirrhosis is said to indicate a poor prognosis.

A certain shortening in the red cell survival time has been noted in most patients with chronic liver disease in whom red cell survival has been measured. Patients with splenomegaly due to portal hypertension often have a profound shortening of red cell survival. The usual compensatory response by

## Table 14–3. ANEMIA OF LIVER DISEASE

1. Defective Erythrocyte Development
   Ineffective erythropoiesis
       Folate deficiency (poor nutrition; alcoholism)
       Iron deficiency (associated gastrointestinal bleeding)
       Pyridoxine deficiency (alcoholism)
       Protein deficiency (hypoproteinemia)
   Hypoproliferative anemia
       "Anemia of chronic disease" (e.g., chronic hepatitis)
       Primary viral suppression (hepatitis B, EBV, CMV)
       Toxic suppression (impaired liver clearance)
       Alcoholic bone marrow suppression
2. Dilutional Anemia
   Elevated plasma volume in cirrhosis
3. Hypersplenism
   Erythrocyte sequestration with congestive splenomegaly
4. Hemolytic Anemia
   Spur cell anemia (abnormal membrane lipids); acanthocytosis
5. Blood Loss Anemia
   Bleeding from esophageal varices—mechanical
   Bleeding associated with coagulopathy of liver disease

the bone marrow, as seen by an elevated reticulocyte count, may be impaired owing to the concurrent presence of folate deficiency or iron deficiency or both. Alcohol ingestion will also blunt the marrow's reticulocyte response. In addition, patients with cirrhosis may have an increased plasma volume, which adds a dilutional factor to the anemia.[12]

Thus, patients with known hepatic disease and anemia should be evaluated for the presence of gastrointestinal blood loss and possible iron deficiency. The folate level should also be assessed. Other factors that will blunt the marrow's responsiveness such as acute alcohol intoxication or infection should also be sought.

## ANEMIA ASSOCIATED WITH ENDOCRINE DISEASE

### Thyroid Disease

Anemia occurs in patients with hypothyroidism more commonly than in those with hyperthyroid states. The anemia found in women with hypothyroidism may be due to iron deficiency, since menorrhagia may be a complicating factor. Patients with macrocytosis and goiter should be screened for folate or vitamin $B_{12}$ deficiency. Patients with autoimmune hypothyroidism have a higher incidence of pernicious anemia. Hypothyroidism per se is also known to lead to a mild increase in the MCV.

Finally, a mild normocytic, normochromic anemia may be found in patients with hypothyroidism uncomplicated by nutritional deficiencies. Thyroid hormone apparently has a minor role in the regulation of erythropoiesis, acting on red cell precursors in a synergistic manner with the major regulating hormone erythropoietin.[13]

### Hypogonadism

Androgens have important roles as stimulants of erythroid activity, both physiologically and therapeutically. The hemoglobin concentration of a healthy adult male is 1 to 2 g/dl higher than that of a healthy adult female. This difference is thought to be due to the effect of androgens, which seem to promote erythropoiesis in at least two ways: (1) by increasing the production of erythropoietin by the kidney; and (2) by a direct stimulatory effect on the marrow in conjunction with erythropoietin.[14] Pharmacologic doses of androgens are often given to patients with anemia due to primary bone marrow diseases with varying degrees of success.

It is not surprising that males with hypogonadism and decreased levels of androgens may have anemias. These anemias are usually mild and may be reversed with administration of androgen.

### Pituitary Dysfunction

A mild to moderate anemia is seen in many patients with hypopituitarism. Since the pituitary secretes both thyroid-stimulating hormone (TSH) and gonadotrophins (which control the production of androgens), the presence of anemia in such patients is not surprising. However, the optimal correction of the anemia in such patients seems to require not only the replacement of thyroid hormone and androgens but also the administration of steroids (for adrenal deficiency).

## ANEMIA ASSOCIATED WITH CONNECTIVE TISSUE DISORDERS

All of the chronic connective tissue diseases may lead to the anemia of chronic disease (see earlier section). However, other factors may complicate the expression of the anemia. One important consideration is gastrointestinal blood loss, from ingesting either aspirin or another nonsteroidal anti-inflammatory medication. All of these drugs share the side effect of irritation of the upper gastrointestinal mucosa, which can lead to gastritis. The cumulative effects of small amounts of daily blood loss may cause an iron-deficiency anemia. In addition, corticosteroids, which have an important place in the management of these disorders, are associated with an increased incidence of peptic ulcer disease, a potential source of blood loss.

### Rheumatoid Arthritis

Anemia is a common but asymptomatic manifestation of rheumatoid arthritis. It is usually mild (hemoglobin 10 to 11 g/dl), and normocytic. The anemia tends to fluctuate in accordance with the clinical severity of the disease: severe disease is generally associated with more profound anemia. When bone marrow from patients with rheumatoid arthritis is cultured, smaller numbers of early precursors to red cells are found than in nonarthritic patients. The level of serum IgM and rheumatoid factor was shown to be inversely proportional to the number of red cell precursor colonies.[15] This suggests that certain immunoglobulins may have a suppressive effect on the marrow's production of red cells.

### Systemic Lupus Erythematosus

As in rheumatoid arthritis, systemic lupus erythematosus is often associated with the anemia of chronic disease, which may fluctuate with the activity of the disease. In addition, a humoral inhibitor (IgG or IgM) has been demonstrated in some patients that will suppress the growth of early red cell precursors, the activity of these antibodies was reduced following steroid treatment or plasmapheresis.[16]

Systemic lupus is associated with the production of numerous autoantibodies, some of which are directed at common antigens on red cells. Thus, another important mechanism that can lead to anemia in this disease is autoimmune hemolytic anemia. This is associated with a direct Coombs test, which detects the presence of IgG of complement adherent to the red cell membrane. As these "coated" cells circulate through the spleen and liver, they undergo either partial or complete phagocytosis by the macrophages. Partial phagocytosis results in the formation of spherocytes—cells in which part of the membrane has been lost, causing a change from the normal, biconcave-disc morphology to that of a sphere.

Unlike the anemia of chronic disease, the autoimmune hemolytic anemia associated with systemic lupus may be severe and symptomatic and can become an indication for treatment. The major treatment is corticosteroid therapy, which results in decreased hemolysis by bringing about a decrease in the titer of the antibodies that adhere to the red cells and by blocking the uptake of antibody-coated red cells by the macrophages of the spleen and liver. In patients who do not respond to steroids or who develop major side effects from these drugs, the addition of alkylating agents such cyclophosphamide or azathioprine may be useful. Splenectomy may be a helpful treatment, since in removing the spleen, a major site of red cell destruction is eliminated.

Renal disease is a frequent manifestation of systemic lupus. The development of chronic renal failure will superimpose the anemia associated with this entity (see earlier section) onto any pre-existing anemia.[17]

## ANEMIA ASSOCIATED WITH MALIGNANCY

The hematologic effects of malignancies are multifactorial and depend on the particular type of cancer as well as the site or sites in the body in which it occurs. The mechanisms of anemia in cancer may be broadly divided as follows: (1) direct effect of a tumor, (2) indirect effect of a tumor, and (3) effect of treatment (Table 14–4).

### Direct Effects

The presence of anemia, either symptomatic or asymptomatic, is often the first clue that a malignancy is present in a patient. Any gastrointestinal malignancy may produce bleeding, and over time this chronic blood loss may lead to an iron-deficiency anemia. Similarly, a tumor in the bladder or

**Table 14–4. MECHANISMS OF ANEMIA IN MALIGNANCY**

1. Direct Effects
   Replacement of marrow by malignant cells
   Primary hematologic malignancy
      Ineffective erythroid production
      Qualitative reduction in erythropoiesis
   Metastatic marrow infiltration
      Quantitative reduction in erythropoiesis
   Replacement of marrow by fibrosis
   Acute and chronic blood loss
2. Indirect Effects
   "Anemia of malignant disease"
   Anemia of associated organ failure (e.g., renal; hepatic)
   Malnutrition and vitamin deficiency
   Microangiopathic hemolytic anemia
   Immune hemolytic anemia
3. Treatment-Associated Anemia
   Immediate
      Chemotherapy
      Radiation therapy
   Late
      Secondary myelodysplasia/leukemia
      Idiopathic    ?Depleted marrow reserve
         —Microangiopathic hemolytic anemia
         (Postmitomycin)

kidney may lead to an anemia through urinary blood loss. In women, endometrial cancer is often associated with abnormal vaginal bleeding.

The infiltration of the bone marrow by a malignant tumor (myelophthisis) can lead to anemia (myelophthisic anemia), which is often accompanied by a decrease in the white blood cell and platelet counts. A typical peripheral blood picture exhibiting "leukoerythroblastosis" frequently accompanies marrow infiltration by tumors **(see Color Figure 131)**. This is characterized by the presence of immature white blood cells and nucleated red cells in the peripheral blood. The red cells show marked morphologic abnormalities. The teardrop-shaped red cell exemplifies this syndrome **(see Color Figure 132)**. Malignancies frequently associated with a leukoerythroblastic blood picture include carcinomas of the breast, prostate, and stomach.

Marrow infiltration is, of course, a central feature of all the primary hematologic malignancies. In the acute leukemias, the marrow is usually completely replaced with abnormal blasts. The lymphomas may be associated with varying degrees of bone marrow invasion, ranging from spotty involvement to a total replacement. Hodgkin's disease is a malignant disorder that often disseminates to the bone marrow. Like the lymphomas, Hodgkin's disease may not involve the marrow at all, may be present in a spotty distribution, or may totally efface the normal marrow architecture.

The chronic myeloproliferative diseases (chronic myelogenous leukemia, polycythemia vera, agnogenic myeloid metaplasia) are often associated with fibrosis of the bone marrow. The fibrosis results in the replacement of viable hematopoietic tissue by pathologic, nonfunctioning connective tissue. This leads to a progressive pancytopenia, including a profound anemia that may require frequent transfusion therapy.

## Indirect Effects

The anemia of chronic disease is a common manifestation of all types of malignancies, and the laboratory features are indistinguishable from the uncomplicated anemias that accompany chronic infections or connective tissue diseases. In general, this type of anemia is more common in patients with advanced stages of malignancy. The hemoglobin level may improve with treatment of the underlying malignancy.

Anemias associated with chronic liver or chronic renal disease can occur in patients with cancer. For example, a patient with advanced prostatic carcinoma may develop bilateral blockage of the ureters, leading to renal failure. Liver failure may occur owing to massive infiltration of that organ, resulting from metastatic or primary malignancies.

Advanced malignancies are associated with cachexia and malnutrition, especially in patients undergoing chemotherapy or radiation therapy or both. These patients are prone to develop folate deficiency. Patients who have had partial or complete removal of the stomach because of gastric carcinoma will lose the ability to produce intrinsic factor and can become vitamin $B_{12}$ deficient.

Certain types of hemolytic anemias can develop in patients with malignancies. Lymphomas (especially those of B-cell lineage) may be associated with autoimmune hemolytic anemia, owing to the production of an IgG antibody that reacts with a basic component of the red cell membrane ("panagglutinin") (see Chapter 12). This is associated with a reticulocytosis, and the peripheral smear will demonstrate the presence of spherocytes and polychromatophilia **(see Color Figure 115)**. The hemolytic anemia associated with lymphomas may decrease in severity or disappear when the lymphoma is treated.

Certain types of advanced malignancies, particularly mucin-secreting adenocarcinomas of the gastrointestinal system, may be associated with uncontrolled activation of the coagulation system, leading to deposition of fibrin in small blood vessels throughout the body. Red cells passing through these partially blocked capillaries undergo mechanical shear-induced damage, causing the formation of fragmented cells, or schistocytes. The concurrent activation of the coagulation system leads to depletion of coagulation factors and platelets (disseminated intravascular coagulation), which in turn is associated with an increased tendency toward bleeding. This clinical entity, microangiopathic hemolytic anemia, may be recognized by a reticulocytosis, with schistocytosis and polychromatophilia present on the peripheral smear. The occurrence of microangiopathic hemolytic anemia is associated with a poor prognosis, as this type of anemia is an indicator of widespread metastatic disease (see Chapter 13).[18]

## Treatment-Associated Anemia

Most combination chemotherapy regimens employ one or more of the class of drugs called alkylating agents, which includes chlorambucil, melphalan, nitrogen mustard, cyclophosphamide, and busulfan. These drugs, when given over a short-term period, can cause an acute decrease in the white blood cell and platelet counts. This bone marrow depression is reversible if drug administration is stopped. However, it is not uncommon for patients who received chemotherapy with one or more of these drugs over an extended period of time to develop an irreversible decline in their blood counts. These patients can develop anemia, leukopenia, or thrombocytopenia, either as an isolated laboratory abnormality, or together, as pancytopenia.

The anemia in this setting may be normocytic, microcytic, or macrocytic. Other causes of anemia, such as recurrent tumor, need to be eliminated. On further investigation, many of these patients will be found to have a primary bone marrow disease called the myelodysplastic syndrome. This term covers a group of disorders that have in common cytopenias of varying severity resulting from bone marrow failure; it is often used synonymously with "preleukemia." The myelodysplastic syndrome may occur de novo or in a patient who has been previously treated with chemotherapy, radiation therapy, or both. This syndrome has a high probability of evolving into acute nonlymphocytic leukemia. The leukemias that arise from these myelodysplastic states are usually much more resistant to treatment than is leukemia that occurs in patients who have never been on chemotherapy.

Ironically, the myelodysplastic syndrome and acute leukemia may occur years after a patient with Hodgkin's disease or a lymphoma has been cured of the primary neoplasm.[19]

## HEMATOLOGIC CHANGES IN PATIENTS WITH THE ACQUIRED IMMUNE DEFICIENCY SYNDROME

The acquired immune deficiency syndrome (AIDS) is a chronic infection caused by a retrovirus, the human T-cell leukemia virus (HTLV) type III, also called lymphadenopathy-associated virus (LAV).[20] This virus brings about profound and irreversible destruction of the immune system. The major target of the HTLV III virus is the group of T lymphocytes called the T4 lymphocytes. T4 cells occupy a central position in the mediation of the immune response in humans. As a result, the virus slowly destroys the T4 cells, causing a lymphopenia and a decreased T4:T8 ratio, which characteristically is less than 1.0 in AIDS patients. This leads to a profound suppression of cell-mediated immunity. The clinical manifestations of this defect result in severe and life-threatening opportunistic infections and unusual neoplasms, such as Kaposi's sarcoma. Over a period of time that probably lasts two or more years, this destructive process results in multiple, recurrent infections, with a discrete group of organisms: Pneumocystis carinii, cytomegalovirus, atypical mycobacteria, Toxoplasma gondii, and herpes simplex, to name some of the most common. These infections tend either to respond poorly to available therapy or, if they respond well, to recur when antibiotic therapy is discontinued.[21]

Hematologic abnormalities are common in patients with AIDS. In many cases it is important to try to differentiate potentially reversible causes of cytopenias from those that may be secondary to the disease process itself. Drug reactions are common, especially to trimethoprim/sulfamethoxazole (which is used to treat Pneumocystis carinii pneumonia); these reactions may lead to neutropenia or thrombocytopenia or both.[22] Severe infections may lead to lowering of the white cell and the platelet counts. Hyperactivity of B lymphocytes is also characteristic. Examination of the peripheral smear reveals atypical immunoblastic lymphocytes, anemia, granulocytopenia, and frequently thrombocytopenia. Peculiar-looking vacuolated monocytes have also been reported on peripheral smears. Bone marrow examination usually reveals phagocytic macrophages, which are filled with cellular debris. This finding is very similar to the "hemophagocytic syndrome," which has been defined.

Spivak and colleagues[23] described hematologic abnormalities in 12 patients with AIDS. Ten patients were anemic, eight leukopenic, and three thrombocytopenic. The anemia was hypoproliferative and normochromic, normocytic in character. Castella and associates[24] described 49 patients; of these, 85 percent were anemic, 40 percent neutropenic, and 29 percent thrombocytopenic. Lymphopenia was present in the vast majority of patients.

In both of these series, bone marrow examinations were performed in all patients. No distinctive marrow histologic finding was present. Spivak noted that an increase in bone marrow histiocytes was present in seven marrow aspirates. In five of these seven, histiocytes were seen engulfing red cells, white cells, and platelets. Focal marrow necrosis was a feature in three marrows, and global necrosis was seen in one. Castella's series included eight bone marrows with noncaseating granulomas

present. When cultured for acid-fast bacilli, four of the eight marrows produced Mycobacterium avium intracellulare, an atypical mycobacterial organism commonly encountered in patients with AIDS.

The precise mechanisms by which the HTLV III virus brings about these marrow changes is not known at present. Nevertheless, bone marrow examinations may be useful in patients with AIDS for two reasons: (1) to obtain tissue to aid in the diagnosis of infections and (2) to assess the amount of functioning marrow in patients who may require chemotherapy for treatment of malignancy. Hypocellular marrows may be predictive of poor hematologic tolerance of chemotherapy.

A subgroup of patients with AIDS have developed non-Hodgkin's lymphomas of aggressive histologic types, which will be fatal unless treatment is undertaken.[25] These lymphomas are often located outside of lymph nodes, in areas such as the central nervous system, bone marrow, and gastrointestinal system. Such patients tend to have a high mortality owing to a combination of factors, including overwhelming infection and recurrent or resistant lymphoma.

Hodgkin's disease has also been described in homosexuals with generalized lymphadenopathy (a prodromal form of AIDS).[26] Too few patients have been reported, however, to ascertain whether Hodgkin's disease is more frequent in this population than in uninfected people in the same age group.

## CASE HISTORIES
### Case 1

A 29-year-old woman came to an emergency room complaining of "not feeling well" for the past five days. On physical examination, she was found to be pale; her pulse rate was 100 bpm, blood pressure 110/80, temperature 100°F. A II/VI holosystolic murmur was discovered at the left lower sternal border. Laboratory data showed Hb 10.0 g/dl, HCT 30 percent, MCV 79 fl, white blood cell count of 10,800 with 90 percent neutrophils and 10 percent lymphocytes, and a normal platelet count.

The physician in the emergency room felt that the patient had mild iron-deficiency anemia secondary to menstrual losses. He prescribed ferrous sulfate, 325 mg three times a day.

The patient continued to feel unwell despite the iron therapy. Four days later she saw a physician in an outpatient clinic. Now she felt that in addition to worsening fatigue she was "feverish." Her appetite was poor. Her recent history was revealing only in that one and a half weeks previously she had had some extensive dental work done. The physician examined the patient and found that she was pale. Her temperature was 101°F. She had a rapid, bounding heart rate. A III/VI holosystolic murmur was heard over the left lower sternal border and the apex. The liver and spleen were not palpable, and the rest of the examination was noncontributory.

A complete blood count showed Hb 9.3 g/dl, HCT 29.5 percent, MCV 77 fl, white cell count of 11,800 with 90 percent neutrophils, 5 percent lymphocytes, and 5 percent bands; the reticulocyte count was 1 percent.

The physician hospitalized the patient. Four out of four blood cultures eventually produced Streptococcus viridans. She was diagnosed as having subacute bacterial endocarditis. It was thought that the patient had a prolapsed mitral valve, which became infected during the transient bacteremia associated with the dental work.

**Comment.** Anemia is a nonspecific laboratory finding and needs to be interpreted in the context of a patient's complaints and physical findings. Both the history and the physical examination done by the first physician were superficial: he thought that the slightly decreased MCV of 79 fl was indicative of mild iron deficiency due to menstrual blood losses, and his diagnostic formulation stopped at this point.

A mild decrease in the MCV can be seen *both* in early iron-deficiency anemia and in the anemias associated with systemic disorders. The second physician who saw this patient took more time to elicit a history of recent dental work and performed a more careful examination. He was concerned that the anemia, when considered in context with the patient's physical examination findings and history of systemic complaints, may be indicative of a serious infection.

## Case 2

A 49-year-old man with a long history of alcohol abuse was admitted to the hospital with the complaint of having vomited "half a glass" of bright red blood. His complete blood count on admission showed HCT 31 percent, Hb 10.5 g/dl, and MCV 95 fl. The next day an upper endoscopic examination was performed, which disclosed a duodenal ulcer, that was still oozing blood. The patient was started on antacid therapy. He swore that he would never drink alcohol again.

During the next few months, the patient's duodenal ulcer healed, and he felt better. Four months later, the HCT was 43 percent. Six months later, he came to his physician's office saying that he felt "lousy." He had alcohol on his breath and was unshaven. He admitted to having been drinking heavily for the past four months. He denied nausea or vomiting. His physical examination was unrevealing. A complete blood count showed HCT 29 percent, Hb 9.5 g/dl, and MCV 110 fl. A peripheral smear revealed macrocytic red cells and hypersegmented neutrophils. Serum folate level was below normal limits. The patient's vitamin $B_{12}$ level was normal. The patient was diagnosed as having folate deficiency, owing to poor nutrition and alcoholism. This time the physician told the patient that if he did not stop drinking, he would sooner or later develop alcoholic cirrhosis of the liver, and die. The patient voluntarily entered an intensive alcoholism rehabilitation program.

One year later, the patient went to his physician for a routine checkup. He claimed that he had not had any alcohol for 10 months and was feeling well. Results of a physical examination were normal. A complete blood count showed Hb 10.0 g/dl, HCT 30 percent, and MCV 74 fl. A stool sample tested positive for occult blood. Serum iron level and TIBC were compatible with iron-deficiency anemia. The physician ordered a barium enema, which revealed a small filling defect in the sigmoid colon. A colonoscopy with biopsy revealed a benign colonic polyp, which was the source of the bleeding. An upper gastrointestinal series was normal.

**Comment.** Patients with a history of alcoholism can have multiple potential causes of anemia. This particular patient first presented with a bleeding duodenal ulcer. However, once this first problem resolved, the patient continued to drink and soon developed folate deficiency. One year later, after he supposedly had completely abstained from drinking, his physician found that he had a mild iron-deficiency anemia, and an investigation of his gastrointestinal tract revealed a benign colonic polyp as the source of blood loss.

This case illustrates how patients may have several different causes of anemia, either simultaneously or sequentially. This patient had two causes of anemia (duodenal ulcer and folate deficiency) that were associated with chronic alocholism and one (the colonic polyp) that was not.

## References

1. Dinarello, CA: Interleukin-1 and the pathogenesis of the acute-phase response. N Engl J Med 311:1413, 1984.
2. Lee, GR: The anemia of chronic disease. Semin Hematol 20:61, 1983.
3. Cook, JD: Clinical evaluation of iron deficiency. Semin Hematol 19:6, 1982.

4. Perrin, LH, Mackey, LJ, Miescher, P, et al: The hematology of malaria in man. Semin Hematol 19:70, 1982.

5. Pruzanski, W, and Shumak, K: Biological activity of cold-reacting autoantibodies. N Engl J Med 297:538, 1977.

6. Murray, HW, Masur, H, Senterfit, LB, et al: The protean manifestations of *Mycoplasma pneumoniae* infection in adults. Am J Med 58:229, 1975.

7. Horwitz, CA, Moulds, J, Henle, W, et al: Cold agglutinins in infectious mononucleosis and heterophil-antibody-negative mononucleosis-like syndromes. Blood 50:195, 1977.

8. Young, N and Mortimer, P: Viruses and bone marrow failure. Blood 63:729, 1984.

9. Fried, W: Hematologic complications of chronic renal failure. Med Clin North Am 62:1363, 1978.

10. Neff, MS, Goldberg, J, Slifkin, RF, et al: A comparison of androgens for anemia in patients on hemodialysis. N Engl J Med 304:871, 1981.

11. Cooper, R: Hemolytic syndromes and red cell membrane abnormalities in liver diseases. Semin Hematol 17:103, 1980.

12. Conrad, ME and Barton, JC: Anemia and iron kinetics in alcoholism. Semin Hematol 17:149, 1980.

13. Golde, DW, Bersch, N, Chopra, IJ, et al: Thyroid hormones stimulate erythropoiesis *in vitro*. Br J Haematol 37:173, 1977.

14. Shahidi, NT: Androgens and erythropoiesis. N Engl J Med 289:72, 1973.

15. Harvey, AR, Clarke, BJ, Chui, DHK, et al: Anemia associated with rheumatoid disease: Inverse correlation between erythropoiesis and both IgM and rheumatoid factor levels. Arthritis Rheum 26:28, 1983.

16. Daniak, N, Hardin, J, Floyd, V, et al: Humoral suppression of erythropoiesis in systemic lupus erythematosus and rheumatoid arthritis. Am J Med 69:537, 1980.

17. Budman, DR and Steinberg, AD: Hematologic aspects of systemic lupus erythematosus. Ann Intern Med 86:220, 1977.

18. Antman, KH, Skorin, AT, Mayer, RJ, et al: Microangiopathic hemolytic anemia and cancer: A review. Medicine 58:377, 1979.

19. Casciato, DA, and Scott, JL: Acute leukemia following prolonged cytotoxic agent therapy. Medicine 58:32, 1979.

20. Broder, S, and Gallo, RC: A pathogenic retrovirus (HTLV-III) linked to AIDS. N Engl J Med 311:1292, 1984.

21. Fauci, AS, Masur, H, Gelmann, EP, et al: The acquired immunodeficiency syndrome: An update. Ann Intern Med 102:800, 1985.

22. Gordin, FM, Simon, GL, Wofsy, CB, et al: Adverse reactions to trimethoprim-sulfamethoxazole in patients with the acquired immuno-deficiency syndrome. Ann Intern Med 100:495, 1984.

23. Spivak, JL, Bender, BS, Quinn, TC, et al: Hematologic abnormalities in the acquired immunodeficiency syndrome. Am J Med 77:204, 1984.

24. Castella, A, Croxson, T, Mildvan, D, et al: The bone marrow in AIDS. A histologic, hematologic, and microbiologic study. Am J Clin Pathol 84:425, 1985.

25. Ziegler, JL, Beckstead, JA, Volberding, PA, et al: Non-Hodgkin's lymphoma in 90 homosexual men. N Engl J Med 311:565, 1984.

26. Schoeppel, SL, Hoppe, RL, Dorfman, RF, et al: Hodgkin's disease in homosexual men with generalized lymphadenopathy. Ann Intern Med 102:69, 1985.

# CHAPTER 15

NEAL ROTHSCHILD, M.D., AND
RONALD A. SACHER, M.D., F.R.C.P.(C)

# The Polycythemias

## TERMINOLOGY AND CLASSIFICATION

The term "polycythemia," as it is commonly applied, refers to an etiologically diverse group of disorders whose principal laboratory manifestation is an increase in the number of red blood cells in the peripheral blood. Although "polycythemia" and "erythrocytosis" are often used interchangeably, the latter term is probably more accurate, as in most of these disorders the primary abnormality is restricted to the red blood cell series. The entity polycythemia vera is the one exception in that, for reasons that will become clear, leukocyte and platelet counts are also commonly elevated.

It is important to remember that the red blood cell count, hemoglobin, and hematocrit determinations all measure the *concentration* of red cells relative to plasma. It follows that a contraction in plasma volume, as might occur with dehydration, will produce an elevation in hemoglobin concentration independent of any change in the actual number of circulating red blood cells. We refer to this as *relative erythrocytosis*, and the clinical conditions with which it is associated are listed in Table 15–1. This condition should be distinguished from *absolute erythrocytosis*, which implies a true increase in the number of circulating red blood cells. The absolute erythrocytoses may be further classified as either primary or secondary, depending on whether the disorder arises from a primary disturbance in bone marrow function (e.g., polycythemia vera) or represents a physiologic response to some abnormal stimulus (e.g., hypoxia, erythropoietin secreting tumor).

## RELATIVE ERYTHROCYTOSIS

A relative erythrocytosis exists when plasma volume is contracted in the face of a normal red cell mass. Clinically, this is most commonly seen in the

**Table 15-1. CLASSIFICATION OF POLYCYTHEMIA**

**Primary Polycythemia**
  Polycythemia vera
**Secondary Polycythemia**
  Appropriate increase in erythropoietin secondary to tissue
      hypoxia
    High altitude
    Chronic pulmonary disease
    Cyanotic congenital heart disease
    Low cardiac output states
    Hypoventilation syndromes (neuromuscular disease,
        pickwickian syndrome, sleep apnea)
    High-affinity hemoglobin variants
    Methemoglobin variants
    Carboxyhemoglobinemia
  Inappropriate increase in erythropoietin
    Neoplasms (hypernephroma, hepatoma, uterine
        myoma, cerebellar hemangioblastoma,
        pheochromocytoma)
    Renal artery stenosis
    Renal transplantation
    Renal cysts
    Hydroephrosis
**Relative Erythrocytosis**
  Dehydration and other secondary causes of volume
      depletion
  Gaisböck's syndrome (stress erythrocytosis)

setting of acute or subacute dehydration from any one of a number of causes, and hematologic parameters can be corrected by replacement of the associated volume deficit. A chronic relative erythrocytosis is occasionally seen in middle-aged men who lack any obvious cause for chronic volume depletion. These patients are frequently hypertensive and obese, and many are smokers. The condition has variously been labeled Gaisböck's syndrome, stress erythrocytosis, or benign polycythemia. The diagnosis requires confirmation of normal red blood cell mass by radionuclide studies. All other hematologic parameters should be within normal limits, and splenomegaly should be absent. The pathogenesis is not well understood. Alterations in aldosterone and antidiuretic hormone secretion have been implicated but are not completely reproducible. Cigarette smoking may be etiologically significant in that smokers have lower plasma volumes in general, but why some individuals exhibit an exaggerated response is unclear. The condition usually follows a benign course, but some investigators have suggested that there may be an increased incidence of thromboembolic complications.[1] The role of therapeutic phlebotomy in this condition is controversial.

## REGULATION OF RED CELL PRODUCTION

Red blood production, like many other biologic systems, is governed by a feedback control mechanism (Fig. 15-1). Under normal circumstances, the bone marrow of an average adult produces in the neighborhood of 200 billion red cells per day. The basal rate of red cell production can be augmented as much as 10-fold when acute blood loss (e.g., hemolysis, hemorrhage) supervenes. Alternatively, production of red blood cells, as measured by the reticulocyte count, can be suppressed by hypertransfusion of packed cells. Red cell destruction, on the other hand, proceeds at a remarkably constant rate unless pathologic hemolysis exists (see Chapter 2).

Under physiologic conditions, the rate of red cell production is closely regulated by the polypeptide hormone erythropoietin, a glycoprotein with a molecular weight of 40,000 daltons. The kidney is the major site of human erythropoietin synthesis, although extrarenal production may assume more importance during fetal life and in the anephric state.

Decreased oxygen supply at the tissue level appears to be the principal stimulus for erythropoietin secretion. Tissue oxygen delivery is directly related to peripheral blood hemoglobin concentration. It follows that when hemoglobin concentration is reduced (i.e., when a patient becomes anemic), the kidney recognizes a condition of reduced oxygen availability and responds by releasing increased amounts of erythropoietin, stimulating the bone marrow to accelerate red cell production. In this manner, peripheral blood hemoglobin concentration is maintained within an optimal range, as long as the bone marrow is functioning normally and its reserve capacity is not exceeded. The location of the renal oxygen sensor and the exact site of renal erythropoietin synthesis have not yet been identified with certainty.

Erythropoietin has several actions on erythroid precursors in the bone marrow. After exposure to erythropoietin, stem cells committed to erythroid development undergo division and maturation at an increased rate. The entire sequence of erythroid development is abbreviated, and hemoglobin synthesis accelerates. Finally, there is early release of reticulocytes from the marrow.

Until recently, erythropoietin could be only measured by cumbersome biologic assays that lacked sensitivity and reproducibility. For example, in the whole animal assay, hypertransfused rats would be injected with a sample of test plasma and some time later would be given a predetermined dose of $^{59}$Fe. Incorporation of radiolabeled iron is measured at a pre-established interval. Erythropoietin levels can then be extrapolated from standard nomograms based on the rate of iron incorporation. In other bioassays, test plasma is applied to in vitro erythroid cell suspensions, and the rate of erythroid colony formation is recorded. With recent purification of erythropoietin, a sensitive radioimmunoassay has become available. Preliminary studies indicate that

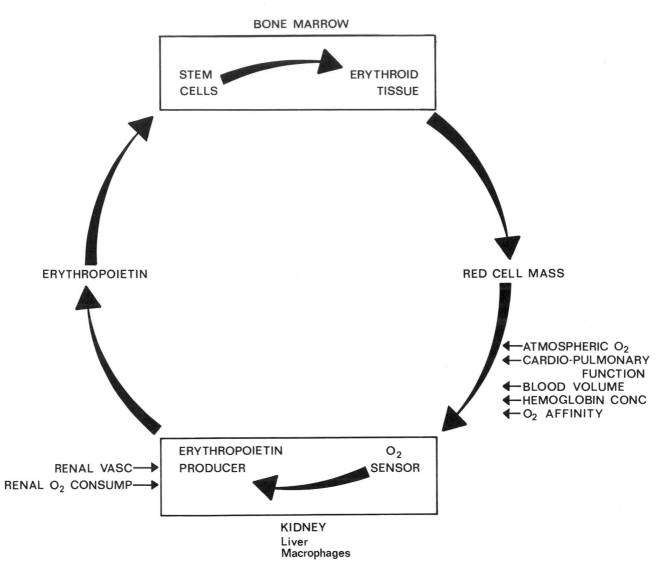

**Figure 15-1.** Feedback control regulation of red blood cell production. (From Williams, WJ, Beutler, E, Erslev, A, et al: Hematology, ed 3. McGraw-Hill, New York, 1983, p. 373, with permission.)

it can be used successfully to discriminate between primary and secondary polycythemia, in which erythropoietin levels are low and high, respectively.[2]

Under normal conditions, the erythropoietin regulatory system will maintain the red blood cell mass within a precise range. Should tissue oxygenation become compromised for reasons unrelated to hemoglobin concentration, erythropoietin secretion will increase, leading to accelerated erythropoiesis and polycythemia. For example, under hypoxic conditions, as might occur at high altitudes or in the setting of severe pulmonary disease, less oxygen is available for binding with hemoglobin. If sufficient deoxygenated hemoglobin is present, clinical cyanosis may be observed. If hypoxemia is sustained, reduced oxygen delivery to the tissues results in enhanced secretion of erythropoietin. After a period

of time, erythrocytosis ensues. Since the bone marrow is responding appropriately to a physiologic signal, the condition is referred to as secondary erythrocytosis. The disorders that give rise to secondary erythrocytosis will be discussed further in the next section.

## SECONDARY ERYTHROCYTOSIS
### Etiology and Pathogenesis

The underlying mechanism common to all cases of secondary erythrocytosis is an increased secretion of erythropoietin. This feature distinguishes these disorders from primary polycythemia (polycythemia vera), in which the bone marrow behaves autonomously, independent of the usual physiologic signals. The secondary polycythemias are conveniently divided into those that arise as an appropriate physiologic response to impaired tissue oxygenation and those that result from inappropriate (pathologic) erythropoietin secretion. The latter situation is most commonly seen as a paraneoplastic syndrome associated with certain tumors capable of elaborating abnormal hormones.

The prototypical case of secondary polycythemia is that which is seen with acclimatization to high altitudes. As one ascends from sea level, the partial pressure of inspired oxygen declines in proportion to the barometric pressure. At 3000 meters the oxygen saturation of hemoglobin approaches 90 percent, and increases in red cell mass become detectable.[3] Hematocrit levels in the 60 to 70 percent range are regularly observed in inhabitants of remote mountain settlements at 5000 meters. The adaptive polycythemia enables such individuals to function normally, despite the fact that inspired air contains less than 60 percent of the oxygen available at sea level. On the other hand, when nonacclimatized individuals rapidly ascend to similar elevations, they invariably develop symptoms of headache, dizziness, insomnia, nausea, and vomiting—a syndrome that has come to be known as acute mountain sickness.

Compensatory polycythemia is only one of several mechanisms involved in human adaptation to high altitudes. Changes in pulmonary mechanics can be demonstrated, along with alterations in oxidative metabolism at the subcellular level. Erythrocyte 2,3-DPG, a substance that modulates the binding of oxygen to hemoglobin, is synthesized in increased quantities. High intracellular levels of this compound favor the dissociation of oxygen from hemoglobin, making more oxygen available to the tissues. However, a reciprocal decreased tendency for oxygen loading in the lungs probably offsets any potential physiologic advantage from this mechanism.

The clinical conditions that can result in impaired oxygen delivery to the tissues and secondary erythrocytosis are enumerated in Table 15–1. In chronic lung disease impaired gas exchange may lead to arterial hypoxemia and compensatory increase in red cell mass. For reasons that have not been fully elucidated, the erythrocytosis is usually not as marked as one would expect for the degree of hemoglobin desaturation. It has been hypothesized that the blunted erythropoietic response may be attributable to the bone marrow suppressive effects of the underlying chronic disease state.

Some of the highest venous hematocrits recorded have been seen in cases of congenital heart disease with right to left shunts. These cardiac anomalies result in the shunting of poorly oxygenated, mixed venous blood into the systemic circulation, leading to clinical cyanosis and polycythemia. A modest increase in red cell mass may also occur in low cardiac output states (e.g., congestive heart failure), but this is usually offset by a concomitant increase in plasma volume resulting in relatively little change in the measured hematocrit.

The alveolar hypoventilation syndromes are an uncommon but fascinating group of disorders characterized by inadequate or ineffective ventilation, usually in the absence of primary pulmonary abnormalities. Arterial blood gas measurements reveal carbon dioxide retention and a proportional degree of hypoxemia. The condition may be seen in severe neuromuscular disorders and chest wall abnormalities or may arise from primary abnormalities in the central mechanisms involved in the regulation of respiratory drive (pickwickian syndrome, central sleep apnea).

Rarely, abnormalities in the hemoglobin molecule itself may be responsible for an otherwise unexplained polycythemia. A single amino acid substitution in a critical region of the hemoglobin molecule may alter the affinity for oxygen binding. The molecular abnormality may reside in the region responsible for interaction among the alpha and beta globin chains (e.g., hemoglobin Chesapeake); the region involved with 2,3-DPG binding (e.g., hemoglobin Little Rock); or, on rare occasions, the heme pocket itself. The unusually avid binding of oxygen by these abnormal hemoglobins leads to impaired release of oxygen to the tissues and a compensatory erythrocytosis ensues. Some of these hemoglobin variants are physically unstable and associated hemolysis may mask full expression of the polycythemia.

To date, more than two dozen high-affinity hemoglobin variants have been characterized. These disorders are usually inherited in an autosomal dominant fashion; therefore, careful investigation into family history may alert one to the diagnosis. In most cases, the mutant hemoglobin will be evident on hemoglobin electrophoresis; however, some variants may be electrophoretically silent. In such cases, reduction in the measured $P_{50}$ (the partial pressure at which hemoglobin is 50 percent oxygenated) may be the only demonstrable laboratory abnormality.

Methemoglobinemia results when heme iron is oxidized to the ferric state. The disorder may occur on either a congenital or toxic basis. The oxidized heme moiety is incapable of binding oxygen, and clinically, cyanosis results. In a small minority of cases, a mild associated polycythemia may be observed.

Heavy cigarette smokers may exhibit a mild erythrocytosis related to elevations in carboxyhemoglobin levels.[4] Carbon monoxide, found in cigarette smoke, in automobile exhaust, and as a product of a wide range of industrial processes, is capable of binding hemoglobin with an affinity some 200 times that of oxygen. The resulting carboxyhemoglobin complex is unavailable for binding with oxygen. The decreased blood oxygen-carrying capacity may result in compensatory erythrocytosis. The arterial oxygen tension measured in an arterial blood gas sample does not reflect levels of carboxyhemoglobin and direct measurement of hemoglobin saturation or carboxyhemoglobin concentration must be performed. Both carboxyhemoglobin and methemoglobin can be measured spectrophotometrically.

In all of the disorders discussed up to this point, the erythropoietic response represents a physiologic compensation by the individual intended to correct a state of tissue hypoxia. In the next group of disorders, excessive elaboration of erythropoietin is clearly inappropriate and autonomous, and the secondary polycythemia confers no physiologic advantages.

A number of renal disorders may give rise to pathologic erythropoietin secretion and secondary erythrocytosis. The common mechanism underlying these cases appears to be selective renal ischemia/hypoxia.[5] Rare cases of renal artery stenosis and erythrocytosis that corrected following nephrectomy have been reported. Erythrocytosis has been seen following renal transplantation, presumably on the basis of small blood vessel disease and disturbance of intrarenal blood flow. Renal cysts and hydronephrosis are also rare causes of erythrocytosis. The mechanism is probably related to local ischemia from pressure effects. The erythrocytosis corrects itself after nephrectomy or decompression.

Erythrocytosis can be seen as a paraneoplastic syndrome associated with certain malignant tumors. Indeed, certain neoplasms have been demonstrated to elaborate erythropoietically active substances. Tumors of the kidney or liver account for the vast majority of these cases. Cerebellar hemangioblastomas, uterine myomas, and adrenal tumors represent less common causes. The hematologic abnormalities usually remit if the tumor can be resected. Reappearance of the erythrocytosis may signal recurrence of the tumor.

## Clinical Consequences

Although an increase in hemoglobin concentration will afford a proportional increase in oxygen-carrying capacity per unit volume of blood, concomitant changes in the viscosity of the blood may limit the effectiveness of the compensatory erythrocytosis and may, in fact, produce deleterious signs and symptoms. Blood viscosity increases exponentially with the hematocrit. Clearly, as blood flow becomes more sluggish, oxygen transport will be compromised. In actual fact, animal studies have shown that if blood volume is kept constant, oxygen delivery is maximal with hematocrits in the normal range and decreases with progressive erythrocytosis.[6] In polycythemic patients, however, erythrocytosis is accompanied by a *net increase* in blood volume with expansion of the vascular bed and increase in cardiac output. Consequently, net oxygen transport is increased despite reduced flow rates.

Clinically, the expanded blood volume results in dilatation of cutaneous blood vessels, giving rise to the ruddy complexion so characteristic of the patient with polycythemia. Hemodynamic alterations secondary to increased viscosity and expanded blood volume are also responsible for the frequent symptoms of dizziness, headache, and tinnitus experienced by these patients. Likewise, capillary distension and sluggish blood flow result in abnormal mucous membrane bleeding. The incidence of thromboembolic events is also probably increased. Clearly, any attempt to phlebotomize a patient with compensatory erythrocytosis may offset any physiologic advantage conferred by the increased blood volume.

## POLYCYTHEMIA VERA

Polycythemia vera is a chronic clonal hematopoietic stem cell disorder characterized by uncontrolled growth and proliferation of predominantly erythroid precursors. It is considered to fall within the spectrum of the chronic myeloproliferative disorders, which also include chronic myelogenous leukemia, agnogenic myeloid metaplasia, and primary thrombocythemia (see Chapter 21). The unregulated nature of the erythroid expansion distinguishes this disorder from the secondary erythrocytoses where the bone marrow response is governed by excessive erythropoietin secretion. In further contrast to the secondary polycythemias, more widespread expression of the unregulated growth is often evident, as about two thirds of patients will exhibit leukocytosis and about half will have thrombocytosis. Manifestations of myeloid metaplasia in other organs (liver, spleen, and occasionally lymph nodes) are also seen. It is this hyperplasia of all three marrow cell lines that led to the original description of this order as a polycythemia rather than an erythrocytosis.

### Etiology, Epidemiology, and Pathogenesis

The etiology of primary polycythemia is not known. It is typically a disease of middle-aged and elderly persons, with a slighly higher incidence in men. The disorder is uncommon among blacks and occurs with increased incidence among Ashkenazy Jews. Familial occurrences are seemingly rare.

Like the other myeloproliferative diseases, there is substantial evidence that polycythemia vera is a clonal disorder arising from a multipotential stem cell.[7] Studies in G-6-PD heterozygotes reveal a single isoenzyme type in cells of myeloid, monocytic, megakaryocytic, and erythroid lineage, whereas both isoenzymes are represented in nonhematopoietic tissues. This suggests that the abnormal hematopoietic elements arise from a single clone. The involvement of all three bone marrow cell lines implies that the primary abnormality resides at the stem cell level. There is similar evidence to support a clonal, stem cell origin for the other myeloproliferative disorders (see Chapter 21).

Further evidence of autonomous growth is the demonstration that urinary erythropoietin levels are low or absent in polycythemia vera. Again, this contrasts with secondary erythrocytosis, in which erythropoietin levels are usually elevated. The reduced levels of erythropoietin in polycythemia vera suggests that the feedback control mechanism is intact and that hormone secretion is appropriately suppressed.

Normal bone marrow progenitor cells require the addition of erythropoietin in order to form erythroid colonies in culture (BFU-E, CFU-E, and erythroid clusters). Cells from polycythemia vera patients will form colonies even in the absence of erythropoietin, again suggesting escape from normal regulatory influences.

## Clinical Features

Most of the clinical manifestations of polycythemia are related to the increased blood volume and blood viscosity attributable to the expanded red cell mass. The patient's face appears plethoric, or suffused with blood. The retinal veins may be engorged on funduscopic examination. Cerebral circulatory disturbances account for the frequent symptoms of headache, dizziness, blurred vision, and tinnitus. Sluggish blood flow in the extremities may result in peripheral cyanosis. Thromboembolic complications are frequent and account for a substantial proportion of the early mortality. Vascular distension and platelet dysfunction lead to mucous membrane bleeding, and occult blood loss from the gastrointestinal tract is common.

Splenomegaly is found in greater than 75 percent of patients with polycythemia, although it may be absent at the time of initial presentation. Hepatomegaly is observed in 40 to 50 percent of patients. For reasons that are not completely understood, there is an increased incidence of peptic ulcer disease among patients with polycythemia vera. Pruritis, particularly after a hot shower, is a frequent complaint. This phenomenon may be related to elevated levels of histamine in the blood.

## Laboratory Findings

At the time of diagnosis, the red cell count, hemoglobin concentration, and hematocrit are all elevated, unless there is significant associated iron deficiency. Direct measurement of the total red cell mass should be undertaken. The most satisfactory method for accomplishing this involves $^{51}$Cr labeling of autologous red blood cells. A value greater than 35 ml/kg in men and 32 ml/kg in women is consistent with an absolute erythrocytosis. The plasma volume can be measured simultaneously using radiolabeled $^{131}$I-albumin and is usually normal or slightly increased.

Examination of the peripheral smear reveals normochromic, normocytic red cells with variable amounts of poikilocytosis and anisocytosis **(see Color Figure 133)**. Red cells become hypochromic and microcytic if iron deficiency supervenes. Abnormal elevation of the leukocyte count is present in approximately two thirds of patients, and thrombocytosis occurs in about one half. Myelocytes and metamyelocytes are occasionally encountered on the peripheral smear, and a modest basophilia is common. Platelets can appear morphologically abnormal, and platelet aggregation studies may reveal associated functional defects (see Chapter 27).

Bone marrow specimens are typically hypercellular with hyperplasia of erythroid, myeloid, and megakaryocytic elements **(see Color Figure 134)**. Stainable iron is reduced or absent on Prussian blue stains, owing to the high incidence of occult blood loss from the gastrointestinal tract and the increased use of available iron by the hyperplastic erythroid compartment. Silver stains of biopsy specimens demonstrate the presence of reticulum fibers in up to one third of patients. In advanced stages of the disease, frank myelofibrosis may be observed.

In contrast to the Philadelphia chromosome in chronic myelogenous leukemia, there are no diagnostic cytogenetic markers in primary polycythemia. Aneuploidy is a frequent finding, however, and trisomy of C-group chromosomes is recognized with increased frequency.

Leukocyte alkaline phosphatase levels are elevated in approximately 70 percent of patients **(see Color Figure 135)**. The enzyme, a constituent of polymorphonuclear granules, is measured by staining peripheral blood films with naphthol, AS-B1 phosphate coupled to an azo dye. Uptake of the dye is evaluated in 100 consecutive leukocytes and scored on a 0 to 4+ scale. Normal values range between 15 and 130, with higher scores found in patients with polycythemia vera or leukemoid reactions. Abnormally low scores are seen in patients with chronic myelogenous leukemia.

Elevated serum vitamin $B_{12}$ and vitamin $B_{12}$ binding capacity are frequent but nonspecific laboratory findings. Vitamin $B_{12}$ binding capacity reflects levels of binding proteins transcobalamin I, II, and III in the plasma. Transcobalamin I is the binding protein most commonly elevated in primary polycythemia. The protein is derived from cells of the granulocytic series, and elevated serum levels are thought to reflect increased myeloid activity.

Hyperuricemia, along with hyperuricosuria, is

seen in many patients with primary polycythemia. It is a frequent finding in a wide array of hyperproliferative disorders in which there is increased turnover of cellular nucleotides. Uncommonly, clinical gout may develop.

Hyperkalemia is sometimes reported in patients who have polycythemia vera with thrombocytosis. It is an artifactual finding related to release of potassium from platelets when the plasma is allowed to clot. Plasma potassium concentrations determined from anticoagulated specimens are invariably normal. Finally, elevated histamine levels may be measured in the blood of polycythemic subjects. The histamine is thought to be derived from circulating granulocytes. It may be etiologically related to the frequent complaint of pruritis.

## Treatment

With appropriate therapeutic intervention, polycythemia vera typically runs a chronic course, and most patients can enjoy a fairly normal existence for many years. Since most of the serious complications of the disease are related to expanded blood volume and hyperviscosity, the principal objective of long-term therapy is reduction of the pathologically increased red cell mass. This may be accomplished either by directly lowering the blood volume through intermittent phlebotomy or by controlling the underlying proliferative process with cytotoxic therapy. The latter approach affords a means of controlling the leukocyte and platelet counts as well.

Phlebotomy provides a safe, effective, and relatively inexpensive means of correcting the erythrocytosis. It is a particularly useful mode of therapy for initial control of symptoms or when there is a pressing need to lower the hematocrit acutely. In many patients, the disease process can be successfully controlled for prolonged periods with phlebotomy alone. Therapy is initiated by removing 300 to 500 ml of blood every few days until the hematocrit approaches the upper limits of normal. Subsequent phlebotomies can be performed on a bimonthly basis to maintain the patient in the near normovolemic state. Caution must be exercised in phlebotomizing elderly patients or those with a history of vascular disease. The potential for serious cardiovascular or cerebrovascular complications from acute hemodynamic alterations precludes the removal of more than 200 ml in a single setting in such patients. If the hematocrit must be lowered more rapidly, it is advisable to infuse plasma or saline simultaneously to maintain intravascular volume.

Since approximately 250 mg of iron is removed with every unit of blood, iron deficiency is a predictable complication of repeated phlebotomy. After a period of treatment, the patient's red cells will become hypochromic, microcytic. Since the deficiency interferes with marrow production of erythrocytes, the frequency of phlebotomy required to maintain the hematocrit at acceptable levels may decrease substantially once iron deficiency develops.

The major limitation of phlebotomy is that it does nothing to control the thrombocytosis present in the majority of cases. Consequently, if it is the only treatment modality employed, a significant incidence of thrombotic and hemorrhagic complications is seen. In those patients particularly susceptible to such complications (high platelet counts, the elderly, pre-existing vascular disease) cytotoxic therapy probably represents a more rational therapeutic approach.

Radioactive phosphorus ($^{32}$P) will produce significant improvement of all hematologic parameters in a substantial majority of patients. Approximately two to three months are required to achieve maximal effect, and a second dose may be necessary to obtain full benefit. Duration of remission is typically on the order of six to 24 months. The treatment is simple to administer and associated with little in the way of toxicity. Unfortunately, an excess risk of acute leukemia is associated with its use (see further on).

A variety of chemotherapeutic agents have been employed in the treatment of polycythemia vera. Chlorambucil, busulfan, melphalan, and cyclophosphamide have all been used successfully. As with radioactive phosphorus, maximal benefit is not realized for several weeks or months. Significant myelosuppression is a predictable toxic side effect of each of these agents, and blood counts must be monitored frequently. In addition, each agent is associated with its own unique toxicities of which the treating physician must be aware (e.g., busulfan and pulmonary fibrosis).

Patients who have polycythemia and are treated with alkylating agents may be particularly susceptible to the late complication of acute leukemia. For this reason, it is not recommended as an initial treatment approach in younger patients. It has been suggested that hydroxyurea represents an effective alternative to conventional alkylator therapy.[8] It is frequently employed in chronic myelogenous leukemia and does not appear to have leukemogenic potential. Longer follow-up is necessary before its widespread use can be advocated.

In 1967, the international Polycythemia Vera Study Group began a long-term prospective trial comparing the various therapeutic modalities available for the treatment of polycythemia vera. Study patients were randomized to three modes of treatment: phlebotomy alone, chlorambucil and phlebotomy as needed, and radioactive phosphorus with phlebotomy as needed. With prolonged follow-up, it is not apparent that survival rates for the three types of treatment are comparable.[9] However, several important differences among the treatment groups were recognized. Those patients treated with phlebotomy alone experienced a significantly higher incidence of thrombotic complications. In contrast, those patients treated with radioactive phosphorus or alkylating agents were subject to a substantially higher risk of their disease terminating in acute leukemia. However, many have argued that the leukemic transformation may be a consequence of prolonged survival in a patient with a chronic myeloproliferative syndrome. Moreover, acute leukemia in a setting of an underlying myeloproliferative disease is usually not responsive to forms of therapy presently available, and survival is short once transformation occurs.

Given the treatment options available, each with its own attendant risks and benefits, the choice of therapy must be individualized for each patient. For example, it would seem sensible to attempt to avoid cytotoxic therapy in younger patients whose disease can be controlled with phlebotomy alone so as to minimize the risk of leukemic transformation. In older individuals — particularly those with pre-existing vascular disease — phlebotomy is less well tolerated, and the risk of thrombotic complications is substantial. A more aggressive approach with cytotoxic therapy would seem justified to such patients.

## Clinical Course and Prognosis

As noted earlier, the disease usually progresses in a relatively indolent fashion, and prolonged survival is common. If the red cell mass can be reduced to satisfactory levels with treatment, thrombotic and hemorrhagic complications can be kept to a minimum. Nevertheless, approximately one third of patients will suffer such a complication during the course of the illness.

After a variable period of time (average 10 years), the erythrocytic phase of the disease will give way to what has been referred to as the "spent phase," in approximately 15 to 20 percent of subjects.[10] The clinical picture of this phase is characterized by progressive anemia and striking hepatosplenomegaly. Indeed, this syndrome resembles agnogenic myeloid metaplasia (see Chapter 21) in many respects, with teardrop cells and nucleated red blood cells evident in the peripheral blood and the development of marrow fibrosis with extensive myeloid metaplasia in the liver, spleen, and other sites. The treatment of this phase of the disease is largely supportive, with many patients requiring ongoing transfusional therapy to correct the anemia. Symptomatic enlargement of abdominal organs secondary to the myeloid metaplasia may become problematic, but splenectomy is fraught with hazard. Life expectancy in this phase of the disease is usually less than three years.

Polycythemia vera will terminate in acute leukemia in as many as 15 percent of patients. As discussed earlier, the rate of leukemic transformation appears to be influenced by the type of therapy employed. Survival in the leukemic phase is brief.

The survival rates for patients with polycythemia vera range from 10 to 14 years in a number of published series. Since the mean age of diagnosis is 60 years, many patients will die of unrelated causes. Clearly, therapy directed at correcting the pathophysiologic abnormalities associated with the disease has had a significant impact on morbidity and mortality.

## DIFFERENTIAL DIAGNOSIS OF ERYTHROCYTOSIS

Diagnostic evaluation of a patient with erythrocytosis should begin with a careful history and physical examination. Special attention should be directed at such items as cigarette smoking, cardiopulmonary function, family history, and the presence or absence of hepatosplenomegaly. Table 15–2 compares primary, secondary, and relative polycythemias. The initial laboratory investigation should include radioisotope determination of red cell mass and plasma volume, to distinguish between absolute and relative erythrocytosis (Fig. 15-2). If the red cell mass is normal and plasma volume is reduced, a diagnosis of relative erythrocytosis can be established. If no secondary cause for the chronic reduction in plasma volume is apparent, these cases presumably fall under the heading of Gaisböck's syndrome, or stress erythrocytosis. If, however, the red cell mass is elevated (absolute erythrocytosis), further workup must be undertaken to determine the cause (primary versus secondary) (Fig. 15-3).

The clinical entities associated with secondary erythrocytosis are presented in Table 15–1. Specific diagnostic studies may be helpful in uncovering or confirming the presence of one of these conditions and are warranted in any patient with an unexplained elevation in red cell mass. An abnormal arterial $pO_2$ or oxygen saturation value will identify those patients in whom erythrocytosis occurs on the basis of chronic pulmonary or cardiac disease. Such patients generally have clinical signs and symptoms referrable to the underlying disorder. Smokers should have carboxyhemoglobin levels measured. If these levels are elevated, correction of polycythemia may occur if smoking is eliminated for several months. Caution must be exercised in interpreting carboxyhemoglobin levels, as they vary considerably relative to the time of the last cigarette smoked.

In the absence of cardiopulmonary disease or smoking history, one must consider the possibility of an inherited hemoglobin abnormality (high oxygen affinity variant). The family history may be particularly helpful in these circumstances, as most of

**Table 15-2. FEATURES OF PRIMARY POLYCYTHEMIA, SECONDARY (HYPOXIC) POLYCYTHEMIA, AND RELATIVE ERYTHROCYTOSIS**

| Manifestations | Primary Polycythemia | Secondary Polycythemia | Relative Erythrocytosis |
|---|---|---|---|
| **Clinical Features** | | | |
| Cyanosis (warm) | Absent | Present | May be present |
| Heart or lung disease | Absent | Present | Absent |
| Splenomegaly | Present in 75% | Absent | Absent |
| Hepatomegaly | Present in 35% | Absent | Absent |
| **Laboratory Features** | | | |
| Arterial oxygen saturation | Normal | Decreased | Normal |
| Red cell mass | Increased | Increased | Normal |
| White count | Increased in 80% | Normal | Normal |
| Platelet count | Increased in 50% | Normal | Normal |
| Nucleated red cells, poikilocytes | Often present | Absent | Absent |
| Leukocyte alkaline phosphatase (LAP) | Elevated | Normal | Normal |
| Bone marrow | Hypercellular; increased erythropoiesis and myelopoiesis; increased megakaryocytes; fibrosis | Increased erythropoiesis | Normal |
| Erythropoietin | Decreased | Increased | Normal |
| Serum vitamin $B_{12}$ | Elevated in 75%* | Normal | Normal |

*Owing to an increase in transcobalamin III.

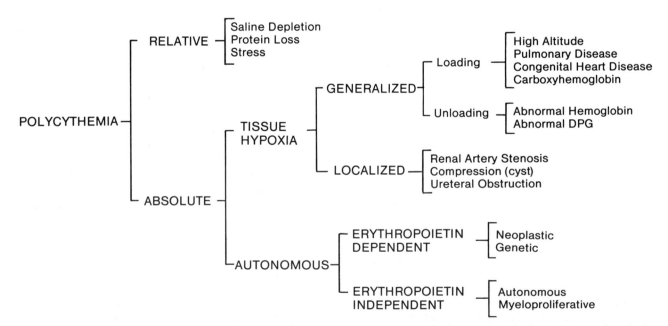

**Figure 15-2.** Classification of the polycythemic disorders. In the differential diagnosis of polycythemia, the first question to be asked is whether the elevated hemoglobin level is an absolute increase or a relative one secondary to plasma volume depletion. The absolute polycythemias may be subdivided on the basis of either a generalized or localized defect in tissue oxygen supply or the appearance of autonomous erythropoietin production or autonomous erythropoiesis. In the patient with hypoxia, studies of oxygen loading, unloading, and renal function can help identify the specific cause of the polycythemia. Patients with autonomous erythropoiesis may be identified on the basis of their clinical presentation or detailed studies of erythropoietin secretion and stem cell growth characteristics. (From Hillman, RS and Finch, CA: Red Cell Manual, ed 5. FA Davis, Philadelphia, 1985, p. 122, with permission.)

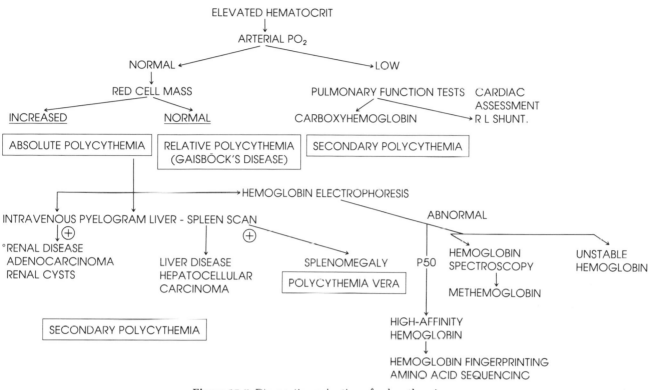

**Figure 15-3.** Diagnostic evaluation of polycythemia.

these variant hemoglobins are inherited in an autosomal dominant pattern. In the majority of such cases, the hemoglobin electrophoresis will be abnormal. An electrophoretic abnormality, however, does not establish abnormal oxygen affinity. The physiologic behavior of the hemoglobin molecule should be characterized by measurement of the $P_{50}$ or the oxygen-hemoglobin dissociation curve. This will also uncover the minority of mutant high-affinity hemoglobins that are electrophoretically silent.

If evidence for tissue hypoxia is lacking, one must raise the possibility of inappropriate secretion of erythropoietin as the mechanism for the erythrocytosis. Renal tumors or other renal structural abnormalities comprise most of the cases in this category. An intravenous pyelogram or abdominal CT scan should disclose the abnormality in most cases.

In patients with fully developed cases of polycythemia vera with splenomegaly and evidence of panmyelosis (leukocytosis and thrombocytosis), the diagnosis is usually clear from the outset. Organ enlargement and pancytosis, common features of primary polycythemia, are always absent in the patient with uncomplicated secondary erythrocytosis. However, if the patient with polycythemia vera is evaluated early enough in the course of the disease, erythrocytosis may be the only hematologic abnormality detected and additional testing is required to secure the diagnosis. An elevated leukocyte alkaline phosphatase score along with a high serum vitamin $B_{12}$ and vitamin $B_{12}$ binding capacity would make the diagnosis of polycythemia vera more tenable. A radioisotope liver/spleen scan might uncover subclinical splenomegaly.

Recent studies have advocated the use of erythropoietin assays to distinguish between primary and secondary polycythemia. These assays have been unreliable in the past, but with newer, radioimmunologic methods available, the role of this test needs to be critically evaluated.

The diagnostic criteria adopted by the Polycythemia Study Group are presented in Table 15–3. The

**Table 15–3. POLYCYTHEMIA STUDY GROUP CRITERIA FOR DIAGNOSIS OF POLYCYTHEMIA VERA***

**Category A (Major Criteria)**
1. Elevated red cell mass
2. Normal arterial oxygen saturation
3. Splenomegaly

**Category B (Minor Criteria)**
1. Leukocytosis
2. Thrombocytosis
3. Elevated leukocyte alkaline phosphatase score
4. Increased serum vitamin $B_{12}$ or vitamin $B_{12}$ binding proteins

*To establish a diagnosis of polycythemia vera, either all three diagnostic criteria from category A or an elevated red cell mass and normal arterial oxygen saturation in addition to two criteria from category B must be present.
(From Beck, WS: Hematology, ed 3. MIT Press, Cambridge, 1982, p. 297, with permission.)

diagnosis of polycythemia vera is considered secure if all three criteria in category A are present. Since splenomegaly is frequently absent at initial presentation, the presence of any two criteria from category B, along with an elevated red cell mass and normal arterial oxygen saturation, is also considered diagnostic.

## CASE HISTORIES
### Case 1

The patient, a 42-year-old white female, is referred for evaluation of an elevated hematocrit. She presented to her private physician one week earlier, complaining of headaches and blurred vision of approximately one month's duration. She denies any abnormal bleeding. She does report generalized pruritus, particularly after taking warm showers. Her past medical history has been unremarkable except for a duodenal ulcer diagnosed one year earlier. Family history is unremarkable for any hematologic disorders. She is a nonsmoker.

On physical examination, the blood pressure was 160/90, pulse 78 and regular. The face appeared plethoric and the retinal veins were engorged. There was no abnormal adenopathy. The lungs were clear. There were no cardiac murmurs or gallops. The spleen tip was palpable three fingerbreadths below the costal margin. The liver was not enlarged. A few small ecchymoses were observed over the lower extremities.

Complete blood count revealed a HCT of 57 percent, Hb 18 g/dl, and an RBC count of 9.5 million/mm³. The MCV was 55 fl, the WBC count was 12,300 with a normal differential, and the platelet count was 375,000.

A diagnostic workup of polycythemia was undertaken. The red blood cell volume, measured by the $^{51}$Cr dilution method, was 41 ml/kg. The plasma volume was 40 ml/kg. Arterial blood gas determination revealed a $pO_2$ of 85 ml Hg. Hemoglobin electrophoresis was normal. The serum iron was 28 and TIBC 419. Uric acid was 9.1. Serum vitamin $B_{12}$ was 900 pg/ml (normal 200 to 800). The serum vitamin $B_{12}$ binding capacity was 2600 pg/ml (normal 1000 to 2000). The leukocyte alkaline phosphatase score was 161. Electrocardiogram and chest roentgenogram were within normal limits. An abdominal CT scan was unremarkable except for the finding of splenomegaly. A bone marrow examination revealed increased cellularity with erythroid hyperplasia, absent iron stores, and increased reticulum on silver stain.

**Comment.** Several findings in the history and physical examination suggest a diagnosis of polycythemia vera. The complaint of generalized pruritus is probably related to the hyperhistaminemia associated with the myeloproliferative process. Furthermore, peptic ulcer disease is recognized with increased frequency in patients with polycythemia vera. On the other hand, headache and blurred vision are nonspecific symptoms of hyperviscosity. The absence of cardiac and pulmonary abnormalities is helpful in excluding secondary causes of erythrocytosis. The palpable spleen tip is highly suggestive of a primary hematologic process. Clinically detectable enlargement of the spleen is generally absent in all secondary causes of polycythemia.

The initial laboratory evaluation revealed a modest elevation of platelet count and white blood cells. Again, evidence of trilineage involvement (panmyelosis) favors a diagnosis of primary polycythemia. Radioisotope studies were obtained to confirm the presence of an absolute erythrocytosis. Normal arterial oxygen saturation, hemoglobin electrophoresis, and abdominal CT scan exclude most of the common causes of secondary erythrocytosis. Abnormal elevation of uric acid levels, leukocyte alkaline phosphatase score, vitamin $B_{12}$, and vitamin $B_{12}$ binding proteins are all consistent with a primary proliferative process. The serum iron studies and bone marrow iron stains suggest associated iron deficiency, probably on the basis of occult gastrointestinal blood loss.

This patient exhibits all criteria set forth by the Polycythemia Study Group for the diagnosis of polycythemia vera. In view of her relatively young age and in the absence of a marked thrombocytosis or a history of thrombotic events, it was elected to phlebotomize the patient as the initial form of therapy. The disturbing pruritus was successfully controlled with cyproheptadine (Periactin).

### Case 2

A 47-year-old white male executive was referred for evaluation of an elevated hematocrit discovered on a routine blood count. He was completely asymptomatic. He stated that he was continually subject to a great deal of stress in his present work environment. The past medical history was remarkable only for a two-year history of mild hypertension. He smoked an occasional cigar.

On physical examination he was mildly obese with a blood pressure of 150/98 and plethoric facies. No hepatosplenomegaly or adenopathy were detected. The HCT was 58 percent, Hb 20 g/dl, WBC count 5400, and platelet count 232,000. The red cell volume was 30.6 ml/kg, the plasma volume 26.9 ml/kg.

**Comment.** In this case, no further workup is necessary. The patient's red cell volume is within normal range. The elevated hematocrit can be explained entirely on the basis of a reduction in plasma volume. In this case, a diagnosis of relative (spurious) erythrocytosis can be made. The finding of relative erythrocytosis in a middle-aged, obese, hypertensive male smoker is consistent with Gaisböck's syndrome. There is some evidence that these patients may be at a higher than normal risk for thromboembolic phenomena. The role of phlebotomy in such cases is controversial.

## References

1. Burge, PS, Johnson, WS, Prankerd, TAJ: Morbidity and mortality in pseudopolycythemia. Lancet 2:1266, 1975.

2. Koeffler, HP and Goldwasser, E: Erythropoietin radioimmunassay in evaluating patients with polycythemia. Ann Intern Med 94:44, 1981.

3. Weil, JV, Jamieson, G, Brown, DW, et al: The red cell mass—arterial oxygen relationship in normal man. J Clin Invest 47:1627, 1968.

4. Smith, JR and Landan, SA: Smokers polycythemia. N Engl J Med 298:6, 1978.

5. Balcerzak, SP and Bromberg, PA: Secondary polycythemia. Semin Hematol 12:353, 1976.

6. Murray, JF, Gold, P, and Johnson, BL: The circulatory effects of hematocrit variation in normovolemic and hypervolemic dogs. J Clin Invest 42:1150, 1963.

7. Adamson, JW, Fialkow, PJ, Murphy, S, et al: Polycythemia vera: Stem cell and probable clonal origin of the disease. N Engl J Med 295:913, 1976.

8. Donovan, PB, Kaplan, ME, Goldberg, JD, et al: Treatment of polycythemia vera with hydroxyurea. Am J Hematol 17:329, 1984.

9. Wasserman, JD: Influence of therapy on causes of death in polycythemia vera. Clin Res 29:573A, 1981.

10. Silverman, MN: The evolution into and the treatment of the late stage of polycythemia vera. Semin Hematol 13:79, 1976.

# CHAPTER 16

RONALD G. STRAUSS, M.D.*

# White Blood Cell Metabolism: Neutrophil Physiology and Metabolism

Three major types of leukocytes are found in blood: granulocytes, lymphocytes, and monocytes. Granulocytes can be subdivided into three types: neutrophils, eosinophils, and basophils based on morphology by light and electron microscopy and on the staining characteristics and contents of cytoplasmic granules. Likewise, despite their fairly uniform appearance on stained blood smears, lymphocytes can be divided into a number of subpopulations that, in turn, can be grouped into three broad categories designated T, B, and null lymphocytes.

In peripheral blood, 65 to 80 percent of the lymphocytes circulating are T lymphocytes and 15 to 30 percent are B lymphocytes. The B lymphocytes are responsible for "humoral" immunity, which involves antibody production. A description of the humoral immune response and the function of B lymphocytes is presented in Chapter 22.

T lymphocytes are responsible for cell-mediated immunity, which is important in protection against intracellular pathogens, delayed type hypersensitivity reactions, and transplantation rejection. Figure 16–1 illustrates the induction of cell-mediated immunity. T lymphocytes circulate throughout the body constantly patrolling and surveying for abnormal or malignant cells. Unlike other white cells, the T lymphocytes are long-lived cells with a half-life estimated between 15 and 30 years. T lymphocytes are thymus derived, being processed and released in total numbers into circulation shortly after birth. It is postulated that T lymphocytes are *not* replaced during adult life.

Various T lymphocyte subpopulations with well-established functions and identifiable surface antigens have been defined. Regulatory T cells are com-

*The author is recipient of Research Career Development Award K04 HD 00255 and Transfusion Medicine Academic Award K07 HL01426 from the National Institutes of Health.

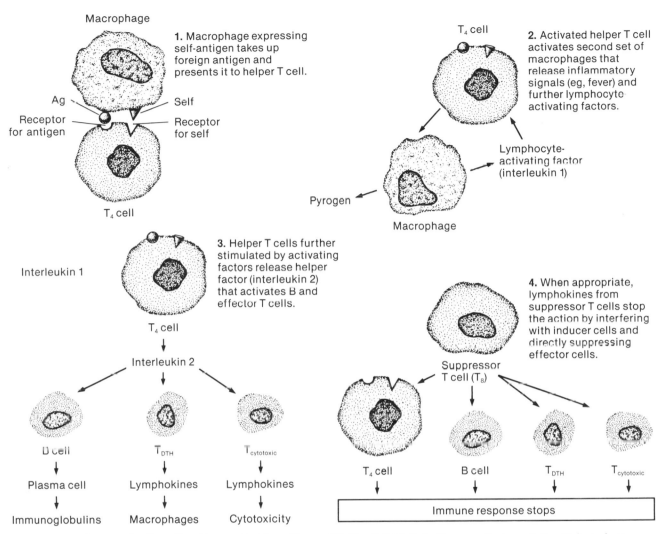

**Figure 16-1.** Induction of cell-mediated immunity. (From Dwyer, JM: The Cell-Mediated Immune System. Cutter Biologicals, Emeryville, CA, 1982, p. 4, with permission.)

posed of T4-helper/inducer and T8-suppressor lymphocytes that function to regulate both humoral and cell-mediated immunity. Both may be identified by the appropriate surface antigen present, namely T4 or T8. A normal T4 : T8 ratio is 1.6 to 2.0.

The effector T lymphocytes include cytoxic T lymphocytes (T-CTL) and delayed hypersensitivity (T-DH) T lymphocytes, which both play major roles in cell-mediated immunity along with macrophages (Fig. 16-1). Table 16–1 summarizes the various subpopulations of T lymphocytes, listing some of their specific functions.

Another population has also been defined of lymphocytes that do not share the same properties as B or T lymphocytes. These lymphocytes have been termed "null cells." The most important type of lymphocyte in this group is the natural killer (NK) cell, which is capable of directly killing a target cell without prior sensitization. NK lymphocytes pos-

**Table 16–1. THYMUS-DERIVED LYMPHOCYTES**

Helper (inducer) T cells
  Aid B-cell maturation in bone marrow
  Supply activating (permissive) signals to B cells
  Activate the generation of different antibody classes
  Activate effector T cells

Effector T cells
  Two types, producing delayed hypersensitivity and
     cytotoxic effects.
    Responsible for:
    1. Immunologic surveillance for malignant cells
    2. Eradication of established viral and fungal infection
    3. Eradication of intracellular bacterial infection
    4. Destruction of parasites

Suppressor (immunoregulatory) T cells
  Control inflammation produced by T cells
  Control antibody production
  Balance ratio of immunoglobulin classes
  Block activation of T- and B-cell clones reactive to "self"

From Dwyer, JM: The Cell-Mediated Immune System. Cutter Biologicals, Emeryville, CA, 1982, p 3, with permission.

sess the ability to lyse tumor cells directly. For a more in-depth discussion of cell-mediated immunity and immune mechanisms, the reader is referred to basic textbooks on immunology.

Information about subpopulations of mononuclear phagocytes is rudimentary at present. However, it is clear that the morphology and functions of these cells is affected greatly by the degree of maturation, by environmental (tissue) factors, and by the state of cellular activation.

Macrophages are required for both kinds of immune response — humoral and cell-mediated. Bone marrow–derived blood monocytes circulate to sites of inflammation and populate various tissues. Monocytes, which migrate from peripheral circulation to tissues, further differentiate into tissue macrophages, which retain the ability to multiply but cannot return back into the blood. Macrophages participate in a wide variety of cellular activities, which may be divided into three general functions: phagocytosis, secretion of chemicals vital to inflammation, and initiation of the immune response (Fig. 16-1). Each function is not performed by all macrophages. A system of fixed macrophages known as the reticuloendothelial system (RES) is located throughout the body and specializes predominantly in phagocytosis. Several of these fixed macrophages are given special designations, such as the "Kupffer's cells" of the liver, "littoral cells" of the spleen, and "dust cells" of the lung. RES cells are also found in the lymph nodes, tonsils, and gut-associated lymphoid tissue. Predominantly nonphagocytic macrophages are also located in many other tissue; one example would be the "Langerhans cells" of the skin.

The metabolism and physiology of granulocytic phagocytes are discussed in this chapter, with major emphasis on neutrophils. Disorders of neutrophils are discussed in Chapter 17.

## PRODUCTION OF NEUTROPHILS AND CIRCULATING KINETICS

All hematopoietic cells arise from a common, self-sustaining pool of pluripotent stem cells that become committed as they mature to one of the designated cell lines (granulocyte-monocyte, erythrocyte, or megakaryocyte). Leukopoiesis is discussed in another chapter and will only briefly be summarized here. The colonal growth of committed granulocyte-monocyte stem cells in vitro is dependent on the presence of growth factors called colony-stimulating activities (CSA); several varieties of CSA have been described in murine and human systems.[1,2] CSA is found in increased quantities in the blood and urine of normal individuals when an increased demand for neutrophils is present; however, CSA produced endogenously in the bone mar-

row may have greater importance than that circulating in the bloodstream.[3] The most important function of CSA seems to be to amplify leukopoiesis (that is, to increase the proliferation of previously committed cells) rather than to recruit pluripotent stem cells into the granulocyte-monocyte differentiation pathway. Many other factors interact with CSA to influence leukocyte production in the bone marrow, but their precise interrelationships and relative biologic importance are incompletely defined.[4-6]

Once committed to the neutrophil cell line, the precursors progress in an orderly manner through stages of proliferation (myeloblast, promyelocyte, and myelocyte) and maturation (metamyelocyte and segmented polymorphonuclear neutrophils). Neutrophils can be stored in the marrow until release into the circulating blood. Once in the bloodstream, neutrophils are equally divided into marginating and circulating pools, between which there is a constant exchange of cells.[7] Marginating cells can be mobilized into the circulating pool during stress by epinephrine. Neutrophils leave the blood in a random fashion after a circulating half-life of approximately seven hours and do not re-enter the blood from the tissue.

Structural development of neutrophil precursors in human marrow has been well studied.[8,9] The myeloblast is the earliest recognized cell committed to neutrophil production. It is a small cell ($10\mu$) with a large nucleus and prominent nucleoli; the cytoplasm is devoid of granules but contains mitochondria and free polyribosomes. The promyelocyte is larger ($15\mu$) with prominent secretory organelles (rough endoplasmic reticulum and Golgi apparatus). The primary (azurophilic) granules arise during this stage from the concave surfaces of the Golgi laminae. They are rounded or slightly elongated and may contain crystalline inclusions. Primary granules are lysosomes containing acid and neutral hydrolases, cationic basic proteins, lysozyme, and myeloperoxidase; myeloperoxidase serves as a convenient marker for these structures. The myelocyte is smaller ($10\mu$) with a prominent secretory apparatus and a mixed population of granules. The secondary (specific) granules, which arise at this stage from the convex surfaces of the Golgi laminae, are seen only in neutrophils and vary considerably in size and shape. Eventually, secondary granules predominate 2:1 over the primary ones. It is likely that there are several subtypes of specific granules, some of which contain lactoferrin, lysozyme, and vitamin $B_{12}$–binding proteins. Metamyelocytes and polymorphonuclear neutrophils are nondividing cells characterized by increasing lobulation and condensation of the nuclear chromatin. The secretory apparatus is inconspicuous by electron microscopy, but organelles present include cytoplasmic granules, aggregates of glycogen, a few mitochondria, and cytoskeletal structures (microtubules and microfilaments).

## LEUKOCYTE COUNTS IN BONE MARROW, BLOOD, AND IN RESPONSE TO INFECTION

Alterations of the number and morphology of leukocytes in the bloodstream and bone marrow have long been used as clinical guides for the diagnosis of many diseases. These alterations may simply reflect the normal physiologic response of leukocytes to an underlying disease or they may indicate a primary disorder of these cells as might be seen in leukemia. Thus, a thorough knowledge of normal values is important so that deviations from normal can be readily recognized.

### Bone Marrow

Although leukocytes are generally regarded to be blood cells, they use the blood primarily as a route of transportation from sites of production in the marrow to sites of function in the tissues. Granulocytes, lymphocytes, and monocytes are leukocytes that are formed in the bone marrow for release into the blood. In addition, lymphocytes can proliferate in extramedullary lymphoid tissue and can be released into the bloodstream from these sites. Just as changes in blood leukocyte composition can furnish important diagnostic information, characteristic changes in bone marrow composition or in cellular morphology can occur with some diseases. Values for the various cell types, as determined by differential cell counting of bone marrow samples from healthy individuals, are presented in Table 16–2. Values are fairly constant except during infancy when they vary according to age.[10]

Erythrocyte precursors decrease shortly after birth and remain low until active erythropoiesis resumes during the second to third month of life. The percentage of granulocyte precursors (predominantly neutrophils) decreases precipitously during the first month of life, owing to a decrease in mature forms. Values are stable during infancy and increase during later childhood to adult levels. Lymphocyte numbers increase sharply during the first month of life, and this cell is the most numerous one

in the marrow throughout infancy. Plasma cells are virtually absent until approximately 6 months of age. Normally, granulocyte precursors outnumber erythroid about 3:1 with the postmitotic neutrophil forms (metamyelocytes and segmented polymorphonuclear neutrophils) predominating to form the storage pool. During bacterial infections the granulocyte to erythrocyte ratio can increase owing to increased granulocyte production.

### Blood

The determination of blood leukocyte concentration is somewhat inaccurate when performed manually using a hemocytometer plus a stained blood smear. This is particularly true when counting leukocytes from one of the less numerous subpopulations; the margin of error can be 10 to 20 percent. However, this range of accuracy is satisfactory for most clinical purposes. Currently, most hospital and clinical laboratories perform total and differential leukocyte counts using electronic, automated equipment, and the margin of error has been reduced considerably.[11] Blood leukocyte counts vary considerably with age; a broad range of acceptable normal counts is provided in Table 16–3. Generally, only mature, nondividing leukocytes are present in the blood of healthy individuals. However, if a large number of leukocytes are counted (for example, by examining stained smears of a buffy coat preparation), immature myeloid cells, atypical lymphocytes, plasma cells, and even nuclear fragments of megakaryocytes can be found. Thus, unusual cells are occasionally found by chance, and a single strange or unexpected leukocyte should not be considered indicative of an abnormality unless other clinical or laboratory findings suggest the presence of disease.

A wide range of blood leukocyte counts exists at birth in healthy infants, and the neutrophil is the predominant cell.[12] Although not apparent in Table 16–3, significant changes in the differential white blood cell count occur during the first few days of life. At birth, the mean neutrophil count is about 8000/$\mu$l. This count rises rapidly to a peak value of about 13,000/$\mu$l at 12 hours of age, but then drops to a mean of about 5000/$\mu$l by 72 hours of age. Thereaf-

Table 16–2. PERCENTAGES OF PRECURSOR CELL TYPES IN THE BONE MARROW

| Cell Type | Birth | 1 mo | 3 mo | 12 mo | Adult |
|---|---|---|---|---|---|
| Erythrocytes | 7–21 | 3–12 | 8–19 | 4–12 | 18–30 |
| Granulocytes | 54–72 | 27–33 | 25–50 | 25–44 | 50–70 |
| Early:Late | 1:12 | 1:9 | 1:9 | 1:10 | 1:5 |
| Lymphocytes | 8–20 | 35–55 | 32–56 | 32–58 | 3–17 |
| Plasma Cells | 0 | 0 | 0 | 0–1 | 0–2 |

Table 16–3. RANGE OF BLOOD LEUKOCYTE COUNTS (ABSOLUTE NUMBER $\times$ 10$^3$/$\mu$l)

| Cell Type | Birth | 6 mo | 4 yr | Adult |
|---|---|---|---|---|
| Total leukocytes | 4–40 | 5–24 | 5–15 | 4–11 |
| Neutrophils | 2–20 | 0.5–10 | 1.5–7.5 | 1.5–7.5 |
| Lymphocytes | 1–9 | 1.5–22 | 1.5–8.5 | 1–4.5 |
| Monocytes | 0–2 | 0–2.5 | 0–1 | 0–1 |
| Eosinophils | 0–1.5 | 0–2.5 | 0–1 | 0–0.5 |
| Basophils | 0–0.3 | 0–0.4 | 0–0.2 | 0–0.2 |

ter, the neutrophil count slowly decreases so that the lymphocyte becomes the predominant cell by the age of two to three weeks ($4000/\mu l$). In addition, during the first few days of life, varying numbers of immature neutrophils such as myelocytes and metamyelocytes can be identified in the blood (so-called left shift). These immature neutrophils have been noted, particularly in the blood of premature infants. When the left shift is carried to extreme in the face of relatively low leukocyte counts—the absolute neutrophil count less than $3000/\mu l$ with greater than 70 percent neutrophils being immature cells such as myelocytes and metamyelocytes— septicemia should be strongly suspected.[13] Finally, the monocyte count during the early days of life may transiently exceed values observed in older children and in adults.

The diurnal variation of neutrophil counts as observed in adults (significantly higher values in the afternoon than in the morning) has not been recognized in infants. No difference in normal values exists between boys and girls during childhood. However, in adults the total leukocyte count is higher in women than in men owing to a significantly higher neutrophil count,[14] a phenomenon apparently related to sex hormones.[15] Presumably, similar findings would be expected in sexually mature adolescents. The mean total leukocyte and neutrophil counts in healthy black children older than one year are lower than those in whites, although no racial differences are apparent in lymphocyte, monocyte, eosinophil, and basophil counts.[16]

## Response of Blood Neutrophils to Infections

The characteristic response of the blood leukocyte count to bacterial infections is neutrophilia with an increased percentage of metamyelocytes, bands, stabs, and high-peroxidase cells. This increase in more immature forms has been traditionally called a left shift. Many investigators have proposed criteria, based on total and differential leukocyte counts, in attempts to accurately distinguish bacterial infections from other disorders causing leukocytosis. Unfortunately, no method can predict the etiology of inflammation with complete accuracy —particularly to document whether or not a bacterial infection is present—and a number of reports have emphasized the lack of specificity and pitfalls of interpreting leukocyte counts.[17-19] With severe infections, atypical features of the leukocyte response can be seen. As mentioned earlier, leukopenia with an absolute neutropenia and marked left shift has been reported, particularly during infancy, to be a bad prognostic feature. It may be a manifestation of increased margination owing to endotoxemia, or it may indicate depletion of neutrophil reserves from the bone marrow and transient failure of leukopoiesis. Only when the results of total and differential leukocyte counts are combined with information from the history, physical examination, and other laboratory studies such as chest roentgenogram, cultures, and sedimentation rate can a rational management decision be made. Certainly, it would be foolish to select or reject antibiotic therapy based exclusively on the leukocyte count.

The kinetics of circulating neutrophils vary greatly depending on the type, duration, and intensity of the infection.[20] The immediate response to infection is transient neutropenia resulting from increased margination and accelerated delivery of neutrophils to the infected site. Within an hour, neutrophils are released from the bone marrow reserve into the bloodstream. In the early phases of infection, the circulating half-life of neutrophils is shortened and cell turnover is accelerated. Later, the blood neutrophil pool is expanded, and the circulating half-life becomes normal. Neutrophil production in the marrow increases by several mechanisms: (1) Pluripotent stem cells are committed to the granulocyte differentiation pathway; (2) the generation (cell cycle) time of myelocytes is shortened; (3) myelocytes undergo an extra division (thus, the proliferative pool of precursors can be expanded independently of an increased input of pluripotent stem cells); and (4) transit time through the bone marrow is accelerated.

In addition to changes in the neutrophil blood count, neutrophil morphology can be altered by infection. Cytoplasmic granules become prominent ("toxic" granulation) owing to altered staining properties of the primary granules (see Color Figure 136), and large, bluish bodies (Döhle) may be seen (see Color Figure 137). Döhle bodies consist of a few strands of rough endoplasmic reticulum that have aggregated.[21] They are basophilic, pyroninophilic, and similar, but not identical, to the inclusions found in the hereditary leukocyte and platelet disorder known as the May-Hegglin anomaly (see Chapter 17 for a description of the May-Hegglin anomaly). Finally, the cytoplasm of circulating neutrophils may become vacuolated (see Color Figure 138) and, occasionally, may contain ingested microorganisms. Although all of these morphologic features suggest the presence of infection, most of them can be seen with severe inflammation due to almost any etiology, including drug reactions.

The function of circulating neutrophils, as well as their number and appearance, can be affected by infection.

The nitroblue tetrazolium (NBT) dye was once used to differentiate certain types of bacterial infection from nonbacterial diseases. The procedure is based on the ability of leukocytes to reduce the NBT dye to large black deposits within the cytoplasm of the neutrophil (NBT positive). Less than 10 percent of the 100 neutrophils counted under oil immersion on the prepared smears are positive in normal, healthy adults. However, the percentage increases drastically during bacterial infections, because the neutrophils undergo metabolic changes during active phagocytosis (see section on biochemistry accompanying phagocytosis). This test has little clinical use currently, because it lacks specificity. Elevated NBT tests have been reported in bacterial infections, tuberculosis, fungal infections, parasitic infections, lymphomas, and in normal newborn infants.

Several neutrophil properties have been studied during infections, and both enhanced and impaired functions have been reported when compared with normal values.[22,23] Although a number of exceptions exist, it is generally accepted that mild infections enhance neutrophil functions,[24,25] whereas neutrophil functions are impaired during severe infections. The role that these acquired functional abnormalities play in the course of infections is unknown. It is important to remember, when investigating patients for qualitative neutrophil defects, that abnormalities of function may be the consequence, and not necessarily the cause, of infections.

## NEUTROPHIL LOCOMOTION

Information pertaining to the in vivo movement of neutrophils in humans has been derived largely from in vitro studies and from experiments in animals.[26-28] Thus, information in this area is somewhat speculative. The three types of neutrophil locomotion that have been identified by in vitro assays are random mobility, chemokinesis, and chemotaxis. Chemokinesis is random mobility that has been enhanced by the mere presence of stimulatory substances (chemotaxins) in the absence of a concentration gradient. Chemotaxis is the oriented or directed locomotion of neutrophils induced by a concentration gradient of stimulatory substances in which the cells move toward the highest concentration of the stimulatory (chemotactic) factors.

To participate in an inflammatory reaction in tissue, the neutrophil first slows its speed in the circulation and rolls along the walls of capillaries and venules. Eventually, the cell adheres to vascular endothelium and emigrates from the bloodstream by penetrating a narrow gap between endothelial cells. Neutrophils are briefly retained by the basement membrane but then enter the tissues by passing through small openings in the vascular basement membrane. This process is dependent on energy (adenosine triphosphate) production from glucose, requires calcium and magnesium, and is enhanced by the presence of chemotactic factors.

A large number of substances generated by the inflammatory response have been demonstrated to be chemotactic factors.[27] Complement-related chemotaxis includes fragments of C5 (C5a and C5a desarg) and the trimolecular complex, $C\overline{567}$. Chemotactic factors that are derived from the kinin-coagulation system include kallikrein, plasminogen activator, fibrinopeptide B, fibrin degradation products, and platelet-derived complement activators. Products of bacterial growth, such as N-formyl-methionyl-oligopeptides and oxidized lipids, exhibit chemoattractant activity. Other substances generated by inflammatory or immune reactions that exhibit chemotactic factor activity are materials released from all types of phagocytic leukocytes, lymphokines, supernatant fluids of virally infected cells, and a variety of denatured proteins.

The first step in the process of neutrophil locomotion is the binding of chemotactic factor molecules to specific receptors located on the plasma membrane of the neutrophil.[28] Depending on experimental conditions, chemotactic factor-receptor interaction can initiate a number of cellular functions in addition to chemotaxis. These functions include neutrophil aggregation (clumping), exocytosis (secretion) of the contents of cytoplasmic granules, and several biochemical changes including an increase in oxidative metabolism. A number of profound cellular effects follow binding of chemotactic factors to the neutrophil plasma membrane to mediate these functions.[26-28] Within seconds of chemotactic factor binding, the neutrophil membrane becomes more fluid, the concentration of cyclic adenosine monophosphate doubles, the electrical charge of the cell changes and calcium is mobilized from the neutrophil membrane into the cytosol. Other findings that have been described within the first few minutes of chemotactic factor-neutrophil interaction include secretion of granular contents, movements of ions (potassium, sodium, and calcium), activation of enzymes, cellular swelling, and an increase in microtubule assembly. At present, the movements of calcium within the neutrophil are considered by most investigators to be a key event. Precisely how calcium controls cell movement is undefined, but it is likely that cooperation with calmodulin (a calcium-binding protein) and interactions with several enzymes and cytoskeletal structures are important.

It is apparent that many humoral and cellular factors promote optimal chemotaxis. Similarly, several processes are involved in suppressing cell locomotion.[29-33] Controlled suppression of neutrophil locomotion is necessary to concentrate these cells at the inflammatory site by halting further migration. In addition, these suppressive mechanisms may protect normal tissues by limiting the inflammatory response. Neutrophils that have interacted with chemotactic factors become refractory or less responsive to subsequent exposure to chemotactic factors, a phenomenon called deactivation. An almost countless number of materials have been identified in normal plasma or serum and in inflammatory exudates and cellular extracts that suppress the chemotactic response in vitro.[32,33] These inhibitors can interact with chemotactic factors simply to inactivate them. Alternatively, some antagonists act directly on neutrophils to render them unresponsive to chemotaxins.

## PHAGOLYSOSOME FORMATION

Phagocytosis, ingestion, or the internalization of particles is the first step in phagolysosome formation. Plasma proteins are necessary for the efficient phagocytosis of most pathogenic microorganisms. These proteins, called opsonins, promote the interaction of the surfaces of microorganisms with receptors on the neutrophil plasma membrane. Heat-stable opsonins are antibodies, most commonly of the IgG and IgM classes, with activity directed against antigens located on the surface of the microorganisms. When alone, specific antibodies are able to function efficiently as opsonins only if they are of the IgG class and are present in great excess (the so-called hyperimmune state). Under these circumstances, the intact immunoglobulin molecule is required, with the antibody simultaneously binding to the microorganism via the $F(ab')_2$ combining site and to the neutrophil surface through the Fc portion of the molecule.

In most clinical situations the opsonic activities of specific antibodies are enhanced by recruiting the complement system.[34] Briefly, the classic complement pathway is initiated by the binding of C1q to the antibody-bacteria complex to eventually induce deposition of opsonically active C3. Another mechanism for opsonization, present in nonimmune individuals, is the heat labile opsonin system. Its activity is destroyed by heating of serum to 56°C, and it depends on an intact alternative pathway of complement activation (complement is discussed further in Chapter 11). Although enhanced by gammaglobulin, it functions independently of specific antibodies. Thus, it is believed to provide an important defense during the early stages of infection (that is, before the appearance of circulating specific antibodies).

The attachment phase of phagocytosis does not require energy but is a surface phenomenon that depends on the presence of receptors on the neutrophil plasma membrane. Human neutrophils will bind, and therefore presumably have Fc receptors for, monomeric IgG1, IgG3, IgA1, and IgA2. Human neutrophils will bind all of these immunoglobulins, plus IgG4, when aggregated, but they will bind neither monomeric nor aggregated IgM, IgE, or IgD.[35] Fc receptors for IgG are important for the ingestion phase of phagocytosis, whereas C3b receptors promote adherence but cannot, by themselves, mediate efficient phagocytosis.[34]

The ingestion of particles that have been bound to the neutrophil surface requires energy (adenosine triphosphate) that is generated via glucose phosphorylation by anaerobic glycolysis. Ingestion is a process of cell locomotion and shares many metabolic requirements with chemotaxis. For example, to ingest a particle that is attached to the neutrophil surface, pseudopodia extend out and around the particle in cup-like fashion until they fuse. This movement requires energy, a functioning cytoskeleton and calcium. Even before ingestion is complete, cytoplasmic granules approach the phagocytic vesicle, fuse with it, and discharge their contents into it (degranulate) to form a phagolysosome (Fig. 16-2). The molecular biology of degranulation in vivo is unknown, but the in vitro process of granule secretion (reverse endocytosis or exocytosis) is believed to be comparable. Secretion involves locomotion of cytoplasmic granules, and much of the molecular biology involved is similar to that pertaining to chemotaxis and phagocytosis.[36,37]

Information from in vitro studies suggests an orderly sequence of events for phagolysosome formation.[38-40] Discharge of secondary (specific) granules precedes that of the primary (azurophilic) ones. In rats and in humans, the timing of degranulation has been coordinated with changes of intravesicular pH. The contents of secondary granules appear within the phagolysosome 30 seconds after ingestion, and the pH at this time ranges between 6.5 and 7.4. Myeloperoxidase, the marker for primary granules, is not detected until approximately three minutes after phagocytosis. The pH begins to fall at this time and reaches a level of about 4.0 ten minutes after particle ingestion. The timing of sequential degranulation and pH changes seems well designed, since the contents of secondary granules function best at neutral pH and those of the primary ones best in the acid range.

## BIOCHEMISTRY ACCOMPANYING PHAGOCYTOSIS

Neutrophils consume glucose and oxygen during phagocytosis.[41-46] Glucose is metabolized via anaerobic glycolysis to provide adenosine triphosphate as energy for the ingestion of particles. A burst of oxidative metabolism accompanies phagocytosis in vitro and is characterized by an increase in oxygen consumption and by the production of a variety of reactive species of oxygen molecules. To date, oxidative metabolism of human neutrophils is only partially defined, and considerable debate exists regarding many of its aspects.[42-47] The sharp increase in oxygen uptake that accompanies phagocytosis was discovered in the 1930s, and the mistaken assumption was made that oxidative metabolism pro-

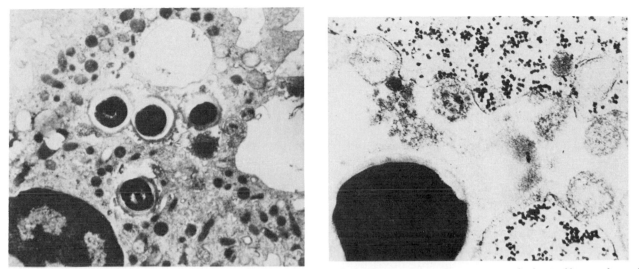

**Figure 16-2.** Electron microscopy of phagolysosome formation. *Left,* Staphylococci lie within phagocytic vesicles limited by sacs formed from inverted pieces of the neutrophil plasma membrane. Cytoplasmic granules are approaching the phagocytic vesicles. *Right,* Higher magnification that shows degranulation with the discharge of granule contents into the vicinity of the staphylococcus.

vided energy for phagocytosis. It is now clear that anaerobic glycolysis, not oxidative metabolism, provides energy for phagocytosis. In the 1960s it was recognized that at least part of the oxygen consumed was converted to hydrogen peroxide ($H_2O_2$), and that increased activity of the hexose monophosphate shunt accompanied phagocytosis. Since the 1970s it has become clear that the oxygen consumed is initially reduced to form superoxide anion ($O_2^-$) and then is reduced further to $H_2O_2$. In addition it has been demonstrated that human neutrophils produce a variety of reactive species of oxygen molecules such as hydroxyl radical ($OH \cdot$) and singlet oxygen ($^1O_2$). A number of other biochemical reactions are associated with the postphagocytic oxidative burst, including the generation of chemiluminescence, reduction of tetrazolium dyes, oxidation and depletion of glutathione, iodination of proteins, production of lipoxygenase and cyclo-oxygenase products of arachidonic acid,[47] and cellular binding of estradiol.

Although the postphagocytic oxidative burst consists of several separate events, all appear to depend on the activity of an intimately integrated, complex enzyme system. This system is insensitive to cyanide and does not require phagocytosis per se for activation but will respond to a variety of surface-active agents such as cardiac glycosides, endotoxin, vitamin C, phorbol myristate acetate, lectins, and many chemotactic factors. Although the key enzyme has not been precisely identified, most investigators agree that the likely candidate is a flavoprotein oxidase located on or intimately related to the plasma membrane.[42–47] Most current evidence suggests that this enzyme is nicotinamide adenine dinucleotide phosphate (NADPH) oxidase, although some investigators favor NADH as substrate. Other

components of this system include a flavoprotein and cytochrome b.[48,49]

Microorganisms within phagolysosomes are killed by a variety of oxygen-dependent mechanisms, the most important of which is the myeloperoxidase-$H_2O_2$-halide system.[46] Myeloperoxidase is present in the primary granules and is delivered to the phagolysosomes by degranulation. $H_2O_2$ is generated during the postphagocytic oxidative burst. Chloride ions are present within the cytosol and serve as the halide, although neutrophils are able to obtain iodide from thyroid hormone. Myeloperoxidase catalyzes the oxidation of halide by $H_2O_2$ to form hypohalite ions, a reaction that greatly increases the bactericidal effects of $H_2O_2$. Bacteria can be killed by a variety of substances generated by this system.[45,46] One is by the formation of singlet oxygen, a highly reactive molecule that can be produced by the reaction of hypochlorite with $H_2O_2$. Other reactions are the halogenation of bacterial cell walls and the decarboxylation of amino acids with their subsequent conversion to aldehydes. The correlation between bacterial killing and either of these last two reactions, however, is only fair. Other oxygen-dependent mechanisms that have been demonstrated in vitro include $H_2O_2$ reacting without myeloperoxidase and the independent actions of $O_2^-$, $OH_2$, and $^1O_2$. The in vivo importance of each of these reactive molecules of oxygen as they act independently remains to be established.

Lipid biochemistry is an area of postphagocytic metabolism that is currently being explored with great interest. Data are incomplete, but it appears certain that phospholipid metabolism, particularly that involving arachidonic acid, plays a crucial role in a number of neutrophil functions.[47] Neutrophils metabolize arachidonic acid to generate products of both the lipoxygenase (derivatives of hydroxyeicosatetraenoic acid) and cyclo-oxygenase (thromboxanes and prostaglandins of the E and F series) pathways when activated by phagocytosis or soluble surface-active agents such as chemotactic factors. Unstimulated (resting) neutrophils either fail to produce these products or do so in much smaller quantities. It has been proposed, largely on the basis of in vitro studies, that arachidonic acid is released from plasma membrane phospholipids of activated cells by a phospholipase. Arachidonic acid is metabolized by neutrophils largely through the lipoxygenase pathway, and the metabolites influence cellular function either directly or by modulating the effects of other agents. For example, certain hydroxyeicosatetraenoic acids mediate enzyme release and cellular locomotion. In addition, certain lipoxygenase products, while having no direct effects of enzyme secretion, enhance this function when neutrophils are stimulated by fragments of C5. The mechanisms by which these lipid products affect or modulate neutrophil functions are only partially defined, although one mechanism defined in rabbit neutrophils is by increasing the influx of calcium. Finally, certain products of arachidonic acid metabolism can inhibit neutrophil functions and, in fact, can suppress further arachidonic acid metabolism (perhaps a means of autoregulation).

Neutrophils, like all aerobic cells, possess antioxidant protective mechanisms against self-inflicted damage (auto-oxidation).[50,51] Two isoenzymes of superoxide dismutase are present in human neutrophils. The majority of superoxide dismutase activity is present as the cytoplasmic copper-zinc enzyme, while the remainder is the manganese-containing enzyme found in mitochondria. Superoxide dismutase catalyzes the dismutation reaction: $2O_2^- + 2H^+ \rightarrow H_2O_2 + O_2$. It protects cells from superoxide anion while generating $H_2O_2$, another potentially damaging molecule. Glutathione peroxidase and catalase detoxify $H_2O_2$. Glutathione peroxidase mediates the reaction: $2GSH + H_2O_2 \rightarrow GSSG + H_2O$. Catalase converts hydrogen peroxide to water: $2H_2O_2 \rightarrow 2H_2O + O_2$. Glutathione peroxidase and catalase are the major enzymes responsible for detoxifying $H_2O_2$. They act, in concert, to protect cells from oxidant damage.

## PHYSIOLOGY AND RESPONSE TO INFECTIONS OF OTHER TYPES OF GRANULOCYTES

It is beyond the scope of this chapter to discuss in great detail all aspects of eosinophil and basophil biology. Information about these two types of leukocytes is scanty when compared with that available for neutrophils, and considerably more controversy exists regarding several aspects of function.

Accordingly, the following discussions are brief and emphasize similarities and differences between these granulocytes and neutrophils.

## Eosinophils

The study of eosinophils in humans has been hampered by difficulties in obtaining sufficient numbers of normal cells for study. Accordingly, most studies of eosinophil physiology and function have employed cells obtained either from patients with eosinophilia or from animals—sources of eosinophils that possibly do not represent normal cells. Indeed, biochemical and functional differences were demonstrated between eosinophils isolated from the blood of normal individuals and those isolated from patients with eosinophilia.[52] These limitations must be remembered.

Eosinophils are formed from committed stem cells in the bone marrow.[53] It is believed that eosinophil development and neutrophil development are similar, although committed stem cells that give rise to eosinophil colonies in vitro can be separated at an early stage of development from those giving rise to neutrophil-monocyte colonies. Moreover, regulatory humoral factors that control eosinophil production in the bone marrow and release to the bloodstream may differ from those involved in neutrophil maturation and release. There is a diurnal variation of blood eosinophil counts, with the highest counts occurring at night.[54] This is believed to be related to the eosinophil suppressive effects of endogenous adrenal corticosteroid levels, which are highest during the morning. Steroids inhibit eosinophil release from the bone marrow and increase the removal of these cells from the blood. The blood eosinophil count is higher in children less than 10 years of age than it is in older individuals.[55] The average eosinophil count for these children ranges from $240/\mu l$ to $740/\mu l$. In children less than age 10, values for boys are slightly higher than those for girls.

The roles that eosinophils play in the body defense mechanisms and in inflammation are only partially understood. Eosinophils are capable of phagocytosis, but it has been suggested that these cells function primarily by secreting granular contents and reactive molecules of oxygen onto extracellular surfaces. Eosinophils possess a single major type of cytoplasmic granule.[56,57] The granules contain a crystaloid core that is composed of the major basic protein (MBP). MBP is an arginine-rich protein with a molecular weight of about 10,000 daltons that accounts for over 50 percent of granule proteins. It can neutralize heparin and is toxic both to organisms (such as Schistoma) and to normal host tissues. Other materials contained in the eosinophil granules include acid hydrolases, arylsulfatase B, phospholipase D, cationic proteins, Charcot-Leyden crystal protein, and a peroxidase that is genetically, chemically, and immunologically distinct from the myeloperoxidase present in neutrophils and mononuclear phagocytes. Eosinophil granules lack lysozyme.

Eosinophils are able to mount a vigorous postphagocytic oxidative burst.[58,59] All aspects of postphagocytic oxidative metabolism are either equal to or in excess of that demonstrated in neutrophils, a finding ascribed to a threefold to sixfold increase in NADPH oxidase activity. Although eosinophils possess the necessary antimicrobial tools, it is generally accepted that their overall microbicidal activities are diminished when compared with those of neutrophils. It is clear, however, that the antimicrobial activities of eosinophils against helminths and other parasites are equal to or exceed those of neutrophils.[60,61]

It is difficult to demonstrate a consistent response of the eosinophil count to infections because of the low numbers of these cells normally present in the bloodstream. Generally, the response to acute infection involves a rapid and persistent decrease that has often been ascribed to an increase in the endogenous levels of adrenal corticosteroids and catecholamines. It is clear that this explanation does not always apply, and eosinopenia may be due to the presence of other inflammatory mediators, such as chemotactic factors.[62] The most frequent cause of eosinophilia is an allergic condition such as asthma or hay fever, although the eosinophil count rarely exceeds $1500/\mu l$ to $2000/\mu l$. Mild eosinophilia can also accompany drug reactions, dermatitis herpetiformis, chronic inflammatory diseases such as ulcerative colitis and vasculitis, and several malignancies, particularly Hodgkin's disease that is being treated by abdominal irradiation. Striking eosinophilia ($>5000/\mu l$) can occur in parasitic infections, particularly those that are characterized by a visceral larva migrans syndrome (Table 16–4).

## Basophils and Mast Cells

Circulating basophils and tissue mast cells are similar in many respects, and they possibly share a common origin. Basophils account for less than 1 percent of leukocytes circulating in the blood, and most of the information available about these cells has been obtained from studies of patients with chronic myelogenous leukemia or from animals. It is becoming increasingly clear that the properties of basophils from animals and humans are not identical. Therefore, much of the following discussion must be considered to be tentative until additional information is available.

Basophilic promyelocytes and myelocytes can be identified in human bone marrow, and it is generally assumed that differentiation parallels the process occurring in neutrophils. The earliest stem cell committed to basophil production has not been identified in normal bone marrow, although colonies grown in vitro from marrow obtained from patients with chronic myelogenous leukemia rarely contain exclusively basophils; rather, colonies contain basophils plus other cells belonging to the granulocyte-monocyte lineage. This suggests that granulocytes, monocytes, and basophils arise from a similar committed precursor in these patients.[63,64]

In many species, the appearance and functional properties of basophils and mast cells are quite similar. In humans, however, the morphology of the two cells is distinctive. Basophils contain a segmented nucleus with a chromatin pattern similar to that of other mature granulocytes, whereas mast cell nuclei are oval, with more widely dispersed nuclear chromatin. Basophil granules contain particulate material, whereas mast granules display crystals, whorls, and lamellae. The finding of transitional cells that exhibit overlapping morphology, such that they cannot be classified as either basophils or mast cells, supports the possibility that human basophils and mast cells arise from the same precursor.[65]

The absolute basophil count in the blood of normal individuals is $30 \pm 10/\mu l$. Basophilia ($>50/\mu l$) occurs in rheumatoid arthritis, allergies, ulcerative colitis, chronic myeloid leukemia, and following estrogen therapy.[66] Basopenia ($<20/\mu l$) has been reported in urticaria and after severe allergic reactions. Since basophils are recognized by their characteristic granules, basopenia in these situations may simply reflect a state of degranulation rather than a true decrease in the number of basophils.

Human basophils and mast cells are characterized by prominent cytoplasmic granules. They are membrane-bound structures that, for the most part, are oval, with a diameter varying in size from 113 to 260 A. These granules contain histamine, which is synthesized within these cells in a reaction mediated by histidine decarboxylase. The metachromatic staining of the granules is due to the presence of sulfated mucopolysaccharides such as chondroitin, dermatin, and heparin sulfates. Basophil granules contain neutral esterases and proteases but apparently lack the acid hydrolases of lysosomes. A number of other substances are released by basophils, although their origin is not always the granules. These substances include platelet-activating factor, eosinophil chemotactic factor, plasminogen

**Table 16–4. CAUSES OF EOSINOPHILIA**

Allergic reactions
Parasitic infections
Asthma
Skin diseases
Brucellosis

activator, peroxidase, and the slow-reacting substance of anaphylaxis. This last material has been identified to be a family of lipid compounds called leukotrienes that are formed from the interaction of arachidonic acid metabolites plus glutathione. Secretion of granule contents can be induced by interactions with cytophilic IgE. It is accomplished by exposing basophils either to antigens to which they are sensitized or to anti-IgE. Basophils and mast cells possess plasma membrane receptors for the Fc fragment of IgE. In addition, a distinct Fc receptor for IgG has been demonstrated on human basophils.[66,67]

Basophils are capable of phagocytosis and pinocytosis, but the major role of these cells in inflammation is related to their release of biologically active materials.[68,69] Mast cells are found in all organs that are rich in connective tissue including the skin, the reticuloendothelial organs, and the submucosal areas of all serous membranes. The consequences of the release of basophil and mast cell mediators are vasodilatation with increased vascular permeability, spasm of smooth muscles, increased secretions, both activation and inhibition of various aspects of blood coagulation, and modulation of the inflammatory response by the recruitment of eosinophils and neutrophils.[66]

## CASE HISTORY

**History of Present Illness.** A 12-year-old girl was admitted with lobar pneumonia. She was perfectly well until two days prior to admission, when she began having fever and cough. Over the previous 48 hours, the temperature had remained at approximately 104°F, and the cough was increasing in intensity. On one occasion, the sputum contained a few flecks of blood. In the past, she had experienced only the usual number of minor respiratory infections, and she had never been this ill before. Approximately six hours prior to admission, she began to breathe rapidly, and her lips became dusky.

**Physical Examination.** She was acutely ill and appeared short of breath. The temperature was 104°F, and she was listless and slightly cyanotic. The only other pertinent findings on the physical examination were confined to the right side of the chest. The right upper chest was dull to percussion, and on auscultation there was very poor air exchange with many fine crackling rales.

**Laboratory Data.** The hemoglobin was 14 g/dl. The total WBC count was 35,000/μl, with 12,000 segmented neutrophils and 18,000 immature neutrophils (bands and stabs and myelocytes); the remainder were mononuclear leukocytes. The neutrophils were filled with toxic granulations and Döhle bodies, and vacuoles were quite abundant. A rare neutrophil contained tiny bodies that appeared on Gram's stain to be gram-positive diplococci. The blood culture subsequently grew Streptococcus pneumoniae.

**Discussion.** This child with lobar pneumonia exhibits the typical picture of a neutrophilic, leukemoid reaction owing to a bacterial infection. Both the absolute and relative neutrophil count were elevated with a marked increase in immature forms (bands, stabs, and myelocytes). Moreover, the alterations of neutrophil cytoplasm (toxic granules, Döhle bodies, and vacuoles) were characteristic of stress leukopoiesis. Obviously, the presence of intracellular microorganisms confirmed that this leukemoid reaction was due to a bacterial infection. However, none of the other features were specific for any single etiology. Other causes that must always be considered include other types of infections (e.g., Staphylococcus, other types of pyogenic bacteria, and leptospirosis), hypersensitivity drug reactions, burns, and other inflammatory diseases such as rheumatoid arthritis. It must also be remembered that at times of overwhelming infection, the leukocyte picture may actually be that of neutropenia, rather than neutrophilia (e.g., Salmonella typhi). Even in this instance, however, the neutrophils that are present are frequently immature forms.

## References

1. Brennan, JK, Lichtman, MA, DiPersio, JF, et al: Chemical mediators of granulopoiesis: A review. Exp Hematol 8:441, 1980.
2. Burgess, AW and Metcalf, D: The nature and action of granulocyte-macrophage colony stimulating factors. Blood 56:947, 1980.
3. Francis, GE, Rhodes, EGH, Berney, JJ, et al: Bone marrow endogenous colony stimulating factor(s): Relation to granulopoiesis in vivo. Exp Hematol 9:332, 1981.
4. Miller, AM, Russell, TR, Gross, MA, et al: Modulation of granulopoiesis: Opposing roles of prostaglandins F and E. J Lab Clin Med 92:983, 1978.
5. Verma, DS, Spitzer, G, Gutterman, JU, et al: Human leukocyte interferon preparation blocks granulopoietic differentiation. Blood 54:1423, 1979.
6. Broxmeyer, HE, DeSousa, M, Smithyman, A, et al: Specificity and modulation of the action of lactoferrin, a negative feedback regulator of myelopoiesis. Blood 55:324, 1980.
7. Cartwright, GE, Athens, JW, and Wintrobe, MM: The kinetics of granulopoiesis in normal man. Blood 24:780, 1964.
8. Bainton, DF, Ullyot, JL, and Farquhar, MR: The development of neutrophilic polymorphonuclear leukocytes in human bone marrow. J Exp Med 134:907, 1981.
9. Bainton, DF: Selective abnormalities of azurophil and specific granules of human neutrophilic leukocytes. Fed Proc 40:1443, 1981.
10. Rosse, C, Kraemer, MJ, Dilon, TL, et al: Bone marrow cell populations of normal infants: the predominance of lymphocytes. J Lab Clin Med 89:1225, 1977.
11. Rosvoll, RV, Mengason, AP, Smith, l, et al: Visual and automated differential leukocyte counts. Am J Clin Pathol 71:695, 1979.

12. Xanthou, M: Leukocyte blood picture in healthy full-term and premature babies during neonatal period. Arch Dis Child 45:242, 1970.
13. Christensen, RD, Bradley, PP, and Rothstein G: The leukocyte left shift in clinical and experimental neonatal sepsis. J Pediatr 98:101, 1981.
14. Bain, BJ and England, JM: Normal haematological values: Sex difference in neutrophil count. Br Med J 877:306, 1975.
15. Bain, BJ and England, JM: Variations in leucocyte count during menstrual cycle. Br Med J 2:473, 1975.
16. Caramihai, E, Karayalcin, G, Aballi, AJ, et al: Leukocyte count differences in healthy white and black children 1 to 4 years of age. Pediatrics 86:252, 1975.
17. Wright, PF, Thompson, J, McKee, KT, et al: Patterns of illness in the highly febrile young child: Epidemiologic, clinical and laboratory correlates. Pediatrics 67:694, 1981.
18. Morens, DM: WBC count and differential. Am J Dis Child 133:25, 1979.
19. Christensen, RD and Rothstein, G: Pitfalls in the interpretation of leukocyte counts of newborn infants. Am J Clin Pathol 72:608, 1979.
20. Walker RI and Willemze, R: Neutrophil kinetics and the regulation of granulopoiesis. Rev Infect Dis 2:282, 1980.
21. Cawley, JC and Hayhoe, FGJ: The inclusions of the May-Hegglin anomaly and Döhle bodies of infection: An ultrastructural comparison. Br J Haematol 22:491, 1972.
22. McCall, CE, Caves, J, Cooper, R, et al: Functional characteristics of human toxic neutrophils. J Infect Dis 124:68, 1971.
23. McCall, CE, DeChatelet, LR, Cooper, MR, et al: Human toxic neutrophils: III. Metabolic characteristics. J Infect Dis 127:26, 1973.
24. Hill, HR, Gerrard, JM, Hogan, NA, et al: Hyperactivity of neutrophil leukotactic responses during active bacterial infection. J Clin Invest 53:996, 1974.
25. van Epps, DE and Garcia, ML: Enhancement of neutrophil function as a result of prior exposure to chemotactic factor. J Clin Invest 66:167, 1980.
26. Becker, EL: Chemotaxis. J Allergy Clin Immunol 66:97, 1980.
27. O'Flaherty, JT and Ward, PA: Chemotactic factors and the neutrophil. Semin Hematol 16:163, 1979.
28. Schiffman, E: Leukocyte chemotaxis. Ann Rev Physiol 44:553, 1982.
29. Nelson, RD, McCormack, RT, Fiegel, VD, et al: Chemotactic deactivation of human neutrophils: Possible relationship to stimulation of oxidative metabolism. Infect Immun 23:282, 1979.
30. Gallin, JI and Wright, DG: Role of secretory events in modulating human neutrophil chemotaxis. J Clin Invest 62:1364, 1978.
31. Goetzl, EJ, Valone, FH, Reinhold, VN, et al: Specific inhibition of the polymorphonuclear leukocyte chemotactic response to hydroxy–fatty acid metabolites of arachidonic acid by methyl ester derivatives. J Clin Invest 63:1181, 1979.
32. Brozna, JP, Senior RM, Kreutzer, DL, et al: Chemotactic factor inactivators of human granulocytes. J Clin Invest 60:1280, 1977.
33. Ginsburg, I and Quie, PG: Modulation of human polymorphonuclear leukocyte chemotaxis by leukocyte extracts, bacterial products, inflammatory exudates, and polyelectrolytes. Inflammation 4:301, 1980.
34. Scribner, DJ and Farhney, D: Neutrophil receptors for IgG and complement: Their roles in the attachment and ingestion phases of phagocytosis. J Immunol 116:892, 1976.
35. Lawrence, DA, Weigle, WO, and Spiegelberg, HL: Immunoglobulins cytophilic for human lymphocytes, monocytes, and neutrophils. J Clin Invest 55:368, 1975.
36. Weissmann, G, Smolen, JE, and Korchak, HM: Release of inflammatory mediators from stimulated neutrophils. N Engl J Med 303:27, 1980.
37. Ignarro, LJ, Lint, TF, and George, WJ: Hormonal control of lysosomal enzyme release from human neutrophils. J Exp Med 139:1395, 1974.

38. Bainton, DF: Sequential degranulation of the two types of polymorphonuclear leukocyte granules during phagocytosis of microorganisms. J Cell Biol 58:249, 1973.
39. Jensen, MS and Bainton, DF: Temporal changes in pH within the phagocytic vacuole of the polymorphonuclear neutrophilic leukocyte. J Cell Biol 56:379, 1973.
40. Jacques, YV and Bainton, DF: Changes in pH within the phagocytic vacuoles of human neutrophils and monocytes. Lab Invest 39:179, 1978.
41. Weisdorf, DJ, Craddock, PR, and Jacob, HS: Glycogenolysis versus glucose transport in human granulocytes: Differential activation in phagocytosis and chemotaxis. Blood 60:888, 1982.
42. Babior, BM: Oxygen-dependent microbial killing by phagocytes. N Engl J Med 298:659, 1978.
43. DeChatelet, LR: Initiation of the respiratory burst in human polymorphonuclear neutrophils: A critical review. J Reticuloendothel Soc 24:73, 1978.
44. Baehner, RL and Boxer, LA: Disorders of polymorphonuclear leukocyte function related to alterations in the integrated reactions of cytoplasmic constituents with the plasma membrane. Semin Hematol 16:148, 1979.
45. DeChatelet LR: Oxidative bactericidal mechanisms of polymorphonuclear leukocytes. J Infect Dis 131:295, 1975.
46. Klebanoff, SJ: Antimicrobial mechanisms in neutrophilic polymorphonuclear leukocytes. Semin Hematol 12:117, 1975.
47. Stenson, WF and Parker, CW: Metabolism of arachidonic acid in ionophore-stimulated neutrophils. J Clin Invest 64:1457, 1979.
48. Gabig, TG, Schervish, EW, and Santinga, JT: Functional relationship of the cytochrome b to the superoxide-generating oxidase of human neutrophils. J Biol Chem 257:4114, 1982.
49. Borregaard, N and Tauber, AI: Subcellular localization of the human neutrophil NADPH oxidase. J Biol Chem 259:47, 1984.
50. Strauss, RG, Snyder, EL, Wallace, PD, et al: Oxygen-detoxifying enzymes in neutrophils of infants and their mothers. J Lab Clin Med 95:897, 1980.
51. Higgins, CP, Bachner, RL, McCallister, J, et al: Polymorphonuclear leukocyte species differences in the disposal of hydrogen peroxide ($H_2O_2$). Proc Soc Exp Biol Med 158:478, 1978.
52. Bass, DA, Grover, WH, Lewis, JC, et al: Comparison of human eosinophils from normals and patients with eosinophilia. J Clin Invest 66:1265, 1980.
53. Quesenberry, P and Levitt, L: Hematopoietic stem cells. N Engl J Med 301:819, 1979.
54. Dahl, R, Venge, P, and Olsson, I: Blood eosinophil leukocytes and eosinophil cationic protein. Scand J Resp Dis 59:323, 1978.
55. Cunningham, AS: Eosinophil counts: Age and sex differences. J Pediatr 87:426, 1975.
56. Butterworth, AE and David, JR: Eosinophil function. N Engl J Med 304:154, 1981.
57. West, BC, Gelb, NA, and Rosenthal, AS: Isolation and partial characterization of human eosinophil granules. Am J Pathol 81:575, 1975.
58. Pincus, SH: Comparative metabolism of guinea pig peritoneal exudate neutrophils and eosinophils. Proc Soc Exp Biol Med 163:482, 1980.
59. DeChatelet, LR, Shirley, PS, McPhail, LC, et al: Oxidative metabolism of the human eosinophil. Blood 50:525, 1977.
60. Baehner, RL, and Johnston, RB: Metabolic and bactericidal activities of human eosinophils. Br J Haematol 20:227, 1971.
61. DeChatelet, LR, Migler, RA, Shirley, PS, et al: Comparison of intracellular bactericidal activities of human neutrophils and eosinophils. Blood 52:609, 1978.
62. Bass, DA, Gonwa, RA, Szejda, P, et al: Eosinopenia of acute infection. J Clin Invest 65:1265, 1980.
63. Aglietta, M, Camussi, G, and Piacibello, W: Detection of ba-

sophils growing in semisolid agar culture. Exp Hematol 9:95, 1981.

64. Denburg, JA, Davison, M, and Beinenstock, J: Basophil production. J Clin Invest 65:390, 1980.

65. Zucker-Franklin, D: Ultrastructural evidence for the common origin of human mast cells and basophils. Blood 56:534, 1980.

66. Dvorak, AM and Dvorak, HF: The basophil: Its morphology, biochemistry, motility, release reactions, recovery and role in the inflammatory responses of IgE-mediated and cell-mediated origin. Arch Pathol Lab Med 103:551, 1979.

67. Ishizaka, R, Sterk, AR, and Ishizaka, K: Demonstration of Fc$\gamma$ receptors on human basophil granulocytes. J Immunol 123:578, 1979.

68. Henderson, WR, and Kaliner, M: Immunologic and nonimmunologic generation of superoxide from mast cells and basophils. J Clin Invest 61:187, 1978.

69. Henderson, WR, Chi, EY, Jong, EC, et al: Mast cell-mediated tumor cell cytotoxicity. J Exp Med 153:520, 1981.

# CHAPTER 17

RONALD G. STRAUSS, M.D.*

# Neutropenia and Qualitative Disorders of Neutrophils

*The author is recipient of Research Career Development Award K04 HD 00255 and Transfusion Medicine Academic Award K07 HL01426 from the National Institutes of Health.

Neutropenia is a quantitative leukocyte disorder defined as a mature blood neutrophil (PMN) count of less than $1500/\mu l$. An increasing number of diseases are being reported with qualitative PMN abnormalities. In these disorders adequate numbers of PMN are usually present, but they function abnormally. Bacterial infections are the consequence of either severe neutropenia or PMN dysfunction. An effective PMN system consists of several processes that must interact in proper sequence to efficiently kill microorganisms. Multiple factors are involved in each of these processes, and PMN dysfunction may be the consequence of an abnormality in any one of them. The pathogenetic mechanisms responsible for the infectious complications and many of the principles of therapy are identical for both quantitative and qualitative PMN disorders. Accordingly, these disorders will be considered together. Conditions associated with neutrophilia and the response to infections and inflammatory disorders are discussed in Chapter 16.

## NEUTROPENIA

Neutropenia is said to exist when the circulating blood contains less than 1500 mature $PMN/\mu l$ (defined as segmented plus band forms). This traditional definition must be qualified, however, because the PMN count transiently decreases to less than $1500/\mu l$ during viral infection; maintains basal level between $500/\mu l$ and $1500/\mu l$ in some healthy blacks, Jordanian Arabs, and Yemenite Jews,[1] and occasionally is reported to be as low as $500/\mu l$ in healthy children less than 4 years of age (see Chapter 16). PMN counts in children are frequently lower without an evident underlying disease. Should counts of 1000 to $1500/\mu l$ be found in apparently well children with normal hemoglobin and platelet values, no further studies are indicated except for periodic blood counts. If the PMN count is less than 1000/$\mu$l, especially if the child has other evidence of disease, an explanation should be sought.

Recurrent, bacterial infections are the hallmark of persistent neutropenia,[2] and the clinical pattern is generally related to the PMN count. For example, excess infections are not a problem if the PMN count is 1000 to 1500/$\mu$l, whereas life-threatening bacterial infections appear spontaneously in patients whose blood counts are less than 200 PMN/$\mu$l. Exceptions occur; for example, severe infections accompany even mild neutropenia if an associated PMN functional defect is present. Infections in patients with severe neutropenia are well controlled if the PMN count increases transiently in response to the stress of infection.

Neutropenia can be present on a congenital or acquired basis, and it is produced by one or a combination of four general mechanisms: (1) decreased production of PMN by the bone marrow; (2) impaired release of PMN from the marrow into the circulating blood with intramedullary cell death; (3) increased destruction of PMN in the peripheral circulation or reticuloendothelial system; and/or (4) maldistribution of PMN resulting in pseudoneutropenia. To demonstrate definitively the mechanisms involved in a particular patient may require laboratory facilities that are generally not available, such as in vitro cultures to document the growth characteristics of bone marrow, radiolabeling to assess circulating kinetics, and immunologic techniques to detect PMN specific antibodies. However, a presumptive diagnosis can usually be made by a few simple studies in conjunction with the clinical findings. Marrow production can be estimated by examining smears of the marrow aspirate and sections of a needle biopsy specimen. Release of PMN from the marrow storage pool can be quantitated following adrenal corticosteroid stimulation, and the distribution of cells within the marginating and circulating pools of blood can be assessed by epinephrine stimulation.[3] It is of additional importance for therapy, prognosis, and family counseling to determine whether the neutropenia is acquired or congenital. Therefore, the physician should obtain a family history and determine if exposure to a myelotoxic agent occurred, if an underlying primary disease is present, or if recurrent bacterial infections are longstanding (suggestive of chronic disease).

## Acquired

Most transient neutropenias in children are acquired rather than congenital, and *viral infections* are a frequent cause. Many children less than 6 years of age will experience neutropenia with a relative lymphocytosis during a viral infection. Sometimes the viral infection is easily identified, as with roseola infantum or rubella, but most times viral infections are presumed to be present by the existence of nonspecific features of an upper respiratory tract or gastrointestinal infection in the absence of a known cause. Bacterial infections can also be associated with neutropenia, at times owing to endotoxemia. In these and in other nonviral infections, such as those due to Mycobacterium tuberculosis and Histoplasma capsulatum, the finding of an associated neutropenia (especially if accompanied by a marked left shift) is somewhat unusual and carries a poor prognosis. Newborns, in particular, are likely to develop severe neutropenia during bacterial infections owing to depletion of the PMN storage pool in the bone marrow.[4]

Acquired neutropenia as a component of pancytopenia occurs in patients who have *bone marrow failure* due to aplastic anemia, invasion with malignant cells, or toxic injury. The last can be either idiosyncratic or predicted as a known consequence of antitumor therapy. Anemia and thrombocytopenia are often associated, and the production failure is quickly identified by bone marrow examination. Isolated neutropenia as a reaction to drugs is uncommon but has been described with a wide variety of agents, particularly antibiotics, and a drug-exposure history should be obtained. Obviously, if a drug is identified as the cause of neutropenia, it should be discontinued and prescribed again only with great caution.

*Acquired immunoneutropenia* can be idiopathic or drug-related, or can develop in association with diseases such as Sjögren's syndrome, systemic lupus erythematosus, rheumatoid arthritis, and infectious mononucleosis. Symptoms of the primary disease are usually present, and immunohemolytic anemia or thrombocytopenia or both may coexist. Autoimmune neutropenia as an isolated feature in a child without an apparent underlying disease is rare; however, patients are being recognized because of improved techniques in identifying PMN-specific antibodies.[5] Antibody in the patient's serum directed at PMN antigens on autologous (patient) PMN must be documented before an irrefutable pathogenic relationship is established. The clinical picture, numbers of PMN in the blood, myeloid maturation, and size of the marrow storage pool are variable, and antibody studies are required. Adrenal corticosteroids may be helpful in some patients. Obviously, this therapy is not without risk in severely neutropenic patients and probably should be employed only when the diagnosis has been firmly made and when response to therapy can be monitored. Very high dose intravenous IgG has been used experimentally in treating patients with immunoneutropenia.

*Isoimmune neonatal neutropenia* that is analogous to isoimmune hemolytic anemia has been described in infants with severe, but transient, neutropenia.[6] Antibodies, demonstrated in both maternal and infant sera, react with infant and paternal PMN but not with maternal cells. PMN specificity is demonstrated by adsorption of the antibody with PMN but not with other blood cells, and by the lack of interaction with cells other than PMN (e.g., an absence of reactivity with lymphocytes). Apparently, the mother becomes sensitized to PMN antigens shared by the infant and father. Once formed, the anti-PMN antibodies cross the placenta. Of note, this probably is not the case with tissue antibodies of broader specificity such as anti-HLA. The latter are adsorbed and removed by the placenta so that isoimmune neonatal neutropenia occurs infrequently despite the presence of leukoagglutinins (anti-HLA, but not anti-PMN) in many multiparous women. Isoimmune neonatal neutropenia is common in the firstborn. Severe neutropenia is present until 6 to 8 weeks of age and can be accompanied by skin and respiratory infections and even sepsis. Myeloid hyperplasia with depletion of the mature storage pool is generally seen in the bone marrow. Therapy is usually supportive and consists of antibiotics when infections occur.

Neutropenia that is associated with *splenomegaly* is rarely severe and, in itself, is generally not a cause for increased susceptibility to infections. Splenomegaly can result from portal hypertension, storage diseases (Gaucher's disease), work hypertrophy (hemoglobinopathies), autoimmune diseases (rheumatoid arthritis), Felty's syndrome, myeloproliferative diseases, cancer, and a variety of chronic infections. Pancytopenia is often present. Generally, the marrow is hypercellular with a depleted storage pool of mature PMN. The depletion of mature cells may give the false appearance of an "arrest in maturation" at the metamyelocyte stage. Traditionally, a true maturation arrest occurs at the earlier promyelocyte-myelocyte level as seen in congenital agranulocytosis. Since the neutropenia is rarely of clinical significance, this finding alone should not be used as an indication for splenectomy.

## Pseudoneutropenia

A few other causes for acquired neutropenia should be considered in the differential diagnosis. Transient neutropenia has been described as a consequence of *complement activation*, with two prime examples being patients undergoing either hemodialysis or filtration leukapheresis. Occasionally, patients receiving long-term parenteral nutrition have been recognized with manifestations of *trace nutrient deficiencies*, such as the neutropenia and anemia that accompany copper deficiency. Finally, a generalized panleukopenia has been described in patients with *anorexia nervosa*. However, serious infections have not been a common occurrence in these patients because, at the time of infection, adequate numbers of PMN are released from marrow stores.

## Congenital

Congenital neutropenias are so rare that estimates of incidence are usually not provided. Although not all authors agree,[7] it seems important to distinguish the various kinds of congenital neutropenias, recognizing their rarity and current limitations of study, to provide more accurate genetic counseling and to better define the pathogenetic mechanisms involved (Table 17–1). Many congenital neutropenias are inherited, and parents must be informed about the possibilities of giving birth to other affected children. Congenital neutropenias are the consequence of decreased production, and several mechanisms could be responsible: absence of PMN precursors; intrinsic cellular defects of PMN precursors prohibiting growth or differentiation or both; deficiency of "leukopoietins," or growth factors; inhibitors directed against either PMN precursors or leukopoietins; or unsuitable marrow microenvironment. In a few patients it has been possible to identify the pathogenetic mechanisms by in vitro marrow culture techniques,[8] but much is to be learned.

*Congenital agranulocytosis* of the Kostmann type

## Table 17–1. CONGENITAL NEUTROPENIAS

| Disorder | Likely Inheritance | Characteristics |
|---|---|---|
| Kostmann agranulocytosis | Autosomal recessive | Neonatal, severe neutropenia. True marrow maturation arrest. |
| Benign neutropenia | Autosomal recessive* | Stress may increase neutrophils. No typical marrow findings. |
| Myelokathexis | Autosomal recessive* | Stress may increase neutrophils. Senescent marrow neutrophils. |
| Cyclic neutropenia | Usually sporadic | 21-day cycles. Associated with immune diseases. |
| Shwachman syndrome | Autosomal recessive | Stress may increase neutrophils. Associated pancreatic insufficiency. |

*Hereditary nature not always firmly established.

is characterized by a severe failure of PMN production with preservation of erythroid and megakaryocytic maturation in the marrow.[9] It usually is inherited as an autosomal recessive trait and is so rare that only about 30 patients were reported having it, in the 20 years following the initial description of the disease.[9] Children with this condition are frequently seen during the first month of life with bacterial infections. The total white blood cell count may be normal, but a severe neutropenia (<200 PMN/$\mu$l) will be present. The differential count may reveal increased monocytes and eosinophils. PMN morphology is normal, but granulated monocytoid cells may be seen, presumably as circulating abortive forms of early PMN precursors. The marrow is normal in cellularity, and myeloid precursors are present. However, rare PMN precursors have differentiated beyond the promyelocyte or early myelocyte stage. Frequently, vacuoles and abnormally large granules are found in the cytoplasm of these cells.[10] In addition to the defect in maturation, proliferation of PMN precursors is decreased and they die in the marrow.

Bone marrow cells from some patients will differentiate in tissue culture systems that contain normal serum, whereas the growth of patient and normal cells often is decreased in the presence of patient serum. An inhibitor has not been identified; rather, patient sera seem simply to lack granulocyte colony-stimulating activity. Occasionally, as a response to severe bacterial infection, PMNs are produced transiently; however, this is most unusual, and persistent, profound neutropenia is the rule. The ability of these patients to contain infections is related to an intact immune system, to the compensatory microbicidal activities of monocytes and eosinophils, and to the careful use of antibiotics.

The major condition to be distinguished from Kostmann's agranulocytosis is a heterogeneous group of disorders called *chronic benign neutropenia*.[7,11] Patients with these disorders have fairly persistent severe to moderate neutropenia with variable marrow findings. Marrow cellularity may be normal or decreased. True maturation arrest at the promyelocyte-myelocyte stage is not seen, but the storage pool may be depleted to give the appearance of an arrest at the metamyelocyte level. Although the pathogenetic mechanisms have been elusive, an evaluation including anti-PMN antibodies should be done to eliminate known underlying diseases. Bacterial infections may occur with increased frequency, but they are often well contained, as the blood PMN count may transiently increase, presumably a response to the stress of infection. The duration of neutropenia is unpredictable, but the prognosis is generally good. The autosomal dominant, moderate neutropenia of blacks, Yemenite Jews, and Jordanians is often included in this category.

A few patients have been described in whom neutropenia is related to an inability to release mature granulocytes into the blood—a disorder called *myelokathexis*.[12,13] At the time of bacterial infections the PMN count is normal or appropriate for the infections. Between infections, however, the PMN count decreases to extremely low values. Myeloid cells are present in the bone marrow, with an excessive number of mature PMN present. These cells are characterized by pyknotic lobes of the nuclei connected by thin, filamentous strands. Granulation frequently is absent, and vacuolization can be identified. Apparently, these cells become senescent and die in the bone marrow without being released into the blood. The mechanism regulating release of mature PMN, particularly under nonstress conditions, is unknown. In one family, this disorder was judged to be inherited in autosomal recessive fashion.

*Organic acidemia* with hyperglycinemia is a rare cause of neutropenia and pancytopenia. Patients with hyperglycinemia have developmental retardation, vomiting, lethargy, dehydration, and ketosis. They have repeated infections, and myeloid cells are decreased in the marrow. The diagnosis is established by the demonstration of hyperglycinemia and hyperglycinuria.

*Cyclic neutropenia* is associated with a variety of conditions and is the consequence of periodic marrow failure.[14,15] Humoral regulators of hematopoiesis may cycle, but by present understanding these changes are probably secondary to a basic defect of bone marrow stem cells. Experiments in gray collie dogs, a model of cyclic neutropenia, support the concept of a stem cell defect because the disease is cured by marrow transplantation from healthy littermates. Moreover, the disease is produced in normal, healthy dogs who receive marrow from affected ones. The molecular defect of the stem cells or in their regulation is unknown.

The clinical symptoms found at the nadir (i.e., the lowest point during the cycle) of the granulocyte count are mouth ulcers and skin or respiratory infections. Occasionally, bacterial infections can be more severe. In the patient who has recurrent episodic periods of fever or infection, it may be necessary to do serial total and differential white blood cell counts two to three times per week for at least two months to demonstrate the cyclic decrease in blood granulocyte concentration. Nadir points are reached about every 21 days. With increasing age, the cycles tend to dampen out. These patients, however, will often have a persisting mild neutropenia. It is important when studying the patient with cyclic neutropenia to determine if the rest of the immune system is also intact, since cyclic neutropenia has been associated with both humoral and cellular immune deficiency.

Pancytopenia may occur in several congenital

disorders in which neutropenia is a prominent feature. *Fanconi's anemia* is one such disorder; it is most likely inherited in autosomal recessive fashion. Marrow failure may not appear until the patient is 5 to 10 years of age.[16] Usually, anemia or thrombocytopenia is the early sign of disease, while neutropenia develops later. Evidence for structural anomalies should be sought. These patients are frequently growth-retarded and may have areas of either hyperpigmentation or hypopigmentation of the skin. Approximately one third have an abnormality of the thumb, while other skeletal anomalies are less frequently found. A complete evaluation should include an intravenous pyelogram, because renal anomalies are common.

Fetal hemoglobin concentration is increased and can precede overt anemia, a fact useful in genetic counseling. Chromosomal breaks and recombination forms can be demonstrated in marrow cells, stimulated lymphocytes, and fibroblasts. The chromosomal abnormalities are probably related to the increased rate of cancer, particularly myeloid leukemia, observed in these patients. Androgenic hormones (combined with adrenal corticosteroids by some) are usually effective, although PMN and platelet counts are less likely to respond than are the erythrocytes. These patients seem particularly susceptible to the toxicities of irradiation and immunosuppressive therapy, and bone marrow transplantation carries an increased risk for them. The prognosis should be guarded because they may fail prolonged androgen therapy (see Chapter 6).

Another form of pancytopenia related to marrow failure is that associated with *dyskeratosis congenita*.[17] Patients with this disorder are frequently studied early in life because of failure to thrive. They have abnormalities of the epithelial surfaces, such as dyskeratosis and poor dental and nail formation. Progressive marrow failure usually occurs during the second half of the first decade. It is not associated with the chromosome abnormalities described in Fanconi's anemia, and it is not as responsive to androgen therapy.

Shwachman and coworkers[18] described a rare form of congenital marrow failure that presents in early life often as failure to thrive with evidence of malabsorption. Patients have recurrent bacterial infections due to neutropenia, although abnormal PMN mobility has been described as an additional defect in some patients. Anemia and thrombocytopenia may occur. Initially the diagnosis may be obscured, particularly if bacterial infection is present, because with the severe stress of infection the PMN count may be normal. As the infection subsides, severe neutropenia becomes apparent. Serial blood leukocyte counts may be necessary to document the neutropenia. The marrow is usually hypocellular without indications of abnormal maturation, although maturation arrest can be seen.

Pancreatic insufficiency is suggested by clinical features of malabsorption and can be documented by the absence of trypsin and other pancreatic enzymes in duodenal juices. The mechanism linking pancreatic insufficiency and marrow failure is unknown. The pancreas appears to be replaced by fatty tissue in a noninflammatory fashion. The process does not seem to be one of pancreatic malformation, but rather one of gradual involution and replacement with fat. Metaphyseal dysostosis can be seen by roentgenographic examination in some patients. There is no known treatment for this condition other than specific therapy for the infections and pancreatic enzyme replacement. The disease varies in severity; some children die within the first few months of life and other children live several years, plagued with recurrent bacterial infections. It is important to identify this disease for family counseling, since it is inherited in an autosomal recessive fashion. Some patients with the Shwachman syndrome have been reported to progress to leukemia.[19]

Additional rare causes of congenital neutropenia or pancytopenia are reticular dysgenesis, cartilage-hair hypoplasia, transcobalamin II deficiency, osteopetrosis, and type 1B glycogen storage disease. The first three have associated immune defects. Those diseases in which neutropenia and PMN dysfunction occur jointly, such as Chédiak-Higashi disease, will be discussed later in this chapter.

## NEUTROPHIL QUALITATIVE DISORDERS

Disorders of PMN dysfunction are characterized by bacterial infections that are due not to decreased numbers of PMN in the blood but to abnormal PMN function. These disorders will be grouped according to the major defect expressed, although it is recognized that multiple abnormalities (including neutropenia) can be detected in some patients.

### Disorders of Mobility

Although these conditions are collectively referred to as chemotactic or leukotactic defects, it must be remembered that PMNs are capable of three major types of movement (chemotactic factor–directed movement known as chemotaxis, nondirected random mobility, and chemotactic factor–stimulated movement [in terms of speed but not necessarily in direction] known as chemokinesis). Detecting an abnormality in one type of movement does not guarantee defects in the other types, particularly when a single patient is being evaluated. Moreover, various in vitro assays of PMN movement may not correlate with each other or with in vivo studies. Finally, the basis for abnormal movement may lie with the PMN itself (intrinsic cellular defect) or with an imbalance of environmental agents promoting (chemotactic factors) and suppressing (cell or chemotaxin-directed inhibitors) movement.

Selected chemotactic disorders ("chemotactic" is used in its broadest sense to refer to PMN mobility of any type) are listed in Table 17-2. The listing is not intended to be all-inclusive and is somewhat tentative as new conditions continue to be reported. Disorders are grouped according to the most acceptable pathogenetic mechanism, although it is realized that multiple mechanisms may be involved.

## Disorders of Cytoplasmic Granules or Their Contents

*Myeloperoxidase (MPO) deficiency* may be congenital or acquired.[20] MPO is present in the primary (azurophilic) granules of PMN, eosinophils, and monocytes-macrophages (located in different intracellular sites in these last cells depending on their degree of differentiation). In congenital MPO deficiency, PMN and monocytes lack MPO, whereas eosinophils are normal.[21,22] This usually is a mild disorder of autosomal recessive inheritance, but patients may have severe Candida infections. MPO-deficient PMNs consume total amounts of oxygen normally after phagocytosis. However, they exhibit prolonged stimulation of the hexose monophosphate shunt and superoxide anion production, plus increased use of hydrogen peroxide via nonmyeloperoxidase mechanisms compared with normal cells.[22,23] Chemiluminescence is decreased, proba-

bly owing to failure of the MPO-dependent reactions important for generating light.

In vitro, MPO-deficient PMNs are unable to kill certain types of Candida, but they eventually kill Staphylococcus and gram-negative enteric bacilli after prolonged incubation. The increased availability of hydrogen peroxide for use in non–myeloperoxidase-catalyzed reactions partially offsets the diminished activity of MPO-dependent microbicidal activities. Thus, the MPO system is important for rapid killing of organisms, especially certain species of Candida. However, alternative antibacterial mechanisms, particularly those with the nonmyeloperoxidase utilization of hydrogen peroxide, can ultimately kill most bacteria if given sufficient time. In addition, it is suggested by the prolonged postphagocytic oxidative burst observed in MPO-deficient PMN that the burst itself may be limited in normal cells by MPO-dependent factors. MPO deficiency can be recognized by either manual or automated histochemical techniques. In these cases, PMNs that are recognized by peroxidase staining will seem to be few in number whereas large, unidentified leukocytes will be increased. However, a Wright-Giemsa stain will reveal many of the large, unidentified cells to be PMNs. Acquired MPO deficiency has been reported in patients with diabetes mellitus, leukemia, myeloproliferative disorders, megaloblastic anemia, and ceroid lipofuscinosis.

*Chédiak-Higashi disease*[24] **(see Color Figure 139)** is an autosomal recessive disorder characterized by

## Table 17-2. SELECTED DISORDERS OF NEUTROPHIL CHEMOTAXIS WITH SELECTED REFERENCES

| | |
|---|---|
| **Intrinsic neutrophil defects** | |
| Lazy leukocyte syndrome | Lancet 1:665, 1971 |
| Monosomy | Blood 54:401, 1979 |
| Burns | Ann Surg 186:746, 1977 |
| Congenital ichthyosis | J Lab Clin Med 82:1, 1973 |
| Chédiak-Higashi disease | Medicine 51:247, 1972 |
| Newborns | Pediatr Res 5:487, 1971 |
| Actin dysfunction | N Engl J Med 291:1093, 1974 |
| Glycoprotein deficiency | Blood 60:160, 1982 |
| Immotile cilia syndrome | Lancet 2:893, 1978 |
| Glycogenosis IB | J Infect Dis 143:447, 1981 |
| **Cell-directed inhibitors** | |
| Cancer | Clin Immunol Immunopathol 9:166, 1978 |
| Surgical patients | Surgery 85:543, 1979 |
| **Chemotactic factor-directed inhibitors** | |
| Anergy (various causes) | J Immunol 113:189, 1974 |
| Cytomegalovirus | J Pediatr 83:951, 1973 |
| Liver cirrhosis | J Lab Clin Med 85:261, 1975 |
| Acute lymphoblastic leukemia | Blood 54:412, 1979 |
| Sepsis | J Surg Res 26:355, 1979 |
| **Undefined mechanisms** | |
| Influenza A virus | Scand J Immunol 6:897, 1977 |
| Marrow transplant recipients | J Clin Invest 58:22, 1976 |
| Hyperimmunoglobulin E | J Lab Clin Med 88:796, 1976 |
| Uremia | J Lab Clin Med 88:536, 1976 |
| Hemophilia | J Immunol 120:1181, 1978 |
| Peridontitis | J Res 28:81s, 1980 |
| Milk intolerance | Pediatrics 67:264, 1981 |

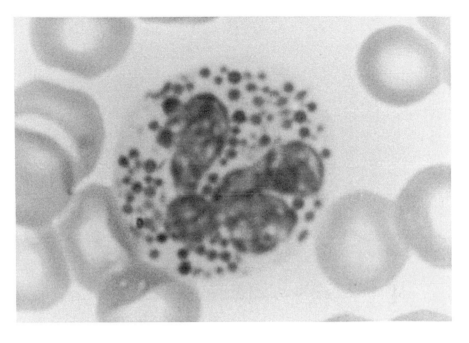

**Figure 17-1**. Neutrophil from a patient with Chédiak-Higashi disease. The cytoplasm is filled with strikingly large primary (azurophilic) granules.

partial oculocutaneous albinism, recurrent pyogenic infections, and the presence of giant lysosomes in most granule-containing cells, including all types of leukocytes (Fig. 17-1). Similar disorders have been described in whales, cattle, mink, and mice. A bleeding diathesis is due to both qualitative and quantitative abnormalities of platelet granules associated with reduced nucleotide and serotonin content. The susceptibility to infections is due to neutropenia, impaired chemotaxis, and delayed killing of ingested bacteria because of abnormal distribution and delivery of lysosomal enzymes. These patients usually die as a result of infection during childhood.

Neutropenia is due to intramedullary granulocyte destruction. It is characterized by normal to increased numbers of precursors in the marrow, vacuolizations and inclusions in the precursors, poor release of PMN from marrow stores, normal half-life of circulating PMN, and increased serum concentrations of lysozyme. At times, splenic sequestration may contribute to the neutropenia. Chemotaxis is impaired and may be related to the inability of abnormal cells to be deformed owing either to cytoskeletal abnormalities or to the presence of the giant cytoplasmic granules. Microorganisms are ingested readily with normal to increased postphagocytic oxidative metabolism, but the delivery of peroxidase to the phagosome is delayed and there is inefficient killing of most bacteria. Although killing is delayed, most bacteria are eventually iodinated and destroyed.

Heterozygotes can be detected by finding the giant lysosomal granules in a small number of circulating leukocytes. Their PMN function is normal. It is known that these giant granules arise from the fusion of lysosomes, and attempts at therapy have been encouraging. Abnormal lysosomal fusion may be related to improper assembly of microtubules that is accompanied by elevated cyclic adenosine monophosphate levels.[25] Clinical and laboratory improvement has been achieved in vivo by the administration of ascorbic acid, bethanechol, lithium, and transfer factor, and by bone marrow transplantation; and in vitro by cyclic guanosine monophosphate. This therapy, however, should be considered experimental.

*Abnormal PMN-specific granules* with impaired function were reported in a patient with recurrent staphylococcal skin and sinus infections but without serious deep tissue infections or sepsis.[26] This disease has been recognized in the United States, Japan, and France. Most circulating PMNs have bilobed nuclei with irregular, finger-like projections (microlobes) and appear to be nearly devoid of cytoplasmic granules on Wright-Giemsa staining (Fig. 17-2). Primary granules are easily seen in PMN stained for myeloperoxidase activity, but stains for secondary (specific) granules are negative (alkaline phosphatase was employed in the initial report). The azurophilic (primary) granules noted on electron micrographs develop normally, but the specific (secondary) granules are deficient in number and abnormal in structure. Most specific granules appear as flattened structures, limited by a trilaminar unit membrane that is in apposition centrally but is separated at the poles to form empty, bulbous enlargements. PMN from the original patient contained less than 8 percent of the normal amounts of the specific-granule proteins lactoferrin and vitamin $B_{12}$ transport protein.[27]

Neutropenia is not a prominent feature but was

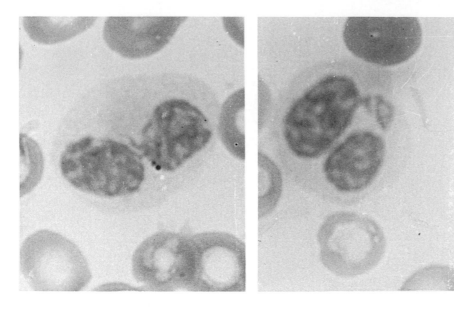

**Figure 17-2.** Neutrophils from a patient with the abnormal specific granule (absent lactoferrin) syndrome. Nuclear lobulation is decreased, and the cytoplasm seems to be devoid of granules.

observed occasionally in some patients. PMN migration was impaired by both skin window and chemotaxis chamber techniques. Random motility was normal, but chemotaxis and adherence both before and after incubation with chemotactic factors were reduced. These defects could be attributed to an inability of PMNs to decrease their surface charge.[27] The PMNs in this disorder aggregate normally in response to chemotactic factors, but they tend to disaggregate unless additional lactoferrin is added to the reaction mixture. In one study,[27] oxygen consumption and superoxide generation were elevated; however, hydroxyl radicals were produced at a significantly decreased rate (another defect probably related to lactoferrin deficiency). Giant abnormal phagolysosomes that contain excessive numbers of bacteria were produced.[26] Many PMNs disintegrated following phagocytosis, and the organisms remained viable.

The nuclear abnormality is reminiscent of that seen in the Pelger-Huët anomaly but differs by the presence of irregular microlobes and the absence of excessive nuclear chromatin condensation. In addition, PMN from the immediate family was normal. Acquired disorders associated with pseudo—Pelger-Huët cells were excluded. The basis of disease is probably a congenital abnormality of specific granule formation with failure to deliver granule contents—particularly lactoferrin—to these granules. Malformation of PMN-specific granules has been reported also in bone marrow cultures of some patients with neutropenia, myeloproliferative diseases, and hairy cell leukemia. Finally, PMN alkaline phosphatase (an enzyme once considered to be a satisfactory marker for PMN-specific granules) deficiency has been detected both in a healthy individual and in a patient with the hyper-IgE syndrome.

## Disorders of the Cytoskeleton

Many PMN functions (chemotaxis, phagocytosis, and phagolysosome formation) are related to movement of all or of parts of the cell. Although the molecular relationships are incompletely defined, it is clear that microtubules, microfilaments, and associated structures are intimately involved.[25] Only a few disorders have been described in which malfunction of the cytoskeleton seems to play a predominant pathogenetic role. Chédiak-Higashi disease was mentioned earlier, and disorders of glutathione will be discussed later. Actin dysfunction was reported in an infant with recurrent bacterial infections and defective PMN functions.[28] Chemotaxis and phagocytosis (ingestion of particles) were greatly impaired. Degranulation, which is probably slowed by actin filament barriers in normal cells, was increased. Equal quantities of actin protein could be isolated from patient and control PMN, but the patient's actin failed to function (polymerize) in a normal fashion. The PMN defect was corrected by bone marrow transplantation, but the patient died of pulmonary fibrosis.

## Disorders of Neutrophil Biochemistry

Energy for particle engulfment is derived largely from anaerobic glycolysis, and maximal microbicidal activity is dependent on oxidative metabolism. The latter is closely related to flavoprotein oxidation, the hexose monophosphate shunt, and the glutathione oxidation-reduction cycle.

## Glycolysis

It is logical to postulate that deficiencies of glycolytic enzymes (Embden-Meyerhof pathway), in a manner analogous to that seen in hemolytic anemias, might result in PMN dysfunction. However, clinically significant disease has not been reported, apparently because alternative metabolic pathways and microbicidal systems are available. Phosphoglycerate kinase is an enzyme in the pathway that regulates one of the two adenosine triphosphate–generating steps. Congenital deficiency of this enzyme is inherited in an X-linked recessive manner and is characterized by hemolytic anemia and progressive central nervous system disease. Infections usually are not a problem. Particle ingestion is normal because of compensatory increase in mitochondrial oxidative metabolism.[29]

## Chronic Granulomatous Disease Syndromes

PMN, monocytes, and eosinophils of children with this disorder are unable to kill certain microorganisms following normal engulfment. The clinical picture of suppurative lymphadenitis, deep tissue infections (osteomyelitis, visceral abscess, perirectal abscess), recurrent pulmonary infections, hepatosplenomegaly, and infected eczematoid rash is characteristic. The basic abnormality is a complete inability to mount a postphagocytic oxidative burst. The molecular defect is incompletely defined and debatable. It is likely that several mechanisms are responsible in different groups of patients.[30,31]

Chronic granulomatous disease was orginally described as an X-linked recessive disease of boys in whom severe bacterial infections appeared by 1 year of age. Neutropenia does not occur. Patients with this disease often die of septicemia or chronic pulmonary disease by 7 years of age. However, much clinical experience has been gained since the description of this disease, and it is now clear that the disease can be much milder and may not be recognized until early adulthood. Moreover, it can occur in girls, and in these patients, it is probably inherited in an autosomal recessive fashion. Pigment-containing macrophages are present throughout the reticuloendothelial system, in the lamina propria of the gastrointestinal tract, and adjacent to the inflammatory areas. Granuloma formation is the characteristic inflammatory lesion.

The failure to reduce oxygen to reactive molecules is responsible for the microbicidal defect.[30] Engulfment of bacteria, with glucose consumption and lactic acid production (anaerobic glycolysis), is generally accepted to be normal, although particle ingestion has occasionally been reported to be slightly impaired. Degranulation and phagolysosome formation are normal. An increase in postphagocytic oxidative metabolism does not occur; there is no increase in oxygen consumption, hexose monophosphate shunt activity, or superoxide anion and hydrogen peroxide production. The diagnosis of chronic granulomatous disease is established by demonstrating a bactericidal defect due to the absence of the postphagocytic oxidative burst. The X-linked recessive inheritance can be confirmed by the presence of disease in male members of the maternal family and by the intermediate performance of PMN from the mothers and sisters of affected boys in certain oxidative assays (the histochemical "slide test" for nitroblue tetrazolium dye reduction). In most cases, these female relatives are clinically well, but occasionally there are reports noting increased susceptibility to infections and a syndrome resembling systemic lupus erythematosus with negative serologic test results.

Some boys with the X-linked form of the disease possess a characteristic abnormality of the Kell antigen system on their erythrocytes or leukocytes or both.[32] The mechanisms involved in expressing Kell antigens on the cell surface are complex. Briefly, the production of standard Kell antigens is mediated by genes located on an autosomal chromosome. Kx is a regulatory glycoprotein antigen that is required for the biosynthesis and full expression of the standard Kell antigens. Its production is controlled by the X chromosome. If the Kx antigen is absent, the expression of the autosomally controlled Kell antigens is markedly diminished. This situation, with regard to erythrocyte typing, is referred to as the McLeod phenotype. Normal PMNs do not possess common Kell antigens. However, in healthy individuals, both leukocytes and erythrocytes are Kx positive. In otherwise healthy persons with the McLeod phenotype (those without chronic granulomatous disease), leukocytes possess Kx but erythrocytes do not. Leukocytes from all patients with the X-linked form of chronic granulomatous disease studied thus far lack the Kx antigen. The relationship of the absence of the Kx antigen to the metabolic defect remains undefined, but it is possible that Kx is a membrane structure present on phagocytic leukocytes of vital importance for initiating the postphagocytic oxidative burst. The erythrocytes from some patients are Kx positive, while others lack the antigen. These latter patients are of the McLeod phenotype and are at great risk of transfusion-induced erythrocyte sensitization (allo anti-Kx). Because these patients are anemic, they frequently receive transfusions. Obviously, transfusions should be considered only after complete erythrocyte typing.

Other patients have been reported with clinical problems similar to chronic granulomatous disease. These disorders may have additional atypical features, such as impaired chemotaxis, low serum concentration of IgA, progressive loss of cellular immunity, and bactericidal defects selective for only single bacteria. Familial lipochrome pigmentation of histiocytes is a similar disorder characterized by hypergammaglobulinemia, recurrent infections (particularly pulmonary), arthritis, splenomegaly,

PMN metabolic abnormalities, and pigment-containing macrophages. Glucose-6-phosphate dehydrogenase (G-6-PD) is the enzyme regulating the flow of glucose into the hexose monophosphate shunt, and PMN function is abnormal only when it is severely deficient. A syndrome similar to chronic granulomatous disease of childhood has been reported in patients with congenital and acquired G-6-PD deficiency.[33]

## Glutathione Metabolism

Interest in the role of the glutathione oxidation-reduction cycle in PMN function has increased since PMN dysfunction has been recognized to be a consequence of disorders of this cycle.[25,34,35] Glutathione peroxidase deficiency is considered by some to produce a variant of chronic granulomatous disease. Glutathione reductase deficiency is characterized by hemolysis and a variety of PMN defects that are not associated with clinical infections.[34] Chemotaxis, phagocytosis, lysosomal enzyme release, and bacterial killing at low bacteria : PMN ratio are normal. Killing at higher bacteria : PMN ratio is impaired. The first few minutes of postphagocytic oxidative metabolism are normal, but the burst stops prematurely. Intracellular levels of reduced glutathione (GSH) drop rapidly, and PMN suffers oxidative damage (auto-oxidation). Several conclusions can be made from the study of this disease: (1) bacterial infections of mild to moderate severity are satisfactorily confined by PMNs, despite their ability to mount only a diminished oxidative burst; (2) the glutathione system provides protection for PMN against oxidative injury (probably in concert with catalase); and (3) the oxidative burst can be terminated by the accumulation of oxidants — a situation that may serve as a type of autoregulation in normal PMN.

Glutathione synthetase deficiency has been described in a patient with a complex condition composed of oxoprolinuria, acidosis, hemolysis, and episodes of severe neutropenia.[35] GSH values in PMN were approximately 25 percent of normal, and hydrogen peroxide levels increased rapidly during phagocytosis. Although early postphagocytic events were normal, irreversible oxidative damage led to decreased iodiation and killing of bacteria.

## Biochemistry of Neonatal Neutrophils

Information on PMN dysfunction in infants is conflicting and incomplete.[36] Abnormal PMN functions have been ascribed to both intrinsic cellular and plasma defects. For example, chemotaxis is decreased, and the generation of chemotactic factors from infant serum is decreased. The responsible mechanisms remain undefined (e.g., chemotactic factor binding by neonatal PMN seems to be normal).[37] In many studies, engulfment and killing of pathogenic bacteria is reported to be inefficient. Reports of oxidative metabolism are perplexing. Certain aspects such as oxygen consumption, hexose monophosphate shunt activity, nitroblue tetrazolium dye reduction, and superoxide anion generation seem to be increased, particularly when nonphagocytic (resting) PMNs are studied. Decreased oxidative metabolism has been reported, however, when other aspects such as postphagocytic chemiluminescence and hydroxyl radical production have been assessed.[38,39] In addition, enzymes responsible for the detoxification of hydrogen peroxide (glutathione peroxidase and catalase) are decreased in neutrophils from newborns.[40] Glutathione levels in neonatal PMN are rapidly depleted by oxidant stress.[41] The increased production of reactive oxygen molecules such as superoxide anion and hydrogen peroxide on the one hand and the decreased activity of oxygen detoxification enzymes on the other suggest that PMN from infants may be prone to oxidant damage. Thus, it is suggested that auto-oxidation contributes, at least in part, to the defective functions of neonatal PMN. However, the precise role of oxidant damage remains to be defined, and other mechanisms undoubtedly are involved.

## Disorders of Neutrophil Glycoproteins

Several patients have been described with abnormal PMN functions that have been ascribed to congenital deficiencies of PMN glycoproteins.[42-46] These missing glycoproteins are believed to be associated with either the PMN plasma membrane of the cytoplasmic granules. Because abnormal function is a consequence of the absence of these glycoproteins, they have been presumed to play crucial roles in normal PMN function. Several glycoproteins have been implicated, largely on the basis of varying molecular weights; and it is unclear how the reported patients may interrelate. Many of the patients have had delayed shedding of the umbilical cord, infection of the umbilical stump, impaired PMN adhesion, decreased chemotaxis, and diminished phagocytosis. Occasionally, abnormalities of other leukocytes have been demonstrated.[45] However, techniques of study have not been consistent among investigators. Much is yet to be learned about these important disorders.

PMN from a 5-year-old boy with recurrent bacterial infections failed to spread on surfaces, which led to a severe defect in chemotaxis and a mild impairment of phagocytosis. Polyacrylamide gel electrophoresis revealed deficiency of a glycoprotein with molecular weight of 110,000 (gp 110) in the plasma membrane – granule fraction of homogenized PMN.[42] PMN movement was abnormal when studied both in vivo (Rebuck skin windows) and in vitro (random migration and chemotaxis were both severely impaired). The phagocytic defect varied with different test particles and was not due to an abnormality of specific immunoglobulin or complement receptors. Anchoring of patient PMN to plastic surfaces was grossly defective, whereas PMNs attached normally to endothelial cells.[43] Degranulation and oxidative metabolic responses to soluble activating agents were fairly normal; oxygen uptake and superoxide production in response to particles were decreased. Similar functional and biochemical defects were found in PMN from the patient's mother and sister. However, PMN from his father and brother was normal, suggesting an X-linked congenital disease. In later studies,[40] the molecular weight of the deficient protein was felt to be 180,000 daltons (deficiency of gp 180).

Another boy with defective PMN function was found to have PMN lacking a glycoprotein with molecular weight 150,000 daltons (deficiency of gp 150), a glycoprotein present in the plasma membrane of normal PMN.[44] The inheritance of this disorder was presumed to be autosomal recessive, because PMN from each parent contained approximately 50 percent of the normal amounts of this glycoprotein. Granulocyte adherence was not studied in this child, but in contrast to the patient described in the preceding paragraph, PMN movement was normal when studied both in vivo by Rebuck skin windows and in vitro by random migration and chemotaxis. Phagocytosis of several types of particles was impaired, but the uptake IgG-coated Staphylococcus aureus was normal. Membrane receptors for immunoglobulins and complement were normal. Oxidative metabolism in response to soluble stimulators was normal, but is was decreased following exposure to opsonized particles. Similarly, degranulation was normal in response to soluble stimulators but was decreased in response to particles.

An 8-year-old boy was found to lack a polypeptide complex of surface proteins that are normally present on PMNs, monocytes, and lymphocytes.[45] Defective adherence, chemotaxis, and particle-induced oxidative metabolism of PMN were present. Lymphocyte proliferation was also decreased.

Finally, a 3-month-old girl with a persistent umbilical stump infection was reported to have decreased PMN adherence, chemotaxis, and phagocytosis.[46] Two PMN membrane proteins were missing with molecular weights of 110,000 and 115,000. The levels of both proteins were decreased in PMN from both parents.

## Hyperimmunoglobulin E Syndrome

The association of recurrent infections (typically with Staphylococcus) of skin and respiratory tract, decreased PMN chemotaxis, and high serum IgE has been called Job's syndrome.[47] Serum IgE is usually more than 2000 IU/ml; and other manifestations of the disorder include coarse facies, eczema, mild eosinophilia, mucocutaneous candida infections, depressed cell-mediated immunity, and the production of a chemotactic inhibitor by mononuclear cells. Many so-called variant patients have been reported, and the full spectrum of this disorder remains to be defined. The cause and optimal treatment are unknown.

## NEUTROPHILS WITH ABNORMAL MORPHOLOGY BUT SATISFACTORY FUNCTION

Several abnormalities of PMN morphology exist in patients without severe infection, in which PMN function is either normal or so slightly defective that the dysfunction has little or no practical importance. Two benign conditions are characterized by abnormalities of the nucleus involving the number of nuclear lobes in the mature PMN. In one of these conditions, giant neutrophilic granulocytes with hypersegmentation have been found to be inherited in a dominant fashion. In these patients 1 to 2 percent of PMN in the blood have five or more segments. A similar hypersegmentation of eosinophilic granulocytes has been described as being inherited in a dominant fashion.

At the other extreme (hyposegmentation) is the Pelger-Huët anomaly (see Color Figure 140).[48] This is a benign familial condition, inherited as a dominant characteristic, in which PMNs are found to be bilobed or to have no lobulation whatsoever. The anomaly can be acquired in some patients with leukemia, and a phase of the leukemia will be characterized by the production of pseudo–Pelger-Huët cells. Clinically, there should be no difficulty in distinguishing leukemia from the benign familial condition. These cells can also be seen as an idiosyncratic response to drugs.

A number of abnormalities demonstrate an alteration of the morphology of PMN cytoplasm. Sometimes these findings can be of diagnostic significance. Alder's anomaly (see Color Figure 141) is the presence of dark-staining and coarse cytoplasmic granules in the cytoplasm of the three major leukocyte types (PMN, lymphocytes, and monocytes). In some patients only one cell line may be involved. This cytoplasmic anomaly, seen in association with the mucopolysaccharidoses, can also be found as an inherited anomaly without other demonstrable defects. On histochemical analysis, the granules are found to contain mucopolysaccharide. In patients with Hurler's disease, mucopolysaccharide inclusions can be found consistently in blood lymphocytes. The inclusions are best demonstrated by to toluidine blue or May-Grünwald–Giemsa staining.

Mucopolysaccharide granules can also be found in the bone marrow. Vacuolated cytoplasm of lymphocytes may be found in patients with Tay-Sachs, Spielmeyer-Vogt, and Niemann-Pick diseases. The finding of these vacuolated lymphocytes may be helpful early in the evaluation of patients suspected of having these diseases (see Chapter 23).

The PMNs of patients with May-Hegglin anomaly (see Color Figure 142) have blue-staining cytoplasmic inclusions that resemble Döhle bodies.[49] On electron microscopy these PMNs are shown to have large granule-free areas in the cytoplasm, which contain fibrils of ribonucleic acid. In addition to the PMN finding, thrombocytopenia exists with the presence of platelets that tend to be large and poorly granulated.

## CASE HISTORY

**History of Present Illness.** A boy 3 years of age was admitted with a liver abscess. He had been ill with many infections since the age of 1 month. Types of infections included recurrent pyoderma, several episodes of pneumonia, perirectal abscess, osteomyelitis of the metacarpals, suppurative lymphadenitis, and mastoiditis. Organisms that were recovered from these sites of infection were Staphylococcus, Serratia, Klebsiella, and Pseudomonas. Despite these episodes of infection, the patient experienced normal growth and development. Immunizations had been given without incident; in particular, he had no difficulties with administration of live virus vaccines. The family medical history was remarkable in that an older brother and a cousin (son of a maternal aunt) had suffered similar chronic infections, and one had died of chronic, gram-negative pneumonia.

**Physical Examination.** The boy appeared to be generally well. His skin was covered with scattered areas of crusted scabs. Gram stain of the moist base of one such scab revealed gram-positive organisms (Staphylococcus). Lymph nodes in all areas were enlarged to 3 to 6 cm, and those in the neck were firm and tender. The tympanic membranes were scarred, and the right one was perforated. The lungs were normal. The liver was enlarged to 8 cm below the lower rib margin, and the spleen was so large that it extended into the pelvis.

**Laboratory Data.** The hemoglobin concentration was 9 g/dl, and the erythrocyte morphology was fairly normal except for slight hypochromia and variation in size. The total white blood cell count was 33,000/$\mu$l, with 28,000/$\mu$l neutrophils. The neutrophils contained toxic granules, Döhle bodies, and vacuoles. The platelet count was 427,000/$\mu$l. Concentrations of serum immunoglobulins and complement components were all increased moderately.

Neutrophilia was consistently found on several occasions when earlier laboratory data were reviewed. Neutropenia was never documented. Neutrophil migration studies were normal when assessed by both in vivo (skin window) and in vitro (chemotaxis chamber) techniques. Phagocytosis (ingestion) of Staphylococcus, yeast organisms, and latex particles was normal. The cytoplasm contained plentiful, prominent granules, and the degranulation process was intact. Oxidative metabolism in response to neutrophil stimulation was completely absent. Specifically, there was no post-phagocytic increase in oxygen consumption, superoxide anion and hydrogen peroxide were not formed, and activity of the hexose monophosphate shunt was not increased. Finally, neutrophils were unable to oxidize and kill staphylococci that had been phagocytized. Neutrophils from the mother were studied, and on some of the assays, they performed at about 50 percent of normal capacity.

**Discussion.** This patient exhibits characteristic features of the X-linked recessive form of chronic granulomatous disease of childhood, with severe and persistent infections caused by Staphylococcus and gram-negative organisms. Anemia and persistent neutrophilia are seen even when these patients are relatively free of infection. Neutrophils from these children are numerous, they migrate normally, they are capable of phagocytosis, and they form phagocytic vesicles. However, they are unable to kill the phagocytized microorganisms because they are unable to generate reactive forms of oxygen. In some families, the X-linked nature of the inheritance pattern can be established by finding disease in male members of the maternal family, and by finding moderate defects in the mother. At present, treatment attempts to diminish the frequency of infections by giving long-term trimethoprim and sulfamethoxazole and to treat established infections promptly. Bone marrow transplantation is an experimental form of more definitive therapy.

## References

1. Shoenfeld, Y, Modan, M, Berliner, S, et al: The mechanism of benign hereditary neutropenia. Arch Intern Med 142:797, 1982.
2. Howard, MW, Strauss, RG, and Johnston, RG, Jr: Infections in patients with neutropenia. Am J Dis Child 131:788, 1977.
3. Dale, DC, Fauci, AS, DuPont, G, IV, et al: Comparison of agents producing neutrophilic leukocytosis in man: Hydrocortisone, prednisone, endotoxin and etiocholanolone. J Clin Invest 56:808, 1975.

4. Christensen, RD, Rothstein, G, Anstall HB, et al: Granulocyte transfusion in neonates with bacterial infection, neutropenia, and depletion of mature marrow neutrophils. Pediatrics 70:1, 1982.

5. Boxer, LA and Stossel, TP: Effects of anti-human neutrophil antibodies in vitro: Quantitative studies. J Clin Invest 53:1534, 1974.

6. Lalezari, P and Radel, E: Neutrophil-specific antigens: Immunology and clinical significance. Semin Hematol 11:281, 1974.

7. Pincus, SH, Boxer, LA, and Stossel, TP: Chronic neutropenia in childhood: Analysis of 16 cases and a review of the literature. Am J Med 61:849, 1976.

8. Amato, D, Freedman, MH, and Saunders, EF: Granulopoiesis in severe congenital neutropenia. Blood 47:531, 1976.

9. Kostmann, R: Infantile genetic agranulocytosis. Acta Paediatr Scand 64:362, 1975.

10. Zucker-Franklin, D, L'Esperance, P, and Good, RA: Congenital neutropenia: An intrinsic cell defect demonstrated by electron microscopy of soft agar colonies. Blood 49:425, 1977.

11. Deinard, AS and Page, AR: A study of steroid-induced granulocytosis in a patient with chronic benign neutropenia of childhood. Br J Haematol 28:33, 1974.

12. Krill, CE, Jr, Smith, HD, and Mauer, AM: Chronic idiopathic granulocytopenia. N Engl J Med 270:699, 1964.

13. Bohinjec, J: Myelokathexis: Chronic neutropenia with hyperplastic bone marrow and hypersegmented neutrophils in two siblings. Blut 42:191, 1980.

14. Andrews, RB, Dunn, CDR, Jolly, J, et al: Some immunological and haematological aspects of human cyclic neutropenia. Scand J Haematol 22:97, 1979.

15. Guerry, D, IV, Dale, DC, Omine, M, et al: Periodic hematopoiesis in human cyclic neutropenia. J Clin Invest 52:3220, 1973.

16. Beard, MEJ, Young, DE, Bateman, CJT, et al: Fanconi's anaemia. Q J Med 42:403, 1973.

17. Inoue, S, Mekanik, G, Mahallati, M, et al: Dyskeratosis congenita with pancytopenia (another constitutional anemia). Am J Dis Child 126:389, 1973.

18. Shwachman, H, Diamond, LK, Oski, FA, et al: The syndrome of pancreatic insufficiency and bone marrow dysfunction. J Pediatr 65:645, 1965.

19. Woods, WG, Roloff, JS, Lukens, JN, et al: The occurrence of leukemia in patients with the Shwachman syndrome. J Pediatr 99:425, 1981.

20. Cappelletti, P and Lippi, U: Hereditary myeloperoxidase deficiency: A rare condition? Diagnostic possibilities of a differential white cell autoanalyzer (Hemalog-D). Haematologica 68:736, 1983.

21. Nauseef, WM, Root, RK, and Malech, HL: Biochemical and immunologic analysis of hereditary myeloperoxidase deficiency. J Clin Invest 71:1297, 1983.

22. Kitahara, M, Eyre, HJ, Simonian, Y, et al: Hereditary myeloperoxidase deficiency. Blood 57:888, 1981.

23. Rosen, H and Klebanoff, SJ: Chemiluminescence and superoxide production by myeloperoxidase-deficient leukocytes. J Clin Invest 58:50, 1976.

24. Root, RK, Rosenthal, AS, and Balestra DJ: Abnormal bactericidal, metabolic, and lysosomal functions of Chediak-Higashi syndrome leukocytes. J Clin Invest 51:649, 1972.

25. Oliver, JM: Cell biology of leukocyte abnormalities: Membrane and cytoskeletal function in normal and defective cells: A review. Am J Pathol 93:221, 1978.

26. Strauss, RG, Bove, KE, Jones, JF, et al: An anomaly of neutrophil morphology with impaired function. N Engl J Med 290:478, 1974.

27. Boxer, LA, Coates, TD, Haak, RA, et al: Lactoferrin deficiency associated with altered granulocyte function. N Engl J Med 307:403, 1982.

28. Boxer, LA, Hedley-Whyte, ET, and Stossel, TP: Neutrophil actin dysfunction and abnormal neutrophil behavior. N Engl J Med 291;1093, 1974.

29. Strauss, RG, McCarthy, DJ, and Mauer, AM: Neutrophil function in congenital phosphoglycerate kinase deficiency. J Pediatr 85:341, 1974.

30. Tauber, AI, Borregaard, N, Simons, E, et al: Chronic granulomatous disease: A syndrome of phagocyte oxidase deficiencies. Medicine 62:286, 1983.

31. Gallin, JI, Buescher, ES, Seligmann, BE, et al: Recent advances in chronic granulomatous disease. Ann Intern Med 99:657, 1983.

32. Marsh, WL, Oyen, R, Nichols, ME, et al: Chronic granulomatous disease and the Kell blood groups. Br J Haematol 29:247, 1975.

33. Cooper, MR, DeChatelet, LR, McCall, CE, et al: Complete deficiency of leukocyte glucose-6-phosphate dehydrogenase and defective bactericidal activity. J Clin Invest 51:769, 1972.

34. Roos, D, Weening, RS, Voetman, AA, et al: Protection of phagocytic leukocytes by endogenous glutathione: Studies in a family with glutathione reductase deficiency. Blood 53:851, 1979.

35. Oliver, JM, Spielberg, SP, Pearson, CB, et al: Microtubule assembly and function in normal and glutathione synthetase-deficient polymorphonuclear leukocytes. J Immunol 120:1181, 1978.

36. Strauss, RG and Mauer, AM: Formed elements of the human blood. In Stave, U (ed): Perinatal Physiology, ed 2. Plenum Press, New York, 1977.

37. Strauss, RG and Snyder, EL: Chemotactic peptide binding by intact neutrophils from human neonates. Pediatr Res 18:63, 1984.

38. Strauss, RG, Rosenberger, TG, and Wallace, PD: Neutrophil chemiluminescence during the first month of life. Acta Haematol 63:326, 1980.

39. Strauss, RG and Snyder, EL: Neutrophils from human infants exhibit decreased viability. Pediatr Res 15:794, 1981.

40. Strauss, RG, Snyder, EL, Wallace, PD, et al: Oxygen-detoxifying enzymes in neutrophils of infants and their mothers. J Lab Clin Med 95:897, 1980.

41. Strauss, RG and Snyder, EL: Glutathione in neutrophils from human infants. Acta Haematol 69:9, 1983.

42. Crowley, CA, Curnette, JT, Rosin, RE, et al: An inherited abnormality of neutrophil adhesion. N Engl J Med 302:1163, 1980.

43. Buchanan, MR, Crowley, CA, Rosin, RE, et al: Studies on the interaction between GP-180-deficient neutrophils and vascular endothelium. Blood 60:160, 1982.

44. Arnaout, MA, Pitt, J, Cohen, HJ, et al: Deficiency of a granulocyte-membrane glycoprotein (gp 150) in a boy with recurrent bacterial infections. N Engl J Med 306:693, 1982.

45. Beatty, PG, Ochs, HD, Harlan, JM, et al: Absence of monoclonal-antibody-defined protein complex in a boy with abnormal leucocyte function. Lancet 1:535, 1984.

46. Kobayashi, K, Fujita, K, Okino, F, et al: An abnormality of neutrophil adhesion: Autosomal recessive inheritance associated with missing neutrophil glycoproteins. Pediatrics 73:606, 1984.

47. Donabedian, H and Gallin, JI: The hyperimmunoglobulin E recurrent-infection (Job's) syndrome. Medicine 62:195, 1983.

48. Johnson, CA, Bass, DA, Trills, AA, et al: Functional and metabolic studies of polymorphonuclear leukocytes in the congenital Pelger-Huet anomaly. Blood 55:466, 1980.

49. Cawley, JC and Hayhoe, FGJ: The inclusions of the May-Hegglin anomaly and Dohle bodies of infection: An ultrastructural comparison. Br J Haematol 22:491, 1972.

## CHAPTER 18

MICHELE LYNNE BEST, B.S., M.T.(ASCP)

# Infectious Mononucleosis and Reactive Lymphocytosis

The cell commonly known as the "atypical" lymphocyte has accumulated a rich history of observations and definitions since it was originally described in 1970 by Turk.[1] There have been as many new terms for this morphologic entity as there have been observations since that time. Turk initially described a deeply basophilic plasmacyte-like cell, later referred to as a Turk cell, in the peripheral blood of a patient who was thought to have acute leukemia. Because the patient later recovered, this probably represents the first recorded case of infectious mononucleosis.

Downey and McKinlay[2] in 1923 described three separate morphologic types of abnormal cells seen in the blood of patients with infectious mononucleosis. The subtypes Downey I, II, and III were initiated. The Downey classification of atypical lymphocytes represents the first description of the spectrum of morphologic observations seen when a T or B lymphocyte is stimulated by antigen. Although Downey's descriptions should be required reading for all students of hematology because of their historic and morphologic insights, the separation of atypical lymphocytes into Downey subtypes has no practical value in today's laboratories.

Over the years, it became common practice to combine all lymphocytes that did not appear morphologically normal under the all-inclusive, vague heading of "atypical." The term "atypical lymphocyte" describes any abnormal lymphocyte morphology seen, regardless of whether the abnormality is benign or malignant. "Atypical" is still used in many laboratories in this way. It is also used occasionally to describe normal variants, because of the morphologic variation in normal lymphocyte populations.

A variety of other terms have cropped up over the

years since Downey to describe these same cell types. The terms "virocyte," "immunoblast," and "transformed," "stimulated," or "reactive" lymphocyte are a few of the more commonly used.

Elucidation of lymphocyte subtypes by advances in cellular immunology has led to a functional appreciation of the morphology of the atypical lymphocyte. These atypical cells represent T or B lymphocytes reacting to an antigenic stimulus and tranforming into immune-responsive blast cells. These blast cells are called immunoblasts. All morphologic changes that occur during this transformation process are now defined as reactive, transformed, or stimulated lymphocytes. The term "reactive lymphocyte" is preferred by many hematologists.

It is my opinion that the vague definition and category of "atypical lymphocytes" should be replaced with the more meaningful and specific categories of (1) reactive, (2) abnormal, and (3) abnormal and immature. "Reactive" is used to describe specific morphologic changes that are nonmalignant and elicited by a variety of antigens. "Abnormal" is used to describe other morphologic abnormalities that do not appear reactive and that are probably due to lymphoid malignancy. If the cells also appear immature, they can be described as "abnormal and immature." For the remainder of the text, "reactive" will be used to describe the atypical mononuclear cells seen in infectious mononucleosis and related syndromes.

## MORPHOLOGY OF REACTIVE LYMPHOCYTES

A difficult morphologic challenge is the interpretation of a huge, deeply basophilic, immature-looking cell on a peripheral smear. The immediate reflex is to think the cell is malignant. Often these large, bizarre cells turn out to be reactive lymphocytes, which can achieve sizes (often greater than 30 $\mu$) and can look quite ominous. These cells are commonly encountered in the hematology laboratory and their recognition is essential.

Reactive lymphocytes range in size from that of a large normal lymphocyte to greater than 30 $\mu$. Nuclear and cytoplasmic mass are increased, both contributing to the overall size. It is the nuclear and cytoplasmic morphology of the reactive lymphocyte that differentiates it from a normal, large lymphocyte or a monocyte. The contrasting morphology of a large normal lymphocyte, a monocyte, and several types of reactive lymphocytes is depicted in **Color Figures 143 through 147**.

The nucleus of a large lymphocyte has a densely stained, clumped chromatin with uneven "streaks" of parachromatin in the nucleus. Chromatin clumping is concentrated around the nuclear edges. The monocyte nucleus, in contrast, has a more

lightly stained chromatin with a more even dispersion of chromatin clumps and parachromatin. The clumps are smaller in size than in the lymphocyte and tend to show less tendency to locate near the nuclear membrane. The nuclear chromatin of a reactive lymphocyte shows distinctive changes from the normal lymphocyte chromatin previously described. The chromatin is less intensely clumped with more evidence of parachromatin and a more even pattern of clumping. Compared with that of a monocyte, the chromatin of a reactive lymphocyte is more densely stained and usually more clumped. The chromatin density of a reactive lymphocyte is usually intermediate between a small lymphocyte and a monocyte. Nucleoli may or may not be visible; when visible, these can be multiple and quite large and irregular. Nuclear shape irregularities are common and often striking, varying from cleaved or convoluted to kidney bean–shaped or oblong. It must be emphasized that there is a wide range of reactive morphology from a very slight change in the nuclear chromatin clumping pattern to a very immature, blast-like nucleus with prominent nucleoli. These changes appear to reflect cells being "caught" in different stages of lymphocyte transformation.

The cytoplasm of a normal large lymphocyte tends to be pale blue and has an even staining quality, whereas the cytoplasm of a reactive lymphocyte is most notable for its increased degree of basophilia, which appears patchy (i.e., the cytoplasm is unevenly stained). There are linear or rod-like clear, unstained areas in the cytoplasm adjacent to the nucleus. Often there is a perinuclear clearing or halo also. The cytoplasm of the reactive lymphocyte has traditionally been described as abundant and "sprawled"-looking with a scalloped, deeply basophilic cytoplasmic edge that tends to be indented by the adjacent red cells.[8] These criteria are not as reliable as the features cited earlier in recognizing reactive lymphocytes, because this scalloping effect will be seen only if the cytoplasm and the red cells are abundant. Prominent cytoplasmic granulation is seen in some reactive lymphocytes, but it is neither a regular nor identifying characteristic. Although frequently described in the literature, cytoplasmic vacuolation also is not a regular feature of reactive lymphocytes.

A distinctive type of reactive lymphocyte that bears special mention is the plasmacytoid lymphocyte **(see Color Figure 148)**. These cells look very similar to plasma cells in the cytoplasm (i.e., intensely basophilic with a developing perinuclear halo or "hof"). However, the nuclear chromatin pattern is intermediate between that of a mature lymphocyte and that of a mature plasmacyte. The nuclear:cytoplasmic ratio is also higher than in a plasma cell. Plasmacytoid lymphocytes represent stimulated B lymphocytes maturing toward the plasma cell. When these cells are present in the peripheral blood, their immature precursor, the immunoblast, will often be seen also. Immunoblasts have plasmacytoid cytoplasms but immature blastic chromatin with prominent nucleoli **(see Color Figure 147)**. The mature end product of B-cell maturation, the plasma cell, often accompanies these other types of plasmacytoid, reactive lymphocytes. The presence of plasma cells in the peripheral blood is much more often reactive than malignant, especially when seen with other types of reactive lymphocytes.

The key point to remember in evaluating an abnormal lymphocyte population is to look for heterogeneity or homogeneity of morphology. It is the heterogeneity of morphologic types in the patient's lymphocyte population that is most striking in infectious mononucleosis and other types of reactive lymphocytosis. The abnormal cell population should be looked at as a group and if quite heterogeneous, a reactive cause for the lymphocytosis should be searched for. In contrast, if the cells look abnormal and the population is homogeneous, malignant lymphoma should be ruled out.

## CAUSES OF REACTIVE LYMPHOCYTOSIS

Reactive lymphocytes, as described in the previous section, are seen frequently on peripheral blood smears in a wide variety of clinical conditions.

How many reactive lymphocytes, if any, are seen on normal smears? This is a frequently asked question, and the answer largely depends on an individual laboratory's criteria for what constitutes "atypical." Sometimes a cell is called "atypical" because the technologist does not recognize the wide morphologic variation in normal lymphocyte populations. Therefore, lymphocytes that appear slightly different from normal are called "atypical." If precise criteria are adhered to in the identification of truly "atypical" cells, the problem of overcalling "atypical" lymphocytes can be reduced. It is logical to assume that occasional lymphocytes reacting to antigen will be encountered in the blood of healthy individuals. While it is rare to see these lymphocytes while doing a 100-cell manual differential, the Technicon H-6000 automated differential, which routinely counts approximately 8000 cells, picks up 1 to 3 percent large, unstained cells (LUCs) on normal, healthy individuals. These LUCs are usually identifiable as large lymphocytes or reactive lymphocytes, or both, on a low-power scan. Therefore, 1 to 2 percent reactive lymphocytes should be regarded as normal. Reactive lymphocytosis is present when the number of reactive lymphocytes exceeds 2 percent of the differential count.

Reactive lymphocytes are most striking in number and in morphology in infectious mononucleosis, cytomegalovirus infection, drug hypersensitivity, viral hepatitis, toxoplasmosis, and after infusion of large amounts of blood during open heart surgery (postperfusion syndrome). Cells of similar morphology but of fewer numbers are seen in any type of viral infection and in states of immunologic reactivity. It is common in our laboratory to see less than 10 percent reactive lymphocytes (usually plasmacytoid) accompanying an elevated white blood count and shift to the left. These cells should be interpreted as simply reactive to infection, not necessarily to a viral infection. A variety of bacterial infections and noninfectious conditions are associated with small numbers of reactive lymphocytes in peripheral blood.[9]

## INFECTIOUS MONONUCLEOSIS
## Historic Perspective

The clinical syndrome of mononucleosis was initially described by a German physician Emil Pfeiffer[3] as "glandular fever." The symptomatology initially described of fever, sore throat, and lymphadenopathy closely correlates with the three most prominent symptoms of infectious mononucleosis. The syndrome was actually named "infectious mononucleosis" in 1920 by Sprunt and Evans,[4] who were first to associate the syndrome with atypical morphology of the white blood cells. The discovery of a heterophile antibody in the serum of a patient with infectious mononucleosis was made by Paul and Bunnell[5] in 1932. A heterophile antibody is defined as an antibody that reacts with an antigen of apparently unrelated animal species that is immunologically cross-reactive. The heterophile antibody described by Paul and Bunnell[5] was found to agglutinate both horse and sheep erythrocytes.

Davidsohn and Walker[6] in 1935 described what is known today as the Davidsohn differential absorption test. They established that the key feature of the heterophile antibody in infectious mononucleosis is that it can be absorbed by beef erythrocytes but not by guinea pig kidney cells. This became the basic principle of various rapid slide differential tests on the market today (Monospot, Monosticon, Monotest).

The causative agent of infectious mononucleosis remained a mystery until 1968 when Henle, Henle, and Diehl[7] described the association of infectious mononucleosis with rising titers of antibody to the Epstein-Barr virus.

## Disease Description and Etiology

The term "infectious mononucleosis" is most often used to describe an acute, benign, febrile infection of lymphoid tissue caused by the Epstein-Barr virus

(EBV), a herpes group virus. The classic disease description includes (1) clinical manifestations of fever, sore throat, and cervical lymph node enlargement; (2) absolute lymphocytosis (greater than 4500/mm³) with at least 10 percent reactive lymphocytes; and (3) a positive heterophile antibody test result. This combination of clinical, hematologic, and serologic evidence is considered essential for the diagnosis.

Over the years it became evident that the third criterion mentioned above was not present in all patients with infectious mononucleosis. Two categories of mononucleosis syndromes are now described: (1) heterophile antibody positive and (2) heterophile antibody negative. Many cases of infectious mononucleosis, especially in children under the age of 10, fit into the second category because they do not have a positive heterophile antibody test. Children less than 3 years of age are rarely heterophile antibody positive.[10] Until recent years, these heterophile-negative cases have been a difficult diagnostic problem. This problem has been reduced with the advent of new specific and more sensitive tests for antibodies to the Epstein-Barr virus, the causative agent of infectious mononucleosis. The third criterion for diagnosis is now amended to a positive heterophile antibody test result or a positive EBV antibody titer.

Many cases of heterophile-negative mononucleosis-like syndromes in the adult are not caused by the Epstein-Barr virus at all. These cases are caused by the cytomegalovirus (CMV), a syndrome called CMV mononucleosis. CMV mononucleosis comprises about 65 percent of all heterophile-negative mononucleosis syndromes in patients 15 years of age or older.[11] CMV and EBV mononucleosis show identical hematologic morphology and somewhat similar clinical symptoms; they can be differentiated only by specific viral antibody titers. The remainder of this chapter will deal with the more common type of infectious mononucleosis, that caused by the Epstein-Barr virus.

A list of strong evidence for the Epstein-Barr virus as the causative agent of the common type of infectious mononucleosis has been compiled and summarized by Henle and Henle.[12] The list includes the fact that only individuals who lack protective antibody to EBV get the disease. Also, individuals with classic heterophile-positive infectious mononucleosis demonstrate rising titers of EBV antibody during the disease course. The most compelling evidence is that continuous EBV-infected lymphoid cell lines can be developed using lymphocytes obtained from the blood of patients with mononucleosis.

The virus is transmitted mainly via the exchange of oral secretions, hence the description the "kissing disease." It afflicts mainly teenagers and college-aged adults who have somehow escaped previous infection by the Epstein-Barr virus, which is ubiquitous in nature. Socioeconomic status seems to affect development of the immune status to this virus. In lower socioeconomic groups, 50 to 80 percent of children achieve immune status by the age of 4, whereas in more affluent children only 14 percent are immune by that age.[13] This appears to explain the fact that middle-class college students are particularly susceptible to this disease.

## Clinical Manifestations

A combination of clinical and laboratory findings is required for the diagnosis of infectious mononucleosis. The clinical presentation of infectious mononucleosis is quite variable, depending on the age of the patient. In childhood, infections are often asymptomatic and go undiagnosed because the typical symptoms and the heterophile antibody are absent. The teenager with infectious mononucleosis typically presents with a sore throat, fatigue, and cervical lymphadenopathy. The clinical manifestations of infectious mononucleosis in teenagers and young adults are summarized in Table 18–1. Rare cases of infectious mononucleosis have been reported in older adults and the elderly. Liver involvement tends to be more striking than lymphadenopathy in older patients.[14]

The usual case of infectious mononucleosis is uncomplicated and resolves in two or three weeks. Common complications that do occur include group A beta-hemolytic Streptococcus infection of the pharynx and a rash if the drug ampicillin is used to treat the sore throat. Rare complications including splenic rupture, immune thrombocytopenic purpura, Guillain-Barré syndrome, and hemolytic anemia have been reported.[15]

**Table 18–1. CLINICAL MANIFESTATIONS OF INFECTIOUS MONONUCLEOSIS**

**Common Manifestations**
  (seen in >50% of patients)
Sore throat
Posterior cervical lymphadenopathy
Fatigue
Fever
Splenomegaly

**Less Common Manifestations**
  (seen in <50% of patients)
Hepatomegaly
Jaundice
Rash
Facial edema
Anorexia
Nausea and vomiting
Generalized lymphadenopathy

Adapted from Schleupner and Overall.[15]

## Laboratory Tests in Diagnosis

Infectious mononucleosis is a disease state in which laboratory testing is essential to the diagnosis. The clinician presented with suggestive clinical manifestations in a patient will most frequently order a complete blood count and heterophile antibody test (often called a Monospot test).

The most important peripheral blood abnormality in infectious mononucleosis is the presence of more than 10 percent reactive lymphocytes. These cells often comprise more than 50 percent of the circulating white blood cells and represent the first detectable laboratory abnormality found in most patients. The morphology of reactive lymphocytes has been described in a previous section. In addition to the abnormality in morphology of the lymphocyte, there is an absolute increase in the number of total lymphocytes per cubic millimeter (greater than 4500/mm³ for adults). The total white blood cell (WBC) count varies according to the clinical stage of infection. It is normal or decreased in the first week of illness and elevated with counts usually between 15,000 and 25,000/mm³ during the second and third weeks. Rarely, the WBC count may exceed 30,000/mm³. The hemoglobin level and platelet count are usually normal; however, mild thrombocytopenia (100,000 to 150,000/mm³) is seen in about one third of all cases. Spherocytosis, erythrophagocytosis, and cold autoagglutination may occasionally be seen as manifestations of an autoimmune hemolytic anemia. Cold agglutinins of anti-i specificity are seen in 20 percent of patients with infectious mononucleosis.

The finding of absolute lymphocytosis with reactive lymphocytes on a patient's peripheral smear necessitates a logical scheme of laboratory testing for correct diagnosis (Fig. 18-1). The first test to be performed is a simple, inexpensive, rapid slide differential absorption test, such as the Monospot (Ortho Pharmaceuticals). This test detects the presence of the characteristic heterophile antibody by the ability of the antibody in the patient's serum to agglutinate horse red cells. It also tests for the differential absorption characteristic of the antibody in infectious mononucleosis by absorbing the serum with guinea pig kidney prior to adding horse red cells. The antibody in infectious mononucleosis is not absorbed by guinea pig kidney cells and thus, if present, agglutinates the horse red cells in the test system. The Monospot test using horse erythrocyte agglutination is a sensitive, rapid test for infectious mononucleosis. The Monosticon (Organon) is another highly sensitive, rapid slide test for infectious mononucleosis. It tests for the differential absorption character of the heterophile antibody by using both beef erythrocytes and guinea pig kidney cells. This kit incorporates a combination horse/sheep erythrocyte stromal antigen instead of just horse

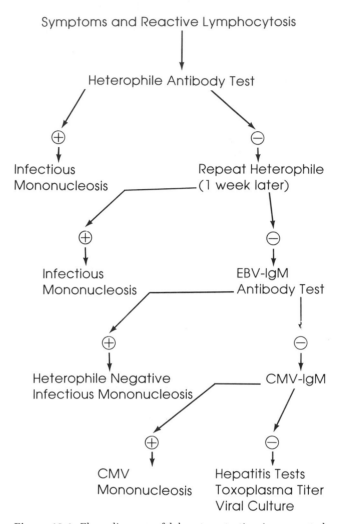

**Figure 18-1.** Flow diagram of laboratory testing in suspected cases of infectious mononucleosis.

erythrocytes to demonstrate the agglutination ability of the heterophile antibody.

It is important to remember that heterophile antibody titers are sometimes not elevated to detectable levels until the second or third week of the disease course. Therefore, it is possible to see greater than 10 percent reactive lymphocytes early in the course of infectious mononucleosis and to have a negative heterophile antibody test result. This test should be repeated in seven to 10 days if the morphology is suggestive of infectious mononucleosis. If the repeat heterophile result is negative, other tests must be performed to determine the cause of the hematologic abnormality (Fig. 18-1).

The tests for antibody response to the Epstein-Barr virus are highly specific and sensitive. A variety of tests for antibodies to Epstein-Barr viral antigens have been described (Table 18-2). These include IgM and IgG antibody tests to viral capsid antigen (EBV-VCA), which are available at larger

**Table 18–2. SUMMARY OF SPECIFIC ANTIBODY TESTS TO EPSTEIN-BARR VIRUS ANTIGENS**

| Test Name | Description | Clinical Significance |
|---|---|---|
| EBV-VCA (IgM) | IgM antibody to viral capsid antigen | Present at detectable levels in first week of infection; the best indicator of *current* infection |
| EBV-VCA (IgG) | IgG antibody to viral capsid antigen | Present at detectable levels about 7 days after exposure; indicates either current or past infection; a rise in titer must be demonstrated on acute and convalescant sera |
| EBNA | Antibody to Epstein-Barr virus nuclear antigen | Appears late in first month of infection and persists indefinitely; indicates a *past* infection |
| EBV-EA | Antibody to Epstein-Barr virus early antigen complex | Seen in less than 5% of normal, healthy subjects; indicates EBV-carrier state |

clinical centers and reference laboratories. These tests are not routinely performed in most hospital laboratories. A rise in the titer of IgM-EBV antibodies occurs initially and parallels the rise in titer of heterophile antibodies during the disease course. The IgM antibody is detectable in 82 percent of the cases in the first week and in 100 percent by the third week.[16] Its presence constitutes conclusive evidence of current infection. IgG-EBV antibody is detectable early also; however, its presence indicates current or past infection. IgG antibody is present in detectable titer in 87 percent of cases during the first week of illness and in 100 percent by the third week.[16] A rise in titer must be demonstrated to be indicative of a current infection. It is advisable to perform the IgG or IgM-EBV antibody titers on all heterophile-negative cases. It is prudent to order these tests immediately for children suspected of having infectious mononucleosis, as there is a high probability that the heterophile test result will be negative. If these specific test results are negative, other tests should be performed to determine the cause of the reactive lymphocytosis (Fig. 18-1 and Table 18-3).

Other laboratory tests with diagnostic significance in infectious mononucleosis are the liver enzyme tests such as the serum glutamic-oxaloacetic transaminase (SGOT), serum glutamic-pyruvic transaminase (SGPT), and alkaline phosphatase tests. Patients with infectious mononucleosis consistently demonstrate abnormal liver function with elevated levels of these enzymes.

## CASE HISTORY

A 25-year-old white male was admitted to the hospital with symptoms of anorexia, fever, malaise, and headache. He had recently noted a darkening of his urine. He has been taking no prescribed medication.

| Physical Exam: | Slight splenomegaly, no lymphadenopathy |
|---|---|
| Laboratory Data: | |
| WBC | 11,000/mm³ |
| RBC | 4,720,000/mm³ |
| Hb | 14.0 g/dl |
| HCT | 42% |
| MCV | 89 $\mu^3$ |
| MCH | 29.7 $\mu\mu$g |
| MCHC | 33% |
| Reticulocyte count | 2% |
| Platelet count | 252,000/mm³ |
| Coomb's test (DAT) | Negative |
| Differential | 31% Segmented neutrophils |
| | 32% Lymphocytes |
| | 31% Reactive lymphocytes |
| | 6% Monocytes |
| | Red cell morphology— normal |
| Serum bilirubin | 1.4 mg/dl (0.2–1.0) |
| SGOT | 257 U/l (0–41) |
| SGPT | 85 U/l (0–45) |
| Monospot test | Negative (initially and on repeat) |
| Hepatitis B antigen | Negative |
| Toxoplasma titer | Negative |

**Table 18–3. DIFFERENTIAL DIAGNOSIS OF LYMPHOCYTOSIS**

**Viral**
Infectious mononucleosis
Measles
Mumps
Chickenpox
Infectious hepatitis
Cytomegalovirus mononucleosis
**Bacterial**
Tuberculosis
Whooping cough
Brucellosis
Typhoid fever
Paratyphoid fever
**During Recovery from Acute Infections**
  (especially in children)
**Neoplasms**
Lymphocytic leukemia
Lymphoma
Macroglobulinemia
**Miscellaneous**
Rickets
Syphilis
Malnutrition
Hyperthyroidism
Acute infectious lymphocytosis
Autoimmune diseases
Allergic reactions

## Questions

1. What is the differential diagnosis?
2. What do the clinical symptoms suggest?
3. What do the laboratory test results indicate?
4. What further laboratory tests should be performed in this case?

## Answers

1. The differential diagnosis in this case includes EBV infectious mononucleosis, CMV mononucleosis, infectious hepatitis, and toxoplasmosis.
2. The clinical findings are fairly nonspecific and can be associated with all of these infections. A darkening of the urine could indicate the presence of increased amounts of urine urobilinogen. Of particular interest is the fact that the classic symptoms of EBV-infectious mononucleosis — sore throat and cervical lymphadenopathy — were not present.
3. Laboratory findings show an absolute lymphocytosis with reactive morphology and evidence of hepatic dysfunction (elevated SGOT, SGPT, and slightly elevated serum bilirubin). Reactive lymphocytosis is seen in all of the aforementioned infections. Liver involvement, while most striking in hepatitis, is also seen in both EBV and CMV mononucleosis.
4. Further tests indicated by the hematology and chemistry findings included a heterophile antibody test, hepatitis B antigen test, and toxoplasma titer. These tests were negative and ruled out hepatitis B infection and toxoplasmosis. Therefore, this case was interpreted as a heterophile-negative infectious mononucleosis syndrome. For accurate diagnosis, EBV and CMV antibody titers had to be performed. The EBV-IgG on this patient showed no change in titer between the acute and convalescent specimens; the CMV-IgM antibody titer was elevated at 1:256. CMV-IgM titers of greater than 1:32 are considered diagnostic of an active cytomegalovirus infection.

   This patient therefore had CMV mononucleosis, which often presents with nonspecific symptoms of fever, malaise, headache, and liver involvement in young adults (20 to 40 years). The blood picture is indistinguishable from that of the classic EBV infectious mononucleosis. This infection should be suspected when the heterophile test result is negative on a patient who lacks the typical symptoms of EBV infectious mononucleosis — sore throat and lymphadenopathy.

## References

1. Turk, W: Septische Erkranhungen bei Verkummerung des Granulozylensystems. Wien Klin Wochenschr 20:157, 1907.
2. Downey, H and McKinlay, CA: Acute lymphadenosis compared to acute leukemia. Arch Intern Med 32:82, 1923.
3. Pfeiffer, E: Drusenfieber. Jarbuch Fur Kinderheilkunde 29:257, 1889.
4. Sprunt, TP and Evans, FA: Mononuclear leukocytosis in reaction to acute infection (infectious mononucleosis). Bull Johns Hopkins Hosp 31:410, 1920.
5. Paul, JR and Bunnell, WW: The presence of heterophile antibodies in infectious mononucleosis. Am J Med Sci 183:80, 1932.
6. Davidsohn, I and Walker, PH: Nature of heterophile antibodies in infectious mononucleosis. Am J Clin Pathol 5:455, 1953.
7. Henle, G, Henle, W, and Diehl, V: Relation of Burkitt's tumor–associated herpes–type virus to infectious mononucleosis. Proc Natl Acad Sci USA 59:94, 1968.
8. Kapff, C and Jandl, J: Blood Atlas and Sourcebook of Hematology. Little, Brown, Boston, 1981, p 122.
9. Miale, JB: Laboratory Medicine Hematology. CV Mosby, St Louis, 1982, p 166.
10. Karzon, DT: Infectious mononucleosis. Adv Pediatr 22:231, 1976.
11. Horwitz, CA, Henle, W, and Henle, G: Diagnostic aspects of cytomegalovirus mononucleosis syndrome in previously healthy persons. Post Grad Med 66:153, 1979.
12. Henle, W and Henle, G: Epstein-Barr virus and infectious mononucleosis. N Engl J Med 288:263, 1973.
13. Henle, G and Henle, W: Observations on childhood infections with the Epstein-Barr virus. J Infect Dis 121:303, 1970.
14. Horwitz, CA, Henle, W, Henle, G, et al: Clinical and laboratory evaluation of elderly patients with heterophile–antibody positive infectious mononucleosis: Report of seven patients ages 40 to 78. Am J Med 61:333, 1976.
15. Schleupner, C and Overall, J: Infectious mononucleosis and Epstein-Barr virus. Postgrad Med 65:83, 1979.
16. Evans, AS, Niederman, JC, Cenabre, LC, et al: A prospective evaluation of heterophile and Epstein-Barr virus–specific IgM antibody tests in clinical and subclinical infectious mononucleosis: Specificity and sensitivity of the tests and persistence of the antibody. J Infect Dis 132:546, 1975.

# CHAPTER 19

MARY LORING PERKINS, M.T.(ASCP), S.H., C.L.S.(NCA)

# Introduction to Leukemia and the Acute Leukemias

## INTRODUCTION TO LEUKEMIA

Leukemia is a malignant disease characterized by unregulated proliferation in the bone marrow of cells derived from one of the blood-forming elements. It may involve any of the hematopoietic cell lines or a stem cell common to several lines of differentiation. The uncontrolled proliferation and accumulation of these cells leads to replacement of normal marrow elements. The leukemic cells commonly infiltrate the reticuloendothelial system including the spleen, liver, and lymph nodes. They may also invade other tissues, infiltrating any organ of the body. If left untreated, leukemia eventually causes death.

## Historic Perspective

The discovery of leukemia as a clinical entity was made simultaneously by John Bennett[1] in Scotland and Rudolf Virchow[2] in Germany who independently published their findings in 1845. Several cases of leukemia were reported in the literature prior to this; however, it was Bennett and Virchow who recognized the significance of their observations and attempted to define this remarkable new disease.[3] Their discovery was made at the autopsy table, each observing a markedly enlarged spleen and purulent-appearing blood in victims of a progressive chronic disease of unknown origin. Microscopic examination of the blood, unstained, showed a striking increase in the number of "colorless" cells. Bennett and Virchow differed on their interpretation of these findings. Bennett concluded that they were due to an inflammation of the blood. Virchow, in contrast, was disinclined to call the condition "pyemia", i.e., blood containing pus; he chose instead to call it, simply, "Weisses Blut" (white blood). This was subsequently translated into Greek as "leukemia."[3] Virchow later published a summary of his studies on the nature of leukemia, classifying the disease into two groups—one with primarily splenic involvement and the other with primarily lymph node involvement. Today these are recognized respectively as chronic myelocytic leukemia and chronic lymphocytic leukemia.[4]

In 1857 Friedreich[5] gave a classic account of an acute form of leukemia characterized by a rapidly fatal course; however, the term "acute" was not used to describe leukemia until 1889, when Epstein first used it.[6] Paul Ehrlich's contribution in 1877 of a triacid stain permitting the differentiation of the various nucleated cell types present in the blood allowed for further classification of leukemia based on cell morphology. It became clear that acute leukemia was characterized by the presence of less differentiated cells than those seen in chronic leukemia.

Naegeli in 1900 described the myeloblast and divided the acute leukemias into myeloblastic and lymphoblastic. A decade later Shilling described a monoblastic variant. By 1930 the main morphologic variants of acute and chronic leukemia had been established.[7] Since then, many details have been elaborated on. Subclassification of the leukemias has been aided by development of cytochemical techniques, immunologic cell markers, cytogenetic techniques, and electron microscopy.

Perhaps the most significant advance in our understanding of leukemia since the time of Virchow has been in the area of treatment. Use of cytotoxic chemotherapeutic agents has improved the survival of many patients with acute leukemia. Acute lymphoblastic leukemia (ALL) in children provides the most striking example of this. Childhood ALL used to be universally fatal; with current treatment programs over one half of children with ALL are potentially cured.[8]

## Etiology

Although the cause of leukemia is still not fully understood, a number of predisposing host factors and several environmental factors have been identified.

### Host Factors

**Heredity.** Leukemia does not appear to be inherited; although some individuals have an increased predisposition for acquiring it. An identical twin of a patient with acute leukemia has a markedly increased risk of developing leukemia. There is also an increased incidence of leukemia, although less dramatic, in other family members of the patient with leukemia.[9]

**Chromosome Abnormalities.** Leukemia has an increased incidence in patients with congenital disorders that have an inherited tendency for chromosomal fragility (e.g., Bloom's syndrome and Fanconi's anemia) or with an abnormality in the number of chromosomes (e.g., Down's syndrome, Klinefelter's syndrome, and Turner's syndrome). An 18- to 20-fold increased incidence of acute leukemia is seen in children with Down's syndrome.[10]

**Immunodeficiency.** An unusually high incidence of lymphoproliferative disease (lymphocytic leukemia and lymphoma) has been found in patients with hereditary immunodeficiency states, including ataxia-telangiectasia and sex-linked agammaglobulinemia.

**Chronic Marrow Dysfunction.** Patients with chronic marrow dysfunction abnormalities have an increased risk of their disorder transforming into acute leukemia. This includes patients with myelodysplastic syndromes, myeloproliferative syndromes, aplastic anemia, and paroxysmal nocturnal hemoglobinuria.

### Environmental Factors

**Ionizing Radiation.** An increased incidence of leukemia is associated with exposure to ionizing radiation. Data collected after the atomic bomb was exploded over Hiroshima and Nagasaki illustrate this fact most dramatically (Fig. 19-1). The incidence of leukemia in survivors exposed to atomic radiation

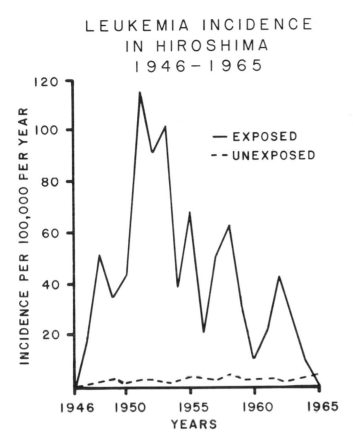

## LEUKEMIA INCIDENCE IN HIROSHIMA 1946–1965

**Figure 19-1.** The leukemia incidence in Hiroshima, 1946–1965 in individuals exposed and unexposed to atomic radiation. (From Gunz,[3] p 528, with permission.)

was many times that of individuals not exposed, and it was highest in those closest to the explosion.[11]

**Chemicals and Drugs.** Numerous chemicals and drugs have been implicated in the etiology of leukemia. In humans, benzene is the most frequently documented.[12] Other agents include chloramphenicol and phenylbutazone. Certain cytotoxic chemotheraputic agents, especially alkylating drugs, are also associated with leukemic development, and the risk in patients receiving alkylators is increased by the use of therapeutic radiation. This has been noted especially in patients with Hodgkin's disease and multiple myeloma.

**Viruses.** In cats (feline leukemia) and other vertebrates, viruses are a proven cause of leukemia; however, no conclusive evidence exists to prove their role in human leukemia. Currently, there is much interest in viral oncogenesis because of the proven etiologic role of viruses in animals, as well as other supporting data on the role of retroviruses in the etiology of human T-cell leukemia and the elucidation of oncogenes with sequences almost identical to viral sequences.

## Classification

Leukemias are classified by cell maturity and by the predominant cell type (Table 19–1). On the basis of the cell differentiation, leukemia is classified as either acute or chronic. The acute leukemias are characterized by a predominance of immature cells (stem cells, blasts, or "pro" forms), whereas the cells in chronic leukemia are primarily differentiated cells. Traditionally, the leukemias were divided into acute and chronic as a means of reflecting the duration of clinical course. Such criteria are no longer valid, because of the increased survival that many acute leukemia patients demonstrate with current therapeutic regimens.

On the basis of predominant cell type, the classification of leukemia has two major categories: lymphoid and myeloid (nonlymphoid). In the past, the identification of cell types was done primarily by morphologic criteria. Now, cytochemistry and immunology are also used and have been incorporated into the current classification systems. Table 19–2 lists the different types of leukemia.

## Incidence

The overall incidence of leukemia in the United States is eight to 10 new cases per 100,000 individuals per year. Approximately half of these cases are acute and half are chronic.

### Age Distribution

Acute leukemia occurs at all ages. Acute lymphoblastic leukemia is most common in children, accounting for approximately 75 percent of childhood leukemias. Acute myeloblastic leukemia occurs more frequently in adults, with an incidence near 80 percent in this group.

Chronic leukemia is generally considered to be a disease of adults. Chronic lymphocytic leukemia is extremely rare in children, and is unusual before

Table 19–1. CLASSIFICATION OF LEUKEMIA: FOUR MAIN CATEGORIES BASED ON CELL MATURITY AND CELL TYPE

| | Cell Maturity | |
| --- | --- | --- |
| Cell Type | Immature (Acute) | Mature (Chronic) |
| Myeloid | Acute myeloid leukemia | Chronic myeloid leukemia |
| Lymphoid | Acute lymphoid leukemia | Chronic lymphoid leukemia |

Table 19-2. CLASSIFICATION OF LEUKEMIA

| Preferred Name | Preferred Abbreviation | FAB* | Alternate Names |
|---|---|---|---|
| Acute | | | |
|   Acute myeloblastic leukemia | AML | M1, M2 | Acute myelocytic leukemia |
| | | | Acute granulocytic leukemia |
| | | | Acute nonlymphocytic leukemia |
|   Acute promyelocytic leukemia | APL | M3 | Acute progranulocytic leukemia |
| | | | Hypergranular promyelocytic |
|   Acute myelomonocytic leukemia | AMML | M4 | Naegeli-type leukemia |
|   Acute monoblastic leukemia | AMoL | M5 | Schilling-type leukemia |
|   Erythroleukemia | EL | M6 | DiGuglielmo's disease |
| | | | Erythremic myelosis |
|   Acute lymphoblastic leukemia | ALL | | Acute lymphocytic leukemia |
| | | L1, L2 |   Common ALL |
| | | L1, L2 |   T ALL |
| | | L1, L2 |   "Null" or "unclassified" ALL |
| | | L3 |   B ALL |
|   Acute undifferentiated leukemia | AUL | | Stem cell leukemia |
| Chronic | | | |
|   Chronic myelocytic leukemia | CML | | Chronic granulocytic leukemia |
| | | | Chronic myelogenous leukemia |
|   Chronic lymphocytic leukemia | CLL | | Chronic lymphoid leukemia |
|   Hairy cell leukemia | HCL | | Leukemic reticuloendotheliosis |

*French-American-British proposal for classification of acute leukemia.
(From Hoffbrand, AV and Lewis, SM (eds): Postgraduate Hematology, ed 2. Appleton-Century-Crofts, New York, 1981, p. 437, with permission.)

the age of 40. Chronic myelocytic leukemia may be seen at any age, but its peak incidence is between 30 and 50 years of age; the disease is rare in children.

## Comparison of Acute and Chronic Leukemias

Acute and chronic leukemias differ in many respects, as summarized in Table 19-3. Although difference in clinical course no longer is the reason for the division into acute and chronic, there are dramatic clinical differences between these groups. Patients with acute leukemia usually have a sudden onset, and if left untreated the disease runs a rapidly fatal course of six months or less. Patients with chronic leukemia typically have an insidious onset and a longer clinical course, usually lasting two to six years.

Chronic leukemia is almost invariably accompa-

Table 19-3. COMPARISON OF ACUTE AND CHRONIC LEUKEMIA

| | Acute | Chronic |
|---|---|---|
| Age | All ages | Adults |
| Clinical onset | Sudden | Insidious |
| Course (untreated) | 6 mo or less | 2-6 yr |
| Leukemic cells | Immature | Mature |
| Anemia and thrombocytopenia | Prominent | Mild |
| WBC | Variable | Increased |
| Lymphadenopathy | Mild | Present |
| Splenomegaly | Mild | Present |

nied by an elevated white blood cell count. In contrast, patients with acute leukemia do not always present with an elevated white blood cell count and may even be leukopenic. It is thought that the immature cells of acute leukemia are more cohesive and have more difficulty escaping into the peripheral blood.[13] The accumulation of these cells in the marrow leads to marrow failure manifested by anemia, thrombocytopenia, and granulocytopenia. These features of marrow failure are typically more prominent in patients with acute leukemia.

Anemia is almost invariably present in patients with all types of leukemia at some time during the course of the disease.[14] Anemia in acute leukemia is usually present from the onset and may be severe. In chronic leukemia the anemia is typically mild at presentation.

The spleen, liver, and lymph nodes may be enlarged in any patient with leukemia, especially in those with chronic leukemia. In adults with acute leukemia, organomegaly is usually less prominent.

## ACUTE LEUKEMIA
## Clinical Features

The leukemic proliferation, accumulation, and invasion of normal tissue are chiefly responsible for the devastating effects of acute leukemia. The most severe complications are those resulting from bone marrow involvement and its subsequent failure. This failure results in anemia, thrombocytopenia, granulocytopenia, and their sequelae.

The majority of patients with acute leukemia typically present with a clinically abrupt onset of signs and symptoms lasting only a few weeks. Patients often seek medical attention because of weakness, flu-like symptoms, or bleeding abnormalities. Table 19–4 summarizes the presenting clinical features of acute leukemia as they relate to pathophysiology.[15] About 5 to 10 percent of cases of acute myeloid leukemia (AML) are preceded by a recognizable "preleukemic" (myelodysplastic) syndrome, but the proportion of patients with this syndrome is higher among the elderly (see section of myelodysplastic syndromes at the end of this chapter).[16]

Infections and bleeding are the leading causes of death in patients with acute leukemia. However, the liberal use of platelet transfusions has reduced the frequency of death from hemorrhage.[17] Other causes of death include hepatic, pulmonary, cardiac, or renal failure resulting from leukemic infiltrates. Leukemic "sludging" (hyperviscosity) due to massive peripheral blood involvement can be fatal when it causes pulmonary or cerebral infarction or an intracerebral hemorrhage.

## Laboratory Evaluation

### Diagnostic Criteria

The laboratory diagnosis of acute leukemia is based on two criteria: (1) substantiating the presence of a significant increase in the number of immature cells (e.g., blasts, promyelocytes, or promonocytes) in the bone marrow, and (2) identification of the cell lineage of these leukemic cells. The percentage of blasts necessary to diagnose acute leukemia is somewhat arbitrary. The French-American-British cooperative group recommends 30 percent.[18]

A preliminary workup of acute leukemia should include a complete blood count (CBC), a platelet count, and a differential in order to assess the peripheral hematologic parameters. Anemia is the most consistent finding; it may be mild to severe and is usually normochromic, normocytic. Typically, the platelets are decreased, although they may be normal. The white blood cell (WBC) count is variable, ranging from decreased to markedly elevated. Review of the blood smear frequently reveals blasts.

The following nomenclature may be used to classify the degree of peripheral involvement: (1) leukemic, (2) subleukemic, and (3) aleukemic. In leukemic leukemia the white blood cell count is elevated owing to numerous blasts in the peripheral blood. Subleukemic leukemia has blasts present without an increase in the total white blood cell count. In aleukemic leukemia no blasts are detectable in the peripheral blood, and white blood cell count is usually decreased.

Features typical of myelodysplastic (preleukemic) syndromes are sometimes present, including pseudo–Pelger-Huët cells and hypogranular neutrophils. These features are more common in elderly patients with acute myeloblastic leukemia.

Once the preliminary studies are done, a bone marrow aspirate and biopsy should be obtained. Evaluation of the marrow is almost always necessary for a definitive diagnosis. Review of the marrow aspirate and biopsy is essential for establishing the extent of marrow involvement. In addition, classification of the leukemic cells is best done on cells obtained from the bone marrow rather than from the peripheral blood.

A definitive diagnosis and proper classification of acute leukemia depends ultimately on the classification of the immature cells involved in the leukemic process. This is accomplished by using some or all of the following laboratory methods: (1) morphology, (2) cytochemistry, and (3) immunologic markers. Occasionally, electron microscopy may be useful. With improvement in cytogenetic techniques this procedure is also becoming useful in diagnosis and prognosis.

### FAB Classification

In the past, acute leukemias have been classified by various systems. The need for a uniform system and nomenclature prompted a group of French, American, and British hematologists to propose a new system in 1976.[19] This system, designated FAB, has proven to be useful in standardizing the classification of acute lymphoid and myeloid leukemias.

The FAB classification is based on morphology and cytochemical evaluation of the leukemic cells. Romanowsky-stained bone marrow and peripheral blood preparations are used to evaluate the morphology. Cytochemical stains are used to identify myeloid and monocytic differentiation. Myeloperoxidase or Sudan black B stains are used to identify myeloid cells, and the nonspecific esterase (NSE) stain is used for identification of monocytic cells. Positive staining with these stains excludes lymphoblastic leukemia.

## Table 19–4. CLINICAL FEATURES OF ACUTE LEUKEMIA

| Clinical Features | Laboratory Abnormalities |
|---|---|
| Weakness and pallor | Anemia |
| Bleeding or bruising | Thrombocytopenia, occasionally DIC |
| Fever, infections | Granulocytopenia, immunosuppression |
| Bone or joint pain | Leukemic infiltrates/ marrow expansion |
| Neurologic symptoms (headache, vomiting, and so on) | Leukemic cells in CSF |
| Lymphadenopathy | Leukemic infiltrates |
| Hepatosplenomegaly | Leukemic infiltrates |

From Kjeldsberg,[15] p. 312, with permission.

Table 19-5. MORPHOLOGIC CLASSIFICATION OF THE ACUTE LEUKEMIAS

1. "Lymphoblastic" (ALL)
    L1: Small, monomorphic
    L2: Large, heterogeneous
    L3: Burkitt-cell type
2. Myeloid (AML)
    M1: Myeloblastic without maturation
    M2: Myeloblastic with maturation
    M3: Hypergranular promyelocytic
    M4: Myelomonocytic
    M5: Monocytic ⟨ a. Poorly differentiated (monoblastic)
                    b. Well differentiated (promonocytic-monocytic)
    M6: Erythroleukemia

Adapted from Bennett et al.[19]

The FAB system separates acute leukemias into two broad groups: lymphoid and myeloid (nonlymphoid). The lymphoid group is divided into three types (L1-L3) and the myeloid group into six main types (M1-M6). These groups, which are summarized in Table 19-5, will be discussed in more detail following a review of laboratory methods for evaluation of acute leukemia.

## Laboratory Methods

**Specimens.** The importance of an adequate specimen and proper handling of material must be kept in mind. Lack of technical excellence may obscure or complicate an otherwise straightforward diagnosis. In fact, technical problems or inadequate specimens or both are the most common causes of an incorrect diagnosis.

Evaluation of the peripheral blood cell morphology should be done using nonanticoagulated fingerstick smears. Anticoagulant (EDTA) causes morphologic artifacts of nucleated cells and platelets. A specimen left in EDTA for over 30 minutes may show artifactual vacuolation of monocytes and neutrophils, nuclear shape changes and swelling, as well as degranulation of platelets.[20,21]

A bone marrow sample, including an aspirate and biopsy, is the specimen of choice for evaluation of acute leukemia. Pulled smears made on cover slips result in thin aspirate smears, which are preferable to thick ones. When an aspirate produces a "dry" tap, touch preps made from the bone marrow biopsy should be made for morphologic evaluation and for cytochemical and immunologic studies.

**Morphologic Evaluation.** The morphologic evaluation of a Romanowsky (Wright-Giemsa)-stained blood or marrow smear is essential for the characterization of leukemic cells. In the hands of an experienced morphologist, the correct classification of cell type is often apparent; however, additional testing is necessary to ensure accurate identification.

A number of morphologic clues, as outlined in Table 19-6, may aid in distinguishing between lymphoblastic and myeloblastic leukemias. These include the size of blast, amount of cytoplasm, nuclear chromatin pattern, presence of nucleoli, and presence of Auer rods. Auer rods are an abnormal fusion of primary granules and are pathognomonic for a myeloproliferative process, in particular AML (and rarely chronic myelocytic leukemia, or CML, in myeloid blast crisis);[17] they have also been described in myelodysplastic (preleukemic) syndromes.[22] On Romanowsky-stained smears, Auer rods appear as pink-staining rods or splinter-shaped inclusions **(see Color Figure 149)**. In acute progranulocytic leukemia (M3), Auer rods appear as "bunches" of cigar-shaped rods ("faggot cells"). They are present in 10 to 40 percent of patients with AML.[17] Their presence rules out acute lymphoblastic leukemia (ALL).

The typical myeloblast is a large cell with a moderate amount of cytoplasm. Its nucleus has a fine reticulated chromatin pattern, and multiple nucleoli are often present. The typical lymphoblast is a smaller cell with scant cytoplasm. The nuclear chromatin often appears more dense than in the myeloblast and usually only one or two nucleoli are present. There is often peripheral condensations of chromatin around the nucleoli. For a review of morphologic descriptions of the blast stage of the blood cell lines, see Chapter 1.

**Cytochemistry.** Cytochemical methods are used

Table 19-6. MORPHOLOGIC CLUES
FOR DIFFERENTIATION OF BLASTS IN AML AND ALL

|  | AML Myeloblast | ALL Lymphoblast |
|---|---|---|
| Blast size | Large blast | Small blast |
| Cytoplasm | Moderate | Scant |
| Chromatin | Fine, lacy | Dense |
| Nucleoli | Prominent (usually more than 2) | Indistinct (usually 2 or less) |
| Auer rods | Present in 10–40% cases of AML | Never present |

to identify specific chemical components of cells, such as enzymes or lipids. They are helpful in distinguishing among the different types of acute leukemia. The following procedures are done by applying staining techniques to bone marrow or peripheral blood smears (see Chapter 31). Fresh smears are preferred. Table 19–7 summarizes the reactions of the cytochemical methods most useful for acute leukemia classification.

***Myeloperoxidase (see Color Figure 150).*** This enzyme is present in the primary granules of granulocytic cells. These primary granules first appear in the early promyelocyte (late blast) and persist through subsequent stages of cell maturation. Monocytes have variable staining with peroxidase and are most often weakly positive. This enzyme is not present in lymphocytes and is therefore useful in differentiating AML from ALL. It is more specific for granulocytic differentiation than the Sudan black B stain.

***Sudan Black B (SBB) (see Color Figure 151).*** Phospholipids and other lipids are stained by Sudan black B (SBB). This is believed to be due to the solubility of the dye in the lipid particles. These lipid particles occur both in primary and secondary granules of granulocytic cells and to a lesser extent in monocytic lysozomal granules. SBB is useful for differentiating AML from ALL, because positivity seldom occurs in lymphoid cells; however, rare cases of SBB-positive ALL are observed.[23] Because it does not stain for enzyme activity, the SBB reaction is useful for staining specimens that are not fresh and have lost their enzymatic peroxidase activity.

***Nonspecific Esterase (NSE).*** The NSE stain is used to identify monocytic cells. It is diffusely positive in these cells **(see Color Figure 152)** and negative in granulocytic cells. T lymphocytes can be NSE-positive but have a focal staining pattern.

Different substrates are available for use in this procedure. Alpha-naphthyl butyrate is the most

specific, while alpha-naphtyl acetate is most sensitive. Another substrate, naphthyl AS-D acetate (NASDA), is less specific and stains both monocytes and granulocytes. It must be used in conjunction with a sodium fluoride inhibition step, which renders monocytic cells negative and thus differentiates them from granulocytic cells, which remain positive. Out of these substrates, the alpha-naphthyl butyrate is the most useful.

***Terminal Deoxynucleotidyl Transferase (TdT).*** This unique DNA polymerase is normally found only in immature lymphoid cells located primarily in the thymus and to a lesser extent in the bone marrow.[24] An indirect immunofluorescence method **(see Color Figure 153)** or an enzyme assay is used to detect TdT. The fluorescence method is done on smears or touch preps. It is particularly important to have fresh material for evaluation of TdT. High levels have been found in 90 percent of cases of ALL, both with non-B, non-T surface phenotype and with T-cell markers (T ALL).[25] The majority of AML cases demonstrate undetectable levels of TdT; thus, it is useful in differentiating ALL from AML. However, 5 to 10 percent of patients with AML have detectable TdT activity in their blasts.[26]

TdT is also present in most cases of lymphoblastic lymphoma and in approximately one third of cases of chronic myelocytic leukemia (CML) in blast transformation.[26,27] Its presence in cases of CML in blast transformation provides a useful predictor of the likelihood of favorable response of the disease to treatment with vincristine and prednisone.[28]

***Periodic Acid–Schiff (PAS).*** The PAS reaction stains for glycogen. Periodic acid ($HIO_4$) oxidizes glycols to aldehydes. The resulting aldehydes react with Schiff's reagent to form a magenta color.

The PAS stain is not very useful for characterizing acute leukemia and is often misinterpreted. Coarse or block positivity in primitive cells has sometimes incorrectly been regarded as necessary and specific for the diagnosis of ALL.[29] The PAS reaction gives variable results in L1 and L2 ALL and in the myeloid leukemias; the result is negative in L3 ALL.[19] Coarse positivity **(see Color Figure 154)**, which was considered specific for ALL, is also present in some cases of AML — especially in the monocytic variants.

Normally, the erythrocytic series does not show detectable amounts of glycogen at any stage of cellular development. In contrast, strong PAS positivity may be present in erythroblasts of some cases of erythroleukemia. This feature, when present, is helpful for differentiating it from pernicious anemia, which is negative except in rare cases.[20] Some of the myelodysplastic syndromes may also have PAS-positive erythroblasts.

**Immunologic Marker Studies.** (See Chapter 31 for procedures.)

***Surface Marker Studies.*** Cell membranes have unique antigens and receptor sites on their surface

**Table 19–7. CYTOCHEMICAL REACTIONS IN IMMATURE HEMATOPOIETIC CELLS**

|  | Perox/Sudan | NSE | TdT |
|---|---|---|---|
| Myeloblast | + | – | –/+ |
| Monoblast | +/– | + | – |
| Lymphoblast | – | –* | + |

*Focal NSE positivity may be seen in T-cell ALL.

that can be identified and used as markers for cell identification and phenotyping. The following are especially useful for immunologic characterization of leukemic cells in ALL: (1) surface immunoglobulins, (2) E-rosette receptors, and (3) specific membrane antigens detected by monoclonal antibodies. Live cell suspensions prepared from a bone marrow aspirate or peripheral blood specimen are preferred for these studies because of the need for cells (blasts) with intact cell membranes.

*Surface Immunoglobulins (SIg).* B lymphocytes produce immunoglobulin, which is first detectable in the cytoplasm (cytoplasmic immunoglobulin or CIg) and, as the cell matures, is detectable on the cell surface (SIg). A direct immunofluorescent method is used to detect SIg **(see Color Figure 155)**. This is useful for characterizing B-cell lymphoid malignancies.

*E Rosettes.* T-cell lymphocytes have receptors on their surface that allow adherence of sheep red blood cells and formation of rosettes **(see Color Figure 156)**. This characteristic is used to help identify T-cell malignancies. It is not, however, as reliable as the use of monoclonal antibodies for T-cell identification, which have now replaced the rosette technique.

*Monoclonal Antibodies.* Certain antibodies produced by hybridoma technology are particularly useful for characterizing ALL. These monoclonal antibodies are used with indirect immunofluorescent methods to detect specific antigens on cell membranes. Examples of these antibodies include anti–T-cell, anti–T-helper, and anti–T-suppressor cells. Another useful antiserum is directed against the common ALL antigen (cALLA), which is present in the majority of cases of childhood ALL. Monoclonal antisera is also available that has specificity for B lymphocytes and myeloid cells. The rapid growth of hybridoma technology will probably make available in the near future additional antibodies that will further aid characterization of leukemic cells.

*Cytoplasmic Immunoglobulins (CIg).* A direct immunofluorescent method is used to detect immunoglobulin within cells that have been fixed to expose their cytoplasm. Fresh blood or marrow smears, touch preps, or cytopreps made from cell suspensions of the leukemia cells are used. CIgM is present in pre–B ALL.

**Cytogenetics.** Cytogenetic methods are currently used to study acute leukemia primarily for prognostic indicators and research interest. Approximately 50 to 55 percent of patients with acute myeloid leukemia and over 65 percent of acute lymphoid leukemia patients exhibit chromosomal abnormalities in their leukemic cells.[30-32]

A number of different chromosome abnormalities have been associated with leukemia including aneuploidy and various translocations. The translocation of a portion of chromosome 17 to 15 is apparently specific for acute promyelocytic leukemia.[33] The Philadelphia (Ph[1]) chromosome, which was thought to be specific for CML (see Chapter 20), has been found in some adult acute leukemias. Its presence in acute leukemia indicates a poor prognosis.

**Electron Microscopy.** Ultrastructural studies are not routinely used for the diagnosis of acute leukemia. However, they are helpful in rare cases of poorly differentiated leukemia when other methods are inconclusive about the identity of the leukemic cell. Ultrastructural examination for the presence of myeloperoxidase or nonspecific esterase may be useful for identifying poorly differentiated myeloblasts or monoblasts. Platelet peroxidase is helpful for identifying megakaryoblastic leukemias.

## Acute Lymphoblastic Leukemia

### FAB Classification

The classification system FAB[19] separates ALL from myeloid leukemia on the basis of the negative staining pattern of lymphoblasts with the myeloperoxidase (or Sudan black B) and NSE stains. It is further subdivided on the basis of the cytologic features of the lymphoblasts, as summarized in Table 19–8.

**Table 19–8. ACUTE LYMPHOBLASTIC LEUKEMIA, FAB CLASSIFICATION**

| Cell Characteristics | L1 | L2 | L3 |
|---|---|---|---|
| Cell size | Predominantly small cells, homogenous | Large, heterogenous | Large, homogenous |
| Nuclear chromatin | Homogenous in any one case | Heterogenous | Stippled, homogenous |
| Nuclear shape | Regular, round, occasional clefting | Irregular, clefting | Regular, round to ovoid |
| Nucleoli | Inconspicuous | One or more, may be large | One or more, prominent |
| Cytoplasm | Scanty | Variable, moderately abundant | Moderately abundant, strongly basophilic |
| Cytoplasmic vacuolation | Variable | Variable | Prominent |

(Adapted from Bennett et al.[19] and from Maslon, WC, Beutler, E, Bell, CA, et al: Practical Diagnosis: Hematologic Disease. Houghton Mifflin, Boston, 1980, p. 332.)

L1 ALL **(see Color Figure 157)** is composed predominantly of a uniform population of small blasts that are characterized by scant cytoplasm, a homogeneous chromatin pattern in any one case, and indistinct nucleoli. The nuclear shape is regular, but occasional clefting or indentation may be present.

L2 ALL **(see Color Figure 158)** is characterized by a heterogeneous group of cells. Some blasts may exhibit features of L1 cells, whereas others are larger and have more abundant cytoplasm, a variable chromatin pattern, and prominent nucleoli. Nuclear clefting and indentation are common. This type may be difficult to distinguish morphologically from certain acute myeloid leukemias.

The recognition of L1 and L2 may be more precisely defined by using a simple scoring system published by the FAB group.[34]

L3 **(see Color Figure 159)** is composed of a uniform population of blasts that are characterized by moderate to abundant dark-blue cytoplasm, usually featuring many vacuoles. The nucleus has a round to oval contour without indentations. L3 ALL is referred to as "Burkitt type," because its morphology is the same as that seen in Burkitt's lymphoma.

## Immunologic Classification

In addition to the FAB classification system, ALL is also classified by immunologic phenotyping. It is divided into four major subgroups using this system: common ALL, "null" or "unclassified" ALL, T ALL, and B ALL. Common ALL is identified by reactivity of the blasts with anti–common ALL antigen (cALLA) and by the lack of activity with T-cell or B-cell markers. The majority of cases of common ALL test positive for TdT. "Null" or "unclassified" ALL has a similar phenotype except that the blasts do not react with cALLA. T ALL is identified by its positive reactivity with monoclonal T-cell antisera. T ALL is also characterized by the spontaneous formation of E rosettes when incubated with sheep red blood cells. Finally, B ALL is defined by the presence of monoclonal surface immunoglobulin; that is, the presence of only one type of light chain immunoglobulin on the surface of the blasts' cell membrane. Pre–B ALL has also been recognized; it has no surface immunoglobulin but is positive for cytoplasmic heavy chain mu (IgM). Pre–B ALL reacts with cALLA antisera and is considered a subgroup of common ALL. Table 19–9 summarizes the immunologic categories of ALL.

## Incidence

The incidence of ALL differs markedly with age. For this reason, and because of the generally poorer prognosis in adults, it is common to divide ALL into the broad groups of childhood ALL and adult ALL. Generally, the childhood group consists of those patients who present with ALL at 15 years of age or younger.

ALL constitutes the single most common malignancy in the pediatric age group. The morphologic type L1 occurs most frequently in this group, whereas the L2 type occurs most frequently in the adult age group. No significant differences occur in the incidence of L3 in children and adults.[34] Differences in incidence of ALL immunologic subtypes also occur in these age groups. T ALL and pre–B ALL are less frequent and "null" ALL subclass has a considerably higher incidence in adults.

## Prognostic Indicators

Prognostic indicators have been identified that are helpful in guiding therapeutic strategies for patients with ALL. The most important indicators are age and white blood cell count. Patients less than 1 year old and those more than 13 years old have a poor prognosis, whereas those between 3 and 7 years of age have a much better prognosis. A white blood cell count of less than $10 \times 10^9/l$ at presentation indicates a good prognosis, in contrast to a count greater than $20 \times 10^9/l$, which is a poor prognostic feature, and those greater than $100 \times 10^9/l$, which are particularly poor.[8] Other presenting features that tend to be associated with a poor prognosis are the finding of a mediastinal mass, early central nervous system (CNS) leukemia, the presence of B-cell or T-cell markers, L2 and L3 type morphology, and male gender.

## Immunologic Subtypes

**Common Acute Lymphoblastic Leukemia.** As the name implies, common ALL is the most frequently encountered form of ALL. It is predominantly seen in the pediatric age group, although it can occur at

## Table 19–9. IMMUNOLOGIC CLASSIFICATION OF ACUTE LYMPHOBLASTIC LEUKEMIA

|  | cALLA | CIgM | SIg | ER | HTA | TdT | FAB |
|---|---|---|---|---|---|---|---|
| Common ALL | + | − | − | − | − | + | L1, L2 |
| Pre–B ALL | + | + | − | − | − | + | L1, L2 |
| B ALL | − | − | + | − | − | − | L3 |
| T ALL | − | − | − | + | + | + | L2, L2 |
| "Null" ("unclassified") ALL | − | − | − | − | − | + | L1, L2 |

cALLA = common ALL antigen; CIg = cytoplasmic immunoglobulin; SIg = surface immunoglobulin; ER = E rosettes; HTA = human T-lymphocyte–associated antigen; TdT = terminal deoxynucleotidyl transferase; FAB = French-American-British classification.

any age. Its peak incidence is between the ages of 3 and 5 years. Common ALL is characterized in most childhood cases by L1 morphology and in adults by L2 morphology. In addition to cALLA positivity, TdT is also present in the majority of cases. The origin of the common ALL leukemia cells has not been fully elucidated; however, recent studies indicate that the majority of cases of non-B, non-T ALL are actually cases of pre B-cell ALL.

Patients with common ALL usually present with disease predominantly localized in the blood and bone marrow. Prominent splenomegaly, hepatomegaly, and lymphadenopathy are infrequently seen at presentation. It is uncommon for patients to present with a markedly elevated white blood count (greater than $100 \times 10^9/l$).

Common ALL, especially in children, has the best prognosis of any of the acute leukemias. The majority of these patients achieve complete remission with current chemotherapy protocols, and 50 percent successfully achieve leukemia-free survivals of five to 10 years and are potentially cured.[8]

**T-Cell Acute Lymphoblastic Leukemia.** T-cell markers are found in approximately 25 percent of all patients with ALL. A small percentage of these patients also test positive for cALLA.[37] Both L1 and L2 morphology are associated with this form of ALL. Using a cytochemical method to stain for acid phosphatase, approximately 90 percent of patients with T, ALL have focal paranuclear staining in the blasts.[38] This, however, is not useful for diagnosis, because in a small percentage of cases non-T, non-B ALL may demonstrate a similar pattern of acid phosphatase staining.

T ALL is associated with several clinical features indicative of a poor prognosis. These include tumoral presentation, mediastinal mass, high peripheral white blood cell count (greater than $100 \times 10^9/l$ in 50 percent of cases), hepatosplenomegaly, early meningeal involvement, male gender, and older age.[39]

T ALL may be difficult to distinguish from lymphoblastic lymphoma, when the patient presents with a mediastinal mass. The cytologic features of this lymphoma are identical to those of T ALL. After a variable time, patients with lymphoblastic lymphoma almost always develop marrow involvement, which then renders their condition indistinguishable from that of patients who have T ALL. In patients who initially present with nodal involvement, the disease is usually diagnosed as lymphoblastic lymphoma, whereas in patients who present with predominant marrow and peripheral blood involvement, the diagnosis of T ALL is made.

**B-Cell Acute Lymphoblastic Leukemia.** B ALL is a homogeneous group that accounts for only a small portion of cases of ALL, with an overall incidence of approximately 4 percent.[40] The majority of these cases are associated with L3 morphology, although rare cases of non-L3 B ALL have been reported.[39] Also rare are cases of ALL with L3 morphology that do not have B-cell markers present. Thus, L3 is the only FAB lymphoid subgroup to accurately predict immunologic type.

Surface immunoglobulin with a monoclonal pattern (only one light chain present) is strongly positive in the majority of cases, with a predominance of IgM lambda.[41] It is thought that the leukemic cell of B ALL likely represents a transformed or stimulated B-cell.[42]

B ALL cells are indistinguishable by cytologic, cytochemical, and immunologic criteria from tumor cells characteristic of Burkitt's lymphoma.[43] Leukemic transformation is extremely rare in African Burkitt's lymphoma, but it does occur in the nonendemic variety.[39] Marrow infiltration is seen in more than half of American patients with Burkitt's lymphoma; however, a leukemic picture is only apparent as a terminal event.[43]

Patients with B ALL respond poorly to current chemotherapy regimens and rarely achieve remission.[44]

**"Null" Cell ("Unclassified") Acute Lymphoblastic Leukemia.** Approximately 10 percent of childhood ALL cases test negative for B-cell and T-cell markers and for cALLA. Most of these are TdT positive.[39] They have an intermediate prognosis that falls between those of common ALL and T ALL.

## ACUTE MYELOID LEUKEMIA (AML)

### FAB Classification

The FAB system divides acute myeloid leukemia into six main types that are defined by the presence of differentiation along one or more cell line and by the degree of differentiation.[19] Myeloid, monocytic, and erythroid types of acute leukemia are included in this group. All of them have a myeloid component except for rare forms of pure monocytic leukemia or pure erythroleukemia (erythremic myelosis). Cytochemical stains (myeloperoxidase, Sudan black B, NSE) are used to identify the type and amount of differentiation of the myeloid and monocytic components. A summary of these cytochemical reactions is found in Table 19–10.

### M1: Myeloblastic Without Maturation (see Color Figure 160)

The leukemic cells are blasts with rare azurophilic granules. The nucleus typically has a fine, lacy pattern, and nucleoli are often multiple and distinct. These blasts have varying amounts of cytoplasm. Three percent of the blasts must stain positive with myeloperoxidase or Sudan black B to rule out lymphoblastic leukemia.

Table 19–10. CYTOCHEMICAL RACTIONS IN ACUTE MYELOID LEUKEMIA

| | FAB Classification | | | | | |
|---|---|---|---|---|---|---|
| | *M1* | *M2* | *M3* | *M4* | *M5* | *M6* |
| Peroxidase or Sudan black | >3% | >50% | Near 100% | 20–80% | Variable | >3% |
| Nonspecific esterase | <20% | <20% | Variable | 20–80% | >80% | Variable |

## M2: Myeloblastic With Maturation (see Color Figure 161)

The leukemic marrow infiltrate resembles M1, except evidence of maturation to or beyond the promyelocyte stage is present. Romanowsky-stained bone marrow smears show that promyelocytes make up greater than 10 percent of the immature cells. More than 50 percent of the immature cells are myeloperoxidase or Sudan black B positive. The NSE activity does not exceed 20 percent. Auer rods are common.

## M3: Hypergranular Promyelocytic (see Color Figure 162)

This form of AML is defined by morphologic criteria. The leukemic infiltrate is composed of abnormal promyelocytes with heavy granulation and often abundant cytoplasm. The primary granules may obscure the nucleus in some cells. Auer rods are frequently seen, and some cells may contain bundles of Auer rods ("faggot cells"). The nucleus varies in size and shape and is often reniform or bilobed. The peroxidase stain is markedly positive in most of the leukemic cells; the NSE stain is variable.[45]

## M3m: Microgranular (Hypogranular) Promyelocytic (see Color Figure 163)

This form of leukemia is similar to hypergranular promyelocytic (M3) form, except that the primary granules are not readily visible on Romanowsky-stained smears. Occasionally some faggot cells are present. The nucleus typically is reniform, bilobed, or "dumb-bell" shaped. Cytochemistry is necessary to identify this variant. As with the hypergranular form, the peroxidase stains positive in nearly all of the leukemic cells, and the NSE stain is variable.

## M4: Myelomonocytic (see Color Figures 164 through 166)

Both granulocytic and monocytic differentiation is present. M4 is identified by 20 to 80 percent of the leukemic cells in the bone marrow staining positive with NSE.

## M5: Monocytic

Greater than 80 percent of the leukemic cells stain positive with NSE. The peroxidase and Sudan black B stains test negative or only weakly positive.

## M5a: Poorly Differentiated (see Color Figure 167)

Poorly differentiated monoblasts predominate. These blasts typically are large with abundant cytoplasm and easily seen nucleoli.

## M5b: Well Differentiated (see Color Figure 168)

Monoblasts, promonocytes, and monocytes are all present, but the number of monocytes is higher in the peripheral blood than in the bone marrow in which the predominant cell is the promonocyte. This cell has abundant cytoplasm. Its nucleus shows folding or lobulation, and nucleoli may be present.

## M6: Erythroleukemia (see Color Figures 169, 170)

The erythropoietic component usually exceeds 50 percent of the marrow elements. Bizarre erythroid morphology is characteristic, including megaloblastic features and multiple nuclear lobulation. Erythroblasts are common in the peripheral blood. Abnormalities of the granulocytic and megakaryocytic lines are also present in varying degrees. The percentage of myeloblasts and promyelocytes exceeds 30 percent of the nucleated cells in the marrow.

### Morphologic Subtypes

**Acute Myeloblastic Leukemia (M1, M2).** Acute myeloblastic leukemias, with and without maturation (M2 and M1, respectively), are the most common types of acute myeloid leukemia. Together, M1 and M2 account for approximately 50 percent of these leukemias.[46] They are characterized by clinical features typical of acute leukemia. Aside from their morphology and cytochemistry, they do not have unique features that set them apart from other myeloid subtypes.

**Acute Promyelocytic Leukemia (M3).** Acute promyelocytic leukemia (APL) is a unique form of acute myeloid leukemia associated with a high incidence of disseminated intravascular coagulation (DIC). It is characterized by an infiltration of the marrow with hypergranular promyelocytes often having multiple Auer rods. The cells are rich in thromboplastic substances that trigger DIC if released.

The majority of patients with APL present with

hemorrhagic manifestations including petechiae, small ecchymoses, hematuria, and bleeding from venipuncture and bone marrow sites.[47] These presenting signs and symptoms may precede the diagnosis by several weeks.

The most consistent coagulation abnormalities include a prolonged prothrombin and thrombin time, elevated fibrinogen degradation products, and decreased amounts of serum fibrinogen and factor V.[48] Thrombocytopenia is almost universally present, and tends to be more severe than in other types of acute leukemia.[49] Schistocytes (RBC fragments) associated with DIC may frequently be seen on the peripheral blood smear.

A particular chromosomal translocation, t(15;17), is also associated with APL. This abnormality has not been reported in any other type of leukemia.[33]

It is important to distinguish APL from other types of AML, because of the complications associated with DIC. Anticoagulant therapy (heparin) is usually indicated in these cases and is most successful when initiated prior to antileukemic therapy.[47]

**Acute Promyelocytic Leukemia, Microgranular (Hypogranular) Variant (M3m).** A microgranular variant form of APL (FAB M3m) (also referred to as hypogranular) has been identified that is characterized by minimal granulation of promyelocytes when observed on Romanowsky-stained smears. These cells do, however, contain many granules that are readily visualized by transmission electron microscopy.[50] This variant behaves clinically in a fashion similar to APL having features of DIC. It is therefore important to recognize it for therapeutic considerations.

Morphologically, this variant of M3 is easily mistaken for a monocytic type of acute leukemia. The leukemic cells are monocytoid appearing with prominent nuclear folding and abundant cytoplasm. The nucleus of most cells in the peripheral blood is bilobed, multilobated, or reniform. Granulation of these cells is scant or absent; however, occasional cells with heavy granulation (faggot cells) are almost always present. The bone marrow aspirate may reveal a morphologic pattern that more closely resembles typical APL.[51]

Cytochemical studies are necessary to distinguish this variant from acute monocytic leukemia. The peroxidase and Sudan black B stains test strikingly positive. Variable results have been reported using the NSE stain.[45,50] Cytogenetic studies of microgranular APL reveal the same abnormal karyotype, t(15;17), that is found in the hypergranular form.

**Acute Monocytic Leukemias (M4, M5).** Monocytic differentiation in acute myeloid leukemia may be present in variable degrees, ranging from none or very little to a moderate amount, as in acute myelomonocytic leukemia (AMML, M4), or a predominance, as in acute monocytic leukemia (AMoL, M5).

AMML (Naegeli-type) accounts for approximately one third of the acute leukemias,[52] whereas "pure" monocytic (M5; Schilling-type) is uncommon with an incidence ranging between 1 and 8 percent of all acute leukemias.[53]

Acute monocytic leukemia (M5) has distinctive clinical manifestations associated with the monocyte's propensity to migrate to extramedullary sites. Skin and gum involvement are particularly characteristic **(see Color Figure 174)**. Lymphadenopathy frequently occurs, and sometimes the spleen and liver are markedly enlarged.[54,55] Central nervous system involvement has an increased incidence in these patients.[56,57]

The white blood cell count is frequently over $10 \times 10^9$/l in AMoL (M5); the median value of $60 \times 10^9$/l was reported in one study.[55] Markedly elevated leukocyte counts in monocytic leukemia (M5) patients have been shown to have a significant correlation with increased lysozyme levels, renal failure, hypokalemia and an increased incidence of disseminated intravascular coagulation.[55,58] DIC has been associated with AMoLs, especially following therapy, although hemorrhagic features are not as prominent as in acute promyelocytic leukemia.

Serum and urine lysozyme levels (muramidase) are frequently high in AMML and AMoL. Lysozyme is a hydrolytic enzyme found in mature granulocytes and in particularly large amounts in monocytes. Serum and urine levels of this enzyme are elevated when there is rapid cell turnover. Such elevations are most striking in the monocytic leukemias and are directly proportional to the amount of monocytic differentiation.[59] These patients with heavy urinary excretion of muramidase may develop a renal tubular defect that results in hypokalemia, hypocalcemia, and azotemia.

**Erythroleukemia (M6).** Erythroleukemia has three sequential morphologically defined phases, which vary in the size of the myeloid component. They are (1) erythremic myelosis, in which there is a preponderance of abnormal erythroblasts; (2) erythroleukemia, in which both increases in erythroblasts and myeloblasts are seen; and (3) myeloblastic leukemia.[60] It is well recognized that many patients who are diagnosed with erythroleukemia will have their disease evolve into a leukemic stage indistinguishable from AML, M1, M2, or M4 type.[19]

Erythroleukemia is characterized by abnormal proliferation of erythroid and myeloid precursors. The bone marrow is hypercellular, showing marked erythroid hyperplasia (greater than 50 percent by FAB criteria)[19] with abnormal forms present. Megaloblastoid changes are seen in the erythroblasts. Other features of dyserythropoiesis are present and may include bizarre multinucleation, markedly vacuolated cytoplasm of proerythroblasts and basophilic erythroblasts, and cytoplasmic budding. Occasionally, erythrophagocytosis by erythroblasts is seen; such phagocytosis is thought to be unique to erythroleukemia.[61] Periodic acid–Schiff (PAS) positive staining of the erythroblasts is consistent with the diagnosis of erythroleukemia; however, negative staining does not rule it out, nor is it specific for erythroleukemia. Myeloblasts and promyelocytes are present in increased numbers (greater than 30 percent by FAB criteria),[19] and Auer rods may be seen. Abnormal megakaryocytes may also be present.

Anemia is invariably present. Lack of a significant increase in reticulocytes is common and is due to ineffective erythropoiesis. Frequently, the peripheral blood has nucleated red blood cells and myeloblasts present, but it is possible to see patients who are anerythremic (no NRBCs) or aleukemic (no blasts), or both.

Caution must be taken when the diagnosis of erythroleukemia is made. The possibility of megaloblastic anemia due to either vitamin $B_{12}$ or folic acid deficiency and sideroblastic anemia must be excluded. These nonmalignant disorders may at times mimic erythroleukemia. Congenital dyserythropoietic anemias and the myelodysplastic syndromes must also be ruled out.[19]

## Acute Megakaryoblastic Leukemia (AMegL)

Acute megakaryoblastic leukemia (AMegL) is a rare disorder characterized by extensive proliferation of megakaryoblasts and atypical megakaryocytes and by thrombocytopenia. Increasing recognition of this entity has been largely aided by the use of platelet peroxidase (PPO) ultrastructural studies. PPO, which is distinct from myeloperoxidase, appears to be specific for the megakaryocytic cell line.[62] It is found in the perinuclear space and endoplasmic reticulum early in the differentiation of these cells.[63]

The blasts observed in AMegL are usually small (10 to 20 microns in diameter), undifferentiated-appearing cells. Cytoplasmic projections may be present. The presence of immature cells with azurophilic granules, resembling early granular megakaryocytes, can be useful in the diagnosis of AMegL.[64] Myeloperoxidase and Sudan black B stain negative, whereas acid phosphatase, PAS, and alpha-naphthyl acetate esterase (ANAE) often stain positive. The combination of a positive ANAE and a negative alpha-naphthyl butyrate esterase is highly suggestive of megakaryoblastic lineage.[65] In addition, demonstration of factor VIII by immunohistochemical techniques is also a useful indicator of AMegL. The diagnosis of AMegL can be confirmed by using ultrastructural studies to demonstrate the presence of PPO.

AMegL is currently not included in the FAB classification, owing partly to the fact that recognition of megakaryoblasts has so far been impossible by routine light microscopic techniques.[65] Because of the increased recognition of AMegL using PPO studies, its inclusion in the FAB classification system may be forthcoming.[66]

AMegL may arise against a background of myelodysplasia or de novo. It has been observed as a transformation of existing hematologic disorders such as sideroblastic anemia, chronic myelocytic leukemia, and myeloid metaplasia. AMegL has also been associated with acute myelofibrosis, which is a myeloproliferative syndrome characterized by diffuse marrow fibrosis and pancytopenia, but which usually lacks the splenomegaly and characteristic red cell morphology changes of classic myelofibrosis. It has been suggested that acute myelofibrosis may be synonymous with AMegL.[67]

## Treatment

The treatment of leukemia has two main goals: to eradicate the leukemic cell mass and to give supportive care. Cures are infrequently realized except in children with common ALL. However, induction of complete remission is a realistic goal for most patients with acute leukemia. Complete remission is defined as the absence of any leukemia-related signs and symptoms, and return of marrow and blood granulocyte, platelet, and red cell values to within normal limits.[17]

Four general types of antileukemic therapy are employed: cytotoxic chemotherapy, bone marrow transplantation, radiotherapy, and immunotherapy. Chemotherapy is the mainstay of treatment, although bone marrow transplantation is being used more frequently. Radiotherapy is used as an adjunct to chemotherapy in patients who have localized tissue involvement that may be targeted with irradiation. The aim of immunotherapy is to stimulate the immune system to help the patient's own defense system mount an immune reaction against the malignant cells. This mode of therapy remains experimental and largely unproven.

The cytotoxic chemotherapeutic agents are a group of diverse drugs having in common their ability to poison dividing cells, usually by blocking DNA or RNA synthesis. Combination chemotherapy is employed, using drugs with different modes of action and different toxicities. The successful treatment of leukemia requires the use of these drugs in dosages that have substantial toxicity, particularly to the marrow. Complications arising from marrow hypoplasia are the leading cause of morbidity and mortality in patients undergoing induction therapy.

Bone marrow transplantation is not in itself a treatment for leukemia. It is a means of rescuing the patient from the consequences of intensive antileukemic therapy used to completely eradicate the patient's marrow.[68] Both normal and leukemic elements in the marrow are destroyed using a regimen of chemotherapeutic agents and total body irradiation. Marrow is collected from an HLA-compatible donor by repeated bone marrow aspirates, is processed, and then is infused into the recipient intravenously. The infused cells travel to the recipient's "empty" marrow, where they begin to multiply and repopulate the patient's marrow with healthy hematopoietic tissue. The complications surrounding bone marrow transplants are numerous and often fatal. It is not suitable therapy for all patients who have leukemia. Infection and hemorrhage are frequent complications. Interstitial pneumonia is the most common cause of death in patients with leukemia undergoing marrow transplantation.[69] Graft-versus-host disease (GVHD) is another serious complication.

## MYELODYSPLASTIC SYNDROMES (MDS), OR PRELEUKEMIA

The myelodysplastic syndromes (MDS) represent a group of primary hematologic disorders associated with abnormal division, maturation, and production of erythrocytes, granulocytes, monocytes, and platelets (dyshemopoiesis). These disorders are characterized by qualitative and quantitative defects of hematopoietic stem cells, which result in ineffective erythropoiesis, granulopoiesis, and thrombopoiesis occurring either singly or in combination. The characteristic cytopenias that commonly accompany myelodysplastic disorders are mainly the result of the intramedullary death of these blood cells. MDS is mainly observed in patients over 50 years old and is associated with a high risk of progressing to acute myeloid leukemia.

Various names, as summarized in Table 19-11, have been used to describe this group of disorders. Recently, the FAB cooperative group has proposed a new classification.[18] They describe five categories: (1) refractory anemia (RA), (2) RA with ring sideroblasts, (3) RA with excess blasts (RAEB), (4) RAEB in transformation, and (5) chronic myelomonocytic leukemia (CMML). Each category represents a constellation of hematologic findings that have been defined by the FAB cooperative group.

MDS has a wide range of morphologic appearances in the peripheral blood and marrow, which are listed in Table 19-12. Anemia is present in the majority of individuals with MDS. It is usually normochromic, normocytic with an MCV in the high normal or slightly macrocytic range, but it may be markedly macrocytic.[70] The reticulocyte response is typically inadequate for the degree of anemia. Circulating nucleated RBCs may be present. Dysgranulopoiesis is manifested by any or several of the following findings: neutropenia, monocytosis, atypical monocytes that are difficult to distinguish from granulocytes, hyposegmentation (pseudo–Pelger-Huët appearance), hypogranularity **(see Color Figure 171)**, low myeloperoxidase and alkaline phosphatase activity, and circulating blasts or other immature forms. Thrombocytopenia is common and platelet morphology may be abnormal, with giant forms present.

The marrow is usually hypercellular despite the associated cytopenia(s) in the peripheral blood. Defects in the red cell precursors include megaloblastic erythropoiesis, ringed sideroblasts, multinuclearity, nuclear fragments, and abnormal cytoplasmic features. The promyelocytes and myelocytes may have abnormal staining of primary granules and secondary granules may be absent or reduced. Abnormalities of the megakaryocytic line include the presence in the marrow of micromega-

Table 19-11. TERMINOLOGY USED IN MYELODYSPLASTIC (PRELEUKEMIC) SYNDROMES

| FAB: Myelodysplastic Syndromes | Other: Preleukemic Syndromes |
|---|---|
| 1. Refractory anemia (RA) | Chronic erythemic myelosis |
| | Refractory megaloblastic anemia |
| 2. RA with ring sideroblasts | Acquired idiopathic sideroblastic anemia |
| 3. RA with excess blasts (RAEB) | Smoldering leukemia |
| | Subacute leukemia |
| | Oligoblastic leukemia |
| 4. RAEB in transformation | Acute myeloproliferative syndrome |
| | Primary acquired panmyelopathy with myeloblastosis (PAMP) |
| 5. Chronic myelomonocytic leukemia | Subacute myelomonocytic leukemia |

Table 19-12. MYELODYSPLASTIC SYNDROMES: COMMON HEMATOLOGIC FINDINGS

| Peripheral Blood | Bone Marrow |
|---|---|
| Dyserythropoiesis | |
| Anemia | Megaloblastic erythropoiesis |
| Macro-ovalocytosis | Ringed sideroblasts |
| Decreased retic count | Binucleated RBCs |
| Nucleated RBCs | |
| Dysmyelopoiesis | |
| Neutropenia | Myeloid hyperplasia |
| Monocytosis | Partial maturation arrest at myelocyte stage |
| Pseudo–Pelger-Huët | Reduced or large granules |
| Hypogranular PMNs | Increase in blasts |
| Circulating metamyelocytes | |
| Decreased myeloperoxidase, and alkaline phosphatase activity | |
| Dysmegakaryopoiesis | |
| Thrombocytopenia | Increased number of bizarre megakaryocytes |
| Large, atypical platelets | Micromegakaryocytes |
| | Abnormal granulation |

karyocytes, large mononuclear megakaryocytes, multiple separate small nuclei, and giant or abnormal granules.

Patients with MDS have a relatively indolent clinical course. However, eventually 20 to 50 percent of patients progress to an acute blastic phase.[71] Standard chemotherapy has been considered by some to be contraindicated in patients with MDS.

## CASE HISTORIES
### Case 1

This 12-year-old boy was originally diagnosed when he was 4 years old. At that time he presented with a three-week history of fatigue, weakness, and a persistent sore throat. His mother noticed also that he was bruising easily. On physical examination he had a palpable spleen but no evidence of lymphadenopathy. A CBC, platelet count, and differential were done, with the following results:

**CBC:**

| | | | |
|---|---|---|---|
| WBC | $2.40 \times 10^9/l$ | MCV | 87.0 fl |
| RBC | $2.41 \times 10^{12}/l$ | MCH | 29.0 pg |
| HCT | 21.0 ml/dl | MCHC | 33.3 g/dl |
| Hb | 7.0 g/dl | Platelets | $6.7 \times 10^9/l$ |

**Differential:**
3% PMN
97% Lymphoid cells

A bone marrow examination was performed that revealed sheets of small blasts having scant cytoplasm and indistinct nucleoli **(see Color Figure 172)**. Cell marker studies revealed:

**T Cells**

| | |
|---|---|
| E rosettes | 3% |
| Human T-cell antigen (HTA) | Negative (pan T cell) |

**B Cells**

| | |
|---|---|
| Surface immunoglobulin (SIg-Total) | Negative |
| Cytoplasmic immunoglobulins (CIgM) | Negative |

**Others**

| | |
|---|---|
| cALLA | 100%, 4+ |

**Cytochemistry**

| | |
|---|---|
| TdT | 95%, 4+ |
| Peroxidase | Negative in blasts |
| NSE | Negative in blasts |

**Diagnosis:** Acute lymphoblastic leukemia, common ALL type, L1.

**Follow-up.** This patient was placed on a protocol for ALL to which he responded very well. His physical examination two months after induction chemotherapy was unremarkable except for some hair loss. His CBC was entirely normal, although his white blood cell count was low-normal. A bone marrow examination at this time was also normal. He was continued on therapy, including one reintensification phase followed by maintenance therapy. Eight years later he is free of any signs of leukemia and is living a normal life.

### Case 2

This 26-year-old woman presented with a two-month history of fatigue and weakness and a two-week history of a sore throat associated with a 15-pound weight loss. No response to antibiotics was obtained and she subsequently developed a peritonsillar abscess. On admission to the hospital she was found to have an elevated white blood cell count with a large number of blasts.

On physical examination the patient was an anxious young female whose vital signs were normal, aside from a slightly elevated temperature of 37.6°C. Her right tonsil was enlarged and erythematous. She had no adenopathy and her liver and spleen were not palpable.

Her hematocrit was 19.5 percent, platelet count $64 \times 10^9/l$, and white blood cell count $79.2 \times 10^9/l$. Examination of the blood showed 80 percent of the white blood cells to be blasts. A bone marrow aspirate was done, which showed virtually total replacement of normal elements with blasts **(see Color Figure 173)**. Approximately 30 percent of the blasts were positive with myeloperoxidase stain, and less than 20 percent were positive with NSE stain. The diagnosis of acute myeloid leukemia, FAB type M1 was made.

HLA matching was performed on the patient's siblings, but unfortunately, no sibling had an identical tissue type. The possibility of a bone marrow transplantation was ruled out. The patient was placed on a therapy protocol for acute myeloid leukemia. During her induction chemotherapy she developed typical problems of anemia, thrombocytopenia, and leukopenia. She required platelets and packed red blood cell transfusions. She also required broad-spectrum antibiotics for fever due to neutropenia, although no specific pathogen could be identified. Three weeks after her induction chemotherapy, a repeat bone marrow showed no residual leukemia. She remained in complete remission for 16 months before relapsing. Attempts to induce a second remission were unsuccessful. She developed progressive hepatomegaly, jaundice, and persistent neutropenia. She also developed multiple infections and was unable to recover.

This case illustrates a typical course of acute myeloid leukemia (AML, M1). Although a cure was not achieved, this patient did survive longer than she would have without treatment.

## References

1. Bennett, JH: Two cases of disease and enlargement of the spleen in which death took place from the presence of purulent matter in the blood. Edinburgh Med Surg J 64:413, 1845.
2. Virchow, R: Weisses Blut. Froriep's Notizen 36:151, 1845.
3. Gunz, FW: The dread leukemias and the lymphomas: Their nature and their prospects. In Wintrobe, MM (ed): Blood, Pure and Eloquent: A Story of Discovery, of People, and of Ideas. McGraw-Hill, New York, 1980, p 511.
4. Virchow, R: Die farblosen Blutkorperchen. In Gesammelte Abhandlungen sur Wissen schaftlichen Medizin. Meidinger, Frankfurt, 1856.
5. Friedreich N: Ein neuer fall von leukamie. Arch Pathol Anat 12:37, 1857.
6. Ebstein, W: Ueber die acute Leukamie und Pseudoleukamie. Deutsches Arch Klin Med 44:343, 1889.
7. Forkner, CE: Leukemia and Allied Disorders. MacMillan, New York, 1938, p 5.
8. Smithson, WA, Gilchrist, GS, and Burgert, EO: Childhood acute lymphocytic leukemia. CA-A Cancer J Clin 30:158, 1980.
9. Gunz, FW, Gunz, JP, Veale, AMO, et al: Familial leukaemia: A study of 909 families. Scand J Haematol 15:117, 1975.
10. Evans, DIK and Stewart, JK: Down's syndrome and leukemia. Lancet 2:1322, 1972.
11. Bizzozzero, OJ, Johnson, KG, and Cicco, A: Radiation-related leukemia in Hiroshima and Nagasaki, 1946–64. I. Distribution, incidence and appearance in time. N Engl J Med 274:1095, 1966.
12. Forni, A and Vigliani, EC: Chemical leukemogenesis in man. Ser Haematol 7:211, 1974.
13. Rapaport, SI: Introduction to Hematology. Harper & Row, New York, 1971, p 162.
14. Gunz, FW and Henderson, ES: Leukemia, ed 4. Grune & Stratton, New York, 1983, pp 197, 247.
15. Kjeldsberg, CK: Acute leukemia. In Maslow, WC, Beutler, E, Bell, CA, et al: Practical Diagnosis: Hematologic Disease. Houghton Mifflin, Boston, 1981, p 311.
16. Geary, CG: Clinical annotation: The diagnosis of preleukaemia. Br J Haematol 55:1, 1983.
17. Wintrobe, MM (ed): Clinical Hematology, ed 8. Lea & Febiger, Philadelphia, 1981, p 1493.
18. Bennett, JM, Catovsky, D, Daniel, MT, et al: Proposals for the classification of myelodysplatic syndromes. Br J Haematol 51:189, 1982.
19. Bennett, JM, Catovasky, D, Daniel, MT, et al: Proposals for the classification of the acute leukaemias. Br J Haematol 33:451, 1976.
20. Shafer, JA: Blood and marrow morphology in acute leukemia patients receiving chemotherapy: A photo-essay. Am J Med Technol 49:77, 1983.
21. Shafer, JA: Artifactual alterations in phagocytes in the blood smear. Am J Med Technol 48:507, 1982.
22. Seigneurin, D and Audhuy, B: Auer rods in refractory anemia with excess blasts: Presence and significance. Am J Clin Pathol 80:359, 1983.
23. Stass, SA, Pui, SM, Rovigatti, U, et al: Sudan black B positive acute lymphoblastic leukemia. Br J Haematol 57:413, 1984.
24. Bearman, RM, Winberg, CD, Maslow, WC, et al: Terminal deoxynucleotidyl transferase activity in neoplastic and non-neoplastic hematopoietic cells. Am J Clin Pathol 75:794-802, 1981.
25. Hoffbrand, AV, Geneshagura, K, Janossy, G, et al: Terminal deoxynucleotidyl transferase levels and membrane phenotypes in the diagnosis of acute leukemia. Lancet 2:520, 1977.
26. Casoli, C, Bonati, A, and Starcich, B: Ph¹-positive acute myelocytic leukemia with high TdT levels. Cancer 52:1210, 1983.
27. Kung, PC, Long, JC, McCaffrey, RP, et al: TdT in the diagnosis of leukemia and malignant lymphoma. Am J Med 64:788, 1978.
28. Marks, SM, Baltimore, D, and McCaffrey, R: Terminal transferase as a predictor of initial responsiveness to vincristine and prednisone in blastic chronic myelogenous leukemia. A cooperative study. N Engl J Med 298:812, 1978.
29. Hayhoe, FGJ and Quaglino, D: Haematological Cytochemistry. Churchill Livingstone, Edinburgh, 1980, pp 130, 243, 265.
30. First International Workshop on Chromosomes in Leukemia: Chromosomes in acute non-lymphocytic leukemia. Br J Haematol 39:311, 1978.
31. Cork, A: Chromosomal abnormalities in leukemia. Am J Med Tech 49:703, 1983.
32. Third International Workshop on Chromosomes in Leukemia: Cancer Genet Cytogenet 4:95, 1981.
33. Rowley, JD, Golomb, HM, and Dougherty, C: 15/17 translocation. A consistent chromosomal change in acute promyelocytic leukaemia. Lancet 1:549, 1977.
34. Bennett, JM, Catovsky, D, Daniel, MT: The morphological classification of ALL: Concordance among observers and clinical correlation. Br J Haematol 47:553, 1981.
35. Abramson, C, Kersey, J, and LeBien, T: A monoclonal antibody BA-1 reactive with cells of human B lymphocyte lineage. J Immunol 126:83, 1981.
36. Nadler, LM, Stashenko, P, Ritz, J, et al: A unique surface antigen identifying lymphoid malignancies of B cell origin. J Clin Invest 67:134, 1981.
37. Thiel, E, Rodt, H, Huhn, D, et al: Multimarker classification of acute lymphoblastic leukemia: Evidence for further T subgroups and evaluation of their clinical significance. Blood 56:759, 1980.
38. Catovasky, D, Greaves, MF, Pain, C, et al: Acid-phosphatase reaction in acute lymphoblastic leukemia. Lancet 1:749, 1978.
39. Peiper, S and Stass, SA: Markers of cellular differentiation in acute lymphoblastic leukemia. Arch Pathol Lab Med 106:3, 1982.
40. Roath, S: Acute lymphoblastic leukemia of B cell origin. Clin Lab Haematol 1:87, 1979.
41. Preud'homme, JL, Brouet, JC, Danon, F, et al: Acute lymphoblastic leukemia with Burkitt's lymphoma cells: Membrane markers and serum immunoglobulin. J Natl Cancer Inst 66:261, 1981.
42. Brouet, JC and Seligmann, M: The immunologic classification of acute lymphoblastic leukemias. Cancer 42:817, 1978.
43. Flandrin, G, Brouet, JC, Daniel MT, et al: Acute leukemia with Burkitt's tumor cells: A study of six cases with special reference to lymphocyte surface markers. Blood 45:183, 1975.
44. Greaves, MF, Janossy, G, Peto, J, et al: Immunologically defined subclasses of acute lymphoblastic leukaemia in children: Their relationship to presentation features and prognosis. Br J Haematol 48:179, 1981.
45. Liso, V, Troccoli, G, and Grande, M: Cytochemical study of acute promyelocytic leukemia: Blut 30:261, 1975.
46. Sultan, C, Deregnaucourt, J, Ko, YW, et al: Distribution of 250 cases of acute myeloid leukemia according to the FAB classification and response to therapy. Br J Haematol 47:545, 1981.
47. Granlick, HR and Sultan, C: Acute promyelocytic leukemia: Hemorrhagic manifestations and morphologic criteria. Br J Haematol 29:373, 1975.
48. Sultan, C, Surender, KJ, and Imbert, M: Variant form of hypergranular promyelocytic leukemia. ASCP Check Sample 25:4, 1983.
49. Jones, ME and Saleem, A: Acute promyelocytic leukemia. A review of the literature. Am J Med 65:673, 1978.
50. Goulomb, HM, Rowley, JD, Vardiman, JW, et al: "Microgran-

ular" acute promyelocytic leukemia: A distinct clinical, ultrastructural, and cytogenetic entity. Blood 55:253, 1980.

51. Bennett, JM, Catovsky, D, Daniel, MT, et al: Correspondence: A variant form of hypergranular promyelocytic leukemia (M3). Br J Hematol 44:169, 1980.

52. Saarni, MI and Linman, JW: Myelomonocytic leukemia: Disorderly proliferation of all marrow lines. Cancer 27:1221, 1971.

53. Shaw, MT: The distinctive features of acute monocytic leukemia. Am J Hematol 4:97, 1978.

54. Rundles, RW: Monocytic leukemia. In Williams, WE, Beutler, E, Erslev, AJ, et al (eds): Hematology. McGraw-Hill, New York, 1972, p 896.

55. Tobelem, G, Jacquillat, C, Chastang, C, et al: Acute monoblastic leukemia: A clinical and biologic study of 74 cases. Blood 55:71, 1980.

56. Meyer, RJ, Ferreira, PPC, Cuttner, J, et al: Central nervous system involvement at presentation in acute granulocytic leukemia: A prospective cytocentrifuge study. Am J Med 68:691, 1980.

57. Petersen, BA and Bloomfield, CD: Asymptomatic central nervous system leukemia in adults with ANLL in extended remission. Proc Am Soc Clin Oncol 18:341, 1977.

58. Cuttner, J, Conjalka, MS, Reilly, M, et al: Association of monocytic leukemia in patients with extreme leukocytosis. Am J Med 60:555, 1980.

59. Catovsky, D, Hoffbrand, AV, Ikoku, NB, et al: Significance of cell differentiation in acute myeloid leukaemia. Blood Cells 1:201, 1975.

60. Pribilla, W: Erythramie und erythroleukamie. In Gross, R and Van de Loo, J (eds): Leukamie. Springer-Verlag, Berlin, 1972.

61. Sondergaard-Petersen, H: Erythrophagocytosis by pathological erythroblasts in the Di Guglielmo syndrome: A study of 18 cases. Scand J Haematol 13:260, 1974.

62. Breton-Gorius, J, Reyes, F, Duhamel, G, et al: Megakaryoblastic acute leukemia: Identification by the ultrastructural demonstration of platelet peroxidase. Blood 51:45, 1978.

63. Breton-Gorius, J and Reyes, F: Ultrastructure of human bone marrow cell maturation. Int Rev Cytol 46:251, 1976.

64. Mirchandani, I and Palutke, M: Acute megakaryoblastic leukemia. Cancer 50:2866, 1983.

65. Koike, T: Megakaryoblastic leukemia: the characterization and identification of megakaryoblasts. Blood 64:683, 1984.

66. Catovsky, D: Educational lecture methods for the study of leukaemic cells. 20th Congress of the International Society of Hematology, 1984, p 59.

67. Bain, BJ, Catovsky, D, O'Brien, M, et al: Megakaryoblastic leukemia presenting as acute myelofibrosis: a study of four cases with the platelet-peroxidase reaction. Blood 58:206, 1981.

68. Navari, RM, Buckner, CD, Clift, RC, et al: Bone marrow transplantation. Lab Med 15:245, 1984.

69. Neiman, PE, Meyers, JD, Medeiros, E, et al: Interstitial pneumonia following marrow transplantation for leukemia and aplastic anemia. In Gale, RP and Fox, CF (eds): Biology of Bone Marrow Transplantation. Academic Press, New York, 1980, p 75.

70. Hanson, GR: Macrocytosis and macrocytic anemia. ASCP Check Sample 26:4, 1984.

71. Greenberg, PL: The smoldering myeloid leukemic states: Clinical and biologic features. Blood 61:1035, 1983.

## Bibliography

Bennett, JM, Catovsky, D, Daniel, MT, et al: Proposals for the classification of acute leukaemias. Br J Haematol 33:451, 1976.

Bennett, JM, Catovsky, D, Daniel, MT, et al: Correspondence: A variant form of hypergranular promyelocytic leukemia (M3). Br J Haematol 44:169, 1980.

Bennett, JM, Catovsky, D, Daniel, MT, et al: Proposals for the classification of the myelodysplastic syndromes. Br J Haematol 51:189, 1982.

Catovsky, D: Acute leukaemia. In Hoffbrand, AV and Lewis, SM: Postgraduate Haematology. Appleton-Century-Crofts, New York, 1981, p 431.

Granlick, HR, Galton, DAG, Catovsky, D, et al: Classification of acute leukemia. Ann Intern Med 87:740, 1977.

Gunz, FW: The dread leukemias and the lymphomas: Their nature and their prospects. In Wintrobe, MM (ed): Blood, Pure and Eloquent: A Story of Discovery, of People, and of Ideas. McGraw-Hill, New York, 1980, p 511.

Hayhoe, FGJ and Quaglino, D: Haematological Cytochemistry. Churchill Livingstone, Edinburgh, 1980.

Jones, ME and Saleem, A: Acute promyelocytic leukemia: a review of the literature. Am J Med 65:673, 1978.

Peiper, S and Stass, SA: Markers of cellular differentiation in acute lymphoblastic leukmeia. Arch Pathol Lab Med 106:3, 1982.

Roggli, VL and Saleem, A: Erythroleukemia: A study of 15 cases and literature review. Cancer 49:101, 1982.

Shaw, MT: The distinctive features of acute monocytic leukemia. Am J Hematol 4:97, 1978.

Smithson, WA, Gilchrist, GS, and Burgert, EO: Childhood acute lymphocytic leukemia. CA-A Cancer J Clin 3:158, 1980.

CHAPTER **20**

ARTHUR J. SILVERGLEID, M.D.

# Chronic Leukemias

## CHRONIC MYELOGENOUS LEUKEMIA

Chronic myelogenous leukemia (CML), also called chronic granulocytic leukemia (CGL), is one of the more distinctive clonal neoplastic syndromes of myeloproliferation. Almost invariably associated with a unique chromosomal abnormality, the Philadelphia (Ph[1]) chromosome, the disease is characterized by unrestrained proliferation of myeloid elements in the bone marrow, spleen, and liver, leading to marked leukocytosis and organomegaly. CML was the first type of leukemia to be described, in 1845,[1] and because of prominent splenomegaly, it was for many years referred to as "splenic leukemia." The Philadelphia chromosome, which characteristically identifies the neoplastic clone in 85 to 90 percent of cases of "typical" CML, was described in 1960.[2]

The clinical course for the patient with CML is well defined and somewhat uniform. At presentation, and for one to four years thereafter, it is generally easy to control the myeloid hyperproliferation and organomegaly with a variety of chemotherapeutic agents. However, sometime during the third or fourth year after presentation, patients almost invariably enter an accelerated, chemotherapy-resistant phase that often terminates in an acute blastic transformation. During this accelerated phase, or "blast crisis," patients are generally unresponsive to all therapeutic agents, including those used to treat acute leukemia. Such patients ultimately die from fever, infection, hemorrhage, or organ infiltration with leukemic cells, or any combination of these.

### Incidence

Chronic myelogenous leukemia accounts for approximately 20 percent of all cases of leukemia in Western countries, with a death rate of roughly one per 100,000 population per year. The disease primarily affects adults between 25 and 60 years old, with a peak incidence among 35- to 45-year-olds. This age of peak incidence, which in recent years has been edging upward, is still approximately 10 years younger than that of chronic lymphocytic leukemia (CLL). CML is seen in its typical form only occasionally among adolescents. On the rare occasion in which it presents in infancy, it tends to display a much more aggressive and acute course.

As with all other types of leukemia, men tend to be affected somewhat more often than women (approximately 57 percent and 43 percent, respectively), but the appearance and course of the disease are identical for both genders.

## Etiology, Pathogenesis, and Pathophysiology

CML, like other human leukemias, is thought to be a neoplastic disease. There is reasonably good evidence to suggest that the primary event is malignant transformation of a pluripotent hematopoietic stem cell, the progeny of which appears to have a growth advantage over normal cell lines. Whereas chromosomal abnormalities are commonly found in all the leukemias, it is only in CML that a consistent abnormality—the Philadelphia chromosome—is found, strongly suggesting that it is directly or indirectly involved in the pathogenesis of the disease.

Etiologic factors that lead to the development of CML are not known with certainty, but most speculation includes ionizing radiation, alkylating agents, and other biologically active chemicals, all of which are capable of inducing chromosomal aberrations in addition to other direct toxic effects. In this respect, the most convincing argument can be made for the role of ionizing radiation. A striking increase in the incidence of leukemia has been documented in several disparate groups of individuals exposed to high doses of radiation. These include radiologists, prior to the advent of careful shielding techniques;[3] patients with ankylosing spondylitis treated with spinal cord irradiation;[4] and survivors of the atomic blasts in Hiroshima and Nagasaki.[5,6] In all of these groups, the incidence of leukemia, which peaked approximately six years after the exposure, was at least 10-fold that of comparable, but unexposed, populations.

The contribution of chemical leukemogens, or toxins, is less readily defined. Although theoretically any chemical capable of producing myelotoxicity is potentially leukemogenic—and that would include most chemotherapeutic agents—the only chemicals that have been clearly identified as having a pathogenic role in myeloid leukemias are benzene and benzol derivatives. This association has generally been described in patients with a history of chronic, occupational exposure, as in the shoe tanners of Iran.[7] Other cytotoxic agents, particu-

larly those associated with neutropenia, may well be implicated, although definitive evidence is unavailable.

Given the association with excessive exposure to irradiation, toxins, or chemotherapeutic agents, it is nonetheless true that the vast majority of patients who develop CML have no known unusual exposure to any of the aforementioned; obviously, other factors are operating that remain to be identified. CML does appear to be an acquired disease, and the regular failure to affect the second member of pairs of identical twins would tend to substantiate this.[8]

### Philadelphia Chromosome

The evidence that CML is a clonal hematopoietic stem cell disorder (that is, that it arises from neoplastic transformation of a single hematopoietic stem cell, the progeny of which have a proliferative advantage over normal stem cells) is based largely on cytogenetic and isoenzyme studies. The Philadelphia (Ph[1]) chromosome arises from the translocation (t) of genetic material from the long arm of chromosome 22 to another chromosome, most often (90 percent) chromosome 9, although occasionally to others, including chromosomes 2, 6, 17, 19, and 22. Since the short arm of a chromosome is designated "p" and the long arm "q," the abbreviation for the most usual Ph[1] chromosome is t (9q+; 22q−) (Fig. 20-1). When the Ph[1] chromosome is present, as it is in 90 percent of cases of CML, it is found in all neutrophil, moncyte, erythrocyte, platelet, and possibly basophil precursors, whereas it is invariably absent from fibroblasts and lymphocytes.[9] Its presence in dividing marrow cells and absence from somatic cells supports the hypothesis that the disease evolves from transformation of a single hematopoietic stem cell, although simultaneous transformation of a number of hematopoietic stem cells is also a somewhat remote possibility.

Additional evidence for the clonal nature of CML is derived from isoenzyme studies of the X-linked glucose-6-phosphate dehydrogenase (G-6-PD) enzyme. Women with CML who are heterozygous for this enzyme and who therefore express both A- and B-type enzymes in all of their somatic cells have

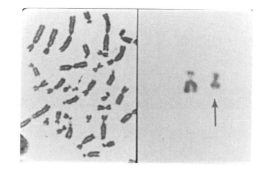

**Figure 20–1.** Philadelphia chromosome A (left), B (right).

been shown to express only one enzyme type (A) on their hematopoietic cells — a pattern that is consistent with the hypothesis that these cells are clonally derived from a common hematopoietic stem cell.[10]

The Ph[1] chromosome is found so exclusively in CML that its presence virtually excludes any other diagnosis, especially those myeloproliferative disorders (polycythemia vera, agnogenic myeloid metaplasia) most likely to appear in the differential diagnosis. It is this extraordinary specificity that makes it reasonable to hypothesize that the Ph[1] chromosome is somehow closely involved in the pathogenesis of the disease. What is unclear, however, is how a simple translocation of genetic material could be oncogenic. Recently, it has been shown that two human homologues of retroviral transforming genes, oncogenes designated c-abl and c-sis, can be mapped to chromosomes 9 and 22, respectively.[11] The viral homologue of c-abl is the transforming gene of a murine leukemia virus that causes B-lymphoid leukemias in mice. The fact that a similar gene is intimately associated with leukemias in both mice and humans may be an early insight into the pathogenesis of CML.

Exactly what induces the leukemic change in a pluripotent hematopoietic stem cell is as yet unknown. It is postulated that the marrow stem cells are subjected to some form of injury (e.g., radiation, chemical, toxic) that leads to chromosomal damage and mitotic abnormalities. Whereas in normal circumstances such mitotic abnormalities would lead to cell death, in certain situations a "defective" (or chromosomally altered) marrow stem cell will be able to survive better, proliferate excessively, or grow independently of normal regulatory forces. Such a cell could transmit enhanced survival and increased growth potential to its progeny, which would continue to proliferate in the marrow until such time (perhaps two to six years) as they replace the normal hematopoietic elements and became predominant. By the time CML is clinically or hematologically detectable, all the myeloid cells in the marrow are Ph[1] positive.

The mechanism by which CML cells gain a proliferative advantage over normal cells is unknown. Suppression of normal hematopoiesis via humoral factors (isoferritin, prostaglandin E) or direct cell contact may be important.[12,13] Studies of cell kinetics have shown that the measurable CML precursors do not divide more rapidly than normal cells. Rather, the defect in the chronic phase of the disease appears to be an expansion of the pools of committed stem cells.[14] As the disease progresses, the unstable Ph[1] chromosome-positive cells undergo additional chromosomal aberrations that lead ultimately to an impairment in precursor cell maturation and differentiation characteristic of acute leukemia. This terminal phase, called the accelerated phase or "blast crisis," usually results from the evolution of a genetically altered clone of neoplastic cells derived from the Ph[1]-positive cells. In fact, the development of additional karyotypic abnormalities (e.g., double Ph[1], trisomy-8, isochrome 17) usually precedes the appearance of any other sign of acute transition.[15,16] The blastic cell lines that evolve from the pre-existing Ph[1]-positive clone have a growth advantage over both normal cells and the chronic-phase Ph[1]-positive clones, a growth advantage that results from their failure to mature into functional end cells and to be removed from the proliferative pool. In addition, these cells are often even more resistant to chemotherapy than are blast cells in patients with acute leukemia.

One interesting feature of the blastic phase of CML is that different cell types may predominate in different patients, a reflection of the pluripotency of the Ph[1]-positive stem cell involved in the pathogenesis.[17] However, 50 to 60 percent of patients will typically have a myeloblastic termination. In 1974, Boggs drew attention to a fascinating observation, which is that the blasts of approximately 30 percent of patients with CML have lymphoblastic rather than myeloblastic morphology.[18] This observation has been substantiated many times and confirmed by additional studies of morphology, cell surface markers, and the presence of cytoplasmic immunoglobulin. The interpretation of these findings is that the Ph[1]-positive pluripotent stem cell involved in the pathogenesis of CML is sufficiently uncommitted or undifferentiated so that it could express either myeloid or lymphoid characteristics, depending on the pathway along which it differentiated.

## Clinical Course

The clinical course of CML can be divided into three fairly discrete stages: an asymptomatic proliferative stage; a symptomatic stage during which hyperproliferation is easily controlled; and an accelerated, or acute, stage in which the cellular proliferation is uncontrollable and the patient appears to have a variant of acute leukemia. Based on a study of atomic bomb survivors by Kamada and Uchino,[19] it is possible to postulate the probable chronologic sequence of events in the evolution of CML. The first event associated with the transition to a leukemic (or preleukemic) state is the appearance of Ph[1]-positive cells in the bone marrow. This occurs while the peripheral leukocyte count is normal. Although basophilia, thrombocytosis, and low leukocyte alkaline phosphatase activity may be found at this point, they are more likely to be present when the peripheral leukocyte count begins to rise, about 6.3 years after the Ph[1]-chromosome first appeared. At this time, immature granulocytes may be found in the peripheral blood for the first time. When the granulocyte count reaches 50,000/mm$^3$, splenomegaly is present and subjective symptoms develop. From the time of development of leukocytosis until the onset of clinical symptoms has been estimated at approximately 19 months. Once the diagnosis of CML has been made, the median survival is three to four years. As mentioned in the beginning of this chapter, patients in the chronic, symptomatic stage of the disease are responsive to a variety of alkylating agents and are often asymptomatic while receiving therapy. When the disease enters an accelerated phase, or becomes frankly blastic, there is a rapid and inexorable progression toward death that is virtually unresponsive to any therapeutic maneuver.

## Symptoms

The most common complaints of patients with symptomatic CML include malaise, fatigue, diminished exercise tolerance, fever, sweating, weight loss, aching in the bones, and fullness in the upper abdomen. The first group of symptoms are the result of anemia and an increase in the basal metabolic rate; the latter two result from marked expansion of the red marrow and hepatomegaly and splenomegaly. Bleeding, in the form of purpura, retinal hemorrhages, or hematuria, may occur in patients with excessive, insufficient, or abnormally functioning platelets. Less common symptoms include chronic and recurring headaches, prolonged or unusual infections, ankle edema, acute "gouty" arthritis, peripheral vascular insufficiency, and priapism.

## Signs

On physical examination, patients with CML manifest warm moist skin, low-grade fever, tenderness to pressure over the sternum, and hepatomegaly and splenomegaly. Pallor or tachycardia or both may be present if anemia is significant. Sternal tenderness is an especially characteristic sign that may be demonstrated in over two thirds of patients with untreated or relapsed CML. Splenomegaly, which may be found in over 90 percent of patients, progresses rapidly in untreated or relapsing patients and often contributes to a reduced food capacity and rapid weight loss. Other physical signs frequently found in patients with CML include punctate retinal hemorrhages and exudates, and bruises or ecchymoses over the extremities. An occasional patient will present with an infiltrating skin tumor, or "chloroma," usually indicative of more advanced disease (e.g., a larger tumor burden) (Table 20–1).

## Laboratory Features

Leukocytosis and anemia are the most common hematologic findings, with three fourths of patients having white blood cell counts in excess of $100,000/mm^3$ and one half of the 80 percent of patients with anemia having hemoglobin levels below

**Table 20–1. CLINICAL SIGNS AND SYMPTOMS OF CHRONIC MYELOCYTIC LEUKEMIA (CML)/CHRONIC GRANULOCYTIC LEUKEMIA (CGL)**

1. **Symptoms Related to Hypermetabolism**
   Weight loss, anorexia, low-grade fever, warm moist skin, night sweats, sternal tenderness (characteristic sign present in ⅔ of patients)
2. **Splenomegaly** (present in >90% of patients and frequently massive)
   Associated discomfort, pain, and indigestion
3. **Symptoms Related to Anemia**
   Pallor, dyspnea, tachycardia
4. **Other Physical Signs or Symptoms**
   Bruising or ecchymoses over the extremities, epistaxis, retinal hemorrhages, menorrhagia in females or hemorrhage from other sites

10 g/dl. The striking feature of the peripheral blood film of the patient with CML is the profusion of relatively normal appearing granulocytes at all stages of development **(see Color Figure 175)**. Although myeloblasts and promyelocytes are present, they usually do not comprise more than 10 percent of the largely mature granulocyte pool. Basophilia and eosinophilia may be present, as may thrombocytosis. However, even in patients with normal platelet counts it is common in CML, as in other disorders of myeloproliferation, to find giant platelets or, more accurately, fragments of megakaryocytes in the circulating blood. Examination of the bone marrow confirms the findings from the peripheral smear **(see Color Figure 176)**, revealing intense cellularity with a marked increase in the myeloid:erythroid ratio to 10 to 50:1 instead of the normal 2 to 5:1.

Cytogenetic studies on peripheral blood and bone marrow will reveal the Philadelphia chromosome (Ph¹, t [22q−; 9q+]) in most metaphases in 85 to 90 percent of patients with CML. Occasionally, other translocations or additional abnormalities (see earlier) may be observed. Rarely, a patient will have normal metaphases.

A characteristic finding in CML is low to absent leukocyte alkaline phosphatase (LAP) activity as demonstrated by both histochemical and biochemical techniques (contrast **Color Figure 177** against **Color Figure 182**, demonstrating increased LAP activity in leukemoid reactions). Enzyme levels may normalize during remissions, and their subsequent reversion to low to absent levels may presage relapse or acceleration of the disease prior to this being reflected in a rising white blood cell count. Interestingly, neutrophils from a patient with CML when harvested by apheresis and transfused into an infected, neutropenic recipient increased their content of LAP to normal, indicating that LAP is to some extent an inducible enzyme, even in a CML neutrophil.[20]

Additional laboratory findings regularly seen in patients with CML include elevated uric acid, LDH, and vitamin $B_{12}$ levels — findings that are related to the hyperproliferation and turnover of granulocytes and that are common to most of the disorders of myeloproliferation.

## Differential Diagnosis

The characteristic clinical picture and peripheral blood smear often leave little question as to the correct diagnosis in the patient with CML. Nevertheless, because marrow fibrosis similar to that found in agnogenic myeloid metaplasia has occasionally been described in patients with CML, or because leukocytosis very often is found in polycythemia vera and essential thrombocythemia, there may be some initial concern about assigning a patient to the appropriate category within the family of disorders of myeloproliferation. However, the Ph[1] chromosome and the low to absent leukocyte alkaline phosphatase levels are virtually unique to CML and clearly distinguish it from any of the aforementioned myeloproliferative disorders. Similarly, leukemoid, or leukoerythroblastic, reactions may be differentiated by their normal to high LAP levels and lack of Ph[1] chromosome. Table 20–2 presents the differential laboratory diagnosis between leukemoid reaction and CML.

## Treatment

### Prognostic Factors

As previously noted, the median survival for patients with CML is roughly three years from the time of diagnosis. The range, however, is quite broad, with a variation of from less than one year to more than 10 years.[21] Although numerous attempts have been made to evaluate various factors for their prognostic importance, it is fair to say that there is as yet no universally accepted formula for quantitat-

ing risk, potential lifespan, or anticipated response to therapy for the individual patient. Nevertheless, there are certain statements that can be made regarding the prognosis of CML patients who present with a particular clinical or laboratory finding.

One of the more important discriminants between "good-risk" and "poor-risk" patients is the presence or absence of the Ph[1] chromosome. Roughly 85 to 90 percent of patients with typical CML are Ph[1]-positive. Analysis of a group of Ph[1]-negative patients indicated that they were older (median age 66 years compared with age 48 years for Ph[1]-positive patients), were male in most cases, had lower initial white blood cell and platelet counts, and responded poorly to antileukemic therapy.[22] The median survival of Ph[1]-negative patients was 8 months, compared with 40 months for Ph[1]-positive patients. Similarly, the time to onset of blast crisis was 6 months for Ph[1]-negative patients, compared with 22 months for Ph[1]-positive patients.

Among the Ph[1]-positive patients, a number of studies have emphasized the role of different prognostic variables.[23-25] Although there is disagreement over some of the findings, there is general agreement that splenomegaly, extreme leukocytosis ($>100,000/mm^3$), a high percentage of blasts ($>1$ percent in peripheral smear; $>5$ percent in marrow), extreme basophilia ($>15$ to 20 percent), thrombocytosis ($>700,000/mm^3$), thrombocytopenia ($<150,000/mm^3$), or the presence of other karyotypic abnormalities in addition to the Ph[1]-chromosome all represent adverse prognostic indicators. Conversely, the absence of any or all of these findings is considered to reflect a greater likelihood of a response to therapy and a more benign clinical course.

Attempts to categorize, or stage, patients according to some of these prognostic criteria have thus far been unrewarding; future efforts will be significant only if it can be demonstrated that such staging accurately and reliably predicts the pace and responsiveness of disease in the individual patient. If that turns out to be the case, we will then be in a much better position to assess the differential results of alternative therapeutic approaches.

### Conventional Therapy

During the chronic phase of "good-risk" patients with CML, it is relatively easy to induce a clinical and peripheral blood remission, using one of several chemotherapeutic agents alone, in at least 75 percent of patients.[26] Remission for these patients involves a decrease in the white blood cell count toward normal, a regression in organomegaly, a normalization of red cell and platelet counts, and the disappearance of clinical symptoms. In some cases, even the LAP levels will normalize as the granulocyte count drops. Although an apparently complete remission is obtained (with normalization of pe-

**Table 20–2. DIFFERENTIAL DIAGNOSIS BETWEEN LEUKEMOID REACTION AND CML**

|  | Leukemoid Reaction | CML |
|---|---|---|
| Toxic vacuoles | 2–4+ | 0–1+ |
| Toxic granules | 2–4+ | 0–1+ |
| Döhle bodies | Frequent | Rare |
| Eosinophilia | 0 | 1–3+ |
| Basophilia | 0 | 1–3+ |
| Pseudo-Pelger-Huët | 0–1+ | Occasional |
| Karyorrhexis | 0–1+ | 1–2+ |
| Giant bizarre nuclei | 1–1+ | 1–3+ |
| Leukemic hiatus | 0 | Occasional |
| LAP score | High | Low (most cases) Normal or high (rare) |
| Ph[1] chromosome | — | + (85% of cases) |

ripheral blood counts and disappearance of clinical symptoms) examination of the bone marrow will continue to reveal granulocytic hyperplasia, and more importantly, the Ph[1]-chromosome is still present in dividing marrow cells. Thus, a true hematologic remission, with disappearance of all traces of the malignant clone, is not obtained with single-agent chemotherapy. Nevertheless, such chemotherapy is easy to administer, is well tolerated by the patient, and can contribute to prolonging survival in addition to improving substantially the patient's quality of life.[27]

The single agents most commonly employed to treat patients with CML, ranked according to popularity and use, are busulfan (Myleran), melphalan (Alkeran), hydroxyurea, and dibromomannitol. Generally, either busulfan or melphalan are used initially at a dosage of 4 to 8 mg orally per day. This regimen is continued until the white blood cell count begins to drop, usually in two to three weeks, at which point the dose is lowered accordingly. Because busulfan can cause prolonged thrombocytopenia, the level and duration of response seemingly out of proportion to the dose, it is therefore very important to monitor blood counts regularly while the drug is being used.[28] Melphalan can also cause cytopenias, but the effect is not nearly as prolonged as that caused by busulfan, which has made it the preferred drug in some institutions.[29] Unlike busulfan and melphalan which are alkylating agents, hydroxyurea is an antimetabolite which acts by inhibiting DNA synthesis. It has an advantage over the other drugs in the rapidity of its action. However, continued daily maintenance therapy is necessary with hydroxyurea, because leukocyte counts will begin to rise almost as soon as the drug is discontinued.[30]

When a clinical and peripheral blood count remission is obtained with busulfan or melphalan, the chemotherapy can be discontinued. A good, stable remission can last from 6 to 18 months, during which no therapy need be given. If necessary, repeated courses of such chemotherapy can be employed, initiating the agent when the white blood cell count rises above 50,000/mm³ and discontinuing it when the count normalizes (or drops below 20,000/mm³ when using busulfan). This approach, employing interrupted courses of chemotherapy, appears to be just as effective as the use of continuous chemotherapy and may be associated with fewer side effects and less toxicity. Neither approach has been found to offer a substantial advantage over the other, in terms of survival or in delaying the inevitable onset of blast crisis.

## Aggressive Chemotherapy

It is primarily because conventional, single-agent chemotherapy cannot prevent the onset of blast crisis, in addition to its inability to eliminate the neoplastic clone, that alternative, marrow-ablative chemotherapy regimens have been evaluated.[31-34] The goal of these studies was to determine whether aggressive chemotherapy of chronic phase CML could result in elimination of the Ph[1]-positive clone, and what impact, if any, that would have on survival. Most of the regimens included cytosine arabinoside and thioguanine (standard agents in the treatment of acute myelogenous leukemia), along with either L-asparaginase, splenic irradiation, or splenectomy. In the four studies mentioned here, a significant reduction in Ph[1]-positive cells was seen in 20 to 50 percent of patients. Unfortunately, the reduction was transient in all patients studied; the Ph[1]-positive clone could be suppressed but not permanently eliminated. These studies also demonstrated that the normal hematopoietic clone is not destroyed by the CML; it can repopulate the marrow, resulting in a partial or complete remission. In fact, studies suggest that survival may be longer in patients who have evidence of decreased percentages of Ph[1]-positive cells in the marrow. Unfortunately, the toxicity associated with the more aggressive chemotherapy regimens and their inability to produce ablation or permanent suppression of the Ph[1]-positive neoplastic clone (i.e., long-term remission or cure) render them unsatisfactory alternatives to the much better tolerated, conventional, single-agent chemotherapy.

## Bone Marrow Transplantation

In the last decade, bone marrow transplantation has established itself as the treatment of choice for patients with acute myelogenous leukemia (AML) in first remission and for those with acute lymphocytic leukemia (ALL) in second remission. Because the subsequent infusion of marrow-reconstituting hematopoietic stem cells allows for delivery of extremely high-dose (potentially curative) chemotherapy, bone marrow transplantation has also been effective in patients with CML in the chronic phase. Initially, only patients who had entered the terminal blastic phase of their disease were given transplants. Unfortunately, both failure to achieve engraftment and recurrent leukemia contributed to poor survival of these patients.[35] Attention was focused next on performing transplants in patients during the less chemotherapy-resistant chronic phase of their disease. Preliminary results in such patients, transplanted with marrow from genetically identical twins, indicated that the Ph[1]-positive clone could be eradicated and long-term remissions (?cures) induced by high-dose chemoradiotherapy followed by infusion of normal hematopoietic stem cells.[36] Additional studies are underway to determine whether similar success can be achieved with nontwin HLA-identical, or even HLA-mismatched, marrow. It should be noted that the transplant data for CML, as for AML and ALL, indicate that the procedure is much better tolerated and the results substantially better in younger patients (≤30 years old). At present, most centers are reluctant to consider transplanting otherwise ideal candidates who are past the age of 40.

An alternative approach to homologous bone marrow transplantation, particularly for patients without appropriate bone marrow donors, has been the use of autologous marrow transplantation.[37] Bone marrow stem cells from such individuals have been harvested during the chronic phase of CML, cryopreserved, and transplanted after intensive chemoradiotherapy when the blast crisis supervened. Unfortunately, in addition to problems created by the failure of chemoradiotherapy completely to eliminate neoplastic cells, such an approach cannot hope to be curative until methods are developed that will enable the Ph[1]-positive cells to be purged from the marrow prior to returning it to the autologous donor. It is hoped that using hybridoma technology, a leukemia-specific antibody could be developed that will allow for the selective removal of neoplastic cells from autologous bone marrow. Such marrow, depleted of malignant cells, would offer the potential for cure when reinfused to the patient in chronic phase CML treated aggressively with intensive chemoradiotherapy.

### Treatment of Blast Crisis

As mentioned earlier, the chronic phase of CML almost inevitably terminates in an accelerated or acute process referred to as the blast crisis. The neoplastic cells at this stage of the disease are extremely resistant to chemotherapy, a major factor in the 10-week median survival for these patients. Aggressive chemotherapy regimens that are successful in AML are ineffective in CML blast crisis, as is bone marrow transplantation. Fortunately, however, there is a subset of patients with CML in blast crisis who are more sensitive to chemotherapy. It appears that the 30 percent of patients who develop a lymphoblastoid transformation, characterized by lymphoid morphology and the presence of the enzyme terminal deoxynucleotidyl transferase (TDT) in their blast cells, have a greater likelihood of responding to chemotherapy than do those with a myeloblastic transformation. In several studies, approximately one half of those patients whose blast cells were TDT positive responded to chemotherapy, most often to vincristine and prednisone, the preferred combination for initial treatment of ALL (see Chapter 19).[38,39] Responding patients had a median survival of 27 weeks, compared with 10 weeks for all patients in blast crisis.

The approach to the individual patient with CML whose disease enters an accelerated phase or blast crisis is to attempt to characterize the blasts and, if there are lymphoid characteristics, to treat the patient with vincristine, 2 mg intravenously each

week, and prednisone, 60 mg/m² of body surface area daily by mouth. Two to three weeks' therapy should be given, at which point the responsiveness to therapy can be gauged. If the patient's disease is judged to be refractory to vincristine and prednisone, one of the regimens for AML may be substituted, albeit with only minimal hope for a response. Patients with refractory disease usually succumb to infection or refractory thrombocytopenic hemorrhage.

## CASE HISTORY

At the time of referral, M.M. was a 36-year-old Caucasian woman, housewife and mother of four teenagers, who was referred to hematology clinic for evaluation of a white blood cell count of 225,000/mm³ and splenomegaly. She had no prior medical problems but had noted two months of increasing malaise, low-grade fevers, and abdominal fullness. When she sought medical attention she was found to have a palpable spleen and marked leukocytosis. Evaluation at clinic confirmed the splenomegaly (8 cm below the left costal margin) and also noted hepatomegaly (14 cm overall). A CBC revealed hematocrit 34 percent, hemoglobin 10.4 g%, platelet count 646,000/mm³, white blood cell count 276,000/mm³, differential 56 PMNs, 6 bands, 4 metamyelocytes, 6 myelocytes, 2 promyelocytes, 1 blast, 6 eosinophils, 8 basophils, 6 monocytes, and 5 lymphocytes. Her blood urea nitrogen (BUN) level was 18 mg%, uric acid 9.6 mg%, vitamin $B_{12}$ markedly increased, leukocyte alkaline phosphatase 0. Bone marrow examination revealed increased cellularity with marked granulocytic hyperplasia, M:E ratio 25:1. Chromosome analysis revealed Ph[1] t (22q−; 9q+) in all metaphases.

The patient was given a dosage of allopurinol 300 mg/day and of busulfan 8 mg/day orally. Her white blood cell count began to drop within two weeks, and after three months she had a normal CBC, a low normal leukocyte alkaline phosphatase level, and no hepatosplenomegaly. The busulfan was discontinued, and she was referred for evaluation for consideration of bone marrow transplantation. Although she was near the upper age limit for transplantation, her general good health was in her favor. In addition, she had five siblings, two of whom had marrow HLA-identical to hers and were therefore ideal potential donors.

The patient did well for nine months without any maintenance chemotherapy, at which point her white blood cell count began to rise and her LAP to drop. When her WBC reached 50,000/μl³, she was started again on allopurinol and busulfan and was in second remission three months later. This second clinical remission lasted six months, at the end of which time she gradually relapsed (over two months), requiring medication for the third time in the course of her disease. On this third occasion, although her blood counts were controlled by chemotherapy, the patient required continuous medication, because each time the chemotherapy was discontinued she sustained a rapid increase in blood counts.

Because the patient was 38 years old by this time and appeared to be entering a somewhat more rapidly paced phase of her disease, it was elected to perform a bone marrow transplantation at that time. The patient was admitted to the hospital, given total body irradiation and high-dose cytoxan, after which 500 ml of marrow from her brother were infused. She tolerated the procedure well, endured two episodes of sepsis, aided by granulocyte and single-donor platelet transfusions, and experienced a successful engraftment with Ph[1]-negative cells from her brother.

After experiencing mild graft-versus-host disease symptoms (skin rash, diarrhea, and weight loss), she gradually recovered and was discharged in hematologic remission three months after hospitalization. Currently it is three years post-transplant, and the patient shows no evidence of disease. Chromosome analysis reveals a male karyotype in her hematopoietic cells with no evidence of the Ph[1] chromosome.

## CHRONIC LYMPHOCYTIC LEUKEMIA

Chronic lymphocytic leukemia (CLL) is included in a heterogeneous group of conditions broadly categorized as lymphoproliferative disorders. Lymphoproliferative disorders are characterized by malignant monoclonal proliferation of relatively mature appearing, although immunologically incompetent, lymphocytes. With few exceptions, the pathologic lymphocytes in CLL are B lymphocytes, characterized by the presence of surface membrane immunoglobulin (SmIg). Patients with CLL manifest a peripheral blood and bone marrow lymphocytosis **(see Color Figures 178 and 179)** and may have lymphadenopathy or splenomegaly. As the disease progresses anemia, thrombocytopenia, and aberrant immunologic phenomena (autoimmune disease, immunodeficiency) almost invariably develop. The time course of the disease is extremely variable; some patients die within a few years of diagnosis, whereas others may have prolonged survival ($\geq$10 years) without receiving any treatment.

CLL is the most common form of leukemia in western Europe and the United States. It is predominantly a disease of the elderly; roughly 90 percent of patients are older than age 50, and nearly two thirds are older than age 60. As with all other forms of leukemia, men are affected more often than women. However, this gender disparity is even more prominent in CLL than in any of the other leukemias, with a male:female ratio of greater than 2:1.

## Etiology and Pathogenesis

A specific cause or etiologic agent of CLL has yet to be defined. Rather, a number of factors that may be related to the appearance of CLL in patients have been identified. Interestingly, radiation exposure, which is a prominent etiologic agent in CML and perhaps in other myeloproliferative disorders, plays no role in CLL. Genetic factors are generally recognized as being important in the etiology of CLL, primarily because of the number of families in which multiple cases of CLL or other lymphoproliferative disorders have been reported.[40] From these reports, it is apparent that relatives of patients with CLL either have an increased tendency to develop the disease or are subject to other aberrations of immune function or immunoglobulin production.[41] Incidences of CLL as high as three times that in the general population have been reported among first-degree relatives; even distant relatives have had roughly twice the incidence of unrelated individuals. There is yet to be defined, however, any clear-cut pattern of inheritance; no relationship to blood group or HLA type has been demonstrated.

A characteristic chromosomal abnormality, akin to the Philadelphia chromosome in CML, has not as yet been described in CLL. Published chromosomal studies have generally reported finding predominantly normal karyotypes, although it is thought that because of the low spontaneous mitotic index of leukemic B cells, this may represent normal residual T cells. Recent studies using polyclonal B-cell mitogens such as pokeweed mitogen and Epstein-Barr virus have indicated that nonrandom chromosome abnormalities in leukemic B cells are present in up to 50 percent of patients with CLL.[42] The most common abnormality was an extra chromosome 12 (trisomy 12), followed by a translocation to the long arm of chromosome 14 (14q+). Deletion of the long arm of chromosome 6 (6q−) has also been described.

Additional factors that appear to be important in the pathogenesis of CLL, although the critical pieces of the puzzle have yet to be fitted, are the aberrant immunologic phenomena that often precede and nearly always accompany the clinical expression of CLL. It is of interest in this regard that not only patients but often also unaffected, presumably healthy relatives of individuals with lymphoproliferative disorders manifest measurable abnormalities in the regulation of antibodies and cellular immune responses. It is clear that many of the immunologic abnormalities in patients with CLL are a direct result of the accumulation of an immunologically inert clone of lymphocytes; nevertheless, the presence of immunoglobulin abnormalities and impairment of lymphocyte immune responses in relatives of patients with CLL suggest that immune incompetence may increase susceptibility to other etiologic factors (e.g., viruses) that, in concert with defective immunologic surveillance, lead to the development of a neoplastic condition.

## Characteristics of Abnormal Lymphocytes and Other Immunologic Abnormalities

In more than 95 percent of patients with CLL the predominant circulating lymphocyte is a leukemic B cell, which has been shown to be monoclonal, with a single antibody specificity and single idiotype (variable region).[43] Because these cells have also been shown to have low levels of surface membrane immunoglobulin (SmIg)[44] and an enhanced capacity to form rosettes with mouse erythrocytes,[45] they are presumed to have an arrest of B-cell development at an early stage. B CLL cells usually have C3 and Fc receptors and B1, BA-1, and Ia antigens. They are functionally deficient, manifesting, in addition to decreased levels of SmIg, decreased migration of immunoglobulin on the cell surface (capping), decreased stimulation capacity in mixed lymphocyte culture (MLC), and decreased antibody-dependent cellular cytotoxicity (ADCC) activity. Clinical studies in patients with CLL reveal these individuals to be unable to produce antibodies to new antigens, to remember old antigens and produce antibodies to them, and to develop a delayed hypersensitivity response.[46]

In approximately 5 percent of patients with CLL, the neoplastic cell is of T-cell, rather than B-cell, origin. These cells, which completely lack SmIg, react with T antisera and anti-T monoclonal antibodies and form E rosettes with sheep erythrocytes.[47] A high percentage of patients with T CLL have diffuse organ and skin involvement. Both categories of T cell, the helper-inducer and the suppressor-cytotoxic variety, have been reported in patients with T CLL.[48]

Despite the known functional abnormalities of the leukemic B lymphocyte described earlier, there remain some functional, normal B cells and a normal T-cell pool in most patients with CLL.[49] How then can one explain the impaired immunologic responses in these patients? One suggestion is that the tremendous expansion of the total lymphocyte pool, an expansion primarily caused by a population of long-lived, immunologically incompetent, leukemic B lymphocytes, so dilutes the populations of nonleukemic B and T cells that normal T-B interactions are virtually prohibited.[46] This would explain the observed inability to produce antibody to new

antigens, as well as the general decrease in antibody production (hypogammaglobulinemia) found in the majority of patients with disease of greater than five years' duration. It might also account for the fact that infection with bacterial agents, especially those requiring antibody for optimal clearance, is the major cause of morbidity and mortality in patients with CLL. That some immune responses, such as standard skin tests and resistance to most intracellular pathogens (viruses), are normal is most likely related to retention of some T-cell function independent of T-B interactions.

## Autoimmune Phenomena

In patients with CLL there is a striking occurrence of autoimmune phenomena. Autoimmune hemolytic anemia, characterized by a positive direct antiglobulin (Coombs') test, occurs in as many as 5 to 10 percent of patients. Other reported associated phenomena include idiopathic thrombocytopenic purpura (ITP), systemic lupus erythematosus (SLE), pure red cell aplasia, rheumatoid arthritis, vasculitis, and membranous glomerulonephritis with nephrotic syndrome. There is a great deal of speculation but unfortunately few data as to the relationship between CLL and these autoimmune phenomena. One possibility, for which there is an animal model, is a genetic susceptibility for both diseases, as determined by an immune response gene linked to the HLA region.[50] Alternatively, the altered immunologic responsiveness of patients with CLL, acting either through widening the range of infectious organisms capable of inducing such phenomena or through a failure of normal regulatory control exerted by suppressor T cells, might be a significant etiologic factor. Confusing the issue even further is the fact that the autoimmune phenomena in CLL can precede or follow the appearance of the disease, and the courses even when simultaneous are independent.

## Clinical Course

The pace of disease in CLL varies considerably from patient to patient and is dependent on the rate of accumulation of abnormal lymphocytes. Although in a given patient the amount of abnormal lymphatic tissue seems to increase at a steady rate, there is tremendous variability among patients. Thus, while the median survival of all patients is three to four years from diagnosis, approximately 10 to 15 percent of patients live for greater than 10 years with little or no therapy, and a slightly greater percentage with aggressive disease die within a year. CLL differs from CML in that there is no tendency for an acute exacerbation, acceleration, or blastic transformation; rather, the complications of advanced disease (impairment of immune responses, hypogammaglobulinemia, organ infiltration, anemia, and thrombocytopenia) result from progressive accumulation of the long-lived, poorly functional lymphocytes that represent the leukemic clone. An additional factor complicating mortality figures in CLL is the fact that this is a disease of the elderly. Many patients with a nonaggressive form of CLL die of age-related, rather than CLL-related, factors.[51]

## Symptoms and Signs

The earliest symptoms noted by patients with CLL are excessive fatigue and reduced exercise tolerance. On initial physical examination, lymphadenopathy characterized by the presence of small, discrete, firm, and freely movable nodes occurs, in 75 percent of patients; splenomegaly occurs in 50 percent. As with other hematologic malignancies, the exact time of onset of the disease cannot be ascertained with certainty. In addition, because CLL progresses in an insidious fashion and is associated with only minimal symptomatology, in somewhat more than 25 percent of patients their disease is discovered incidental to a routine physical examination or complete blood count. In these settings, it has been possible to follow disease progression, usually dominated by increasing adenopathy, splenomegaly, and nonlymphatic organ infiltration. Treatment, when instituted (see further on), can effectively reduce the tumor burden and relieve many of the systemic symptoms. Patients with end-stage, or aggressive, disease often have severe and incapacitating fatigue, recurrent or persistent infection, bruising, pallor or jaundice associated with anemia, fever, weight loss, increased bone tenderness, and edema or thrombophlebitis from node obstruction.

## Laboratory Features

An absolute lymphocytosis in the peripheral blood, usually between 10,000 and 150,000/mm³, is the basis for diagnosis in CLL. Depending on the aggressiveness of the disease in a given patient, the lymphocytes can appear either quite mature and virtually normal or quite immature and obviously abnormal. Even the relatively mature appearing lymphocytes, however, are somewhat larger than normal. Despite marked interpatient variability in lymphocyte morphology, the malignant lymphocytes in an individual patient tend to be fairly homogeneous. An additional characteristic of CLL lymphocytes is their marked fragility; this accounts for the large number of smudge cells characteristically seen on the peripheral smear **(see Color Figure 178)**.

A bone marrow examination is not required for the diagnosis of CLL, because the peripheral smear is so characteristic. When the marrow is examined, the extent of involvement tends to reflect the stage of the disease as evidenced by the lymphocyte count and other organ infiltration. Early marrow involvement may be characterized by sporadic aggregates of lymphocytes; more advanced disease is associated with extensive marrow infiltration. When lymphoid tissue comprises 50 percent or more of the bone marrow, patients generally have cytopenias in one or more cell lines **(see Color Figure 179)**.

Anemia is often seen in patients with more aggressive or advanced CLL. The basis for the anemia may be decreased red blood cell production secondary to marrow infiltration, hypersplenism, or an autoimmune process.[52] Autoimmune hemolytic anemia may be found in as many as 10 percent of patients with CLL. A similar range of possibilities, marrow crowding, hypersplenism, or autoimmunity may be invoked to explain neutropenia or thrombocytopenia in CLL patients.

Other laboratory features of importance in CLL include hypogammaglobulinemia, which is progressive, is unaffected by therapy, and may be found in approximately 50 percent of patients; monoclonal immunoglobulin spikes, which can occur in 5 to 10 percent of patients; and cryoglobulins or cryofibrinogens, which are found also in a small percentage of patients. As in all lymphoproliferative disorders, uric acid levels may be elevated.

## Differential Diagnosis

In the patient with sustained, or progressive, lymphocytosis in the peripheral blood and bone marrow, lymphadenopathy, and splenomegaly the diagnosis of CLL is relatively straightforward. Viral infections or hypersensitivity reactions, which may be associated also with lymphocytosis, are usually transitory and rarely produce infiltration of the bone marrow (see Chapter 18). Fortunately, there is usually little urgency to make the diagnosis in a patient with suspected CLL, and it is often possible to observe such a patient for several weeks or months in order to confirm one's suspicions. In the rare situation when a more rapid assessment is desirable, one may differentiate CLL from other causes of lymphocytosis by demonstrating that the patient has a monoclonal proliferation of B lymphocytes (see Chapter 22).

One aspect of the diagnosis of CLL that occasionally may be of concern is the differentiation between CLL and well-differentiated lymphocytic lymphoma (WDLL), when the latter enters a leukemic phase. This entity, which has also been called lymphosarcoma cell leukemia, is exceedingly difficult to differentiate from CLL purely on clinical or morphologic grounds.[53] In fact, since both entities are monoclonal proliferations of small B lymphocytes,[54] and since their response to therapeutic agents appears to be much the same, it is believed that these may not even be different diseases, but rather different variants of a similar pathologic process. The major difference between CLL and WDLL may simply be the anatomic distribution: CLL is diffuse and generalized, whereas WDLL is more or less localized. If distinction is necessary, it has been shown that WDLL cells demonstrate more intense anti-immunoglobulin surface fluorescence and better mobility (capping) of that surface fluorescence than do CLL cells[55] and thus may be derived from a slightly less mature B lymphocyte, although the practical importance of this distinction has yet to be defined.

### Hairy Cell Leukemia

Another disease entity, the differentiation of which from CLL is critically important, is hairy cell leukemia (HCL). This uncommon disorder, also known as leukemic reticuloendotheliosis, is a disease of elderly men and is characterized by malaise and fatigue, marked splenomegaly (although only minimal adenopathy), pancytopenia, and the presence of atypical mononuclear, lymphocytoid cells in the circulating blood (see Color Figure 180). The disease takes its pseudonym from the unique hair-like projections on the cell surface of the malignant cell, visible on routinely stained smears but best appreciated in supravital preparations and with phase microscopy. Although the peripheral blood picture may resemble CLL, unique to HCL is a fibrotic, difficult to aspirate bone marrow (see Color Figure 181), and the presence of a tartrate-resistant acid phosphatase in the malignant cells.[56]

The reason the distinction between CLL and HCL is considered critical is the vast difference in the appropriate management of patients with these disorders. The primary difference is that unlike patients with CLL, those with HCL respond very poorly to chemotherapy or radiotherapy, either of which can produce severe, often life-threatening cytopenias. Instead, it has been shown that many HCL patients with severe pancytopenia respond to splenectomy and also to interferon, often with sustained remission. Thus, although superficially similar, CLL and HCL are clearly distinct entities that require accurate classification in order to allow the clinician to make appropriate management decisions.

## Staging and Prognosis

As noted earlier, there is marked variability in length of survival among patients with CLL, from less than one year to greater than 20 years. Based on empirical observations that patients with the shortest survival tended to have more abnormal findings at the time of diagnosis, a clinical staging system denoting five clinical stages was proposed in 1975.[57]

In that original system, which was widely accepted and verified, although subsequently modified, the five clinical stages were Stage 0, bone marrow and blood lymphocytosis only; stage I, lymphocytosis with enlarged nodes; stage II, lymphocytosis with enlarged spleen or liver or both; stage III, lymphocytosis with anemia (hemoglobin <11 g/dl); stage IV, lymphocytosis with thrombocytopenia (platelets <100,000/mm³) (Table 20-3). Patients with CLL staged according to this system tended to fall into three categories of risk: (1) a "high-risk" group (stages III and IV), with very short survival times; (2) a "low-risk" group (stage 0), with very long survival times; and (3) an "intermediate" group (stages I and II) with intermediate survival times.

In 1981, a modification of the five-stage system was proposed[58] that was subsequently adopted by the International Workshop on CLL.[59] In this system, only three stages were distinguished and the prognostic value of the number of involved lymphatic areas was recognized. The three stages in this system are stage A, lymphocytosis without anemia or thrombocytopenia and fewer than three areas of lymphoid involvement (which would include stages 0, I, and II of former system); stage B, lymphocytosis without anemia or thrombocytopenia but with more than three areas of lymphoid involvement (which would also include stages I and II of former system); and stage C, lymphocytosis with anemia or thrombocytopenia or both (which would include stages III and IV of former system) (Table 20-4). The three-stage system is reproducible and its prognostic value has been confirmed in large series of patients. Its value lies not only in allowing for more accurate comparison of treatment protocols but also in enabling one to make rational decisions as to whether any treatment is appropriate. It is generally believed that patients in stage A should be observed only. Similarly, there is no evidence that treating asymptomatic patients in stages A or B would be beneficial. Symptomatic patients in stage B and all patients in stage C should receive therapeutic intervention.

Recently, two additional prognostic variables, not previously recognized, have been reported. These are the presence and specific type of cytogenetic abnormalities[60] and the histologic pattern of bone

### Table 20-3. CLINICAL STAGES OF CHRONIC LYMPHOCTIC LEUKEMIA (CLL)

| | |
|---|---|
| Stage 0 | Bone marrow and blood lymphocytosis only |
| Stage I | Lymphocytosis with enlarged nodes |
| Stage II | Lymphocytosis with enlarged spleen or liver or both |
| Stage III | Lymphocytosis with anemia (hemoglobin <11 g/dl) |
| Stage IV | Lymphocytosis with thrombocytopenia (platelets <100,000/mm³) |

**Table 20-4. CLINICAL STAGING SYSTEM ADOPTED BY THE INTERNATIONAL WORKSHOP ON CLL**[59]

| | |
|---|---|
| **Stage A** | Lymphocytosis without anemia or thrombocytopenia and with fewer than 3 areas of lymphoid involvement (includes stages, 0, I, and II of former system) |
| **Stage B** | Lymphocytosis without anemia or thrombocytopenia but with more than 3 areas of lymphoid involvement (includes stages I and II of former system) |
| **Stage C** | Lymphocytosis with anemia or thrombocytopenia or both (includes stages III and IV of former system) |

marrow involvement.[61] With respect to cytogenetic analysis, it appears that patients with abnormal karyotypes, other than trisomy 12 as the sole abnormality, may have a shorter median survival time from cytogenetic study than those with either normal karyotypes or trisomy 12 as the sole abnormality.[60] If this finding is confirmed in a larger number of patients, the current staging system may need to be modified to accommodate results of cytogenetic analysis. With respect to bone marrow histologic pattern, it appears that patients with a diffuse pattern of bone marrow lymphocytic infiltration have a substantially poorer outlook than do those with either a nodular or interstitial pattern of involvement, independent of clinical stage as currently classified.[61] Again, if this finding can be confirmed by additional studies, it may add yet another modification to the clinical staging of patients with CLL.

## Treatment

As previously mentioned, CLL is a chronic, progressive disease, the pace of which may vary markedly from patient to patient. It is also, unfortunately, incurable. Even terms such as "remission" or "relapse" are not applicable, since they usually imply an all-or-none type of phenomenon not accurately descriptive of the impact of therapy in CLL. Therapy can reduce symptoms and disability; there is no convincing evidence, however, that treatment of asymptomatic disease can prolong life. The major goal of therapy is to relieve signs and symptoms of disease with the least amount of discomfort or risk to the patient. Many patients are not treated initially; some are never treated. In general, indications for treatment include bulky lymphadenopathy, symptomatic splenomegaly, autoimmune hemolytic anemia or idiopathic thrombocytopenic purpura, marrow failure (neutropenia, anemia, thrombocytopenia), or a hypermetabolic state (weight loss, sweating, and so on).

When therapy is indicated, the most usual first approach is the use of chlorambucil (Leukeran), an oral alkylating agent, given at a dosage of 0.1 to 0.2 mm/kg/day adjusted to the white blood cell count.

Intermittent chlorambucil at a higher dosage, 0.4 mg/kg every two weeks, either alone or in combination with prednisone, can produce equivalent results to daily administration and may be less toxic.[62] Whether given continuously or intermittently, the drug is usually given until bone marrow suppression develops or evidence of active disease decreases. When disease activity subsides, as it will in two thirds to three fourths of patients within two to three months, most clinicians discontinue the drug and withhold therapy for as long as the clinical remission lasts. In this manner, patients may be kept relatively symptom free for a period of months to years, depending on the pace of their disease and their response to chemotherapy.

A second well-tolerated oral alkylating agent used to treat CLL is cyclophosphamide (Cytoxan), which may be substituted for chlorambucil, although there are no studies demonstrating its superiority or even equivalence to chlorambucil. It is claimed, however, that cyclophosphamide may have more activity against more immature lymphocytes and that it may be less toxic to platelets than chlorambucil.

Corticosteroids are an additional class of agent sometimes useful in managing patients with CLL. Steroids are lympholytic and have occasionally been used as single agents in patients with marked adenopathy or splenomegaly. They are also immunosuppressive, however, and, given the immunocompromised state of CLL patients, most clinicians avoid using steroids except in combination with other alkylating agents or for patients with autoimmune phenomena.

For patients with resistant or advanced disease, several different combinations of chemotherapeutic agents have been evaluated, including cyclophosphamide, vincristine, and prednisone (CVP); cyclophosphamide, doxorubicin, vincristine, and prednisone (CHOP); and most recently, vincristine, carmustine (BCNU), cyclophosphamide, melphalan, and prednisone (M-2 protocol).[63] Although response rates of greater than 60 percent have been achieved in patients with advanced disease, few if any of the responders achieve a true hematologic remission. In addition, the aggressive regimen is toxic and expensive, and it only minimally prolongs survival. Thus, many centers have discontinued intensive therapy for all but a few patients with CLL.

In addition to the more conventional chemotherapy regimens discussed here, there are alternative therapeutic approaches that may be applicable to patients with particular clinical problems. One such approach is radiation therapy. Local irradiation may be very effective in reducing bulky adenopathy or splenomegaly; some have advocated total body, or mediastinal, irradiation as a means of inducing a more generalized remission.[64] Because the effects of irradiation on blood counts are unpredictable and in some cases have led to such severe depression of both neutrophil and lymphocyte counts that fatal infections resulted, radiation therapy is not nearly as popular as is chemotherapy, particularly in diffuse disease.

Two additional therapeutic maneuvers with limited applicability are splenectomy and leukapheresis. Splenectomy is useful for the patient with cytopenias secondary to hypersplenism or with splenomegaly and intractable pain. Leukapheresis is a relatively nontoxic way to decrease the tumor burden by removing large numbers of malignant lymphocytes.[65] Unfortunately, although it has a good therapeutic index and is generally well tolerated by the patient, leukapheresis is very expensive, is unable to achieve anything more than limited and temporary control of symptoms, and has no affect whatever on the basic proliferative process.

Several additional treatment approaches are currently in an experimental stage. These include interferon, which has been shown to produce transient responses in advanced CLL; and monoclonal antibodies, which, when directed against idiotypes of B CLL cells and combined with potent immunotoxins such as ricin or diphtheria toxin, have been shown to achieve an effective leukemia-cell kill.

Finally, it should be pointed out that hypogammaglobulinemia, which affects most patients with disease of greater than five years' duration, is irreversible, despite improvement in other factors with therapy. Thus, susceptibility to infection remains a serious problem for the patient with advanced CLL. In this setting, routine administration of immunoglobulin, now available in an intravenous form, has been shown to be effective in controlling both lymphocyte counts and infections.[66] In addition, it is possible that there is also a role for intravenous immunoglobulin in the management of such complications as autoimmune hemolytic anemia or idiopathic thrombocytopenic purpura.[66]

## CASE HISTORY

R.C. was 64 years old in 1960 when he sought medical attention because of malaise and swollen lymph glands in his neck. Physical examination revealed bulky adenopathy in all lymph-bearing areas, as well as a palpable spleen tip. A CBC revealed hematocrit 38 percent, hemoglobin 12.6 g%, platelets 220,000/mm³, WBC count 46,000/mm³, differential 6 PMNs, 1 band, 93 lymphocytes. Examination of the peripheral smear revealed that all of the intact lymphocytes were somewhat enlarged and atypical; there were also numerous smudge cells. A bone marrow examination revealed a diffuse lymphocytic infiltrate with good preservation of normal marrow elements. Additional laboratory data included uric acid

9.8 mg%; immunoglobulin levels, low normal; direct antiglobulin (Coombs') test, negative.

Because the patient was asymptomatic, no therapy was initiated; he was followed in clinic at regular intervals. In 1962, in response to a dramatic increase in the size of his lymph nodes and the development of painful splenomegaly, R.C. was given a course of chlorambucil (6 mg/day). When chlorambucil regimen was started, his white blood cell count was 162,000/mm³ with 98 percent atypical lymphocytes. Within three months, the patient's white blood cell count had dropped to 18,000/mm³ (91 percent lymphocytes), and his splenomegaly and lymphadenopathy had disappeared. At that point, the chlorambucil was discontinued.

For the next eight years, R.C. was seen at regular intervals, although no treatment was administered. In 1970 he had an acute hemolytic episode and presented with jaundice, anemia, and symptoms of congestive heart failure. His CBC revealed hematocrit 21 percent, hemoglobin 6.2 g%, WBC count 62,000/mm³ (94 percent lymphocytes), platelets 122,000/mm³, reticulocytes 8 percent. A direct antiglobulin test result was strongly positive, indicating that the patient's red cells were coated with IgG and C3. A diagnosis of autoimmune hemolytic anemia was made; he was then given a course of steroids. Although he had a good initial response to the steroids, the patient could not have his dose tapered without suffering a relapse; he therefore underwent splenectomy in 1971. With the removal of his spleen, his hematocrit normalized, although he continued to have a strongly positive direct antiglobulin test result.

R.C. remained asymptomatic until 1973, at which point bulky adenopathy led to obstruction of his left ureter. He received emergency radiotherapy, which successfully relieved the obstruction, and he was started on CVP. At that time his WBC count was 184,000/mm³ (97 percent lymphocytes), and he was mildly anemic and thrombocytopenic (hematocrit 28 percent, platelets 88,000/mm³). After four months of CVP therapy, his adenopathy had resolved only minimally, but his WBC count remained high (124,000/mm³), and his platelet count had dropped to 42,000/mm³. The CVP regimen was discontinued at that time.

Over the next six months the patient was admitted to the hospital on four different occasions with pneumonia. He was found to have marked hypogammaglobulinemia and was given prophylactic intramuscular gammaglobulin. In early 1974, R.C., who was then 78 years old and who had had CLL for 14 years, was admitted to the hospital for the last time with a bout of pneumonia from which he did not recover.

# References

1. Craigie, D: Case of disease of the spleen, in which death took place in consequence of the presence of purulent matter in the blood. Edinburg Med Surg J 64:400, 1845.
2. Nowell, PC and Hungerford, DA: Chromosome studies in normal and leukemic human leukocytes. JNCI 25:85, 1960.
3. March, HC: Leukemia in radiologists, ten years later. Am J Med Sci 242:137, 1961.
4. Court Brown, WM and Abbatt, JD: Mortality from cancer and other causes after radiotherapy for ankylosing spondylitis. Br Med J 2:1327, 1965.
5. Lange, RD, Moloney WC, and Yamawaki, T: Leukemia in atomic bomb survivors. I. General observations. Blood 9:574, 1954.
6. Heyssel, R, Brill, AB, Woodbury, LA, et al: Leukemia in Hiroshima atomic bomb survivors. Blood 15:313, 1960.
7. Askoy, M, Erdem, S, and Din, G: Leukemia in shoeworkers exposed chronically to benzene. Blood 44:837, 1974.
8. Jacobs, EM, Luce, JK, and Caileau, R: Chromosome abnormalities in human cancer: Report of a patient with chronic myelocytic leukemia and his nonleukemic monocygotic twin. Cancer 19:869, 1966.
9. Whang, J, Frei, E III, Tjio, JH, et al: The distribution of the Philadelphia chromosome in patients with chronic myelogenous leukemia. Blood 22:664, 1963.
10. Fialkow, PJ, Jacobson, RJ, and Papayannopoulou, T: Chronic myelocytic leukemia: Clonal origin in a stem cell common to the granulocyte, erythrocyte, platelet and monocyte/macrophage. Am J Med 63:125, 1977.
11. Yoshida, M, Miyoshi, I, and Hinuman Y: Isolation and characterization of retrovirus from cell lines of human adult T-cell leukemia and its implication in the disease. Proc Natl Acad Sci 79:2031, 1982.
12. Olofsson, T and Olsson, I: Suppression of normal granulopoiesis in vitro by a leukemia-associated inhibitor (LAI) of acute and chronic leukemia. Blood 55:975, 1980.
13. Kurland, JI, Broxmeyer, HE, Pelus, LM, et al: Role for monocyte-macrophage-derived colony-stimulating factor and prostaglandin E in the positive and negative feedback control of myeloid stem cell proliferation. Blood 52:388, 1978.
14. Golde, DW, Byers, LA, and Cline, MJ: Chronic myelogenous leukemia cell growth and maturation in liquid culture. Cancer Res 34:419, 1974.
15. Spiers, ASD and Baikie, AG: Cytogenic evolution and clonal proliferation in acute transformation of chronic granulocytic leukaemia. Br J Cancer 22:192, 1968.
16. Rowley, J: The role of cytogenetics in hematology. Blood 48:1, 1976.
17. Shaw, MT, Bottomley, RH, Grozea, PN, et al: Heterogeneity of morphological, cytochemical, and cytogenetic features in the blastic phase of chronic granulocytic leukemia. Cancer 35:199, 1975.
18. Boggs, DR: Hematopoietic stem cell theory in relation to possible lymphoblastic conversion of chronic myeloid leukemia. Blood 44:449, 1974.
19. Kamada, N and Uchino, H: Chronologic sequence in appearance of clinical and laboratory findings characteristic of chronic myelocytic leukemia. Blood 51:843, 1978.
20. Schiffer, CA, Aisner, J, Daly, PA, et al: Increased leukocyte alkaline phosphatase activity following transfusion of leukocytes from a patient with chronic myelogenous leukemia. Am J Med 66:519, 1979.
21. Feinleib, M and MacMahon, B: Variation in the duration of survival of patients with the chronic leukemias. Blood 15:332, 1960.
22. Ezdinli, EZ, Sokal, JE, Crosswhite, L, et al: Philadelphia-chromosome-positive and -negative chronic myelocytic leukemia. Ann Intern Med 72:175, 1970.
23. Tura, S, Baccarani, M, Corbelli, G, et al: Staging of chronic myeloid leukaemia. Br J Haematol 47:105, 1981.
24. Cervantes, F and Rozman, C: A multivariate analysis of prognostic factors in chronic myeloid leukemia. Blood 60:1298, 1982.
25. Sokal, JE, Cox, EB, Baccarani, M, et al: Prognostic discrimination in "good-risk" chronic granulocyte leukemia. Blood 63:789, 1984.
26. Koeffler, HP and Golde, DW: Chronic myelogenous leukemia — new concepts. N Engl J Med 304:1269, 1981.
27. Sokal, JE, Evaluation of survival data for chronic myelocytic leukemia. Am J Hematol 1:493, 1976.
28. Galton, DAG: Chemotherapy of chronic myelocytic leukemia. Semin Hematol 6:323, 1969.
29. Hauch, T, Logue, G, Laszlo, J, et al: Treatment of chronic granulocytic leukemia with melphalan. Blood 51:571, 1978.
30. Kennedy, BJ: Hydroxyurea therapy in chronic myelogenous leukemia. Cancer 29:1052, 1972.
31. Smalley, RV, Vogel, J, Huguley, CM Jr, et al: Chronic granulocytic leukemia: Cytogenic conversion of the bone marrow with cycle-specific chemotherapy. Blood 50:107, 1977.
32. Cunningham, I, Gee, T, Dowling, M, et al: Results of treatment of Ph¹ + chronic myelogenous leukemia with an intensive treatment regimen (L-5 protocol). Blood 53:375, 1979.
33. Brodsky, I, Fuscaldo KE and Kahn, SB: Myeloproliferative disorders. II. CML: Clonal evolution and its role in management. Leukemia Res 3:379, 1979.
34. Sharp, J, Joyner, MV, Wayne, AW, et al: Karyotypic conversion in Ph¹-positive chronic myeloid leukaemia with combination chemotherapy. Lancet 1:1370, 1979.
35. Doney, K, Buckner, CD, Sale, GE, et al: Treatment of chronic granulocytic leukemia by chemotherapy, total body irradiation and allogeneic bone marrow transplantation. Exp Hematol 6:738, 1978.
36. Fefer, A, Cheever, MA, Thomas, ED, et al: Disappearance of Ph¹-positive cells in four patients with chronic granulocyte leukemia after chemotherapy, irradiation and marrow transplantation from an identical twin. N Engl J Med 300:333, 1979.
37. Goldman, JM, Catovsky, D, Hows, J, et al: Cryopreserved peripheral blood cells functioning as autografts in patients with chronic granulocytic leukaemia in transformation. Br Med J 1:310, 1979.
38. Rossenthal, S, Carnellos, GP, Whang-Peng, J, et al: Blast crisis of chronic granulocytic leukemia. Am J Med 63:542, 1977.
39. Marks, SM, Baltimore, D, and McCaffrey, R: Terminal Transferase as a predictor of initial responsiveness in vincristine and prednisone in blastic crisis myelogenous leukemia: A co-operative study. N Engl J Med 298:812, 1978.
40. Gunz, FW and Veale, AMO: Leukemia in close relatives — accident or predisposition. J Natl Cancer Inst 42:517, 1969.
41. Fraumeni, J Jr, Wertelecki, W, Blattner, W, et al: Varied manifestations of a familial Lymphoproliferative disorder. Am J Med 59:145, 1975.
42. Gahrton, G, Robert, KH, Friberg, K, et al: Nonrandom chromosomal aberrations in chronic lymphocytic leukemia revealed by polyclonal B-cell mitogen stimulation. Blood 56:640, 1980.
43. Schroer, K, Briles, DE, Van Boxel, JA, et al: Idiotypic uniformity of cell surface immunoglobulin in chronic lymphocytic leukemia (evidence for monoclonal proliferation). J Exp Med 140:1416, 1974.
44. Slease, RB, Wistar, R, and Scher, I: Surface immunoglobulin density on human peripheral blood mononuclear cells. Blood 54:72, 1979.
45. Koziner, B, Filippa, DA, Mertelsmann, R, et al: Characterization of malignant lymphoma in leukemia phase by multiple differentiation markers on leukemic cells. Correlation with clinical features and conventional morphology. Am J Med 63:556, 1977.
46. Abrahm, JL and Smith, LH Jr: Chronic lymphocytic leukemia. West J Med 127:221, 1977.
47. Brouet, JC, Flandrin, G, Sasportes, M, et al: Chronic lymphocytic leukaemia of T-cell origin. Immunologic and clinical evaluation in eleven patients. Lancet 2:890, 1975.
48. Saxon, A, Stevens, RH, and Golde, DW: Helper and suppres-

sor T-lymphocyte leukemia in ataxia telangiectasia. N Engl J Med 300:700, 1979.

49. Fudenberg, HH, Wybran, J, and Chantler S: Isolation of normal T cells in chronic lymphocytic leukemia. Lancet 1:126, 1973.

50. Fudenberg, HH: Basic and Clinical immunology. Lange Medical Publications, Los Altos, 1976, p 653.

51. Boggs, DR, Sofferman, SA, Wintrobe, MM, et al: Factors influencing the duration of survival of patients with chronic lymphocytic leukemia. Am J Med 40:243, 1966.

52. Wasi, P and Block, M: The mechanism of the development of anemia in untreated chronic lymphatic leukemia. Blood 17:597, 1961.

53. Zacharski, LR and Linman, JW: Chronic lymphocytic leukemia versus chronic lymphosarcoma cell leukemia. Am J Med 47:75, 1969.

54. Aisenberg, AC: Cell lineage in lymphoproliferative disease. Am J Med 74:679, 1983.

55. Cohen, HJ: B-cell lymphosarcoma cell leukemia: Dynamics of surface membrane immunoglobulin. Ann Intern Med 88:317, 1978.

56. Yam, LT, Li, CY, and Lam, KW: Tartrate-resistant acid phosphatase isoenzyme in leukemic reticuloendotheliosis. N Engl J Med 284:357, 1971.

57. Rai, KR, Sawitsky, A, Cronkite, EP, et al: Clinical staging of chronic lymphocytic leukemia. Blood 46:219, 1975.

58. Binet, JL: A new prognostic classification of chronic lymphocytic leukemia derived from a multivariate survival analysis. Cancer 48:198, 1981.

59. International Workshop on CLL: Chronic lymphocytic leukaemia: Proposals for a revised prognostic staging system. Br J Haematol 48:365, 1981.

60. Han, T, Ozer, H, Sadamori, N, et al: Prognostic importance of cytogenetic abnormalities in patients with chronic lymphocytic leukemia. N Engl J Med 310:288, 1984.

61. Rozman, C, Montserrat, E, Rodriguez-Fernandez, JM, et al: Bone marrow histologic pattern—the best single prognostic parameter in chronic lymphocytic leukemia: A multivariate survival analysis of 329 cases. Blood 64:642, 1984.

62. Sawitsky, A, Rai, KR, Glidewell, O, et al: Comparison of daily versus intermittent chlorambucil and prednisone therapy in the treatment of patients with chronic lymphocytic leukemia. Blood 50:1049, 1977.

63. Kempin, S, Lee, BJ III, Thaler, T, et al: Combination chemotherapy of advanced chronic lymphocytic leukemia: The M-2 protocol (vincristine, BCNU, cyclophosphamide, melphalan, and prednisone). Blood 60:1110, 1982.

64. Richards, F, Spurr, CL, Ferree, C, et al: The control of chronic lymphocytic leukemia with mediastinal irradiation. Am J Med 64:947, 1978.

65. Curtis, JE, Hersh, EM, Freireich, EJ, et al: Leukapheresis therapy of chronic lymphocytic leukemia. Blood 39:163, 1972.

66. Besa, EC: Use of intravenous immunoglobulin in chronic lymphocytic leukemia. Am J Med 209:218, 1984.

# CHAPTER 21

ROBERT J. JACOBSON, M.D., F.A.C.P.

# Myeloproliferative Disorders

In 1951, Dr. William Damashek[1] used the term "myeloproliferative disorders" to describe a group of hematologic diseases that were distinct from acute leukemia and that shared several clinical and hematologic features. These diseases included chronic granulocytic leukemia, polycythemia rubra vera, agnogenic (idiopathic) myeloid metaplasia, and primary or essential thrombocythemia. He speculated then that these diseases were interrelated and had in common proliferation of bone marrow (stem) cells. These marrow cells could be "affected diffusely or irregularly with the result that various syndromes either clear cut or transitional result."[1] Thus, he cited in polycythemia vera, for example, a proliferation not only of the erythroid series but also of granulocytes and platelets, producing a marrow panmyelosis. In addition, he recognized that each of the clinical definable entities has the potential of terminating in acute leukemia.

Today, Damashek's concept is widely accepted, and the myeloproliferative disorders are considered a group of clonal neoplastic diseases that involve the pluripotent hematopoietic stem cell. These disorders can be further subdivided into acute and chronic types. The acute myeloproliferative disorders are the various types of acute nonlymphocytic leukemias; and the chronic diseases are chronic granulocytic leukemia, polycythemia vera, essential thrombocythemia, and agnogenic myeloid metaplasia (Table 21–1).

The pluripotent stem cell is capable of proliferating and differentiating into progenitors that give rise to granulocytes, erythrocytes, and platelets. The evidence for the involvement of the stem cell and the clonal nature of the myeloproliferative disorders is derived from cytogenetic and isoenzyme markers such as glucose-6-phosphate dehydrogenase (G-6-PD). In chronic granulocytic leukemia a specific chromosome marker, the Philadelphia chromo-

## Table 21-1. MYELOPROLIFERATIVE DISORDERS

**Acute**
  Acute nonlymphocytic leukemia
    Acute myeloblastic
    Acute progranulocytic
    Acute myelomonocytic
    Acute monocytic
    Erythroleukemia
  Unusual variants
    Megakaryocytic leukemia/acute myelofibrosis
    Eosinophilic leukemia
    Basophilic leukemia
**Chronic**
  Chronic granulocytic leukemia
  Polycythemia vera
  Agnogenic myeloid metaplasia with myelofibrosis
  Primary or essential thrombocythemia

some, has been found in erythroid, granulocytic, and megakaryocytic precursors. This suggests that a cell common to these lines is affected in this disease. The other source of evidence for the clonal origin of cells in the myeloproliferative disorders comes from studies of blood and marrow cells using the X-linked isoenzyme G-6-PD.[2] The X chromosome is randomly inactivated early in embryogenesis. Thus, females who are heterozygous (with two X chromosomes) for an X-linked characteristic such as G-6-PD, will have both A and B type enzymes demonstrable in their normal tissues. In individual cells in these heterozygote women there is only one active X chromosome and only one enzyme produced (Fig. 21-1). If a tumor arises from many cells (i.e., is multicellular in origin), both A and B enzymes will be found in tumor lysates. In contrast, if a neoplastic cellular population originates from a single cell then only one isoenzyme will be found, either A or B. Studies in black female G-6-PD heterozygous patients with chronic granulocytic leukemia, polycythemia vera, and essential thrombocythemia have shown a single isoenzyme in red cells, granulocytes, and platelets, indicating the clonal nature of these myeloproliferative disorders and the involvement of a pluripotent stem cell. In patients with myelofibrosis complicating these dis-

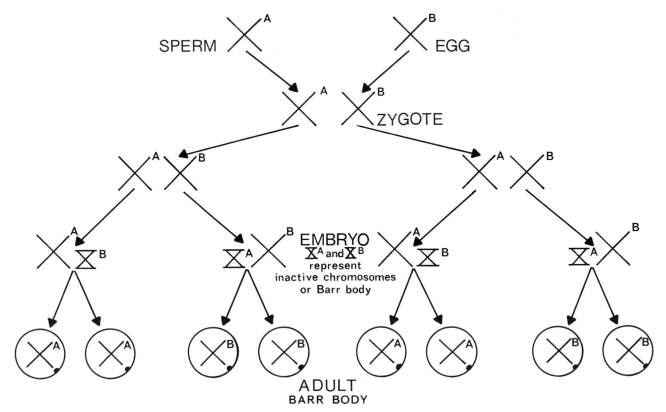

**Figure 21-1.** The enzyme glucose-6-phosphate dehydrogenase (G-6-PD) is present on the X chromosome, and in black populations two types of enzymes are commonly encountered, designated type A and type B. At conception, in a female who is a G-6-PD heterozygote, the paternal X chromosome will have one enzyme (e.g., type A) and the maternal X chromosome the other (e.g., type B). During embryogenesis in each somatic cell, one X chromosome becomes inactive and can be recognized in adult cells as condensed nuclear chromation or Barr body.

Normal tissues in a G-6-PD heterozygote when lysed and subjected to electrophoresis will show the presence of both types of enzyme, even though individual cells contain a single enzyme. If a tumor arises from many cells (is multicellular in origin), both A and B enzymes will be present in the tumor tissue. In contrast, if a tumor arises from a single cell (is of clonal origin) then only a single enzyme—either A or B—will be found in the tumor.

orders or in whom the fibrosis is associated with agnogenic myeloid metaplasia, G-6-PD marker studies have shown the marrow fibroblasts to have both enzymes. This finding, therefore, indicates that the fibroblasts are not derived from the neoplastic clone and the fibrosis most likely represents a reactive response or hyperplasia.[3]

Isoenzyme marker studies in acute myeloproliferative disorders have revealed the clonal yet heterogeneous nature of acute nonlymphocytic leukemia. In some patients the leukemia involves a multipotent stem cell, whereas in other (usually young) patients the disease involves a progenitor already committed to granulocyte/macrophage differentiation.[4]

## ACUTE MYELOPROLIFERATIVE DISORDERS

Acute nonlymphocytic leukemia (ANLL) can be morphologically divided into several subtypes, depending on the predominant cell. Hence, there is acute myeloblastic leukemia and acute myelomonocytic leukemia (the two most common subtypes), acute progranulocytic, acute monocytic, and erythroleukemia. The most widely used classification is the French-American-British (FAB) one. ANLL occurs predominantly in adults. The classification and nature of the acute leukemias are discussed in Chapter 19.

An unusual variant is acute megakaryocytic leukemia, in which the blast cells contain platelet peroxidase rather than myeloperoxidase. Intensive marrow fibrosis may be associated with this leukemia, and the disease may present as acute myelofibrosis. The prognosis is poor, with survival not exceeding one year in most cases.

## CHRONIC MYELOPROLIFERATIVE DISORDERS
### Common Clinical and Hematologic Features

The chronic myeloproliferative disorders are predominantly diseases of the middle-aged and older age groups. In chronic granulocytic leukemia (CGL) (also called chronic myelogenous leukemia, or CML), the peak incidence is in the 40- to 50-year age group, in polycythemia vera the 50- to 60-year age group, and in agnogenic myeloid metaplasia and essential thrombocythemia the 50- to 70-year age group. All of these diseases are usually insidious in onset, and some patients may be asymptomatic and the diagnosis made at the time of a routine physical examination. A few patients may present in blast crises or with a frank leukemic blood picture, and the diagnosis of an underlying chronic myeloproliferative disease may not be obvious. Splenomegaly is the most consistent physical finding, and a common but less frequent occurrence is hepatomegaly. Laboratory studies may reveal a normochromic, normocytic anemia (except in polycythemia vera); basophilia; hyperuricemia; markedly elevated serum vitamin $B_{12}$ levels; and abnormal leukocyte alkaline phosphatase (LAP) values. In patients with CGL the LAP value is depressed, whereas in those with polycythemia vera it is elevated. When a patient with CGL enters an accelerated phase of the disease, the LAP value rises. The LAP values in patients with agnogenic myeloid metaplasia and essential thrombocythemia are variable. Cytogenetic abnormalities are found in marrow and blood metaphases in patients with myeloproliferative disorders. The Philadelphia chromosome t(9;22) is present in about 90 percent of patients with CGL.[5] Other karyotypic abnormalities have been noted in polycythemia vera and agnogenic myeloid metaplasia, yet none are consistently found or are unique to these diseases.

Myelofibrosis can complicate any of the myeloproliferative disorders and is usually present at the time of diagnosis of agnogenic myeloid metaplasia. When myelofibrosis occurs in the course of polycythemia vera or essential thrombocythemia, it may render these diseases indistinguishable from agnogenic myeloid metaplasia. In patients with CGL complicated by myelofibrosis, the detection of the Philadelphia chromosome will reveal that the underlying disease is indeed CGL. A comparison of cellular proliferation, LAP, and cytogenetic findings in the myeloproliferative disorders is provided in Table 21–2.

### Specific Chronic Myeloproliferative Disorders

The chronic myeloproliferative disorders comprise chronic granulocytic leukemia (see Chapter 20), polycythemia vera (see Chapter 15), agnogenic myeloid metaplasia, and essential thrombocythemia. To avoid redundancy, only the latter two entities will be discussed here.

#### Agnogenic Myeloid Metaplasia

**Etiology and Pathology.** The etiology of agnogenic myeloid metaplasia is unknown. The disease has two major components. The first is extramedullary hematopoiesis in the spleen and liver (and other organs, in some instances). The second is marrow fibrosis or myelofibrosis, which can be severe with marked fibroblastic proliferation and calcification (osteosclerosis). Studies of women heterozygous for isoenzymes A and B G-6-PD have shown that peripheral red cells, white cells, and platelets (derived from marrow or extramedullary sources or both) have a single enzyme and therefore presumably arise from a single, multipotential stem cell.[3] In contrast, the marrow fibroblasts contain both enzymes,

Table 21-2. COMPARISON OF CELLULAR PROLIFERATION, LAP, AND CYTOGENETIC FINDINGS IN MPD

| Diagnosis | RBC | Granulocytes | Platelets | Fibroblasts | LAP | Chromosomal Abnormality |
|---|---|---|---|---|---|---|
| Chronic granulocytic leukemia | 0–↓ | 4+ | 0–3+ | 0–2+ | ↓ | Ph¹ 90% |
| Polycythemia vera | 4+ | 1–2+ | 1–3+ | 0–2+ | ↑↑↑ | Aneuploidy 25% |
| Agnogenic myeloid metaplasia | 0–↓ | ↓1–2+ | ↓0–3+ | 2–4+ | N–↑ | Monosomy or trisomy; group C chromosomes |
| Essential thrombocythemia | 0–1+ | 0–1+ | 4+ | 0–2+ | N–↑ | Normal |
| Cellular proliferation | Clonal proliferation | Clonal proliferation | Clonal proliferation | Nonclonal proliferation | — | — |

indicating that they are not derived from the abnormal clone. Additional evidence to support the argument that the marrow fibroblasts represent a secondary effect comes from cytogenetic studies in patients with agnogenic myeloid metaplasia. Chromosomal abnormalities detected in blood cells have not been present in the fibroblasts. If the myelofibrosis is secondary or reactive, what then is the provoking stimulus? Platelets and megakaryocytes contain a potent growth factor, which stimulates fibroblastic proliferation.[6] Serial bone marrow biopsies in patients with agnogenic myeloid metaplasia reveal that as the fibrosis progresses, megakaryocytes are the last cells to be eliminated from the marrow. Thus, it may be that megakaryocytes and platelets abnormally release platelet derived growth factor, which stimulates fibroblast proliferation.

Exposure to benzene or its derivatives and ionizing radiation has been associated with an increased frequency of myeloid metaplasia and myelofibrosis. An increased incidence of myelofibrosis has been reported in survivors of the Hiroshima atomic bomb blast and in patients with polycythemia vera treated with [32]P. Immunologic mechanisms have also been entertained as pathogenetic factors in agnogenic myeloid metaplasia. A high incidence of immune complexes has been demonstrated in patients with myelofibrosis.[7]

**Clinical Features.** The disease affects men slightly more frequently than women, and the majority of patients are between 60 and 70 years of age at the time of diagnosis. Patients present with symptoms and signs of anemia such as weakness, palpitations, dyspnea on exertion, and pallor. As the spleen enlarges, patients become aware of a fullness or mass in the left upper quadrant. Early satiety results from pressure of the spleen on the stomach. Occasionally, patients present with acute left-sided abdominal pain due to splenic infarction. Bleeding manifestations occur as a result of thrombocytopenia, qualitative platelet defects, and coagulation abnormalities. Patients may have petechiae, ecchymoses, and gastrointestinal or urogenital bleeding.

About one third of patients are asymptomatic at presentation, and peripheral blood findings or splenomegaly leads to the diagnosis.

Splenomegaly is the most common and striking physical finding **(see Color Figure 183)**. It has been estimated that the spleen enlarges approximately 2 cm per year. The spleen is mildly enlarged in one third of patients, palpable 5 cm below the left costal margin in another third, and massively enlarged in the remaining third.[8] The splenic enlargement is due to extramedullary hematopoiesis as well as congestion from increased blood flow through the celiac axis. Hepatomegaly is present in the majority of patients and results from both extramedullary hematopoiesis and increased blood flow **(see Color Figure 184)**. In splenectomized patients the liver enlarges to a much greater degree and can fill the entire right side of the abdomen. Extramedullary hematopoiesis can occur in other organs, and lymphadenopathy and renal and pulmonary manifestations have been reported in some patients with myelofibrosis. Ascites and pleural effusions have been seen in patients in whom extramedullary hematopoiesis develops on the pleural and peritoneal surfaces.

Progressive weight loss, worsening anemia and thrombocytopenia, and increasing organomegaly herald the terminal phase of the disease. The five-year survival is about 50 percent of that expected for age- and sex-matched controls.[8] The common causes of death are degenerative cardiovascular disease in 35 percent, hemorrhage in 25 percent, acute leukemia in 25 percent, and infection in 15 percent.[9]

**Laboratory Features.** In nearly all patients there is ineffective erythropoiesis, and with progressive splenomegaly there is increasing splenic sequestration and shortened red cell survival. About 70 percent of patients develop a normochromic, normocytic anemia; and in patients with gastrointestinal or other chronic bleeding, iron deficiency results in a hypochromic-microcytic anemia. Red cell mass and plasma volume measurements using radioisotypes may show an expanded plasma volume and hemoconcentration in a massively enlarged spleen (splenic pooling). Ferrokinetic studies using $^{59}$Fe may be of value in demonstrating reduced sacral marrow activity and increasing hematopoiesis in the spleen and liver. Thrombocytopenia occurs in about one third of the patients, and thrombocytosis in excess of 800,000/$\mu l^3$ in about 12 percent.[8] Qualitative platelet abnormalities can be detected by a prolonged bleeding time and an abnormal second wave of platelet aggregation in response to collagen and epinephrine. The white cell count may be within the normal range, elevated, or decreased. The peripheral blood smear reveals characteristic morphologic abnormalities **(see Color Figure 185)**. There are teardrop-shaped erythrocytes and a leukoerythroblastic reaction (i.e., nucleated red cells and early myeloid precursors circulating in the blood) **(see Color Figure 131)**. Giant platelets and megakaryocytic fragments can also be seen.

The bone marrow aspirate usually gives a "dry tap," and the bone marrow biopsy shows varying degrees of reticulin or collagen fibrosis. Islands of hematopoiesis can be found early in the disease within the marrow. Megakaryocytes may be the most prominent hematopoietic cells seen. The megakaryocytes may also exhibit atypical morphologic features, being large and having abnormal nuclear ploidy. The leukocyte alkaline phosphatase score is variable; it is usually normal but may be elevated or lowered. When patients develop osteosclerosis, there may be radiographic evidence of increased bone density.

No specific chromosomal abnormality has been found in patients with agnogenic myeloid metaplasia. Trisomy and monosomy of C group chromosomes are the most commonly encountered. In one study the presence of chromosomal abnormalities was associated with a worse prognosis but was not predictive of an acute leukemic outcome.[10]

**Treatment.** According to Silverstein,[8] approximately 80 percent of asymptomatic patients with agnogenic myeloid metaplasia seen at diagnosis will remain stable for five years. Patients who are asymptomatic are best left untreated. When patients present with or develop symptomatic anemia, they may require periodic blood transfusions. Trials with androgens (oxymethalone 50 to 200 mg/day orally) or glucocorticoids (prednisone 30 to 60 mg/day for 1 to 4 weeks) are worth trying, because occasionally patients will respond to such treatment, thus lessening transfusion needs. Patients receiving oxymethalone require close monitoring of liver function, and prednisone in therapeutic dosages is poorly tolerated by older patients if continued for several weeks. Folic acid 1 mg/day should be administered to those patients who have chronic hemolytic components to their anemia. Similarly, oral iron supplementation should be given to those patients who develop hypochromic, microcytic anemia secondary to blood loss.

Splenectomy may be indicated in patients with agnogenic-myeloid metaplasia who have (1) painfully enlarged spleen; (2) severe refractory hemolytic anemia; (3) severe thrombocytopenia; and (4) portal hypertension. In patients with severe preoperative thrombocytopenia or qualitative platelet defects (particularly prolonged bleeding time), platelet transfusions may be necessary before and during surgery. In patients in whom surgery is contraindicated because of other medical conditions, radiation therapy in doses of 50 to 200 rads will reduce the spleen size and ameliorate splenic pain. However, within three to four months, splenomegaly recurs. Abdominal radiation is of value in patients with ascites due to peritoneal myeloid metaplasia, and bone radiation is recommended for those patients with severe bone pain due to localized leukemic infiltrates or granulocytic sarcomas.

The alkylating agents busulfan or chlorambucil can be prescribed to lower markedly elevated leukocyte (>50,000/mm³) and platelet counts (>1,000,000/mm³). Hydroxyurea is another chemotherapeutic agent of value in treating patients with myeloid metaplasia with marked organomegaly. When the disease terminates in acute leukemia, intensive chemotherapy is not recommended and only supportive care should be provided.

**Differential Diagnosis.** Besides differentiating it from the other chronic myeloproliferative diseases, agnogenic myeloid metaplasia must be differentiated from metastatic carcinoma, tuberculosis, and fungal infections—all of which can be associated with myelofibrosis. Carcinoma of the prostate in particular may cause myelofibrosis, associated with the development of splenomegaly due to myeloid metaplasia. The osteosclerotic bone lesions in this type of metastatic cancer may be radiologically difficult to distinguish from osteosclerosis associated with agnogenic myeloid metaplasia.

In Table 21–2, the major distinguishing features of the four myeloproliferative disorders are listed. However, patients with previous histories of polycythemia vera and essential thrombocythemia may develop the clinical and hematologic features of agnogenic myeloid metaplasia. Without the antecedent history, the underlying disease will not be apparent. In chronic granulocytic leukemia with myelofibrosis, the presence of the Philadelphia chromosome and the low leukocyte alkaline phosphatase score are the strongest differentiating features that distinguish these disease from agnogenic myeloid metaplasia.

### Essential Thrombocythemia

Also known as primary thrombocythemia or primary thrombohemorrhagic thrombocythemia, essential thrombocythemia is characterized by a sustained platelet count of greater than 1,000,000/$\mu l$, megakaryocytic hyperplasia, adequate marrow iron stores, and the absence of an increased red cell mass or the Philadelphia chromosome. Like the other chronic myeloproliferative diseases, essential thrombocythemia is a clonal disorder originating in a multipotent stem cell.

**Clinical Features.** Most patients are more than 50 years old at diagnosis, but the disease has also been described in young adults. About 20 percent of patients are asymptomatic at the time of diagnosis, which usually follows the incidental finding of a markedly elevated platelet count. Patients who are symptomatic present with symptoms of anemia or with hemorrhagic or thrombotic episodes. The gastrointestinal tract is the most common site of bleeding; skin, mucous membranes, and nose are less common sites. Following trauma or surgery, protracted bleeding may be the first sign of thrombocytosis. Bleeding is mainly due to abnormal platelet function. Thrombosis is the other major manifestation of the disease and is related to thrombocytosis and platelet hyperaggregability. Peripheral arterial occlusion, cerebrovascular thrombosis, transient cerebral ischemic attacks, and occlusion of visceral vessels can all occur. Venous thrombosis can involve veins of the lower extremities, renal veins, and other abdominal veins. In older patients, the combination of increased platelets, platelet functional defects, and degenerative vascular disease all contribute to the hemorrhagic and thrombotic complications.

About half the patients have splenomegaly, which is usually not as prominent as in the other myeloproliferative diseases. According to Silverstein,[11] silent infarction of the spleen occurs in over 20 percent of patients. This is thought to contribute to splenic atrophy. Patients with essential thrombocythemia who have an enlarged spleen have a longer survival than those who do not, perhaps, as Silverstein suggests, because sequestration of platelets in the spleen is beneficial to them.[11] At least 50 percent of patients live five years from diagnosis. In younger patients (under 50 years old) the prognosis appears excellent, but for older patients the bleeding and thrombotic complications pose a constant threat. Of all the chronic myeloproliferative disorders, essential thrombocythemia has been least frequently reported to terminate in acute leukemia.

**Laboratory Features.** The platelet count is markedly elevated usually above $1,000,000/\mu l$. Peripheral blood smear reveals numerous platelets, platelet aggregates, giant platelets (megathrombocytes), and megakaryocyte cytoplasmic fragments **(see Color Figure 186)**. The bone marrow aspirate may be difficult to obtain, as the specimen may clot rapidly. Megakaryocytic hyperplasia and numerous platelets and platelet clumps are found **(see Color Figure 187)**. Megakaryocytes may appear atypical; they may be large, with multiple nuclear lobes or a single nucleus. There may be mild erythroid and myeloid hyperplasia, and the iron stores are adequate. In some patients bone marrow biopsy reveals an increase in reticulin-staining fibers. The red cell count may be normal on presentation, but during the course of the disease, because of bleeding, hypochromic, microcytic anemia occurs in many of the patients. There is a mild neutrophilic leukocytosis with the white blood count ranging from 10,000 to $20,000/\mu l$. The leukocyte alkaline phosphatase score is usually normal. In patients who have sustained splenic atrophy, the peripheral blood may show nucleated red cells and Howell-Jolly bodies. The marrow karyotype is usually normal and the absence of the Philadelphia chromosome distinguishes it from chronic granulocytic leukemia. Platelet function studies reveal abnormalities in the response of platelets to epinephrine and collagen and prolonged bleeding times.

**Differential Diagnosis.** Essential thrombocythemia is to be differentiated from secondary causes of thrombocytosis and the other chronic myeloproliferative diseases in which the platelet count is markedly elevated. Secondary or reactive thrombocytosis seldom causes platelet counts to exceed $1,000,000/\mu l$, and the value most commonly encountered in clinical practice is between 500,000 and $750,000/\mu l$. The causes of secondary thrombocytosis are chronic iron deficiency, gastrointestinal bleeding, inflammatory bowel disease, malignancies, and complications following splenectomy, severe hemorrhage, or hemolysis. When the platelet count rises in reaction to another condition, it is not associated with an increased tendency toward thrombosis or hemorrhage, and functionally the platelets are normal.

Of the myeloproliferative disorders, polycythemia vera may be the most difficult to differentiate from essential thrombocythemia. When patients with polycythemia vera have a normal or decreased red cell mass due to iron deficiency, the platelet count may be markedly elevated. The absence of marrow iron stores excludes the diagnosis of essential thrombocythemia. Agnogenic myeloid metaplasia may be accompanied by extreme thrombocytosis, and without an antecedent history of essential thrombocythemia it is not possible to determine whether it represents a transition from one condition to the other.

**Treatment.** There is considerable controversy regarding the treatment of asymptomatic patients with essential thrombocythemia. Most hematologists would agree that in young patients (less than age 50 years), no treatment is needed for asymptomatic patients regardless of the platelet count. Prior to childbirth or elective surgery in young patients, platelet pheresis is most useful in controlling the extreme platelet count. In patients older than age 50 years who are asymptomatic, some authorities recommend lowering the platelet count by treating the patient with chemotherapeutic agents or $^{32}$P. However, there are studies that indicate that irrespective of the platelet count, there is no increased risk of hemorrhage or thrombosis to these patients.[12] My approach has been not to treat asymptomatic patients unless there is a steady and progressive rise in the platelet count. I favor the use of busulfan or hydroxyurea to lower the platelet count to about 600,000/$\mu$l. Busulfan can be administered for two to three months and then discontinued, and its effect may last for three to nine months before the platelet count again rises to pretreatment levels. Hydroxyurea administration must be continued daily, as once it is stopped the platelet count rapidly rises again. $^{32}$P in doses of 2 to 3 Ci/m intravenously is an effective as an alkylating agent (like busulfan).

In patients who present with gastrointestinal or other bleeding, the platelet count can be rapidly lowered by platelet pheresis or by administering hydroxyurea. Patients who have experienced thrombotic episodes are also treated with platelet count–lowering and antiaggregating agents, such as acetylsalicylic acid and dipyridamole.

## CASE HISTORIES
### Case 1: Essential Thrombocythemia

A 68-year-old woman presented in November 1979 with acute onset of left upper abdominal pain. Her previous medical history was unremarkable. She was a cigarette smoker (up to one pack per day for 25 years). The spleen was palpable 6 cm below the left costal margin, and splenic rub was heard on auscultation. She had no bleeding manifestations in her skin or mucous membranes. Her hematocrit was 45 percent, white cell count 18,200/$\mu$l with 3 percent basophils, and the platelet count was 1,369,000/$\mu$l. A bone marrow aspirate revealed myeloid and megakaryocytic hyperplasia with adequate iron stores. The bone marrow biopsy had an increase in reticulin-staining fibers. The cytogenetic analysis of marrow cells showed a normal karyotype. The leukocyte alkaline phosphatase score was 78 (normal range, 20 to 130). The bleeding time was normal at 6 min, and platelet aggregation studies displayed a loss of the second-phase aggregation response to ATP. The patient was treated with bed rest and analgesics, and when the pain of the splenic infarction resolved she was discharged from the hospital. Aspirin 10 grains/day was prescribed.

Over the next two months the patient's platelet count was found to increase to 1.6 million/$\mu$l, and she complained of pain and cramping in her feet and toes. Her toes were cyanosed, and

there was dependency rubar and elevation pallor. She stopped smoking and was started on a regimen of hydroxyurea 1 g/day, to lower the platelet count. Aspirin was continued at 10 grains/day. The hydroxyurea was continued in dosages varying from 1 g/day to 500 mg five times per week, depending on the blood counts, until the drug was stopped in October 1983. The patient's platelet count during this four-year period varied from 600,000 to 900,000/$\mu$l, and she remained relatively well. In January 1984, she sustained a right-sided transient cerebral ischemic attack and her platelet count had risen to 1.2 million/$\mu$l. The hydroxyurea regimen was started again, and for the past year she has continued with this medication (500 mg/day) and aspirin (5 grains/day). In March 1985, her hematocrit was 40 percent, white cell count 6200/$\mu$l, and platelet count 614,000/$\mu$l.

This 75-year-old woman has a six-year history of essential thrombocythemia. She has had symptoms due to splenic infarction and vascular occlusions. Her platelet count untreated is well in excess of 1,000,000/$\mu$l and responds to the daily oral administration of hydroxyurea. It appears that her arterial insufficiency is most manifest when her platelet count is uncontrolled.

### Case 2: Agnogenic Myeloid Metaplasia

The patient is a 67-year-old retired teacher who was referred for evaluation of pancytopenia. He had noticed progressive exertional dyspnea over the preceding three months and had had two episodes of epistaxis the previous week. He denied any exposure to benzene or petroleum products. His appetite was good, but he noticed early satiety and he had lost about 10 lb over a 12-month period. His previous medical history was unremarkable; he took occasional alcoholic beverages and did not smoke. On examination he was pale and thin, and ecchymoses were present on his upper and lower extremities. His spleen was palpable 8 cm below the left costal margin, and the liver was palpable just below the right costal margin. He had a mild tachycardia (pulse rate 104/min), and had no signs of cardiac failure. His chest and neurologic examinations were normal. Stool specimens did not contain occult blood.

Laboratory evaluations revealed a hematocrit of 23 percent, hemoglobin 7.5 g/dl, MCV 93 fl, MCH 30 pg, MCHC 34.3 g/dl, white cell count of 2500/mm³, with a differential count of neutrophils 50 percent, bands 6 percent, lymphocytes 20 percent, monocytes 9 percent, eosinophils 3 percent, basophils 3 percent, metamyelocytes 4 percent, myelocytes 3 percent, progranulocytes 2 percent, and platelet count 70,000/mm³. Reticulocyte count was 3 percent. The leukocyte alkaline phosphatase score was 64 (normal range, 20 to 120), serum acid 8.5 ng/dl, serum ferritin 132 ng/ml, serum vitamin $B_{12}$ 860 pg/ml, and serum folic acid 4 ng/ml. Chest radiograph was normal, and an abdominal radiograph confirmed the presence of an enlarged spleen. Examination of peripheral blood smear revealed anisocytosis, poikilocytosis, teardrop-shaped erythrocytes, nucleated erythrocytes, large platelets, and immature white cells. A bone marrow aspirate was unsuccessful because of a dry tap, and a bone marrow biopsy revealed large platelets, extensive fibrosis on routine hematoxylin, and easier reticular staining. A diagnosis of myelofibrosis with myeloid metaplasia was made.

The patient received 2 units of packed red cells and was begun on folic acid 1 mg/day and an anabolic steroid (Danazol) 200 mg three times daily. Over the next year, he required blood transfusions every three to four weeks, and epistaxis did not recur.

This patient presenting with pancytopenia and splenomegaly was found to have myelofibrosis in the marrow. The spleen can be expected to enlarge progressively over time, and with worsening of the cytopenia he may benefit from splenectomy. This surgical procedure in elderly patients is not without significant morbidity and mortality. The decision to perform splenectomy should be delayed unless the severity of leukopenia, refractory anemia, or thrombocytopenia makes it essential.

## References

1. Damashek, W: Some speculations on the myeloproliferative syndrome. Blood 6:372, 1951.
2. Fialkow, PJ: The origin and development of human tumors studied with cell markers. N Engl J Med 291:26, 1974.
3. Jacobson, RJ, Salo, A, and Fialkow, PJ: Agnogenic myeloid metaplasia: A colonal proliferation of hemopoietic cells with secondary myelofibrosis. Blood 51:189, 1978.
4. Fialkow, PJ, Singer, JW, Adamson, JW, et al: Heterogeneity of stem cell origin. Blood 57:1068, 1981.
5. Lawler, SD: The cytogenetics of chronic granulocytic leukemia. Clin Haematol 6:55, 1977.
6. Ross, R and Vogel, R: The platelet-derived growth factor. Cell 14:203, 1980.
7. Lewis, CM and Pegrum, GD: Immune complexes in myelofibrosis: A possible guide to management. Br J Haematol 39:233, 1978.
8. Silverstein, MN: Agnogenic Myeloid Metaplasia. Publishing Science Corp, Boston, 1975.
9. Silverstein, MN and Linman, JW: Causes of death in agnogenic myeloid metaplasia. Mayo Clin Proc 44:36, 1969.
10. Nowell, PC and Finan, JB: Cytogenetics of acute and chronic myelofibrosis. Virchows Arch Cell Pathol 29:45, 1978.
11. Silverstein, MN: Primary thrombocythemia. In Williams, WJ, Beutler, E. Erslev, AJ, et al (eds): Hematology, ed 3. McGraw-Hill, New York, 1983, p 218.
12. Kessler, CM, Klein, HG, and Havlik, RJ: Uncontrolled thrombocytosis in chronic myeloproliferative disorders. Br J Haematol 50:157, 1982.

# CHAPTER 22

RONALD A. SACHER, M.D., F.R.C.P.(C)

# Monoclonal Gammopathies and Plasma Cell Dyscrasias

The group of disorders collectively classified as monoclonal gammopathies have one major common denominator; they represent excessive production of an immunoglobulin molecule or parts of an immunoglobulin molecule caused by uncontrolled proliferation of cells of B lymphocyte or plasma cell origin. Because these cells result from the abnormal growth of a single clonal population, the term "monoclonal" refers to the cellular abnormality. The term "gammopathy" refers to an abnormal excess of immunoglobulin proteins, which are, of course, gamma globulins. As these disorders represent uncontrolled cellular growth and abnormal, aberrant immunoglobulin secretion, the principles of each of these will be discussed in sequence.

267

## B LYMPHOCYTE AND PLASMA CELL DEVELOPMENT

As discussed in Chapter 1, lymphocyte development occurs along two major cell lines: (1) T lymphocytes, which are responsible for the complex interactions of cell-mediated immunity; and (2) B lymphocytes, which are concerned with humoral immunity. Both cell types are derived from a single bone marrow stem cell. The disorders discussed in this chapter apply specifically to cells of B lymphocyte origin and to the differentiated B cell—namely, the plasma cell. The development of cells of the B cell lineage and their interactions with T cells are diagrammatically represented in Figure 22-1.

The major characteristic of B lymphocytes and indeed of plasma cells is the ability to produce antibody (i.e., immunoglobulin), and these cells are identified by the presence of cell surface membrane–bound immunoglobulin. Ordinarily, the physiologic mechanisms controlling the cell growth and orderly synthesis of immunoglobulin are regulated by a complex set of interactions that result in the release of specific antibody in response to initiating antigen. Under certain circumstances, this normal response may become uncontrolled, and the process of antibody production may become excessive, leading to the production of a single abnormal immunoglobulin type, as will be described in the disorders classified under the monoclonal gammopathies. Uncontrolled cellular proliferation at any of B lymphocyte development may produce diseases capable of such abnormal antibody production. A brief discussion of immunoglobulin structure, function, and secretion is essential to an understanding of these diseases.

## IMMUNOGLOBULIN STRUCTURE AND FUNCTION

The basic unit of an immunoglobulin molecule is the 7S unit, and all immunoglobulin molecules have variations of this simple unit. The unit consists of two light and two heavy chains, arranged as outlined in Figure 22-2. A specific spatial orientation is achieved by interchain disulfide bonds. Each of the light chains and heavy chains are arranged into domains, or regions.

Within the two identical light chains there are two domains, and within the two identical heavy chains there are four domains consisting of specific amino acid sequence. As indicated in Figure 22-2, the structure has an amino terminal and a carboxy terminal. The molecular orientation toward the amino terminal consists of the antigen binding sites comprising approximately 107 amino acids in the light chains. This region is termed variable, because the amino acid sequences vary in accordance with the initiating antigen. Therefore, it is this sequential arrangement that determines the antibody specificity. The light chains comprise 214 amino acids with a molecular weight of approximately 24,000 daltons. The remaining 107 amino acids oriented toward the carboxy terminal comprise the C, or constant, region of the molecule. These sequences are constant for all specific light chains. Within the V domain, some areas show extreme variability and are termed "hypervariable regions." It is these points that are probably the contact points of antigen binding. The constant region sequences determine the properties of the molecule and, specifically with regard to the heavy chain molecule, determine the effector functions. In this regard the

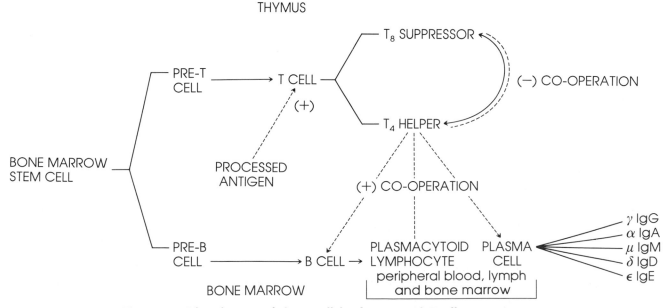

**Figure 22-1.** B lymphocyte and plasma cell development with T cell cooperation.

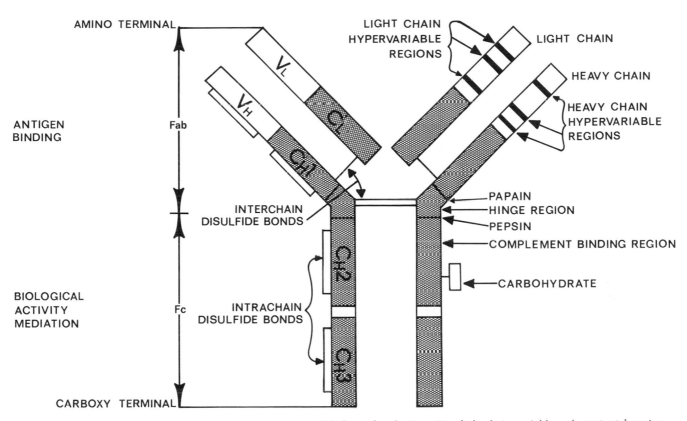

**Figure 22-2.** Diagram showing basic structure of the immunoglobulin molecule. $V_L + C_L$ = light chain variable and constant domains, respectively, $V_H + C_H1$; $C_H2$; $C_H3$ = heavy chain variable and constant domains, respectively.

constant regions for the heavy chains determine whether the molecule is complement binding, neutrophil binding, and so forth. It is these regions that are oriented toward cellular receptors.

There are two types of light chains, designated kappa ($\kappa$) and lambda ($\lambda$). The molecular differences are based on specific differences in the constant region structure that are the same for the specific light chain (e.g., kappa or lambda). The ratio of kappa to lambda chains in plasma immunoglobulins is 2:1.

Each heavy chain has a molecular weight varying between 50,000 and 70,000 daltons, the weight being proportional to the length of the constant region. The variable region of the heavy chain has an amino acid structure similar to that of the variable region of the light chain. For the heavy chain, then, this region also imparts antigen specificity. As shown in Figure 22-2, the constant region of the heavy chain has three domains, each 110 amino acids in length and designated $C_{H1}$, $C_{H2}$, and $C_{H3}$. There are five major classes of heavy chains; gamma ($\gamma$), alpha ($\alpha$), mu ($\mu$), delta ($\delta$), and epsilon ($\epsilon$). These correspond to the immunoglobulin types IgG, IgA, IgM, IgD, and IgE, respectively. The complete immunoglobulin molecule consists of two chains of a specific type of heavy chain (either gamma, alpha, mu, delta, or epsilon) and two chains of a specific light chain (either kappa or lambda, but not both).

As shown in Figure 22-2, the hinge region represents the site of proteolytic cleavage. Under the influence of certain proteolytic enzymes, the immunoglobulins are broken up into fragments. Specifically, two enzymes have been useful in identifying physical and functional fragments. Following papain digestion of the immunoglobulin molecule, three fragments are produced. There are two identical Fab fragments (containing the antigen-binding sites) and one Fc fragment (containing crystallizable and constant binding sites). The Fab portion contains the whole light chain plus the variable portion of the heavy chain. Therefore, with papain digestion, the antigen binding sites may be removed from the constant region of the heavy chain. Following pepsin digestion, however, several fragments are produced, including one large Fab fragment that contains the two joined Fab fragments of the immunoglobulin molecule designated F(ab$^1$)2 and several digested small fragment products of the Fc region. In both cases, following digestion, intact light chains and portions of the heavy variable chain region are obtained. The Fab fragment represents antibody specificity, whereas the Fc fragment represents the portion of the molecule containing biologic activity (such as complement activation, placental transfer, and macrophage attachment.

## IMMUNOGLOBULIN CLASSES

As mentioned, the immunoglobulin classes are distinguished by molecular differences within the Fc portion of the heavy chain. Subclasses of the immunoglobulins also exist. There are four subclasses of IgG, designated 1 through 4, and two subclasses of IgA. Other subclasses also exist and impart different physical and biologic activity. The characteristics of the immunoglobulin classes are outlined in Table 22–1. Certain points, however, are worthy of highlighting. As can be seen, IgG is generally a monomeric immunoglobulin; however, IgG3 subclass may undergo polymerization and when present in excess may contribute to increased plasma viscosity. IgA represents 13 percent of the total immunoglobulin level. It generally exists in a dimeric form, bound to a J (joining) chain polypeptide and a secretory peptide (which imparts functional and protective properties). It is the major immunoglobulin found in body secretions.

IgM forms 6 percent of the total immunoglobulin content and is a pentamer of 5 units of monomeric chains joined by disulfide bonds. IgD and IgM are the main surface immunoglobulins present on B cells. The characteristics of IgD and IgE are listed in Table 22–1.

## INTRACELLULAR SYNTHESIS AND EXCRETION OF IMMUNOGLOBULINS

Genetic coding for light chains are found on chromosomes 2 (kappa) and 22 (lambda). The coding for heavy chains are believed to be found on chromosomes 14 and 8. The DNA sequences that are responsible for coding of the amino acid composition of the immunoglobulins exist in unprimed B lymphocytes in a germ line fashion. During the differentiation of the B lymphocytes, the immunoglobulin genes become rearranged in an apparently orderly fashion, although the actual control mechanisms are uncertain.

Light chain immunoglobulin rearrangement appears to occur first, followed by heavy chain rearrangement. The variable and constant DNA sequences are subsequently oriented facilitating translation by messenger RNA. Synthesis of complete heavy and light chains occurs on the polyribosomes, in the rough endoplasmic reticulum of the cell cytoplasm. The synthesis of heavy and light chains takes place at different sites on the endoplasmic reticulum. The synthesized heavy and light chains are released into the cisternal space of the rough endoplasmic reticulum and are then combined to form a four-chain product. Within the Golgi apparatus of the cell, carbohydrate moieties are attached and the immunoglobulin secreted from the cell by reverse pinocytosis (Fig. 22-3). It remains attached to the cell membrane for an uncertain length of time. The full regulation mechanism is uncertain. It appears that the synthesis of heavy and light chains is not exactly balanced, and often excess light chains are synthesized. Furthermore, even though two genes exist (from both parents) that are each capable of rearranging their DNA sequences from germ line to committed DNA arrangement, only one species of light chain and heavy chain is synthesized by the cell, even though the cell has the capacity to synthesize all species. Thus, it appears that the expression of the other alleles is excluded, and this process of exclusion is termed "allelic exclusion." Nevertheless, the marked variation in the variable regions and the potential for variable expression enhance the cell's capabilities of manufacturing an immunoglobulin that is complementary to the initiating antigen, of which there is tremendous diversity.

## CLINICAL LABORATORY EVALUATION OF IMMUNOGLOBULIN DISORDERS

### Serum

#### Serum Protein Electrophoresis

Serum protein electrophoresis is the process whereby the patient's serum proteins are separated by electrical charge and molecular size when ex-

### Table 22–1. IMMUNOGLOBULIN CLASSES: PHYSICAL AND BIOLOGIC PROPERTIES

|  | IgG | IgA | IgM | IgD | IgE |
|---|---|---|---|---|---|
| Heavy chain class | $\gamma$ | $\alpha$ | $\mu$ | $\delta$ | $\epsilon$ |
| Subclass | $\gamma^1\gamma^2\gamma^3\gamma^4$ | $\alpha^1\alpha^2$ | $\mu^1\mu^2$ |  |  |
| Molecular weights | 150,000 | 160,000 (monomer) 400,000 (secretory) | 900,000 | 180,000 | 196,000 |
| Sedimentation coefficient | 6.7 | 7–15 | 19 | 7 | 8 |
| Serum concentration (mg/ml) | 8–16 | 1.4–4.0 | 0.5–2.0 | 0–0.4 | 17–450 ng/ml |
| Biologic half-life (days) | 23 | 6 | 5 | 2.8 | 2.4 |
| Intravascular distribution (%) | 45 | 42 | 76 | 75 | 51 |
| Complement fixation | + (variable) | — | ++++ | — | — |
| Placental transfer | + ($\gamma^1\gamma^3$) | — | — | — | — |
| Basophil/mast cell receptors | — | — | — | — | ++++ |
| Percent of total Ig | 80 | 13 | 6 | 1 | 0.002 |

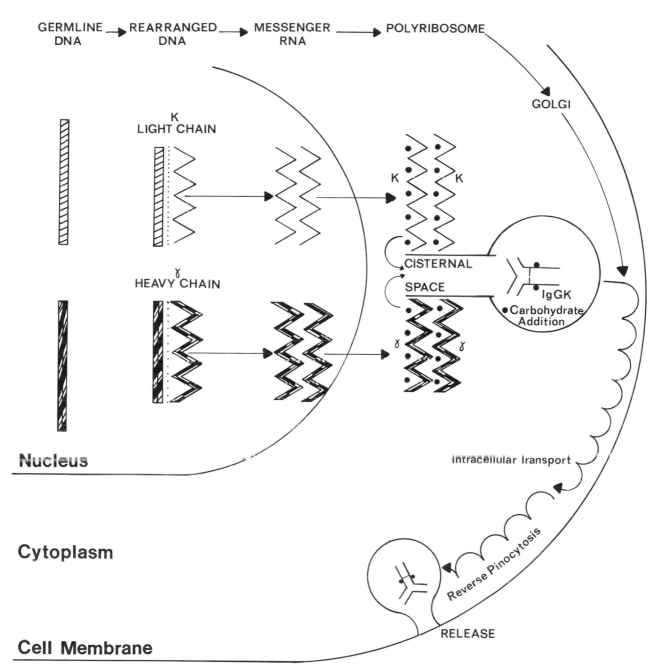

**Figure 22-3.** Schematic representation of IgGκ immunoglobulin synthesis at a cellular level.

posed to an electrical current. The serum is placed on a support medium, most commonly cellulose acetate, within an electrostatic medium. An electrical charge is applied to the medium, and as a consequence, the serum proteins separate. Figure 22-4 shows the major serum protein components separated into the albumin and the globulin fractions. Immunoglobulins separate electrophoretically as the gamma globulins. Following separation, the cellulose acetate is stained with a protein stain (e.g., Ponceau red), the intensity of the stain reflecting the

amount of protein present. This may then be scanned by a densitometer, and a tracing pattern is obtained. Several different patterns may be seen, depending on the amount of the specific proteins and whether immunoglobulin production is excessive or depleted. Differing profiles are outlined in Figure 22-4. In situations of monoclonal production of an abnormal protein, a so-called monoclonal spike, or M spike, is obtained. In this disorder, a single population of immunoglobulin-producing cells synthesizes a homogeneous immunoglobulin

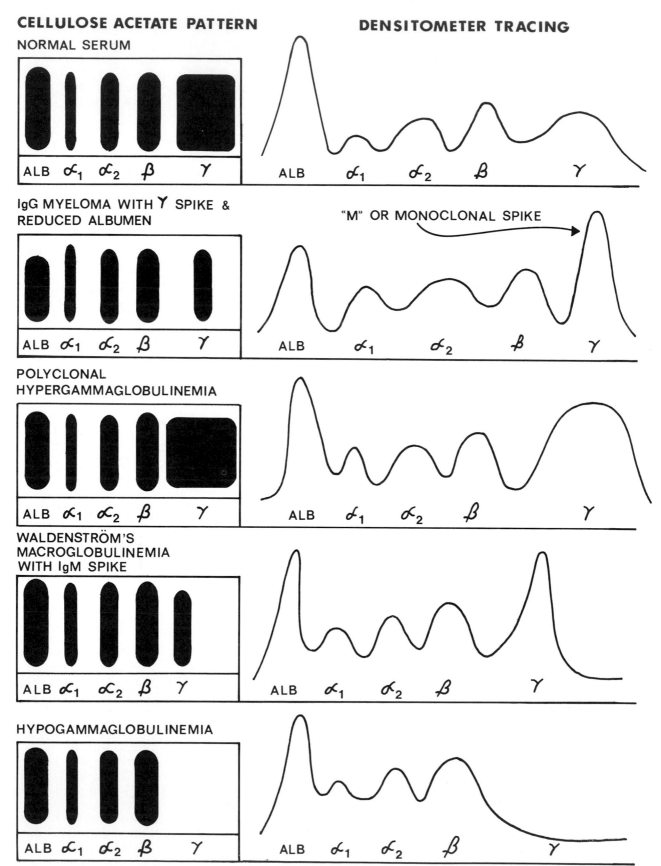

**Figure 22-4.** Serum protein electrophoretic profiles in differing medical conditions.

that has monospecific physical properties. Therefore, upon electrophoresis this protein separates from other serum proteins in a uniform manner. In circumstances when many immunoglobulin-producing cells proliferate in response to an infectious or inflammatory stimulus, heterogeneous immunoglobulin molecules are produced, each with different physical properties that, when separated by this procedure, exhibit a broad-base gamma globulin pattern (Fig. 22-4). This test, therefore, can serve as a screen to differentiate monoclonal from polyclonal hypergammaglobulinemia, as well as to differentiate other qualitative protein abnormalities occurring in the patient's serum.

Serum protein electrophoresis (SPEP) does not identify the class of the immunoglobulin but indicates the relative percentage of the separated proteins and whether in conditions of gamma globulin excess the process is likely to be monoclonal or polyclonal.

Certain clues can be present that may help distinguish whether the abnormal immunoglobulin is IgG or IgA. Because IgA contains more carbohydrate and therefore a more negative charge, it tends to migrate faster toward the anode. Light chains also tend to migrate faster toward the anode, by virtue of their charge and smaller size. Examples of the different SPEP patterns are shown in Figure 22-4.

It is apparent that the SPEP and densitometer scan profile can differentiate a monoclonal gammopathy from a polyclonal gammopathy (Fig. 22-4), but that it does not elucidate the type or nature of the monoclonal paraprotein. Although a quantitative value is given, the value neither accurately reflects the level of immunoglobulin nor differentiates the immunoglobulin class.

## Immunoelectrophoresis

Immunoelectrophoresis (IEP) couples electrophoretic separation with a two-dimensional immunodiffusion reaction and is used for specific identification and semiquantitative estimation of immunoglobulin class. The technical process requires the placement of the serum sample in agar followed by subsequent electrophoresis. Following the completion of electrophoresis, a lateral well is prepared along one margin of the slide or gel. The following specific antiserum is then applied to the individual wells; anti–whole blood human serum; anti-IgG (gamma chains); anti-IgM (mu chains); anti-IgA (alpha chains); anti-kappa; and anti-lambda (Fig. 22-5). Diffusion is then allowed to proceed, and the precipitant lines form. The relative thickness of the individual bands is proportional to their concentrations. The relative positions of the electrophoretic migration can also aid in their identity. This approach is the definitive method for identifying monoclonal immunoglobulins. Immunoelectrophoresis allows for identification of specific heavy and light chains but cannot verify the existence of an entire immunoglobulin molecule containing both two heavy and two light chains.

If protein excretion occurs in the urine, the urine may be concentrated, and the protein may also be analyzed by IEP. The urine sample would then be substituted for the patient's serum.

## Immunoglobulin Quantitation

Immunoglobulin quantitation is usually performed using the radial immunodiffusion technique. Antibody to the immunoglobulin is incorporated into the agar gel, which is then poured onto a plate or a glass slide. Wells are cut into the agar, and the test material—usually patient serum—is applied to the wells. The concentration of the immunoglobulin in milligrams per deciliter is proportional to the diameters of the precipitin rings.

# Urine: Tests for Light Chains

## Urine Immunoelectrophoresis

This is the definitive test and allows for differentiation between kappa and lambda light chains in the urine (Fig. 22-5D).

## Sulfosalicylic Acid Test

This precipitation procedure quantitates of the total amount of protein present in a 24-hour concentrated urine sample.

## Heat Precipitation Test

This procedure is based on the original test for detection of Bence-Jones proteins and is a qualitative test for the presence of urinary light chains. Upon heating the urine sample to 56°C, Bence-Jones proteins will precipitate. This precipitate will resolubilize upon heating beyond 56°C. The reciprocal events occur on cooling from above 56°C.

# CLASSIFICATION OF MONOCLONAL GAMMOPATHIES

Monoclonal gammopathies are generally classified according to the clinical course (benign or malignant), the proliferating cell type (lymphomas,[1] macroglobulinemia, or multiple myeloma), and the nature of the abnormal immunoglobulin produced (IgG, IgA, light chain, and so on). An outline of the classification is given in Table 22–2.[8,9,10]

## Malignant Monoclonal Gammopathies

### Multiple Myeloma

**Subtypes of Myeloma.** Multiple myeloma represents an uncontrolled growth and proliferation of plasma cells in a progressive manner, leading ulti-

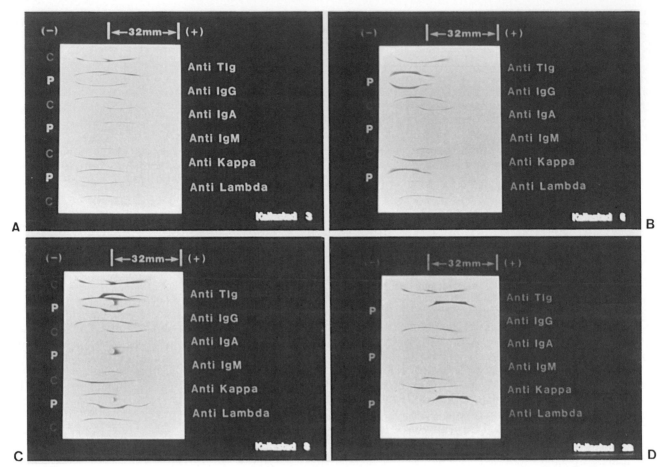

**Figure 22-5.** *A*, IEP: normal polyclonal pattern. This demonstrates a normal polyclonal pattern. Evaluation of IEP patterns begins by observing reactions to the patient's serum with antiserum to total immunoglobulins (anti-TIg) and then identifying the individual components of the reaction with each monospecific antiserum. The anti-TIg is a polyvalent antiserum with specificity to IgG, IgA, IgM, kappa (K), and lambda (L) antigens. The precipitin arcs of the patient sample (P) are evaluated according to shape, density, and position and compared with those of a normal serum control (C). The electrophoretic migration of an immunoglobulin depends on its amino acid composition. After separation by electrophoresis, the antigens (immunoglobulins) diffuse through the agarose radially, depending on the concentration and size of the molecules and react with the antibodies that have diffused linearly from the trough. This reaction generates elliptical precipitin arcs. Note the kappa arc mimics a composite of the IgG and IgA precipitin arcs and is symmetrical to the lambda precipitin arc. This symmetry reflects both the normal kappa : lambda ratio and the polyclonal nature of the immunoglobulins. IgM, which exists as a pentamer, diffuses more slowly through the gel than IgG or IgA does. Consequently, the light chains attached to IgM are not represented in the K and L light chain reactions in a normal pattern.

*B*, IEP: IgG kappa monoclonal protein. The use of a standard protocol and established criteria facilitates interpretation of IEP patterns. Monoclonal immunoglobulins are the product of single clonal proliferations of plasma cells. The criteria that define a monoclonal protein are (1) limited electrophoretic mobility of a single immunoglobulin class and (2) a deviation in the kappa : lambda ratio in the area of restricted mobility. Both of these criteria are demonstrated in this part of the figure. This pattern presents a typical laboratory finding for a patient with plasma cell myeloma. The dense IgG arc shows restricted electrophoretic mobility, which is duplicated by the kappa reaction. The weak lambda reaction reflects the lowered concentration of normal immunoglobulins. IgA and IgM are markedly reduced. The presence of a serum or urine monoclonal protein may be used as one of the criteria for the diagnosis of plasma cell myeloma or other B cell malignancies. These laboratory findings, along with radiologic data and bone marrow pathology, contribute the the diagnosis of plasma cell myeloma.

*C*, IEP: monoclonal IgG lambda with free lambda monoclonal light chains. Here the patient's serum reaction with anti-TIg IgG shows two atypical precipitin arcs. The very dense arc seen with the antiserum is duplicated in the lambda reaction, typing the protein as a monoclonal IgG lambda. The IgA and IgM precipitin reactions appear reduced, indicating their decreased concentrations. The second arc seen with the anti-TIg migrating anode to, or faster than, the IgG reaction is also duplicated in the lambda light chain reaction. The absence of a corresponding reaction with IgG, IgA, or IgM aligning with this faster lambda arc suggests two possibilities: (1) a monoclonal protein of a minor immunoglobulin class — IgD or IgE — or (2) free lambda monoclonal light chains (i.e., lambda Bence-Jones protein).

*D*, IEP: urine kappa monoclonal light chains. A protein electrophoresis of this urine demonstrated a single discrete band in the beta-gamma area. Because the protein level was significant, the urine was only concentrated 25 times and evaluated by IEP to identify the band. The kappa precipitin reaction parallels the reaction in the anti-TIg identifying a kappa monoclonal protein. Notice that the arc is quite close to the trough, indicating the rapid diffusion typical of low molecular weight light proteins. The absence of corresponding precipitin reactions with any class-specific antisera implies the presence of kappa Bence-Jones protein in the urine.

**Table 22–2. CLASSIFICATION OF MONOCLONAL GAMMOPATHY**

I. Monoclonal gammopathy of uncertain significance (MGUS)
   Tumor-associated gammopathy
   Biclonal gammopathy
   Monoclonal gammopathy associated with miscellaneous disorders
II. Malignant monoclonal gammopathy
   Multiple myeloma
      Smouldering myeloma
      Nonsecretory myeloma
      Plasma cell leukemia
   Plasmacytoma
      Localized (solitary)
      Diffuse
      Extramedullary
   Monoclonal gammopathy associated with
      lymphoproliferative disease
      Malignant lymphoma
      Waldenström's macroglobulinemia
   Heavy chain disease
   Primary systemic amyloidosis

mately to the death of the patient. It is a disease of the elderly, generally those past the age of 40, and may be characterized by diffuse plasma cell involvement of the marrow **(see Color Figures 188 and 189)** and overproduction of either intact monoclonal immunoglobulins (IgG, IgA, and rarely IgD) or light chains only. The more typical presentation of cell proliferation is as a diffuse disorder. However, occasionally the disorder may be focal and may present as tumor masses of plasma cells (plasmacytomas). There are several other variant forms of multiple myeloma that will be discussed; these are smouldering myeloma, nonsecretory myeloma, plasma cell leukemia, and plasmacytomas.

***Smouldering Myeloma.***[12-14] This form of the disease assumes a far more indolent clinical course, which, in the early stages, resembles that of a monoclonal gammopathy of uncertain significance. In this situation there are few symptoms associated with the uncontrolled synthesis of the immune protein. However, with time, neoplastic plasma cells progressively invade the bone marrow parenchyma **(see Color Figures 188 and 189)**. Smouldering myeloma usually does not develop into full-blown multiple myeloma immediately; rather there is a progressive development of clinical symptomatology over the course of several years. Most cases of smouldering myeloma do ultimately terminate into some form of multiple myeloma.[12]

***Nonsecretory Myeloma.***[13] This variant constitutes less than 1 percent of all multiple myeloma cases. In this disorder, the neoplastic cells are highly dedifferentiated and are incapable of secreting any intact immune protein. These immature plasma cells are nonetheless neoplastic and have marked invasive potential of the bone marrow; they pro-

duce lytic lesions as well as the other stigmata of multiple myeloma, except for secretion.

***Plasma Cell Leukemia.***[13] This particular disorder occurs when the neoplastic cells spill over from the overcrowded bone marrow into the general circulation **(see Color Figure 191)**. In these instances, there are greater than 5 to 10 percent plasma cells in the peripheral blood, and in many instances the peripheral blood shows a leukoerythroblastic blood picture. This implies that there are immature white cells as well as nucleated red blood cells in the peripheral blood **(see Color Figure 131)**.

***Plasmacytoma.*** As already mentioned, a plasmacytoma refers to a tumor mass of plasma cells. Plasmacytomas may be localized or generalized **(see Color Figure 192)**. If localized, an actually palpable tumor mass of plasma cells may be present either within the bone marrow (intramedullary) or without (extramedullary). In the case of generalized plasmacytomas, the systemic spread of localized plasmacytomas may evolve, or progeny of the original clone may grow and populate other areas of the bone marrow, thereby producing multiple lytic areas or multiple masses. In most instances, patients with generalized plasmacytomas progress in a fashion similar to that of patients with multiple myeloma.[7,9]

As mentioned, occasionally localized plasmacytomas may be present in an extramedullary situation outside of the bone marrow; they may develop in other organs and tissues systems. The most common site for such involvement is the upper respiratory tract. These patients generally present with localized symptoms, and these disorders may or may not exhibit immunoglobulin secretory manifestations.[7,9]

**Epidemiology.** Multiple myeloma occurs more commonly in blacks than in whites. It is one of the most common malignancies of elderly black people. The incidence of multiple myeloma in whites is approximately two per 100,000. The incidence of the disease increases with age. The higher incidence in blacks suggests that genetic factors may play a role.[3]

Other potential factors that appear to be involved in the pathogenesis of multiple myeloma include radiation exposure. There is a five times greater incidence of multiple myeloma in survivors of the atomic bombs in Hiroshima and Nagasaki than in the unexposed population.

Other theories include the possible association between multiple myeloma and chronic antigenic exposure, such as seen in patients with rheumatoid arthritis or Gaucher's disease. Chronic antigenic exposure in patients with asbestosis has also been associated with multiple myeloma.

Plasma cell myeloma is the most common plasma cell neoplasm.

**Clinical Features.**[7,9,13,14] Patients may be entirely

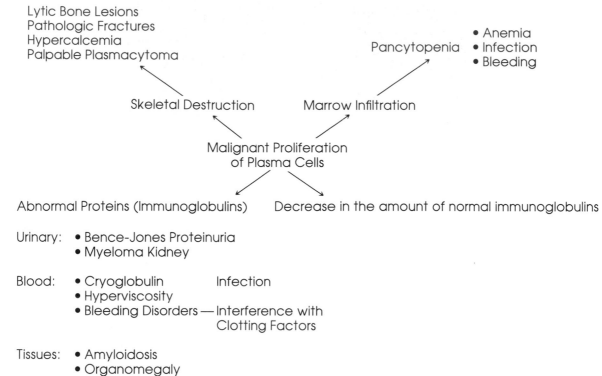

**Figure 22-6.** Diagram outlining the clinical features and complications in multiple myeloma.

asymptomatic on initial presentation. More usually, they present with multiple symptoms (Fig. 22-6).

Bone pain is the major symptom, occurring in about 60 percent of all patients at presentation. Approximately 25 percent of patients present with anemia and renal insufficiency; about 10 percent present with infection; and the remainder present with less common clinical presentations.

The constellation of clinical features presented in multiple myeloma is variable but can be systematically evaluated as follows.

1. Cell Mass
   a. *Localized.* Proliferating cell populations may produce space-occupying lesions that impinge on neighboring structures and cause local effects (for example, compression of the spinal cord).
   b. *Generalized.* Uncontrolled growth of the cell populations may cause repopulation of the bone marrow by the neoplastic plasma cells or B lymphocytes, causing a pancytopenia or even failure of the bone marrow.
2. Activity
   a. *Osteoclastic Activity.* Certain neoplastic plasma cells elaborate osteoclast-activating factor (OAF), which stimulates resorption of bone and the development of depleted, demineralized bone (osteopenia) and areas

of bone rarefaction (osteolysis) (Figs. 22-7, 22-8).[5]
   b. *Protein Properties.*
      (1) Type: The monoclonal immunoglobulin may possess antigen-binding capabilities. The capacity to bind antigen could conceivably cause the patient significant clinical symptomatology. In most cases, however, the immunoglobulin lacks any defined specificity and produces its clinical symptoms according to the amount and physical properties of the protein.
      (2) Quantity: The absolute quantity of protein produced by the neoplastic cells may cause an elevated plasma viscosity with interference in blood flow and nonspecific interference of platelets and/or coagulation factors. This results in the hyperviscosity syndrome, which will be discussed later.
3. Physical Properties
   a. *Cryoprotein.* A protein circulating in the plasma or demonstrable in serum testing that precipitates on exposure to cold temperatures is termed a "cryoprotein." Often when this protein is reheated to normal body temperatures, or on exposure to warm environments, it resolubilizes. Many cryoproteins are cryoglobulins and may be seen

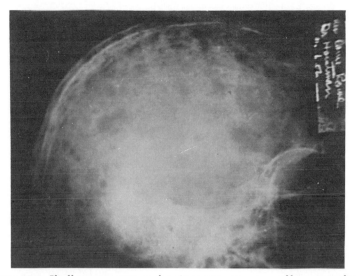

**Figure 22-7.** Skull roentgenogram showing numerous areas of bone osteolysis.

in patients with multiple myeloma, Waldenström's macroglobulinemia, or monoclonal cryoglobulinemia. Patients with large amounts of cryoproteins may, on exposure to the cold, develop significant impairment of vascular flow sufficient to produce ischemic necrosis of digits or exposed tissue **(see Color Figure 190)**.

b. *Polymerization.* Certain paraproteins—particularly IgA and IgG3—may polymerize, producing, in effect, macroglobulins that also interfere with blood flow. These proteins may produce characteristic features of the hyperviscosity syndrome.

c. *Entire Proteins or Partial Proteins.* Proliferating cells may synthesize any single component of an immunoglobulin molecule in excessive amounts, such as light chains, heavy chains, or protein fragments. Free light chains in the plasma may be filtered out in the kidney and be excreted in the urine as Bence-Jones proteins (see Fig. 22-5 *D*). Bence-Jones proteins, therefore, are monoclonal light chains consisting of either kappa or lambda chains. These free light chains may also precipitate in the kidney, particularly in the renal tubules following urinary concentration, and may produce blockage or impairment of renal tubular function or renal damage.

The foregoing processes may cause common complications of monoclonal gammopathies that include bone marrow failure, amyloidosis, hypercalcemia, hyperurice-

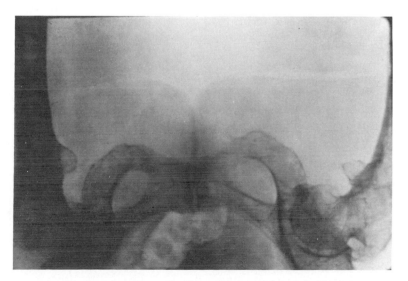

**Figure 22-8.** Roentgenogram of pelvis showing marked bone demineralization and lytic lesions in the left femur.

mia, demineralization of bone, and renal failure.

4. Immunologic Impairment

The normal humoral immune response may be depressed, rendering the patient susceptible to bacterial infections. This phenomenon is to be contrasted with the lymphoproliferative disorder chronic lymphocytic leukemia (CLL), in which both humoral and cell-mediated limbs of the immune response are abnormal. In the monoclonal gammopathies, excess production of "nonsense" paraprotein is associated with increased immunoglobulin catabolism; therefore, there is often depletion of the normal immunoglobulins. In addition, with extensive crowding of the marrow and of normal populations of plasma cells, the humoral limb of the immune response is quantitatively depleted.

## Laboratory Features

*Hematologic.* As already mentioned, many patients present with anemia that is generally normochromic and normocytic but that can be macrocytic. The hemoglobin is usually below 10 g/dl and hematocrit below 30 percent. Red cell morphology is usually unremarkable, with the exception of rouleau formation **(see Color Figure 193)**. Rouleau formation results from protein coating of the red cells, which also contributes to the markedly elevated erythrocyte sedimentation rate. Sedimentation rates in excess of 100 mm/hr are common in patients with multiple myeloma.

At initial presentation, the white cell count and platelet count are usually not depressed; however, patients may have neutropenia, which depends on the extent of marrow plasma cell infiltration. Similarly, patients can have a marked pancytopenia. Some patients may show a leukoerythroblastic blood picture, with plasma cells occasionally seen on the peripheral blood smear **(see Color Figure 131)**.

The bone marrow is usually markedly hypercellular with normal numbers of megakaryocytes. The increase in marrow cellularity is due to plasma cell infiltration **(see Color Figures 188 and 189)**. Many of the plasma cells seen in multiple myeloma are large and binucleated with prominent nucleoli **(see Color Figure 188)**. These nucleoli have been referred to as having a "punched-out" appearance. The cytoplasm of myeloma plasma cells is usually abundant and less basophilic than the cytoplasm of normal plasma cells. Although these cells are termed "myeloma cells," they are not pathognomonic for multiple myeloma. Morphologic variations have been described for myeloma cells, including multinucleation and intracytoplasmic inclusions. The appearance of eosinophilic intracytoplasmic material (aggregated immunoglobulin) in

plasma cells has been referred to as Russell bodies **(see Color Figure 188)**. Plasmocytes with a red-staining cytoplasm have been termed "flame cells" **(see Color Figure 197)**. Some consider flame cells to be associated with IgA myeloma; however, these morphologic abnormalities have been described both in benign inflammatory disorders and in malignant myelomas. Neoplastic plasma cells almost invariably comprise more than 20 percent of the marrow cell population in multiple myeloma, a feature that is essential for diagnosis. The other cell lines are usually relatively decreased, but their proportions may vary. Occasionally an increase in osteoclastic activity may be seen, however, which is more usually apparent upon bone marrow biopsy. Bone marrow biopsy shows areas of bone resorption and often a decrease in cancellous bone. In many instances, the bone marrow is almost totally replaced by abnormal plasma cells, and it is quite surprising how many of these patients have normal leukocyte and platelet counts.

*Biochemical Parameters.* In patients who have renal insufficiency, levels of blood urea nitrogen, and creatinine will be elevated. Concomitant with this is an elevation in uric acid, a purine nucleotide breakdown product. The serum calcium may be increased owing to bone resorption; if so, this is an adverse prognostic feature (see further on). In the majority of cases, the serum protein level is elevated, and on serum protein electrophoresis the M protein is identified. More often, the M spike is greater than 2 g/dl. The frequency of the different types of immunoglobulins in multiple myeloma is shown in Table 22–3. Additional tests may be performed to demonstrate the presence of cryoglobulins or hyperviscosity.

Protein may be identified on routine urinalysis and quantitated with a 24-hour urine specimen. Occasionally, protein levels in excess of 4 g/24 hr may be seen; in this situation, one must consider the possibility of associated amyloidosis. Examination of the urine sediment may reveal the presence of hyaline casts or uric acid crystals.

*Radiologic Features.* The presence of lytic bone lesions are often demonstrated in multiple myeloma. These areas appear as lucent areas on roentgenogram within the axial skeleton and particularly in the skull (Fig. 22-7) and pelvis (Fig. 22-8). In situations of solitary plasmacytoma or multiple plasmacytomas, large lucent areas may be demonstrated

**Table 22–3. MONOCLONAL PARAPROTEIN FREQUENCIES IN MULTIPLE MYELOMA**

| | |
|---|---|
| IgG | 52% |
| IgA | 25% |
| Bence-Jones (light chain myeloma) | 22% |
| IgD, IgE, IgM | 1% |

**Table 22-4. CLINICAL STAGING AND PROGNOSTIC FACTORS IN MULTIPLE MYELOMA**

1. High Tumor Mass (Stage III)
   One or more of:
   Hemoglobin <8.5 g/dl
   Serum calcium >12 mg/dl
   Advanced lytic bone lesions
   IgG M protein spike >7 g/dl; IgA >5 g/dl
   Urine light chain M component >12 g/24 hr
2. Low Tumor Mass (Stage I)
   All of the following:
   Hemoglobin >10 g/dl
   Serum calcium <12 mg/dl
   Normal skeletal survey or one lytic bone lesion
   IgG <5 gm/dl; IgΛ <3 g/dl
   Urine light chain M component <4 g/24 hr
3. Intermediate tumor mass (Stage II)
   Laboratory parameters fitting neither low nor high
   categories

on roentgenogram. The best test for detecting the lytic bone lesions is a skeletal survey. Bone scans do not aid in the detection of these osteolytic lesions associated with multiple myeloma.

**Diagnosis and Staging.** It may sometimes be difficult to distinguish among monoclonal gammopathy of uncertain significance, myeloma in evolution, and frank multiple myeloma. If patients have two or three of the major criteria — namely, a monoclonal paraprotein, a marrow plasmacytosis of greater than 20 percent, and lytic bone lesions — the diagnosis can then be established with some certainty. A staging system has been developed in an attempt to quantitate the degree of plasmacytosis and prognostic implications. The staging system, listed in Table 22-4, is classified according to the estimation of tumor mass. This system correlates the major prognostic clinical parameters with the measured multiple myeloma cell mass. Patients may be classified into stage I, II, or III, based on routine clinical parameters. This system allows for a reasonable estimate of anticipated duration of survival.[4]

**Treatment.** Multiple myeloma is not a curable disease, and therapy is associated with cost, morbidity, and the likelihood of drug resistance.[6,11] As a consequence, therapy is generally not instituted in the more benign presentations and is certainly not instituted in monoclonal gammopathy of undetermined significance. Establishment of the diagnosis of multiple myeloma is generally associated with implementation of treatment, and, although treatment has not dramatically prolonged patient survival, treatment has improved the morbidity of the disease. Treatment, however, is reserved for the symptomatic patient.[6] The principles of treatment may be classified as follows:

1. Definitive Treatment (treatment of the primary disease)
   a. *Radiation treatment.* Radiation is generally administered for local plasmacytomas or for symptomatic relief of bone pain.
   b. *Chemotherapy.* Chemotherapy is preferred for the initial treatment of multiple myeloma. The most common drugs used are alkylating agents such as melphalan, which are given together with prednisone for four days every four to six weeks. This regimen produces objective responses in approximately 60 percent of patients. Various other treatment protocols have also been implemented, but the median duration of survival is still only two years from the date of diagnosis. These survival statistics remain essentially the same, irrespective of what treatment regimens are used. Treatment is continued for at least one and a half to two years, should the patient show response or benefit. There are, however, reports of an increasing incidence (approximately 6 percent of acute leukemia developing in long-term survivors following the use of alkylating agents.[2,10,15] Because of this, long-term responders may have discontinuation of therapy after 18 months. In general, most of these patients do relapse. Patients relapsing on treatment or failing to respond to initial treatment are usually resistant to further therapy. Newer combination chemotherapy and agents such as interferon have been tried, with limited reports of success.

2. Supportive Treatment (treatment of the complications and symptoms secondary to the primary disease)
   a. *Skeletal destruction and bone lesions.* Radiation therapy is used to treat solitary plasmacytomas. In the case of pathologic fractures, a combination of orthopedic fixation and local radiation treatment is generally given.
   b. *Hypercalcemia.* The elevated calcium, as a result of osteoclastic activity, is generally treated with fluid and diuretic therapy. Antihypercalcemic agents such as prednisone, calcitonin, and mithramycin are used.
   c. *Bone marrow infiltration and resultant failure.* Depending on the degree of involvement and symptoms, blood transfusion therapy is given. This may include red cell replacement for symptomatic anemia and platelet transfusions occasionally for patients who have symptomatic thrombocytopenia. Infections are vigorously treated with antibiotics, as these patients have disturbed humoral immunity.
   d. *Renal insufficiency.* Patients with renal failure may require dialysis and occasionally plasmapheresis has been tried with limited success.

e. *Cryoglobulinemia, hyperviscosity syndrome, and bleeding disorders.* These may all be treated by plasmapheresis to remove the abnormal protein. This is, however, only a temporary means of therapy.

f. *Amyloidosis.* This condition will be discussed in the following section but represents the extracellular deposition of light chains in the tissues. When this occurs as a complication of multiple myeloma, it is generally refractory to treatment and causes organ failure.[7]

The state of hyperuricemia that results is treated with the use of agents such as allopurinol.

## Waldenström's Macroglobulinemia

Macroglobulinemia refers to an elevation in the macroglobulin IgM in the plasma or serum or both. There are several disorders associated with increased macroglobulins (Table 22–5). Most of these conditions are polyclonal.

Waldenström's macroglobulinemia occurs as the result of an uncontrolled proliferation of cells that are intermediate between mature B lymphocytes and plasma cells **(see Color Figure 194)**. These cells are described as plasmacytoid lymphocytes and have the capability to manufacture excessive amounts of macroglobulin (IgM). IgM paraproteins can occur in a wide spectrum of other disorders, many of which are secondary to other conditions such as malignant lymphomas, chronic lymphocytic leukemia, and the extremely rare IgM multiple myeloma. Most usually an elevated monoclonal IgM occurs in association with the lymphoproliferative disorder called Waldenström's macroglobulinemia.[16,18,19] Occasionally, elevated IgMs may occur in patients without any abnormalities. The differential diagnosis of macroglobulinemia is listed in Table 22–5.

**Clinical Features.** In contrast to multiple myeloma, Waldenström's macroglobulinemia is more like a lymphomatous process than myeloma.[16–18] As a consequence, the clinical features exhibit both reticuloendothelial cell proliferation in addition to consequences of the abnormal paraprotein. Because the abnormal protein is a macroglobulin, the whole blood viscosity may increase and a hyperviscosity syndrome often predominates. Patients usually present with weakness, weight loss, and fatigue but may also present with bleeding abnormalities. Hyperviscosity syndrome with its associated clinical features occurs in approximately 17 percent of cases.[18] On physical examination, patients may manifest hepatomegaly, splenomegaly, and lymphadenopathy. Ocular changes are commonly seen. Examination of the fundus of the eye often shows tortuous veins with the sausage-linked appearance **(see Color Figure 196)**. Occasionally, retinal hemorrhages may be seen.

**Hyperviscosity Syndrome.** Hyperviscosity develops from an elevated blood viscosity, the clinical features of which are quite varied (Table 22–6). They usually include vague neurologic changes, tinnitus (buzzing in the ears), retinopathy (as mentioned earlier), and clinical effects of fluid overload. This hypervolemia may cause congestive cardiac failure, since the huge amounts of protein in the serum exert an osmotic pressure drawing fluid into the intravascular fluid compartment. Patients may also present with a bleeding diathesis when the abnormal protein interferes with clotting factors or platelets or both.

**Treatment.** The treatment of Waldenström's macroglobulinemia consists of chlorambucil (Leukeran), a drug often used in treating chronic lymphocytic leukemia. The hyperviscosity syndrome that arises secondary to Waldenström's macroglobulinemia is generally treated by plasmapheresis to remove the excess macroglobulin. This procedure is efficient in this situation, because the bulk of the macroglobulin is distributed intravascularly.

Waldenström's macroglobulinemia is associated with a five- to seven-year median survival and a more benign clinical course than that seen in multiple myeloma. Table 22–7 compares the clinical features of Waldenström's macroglobulinemia with those of multiple myeloma.

## Heavy Chain Diseases

These disorders are characterized by an uncontrolled production of excess heavy chain compo-

**Table 22–5. CLASSIFICATION OF MACROGLOBULINEMIA**

Malignant
  B cell malignancies
    Waldenström's macroglobulinemia
    Chronic lymphocytic leukemia
    Lymphomas
    Other malignancies
Benign
  Parasitic infections (trypanosomiasis, kala-azar)
  Rheumatoid arthritis
  Cirrhosis
  Cold agglutinin disease
  Tropical splenomegaly syndrome
  Idiopathic

**Table 22–6. CLINICAL FEATURES OF HYPERVISCOSITY SYNDROME**

| | |
|---|---|
| Neurologic changes | 20% |
| Retinopathy | 35% |
| Hypervolemia/congestive heart failure | 20% |
| Bleeding diathesis | 20% |
| Hepatosplenomegaly | 35% |
| Lymphadenopathy | 45% |

Table 22–7. RELATIVE COMPARISON OF CLINICAL FEATURES IN MULTIPLE MYELOMA AND MACROGLOBULINEMIA

|  | Macroglobulinemia | Myeloma |
|---|---|---|
| Organomegally | +++ | + |
| Hyperviscosity | +++ | + |
| Lytic bone lesion | + | +++ |
| Azotemia | + | +++ |
| Length of survival | ++ | + |

nents of immunoglobulins.[25,26] These proteins are elaborated by monoclonal B lymphocytes.

**Gamma Chain Disease.** This is a rare disorder restricted to older men. Clinically, the disease resembles malignant lymphoma, with hepatosplenomegaly and lymphadenopathy the usual physical findings. Fever, anemia, and recurrent infections are common symptoms. Survival ranges from one month to five years, with death resulting from infection or malignancy. Chemotherapy is generally ineffective.

**Alpha Chain Disease.** This disease entity is also known as "Mediterranean lymphoma." It is the most common heavy chain disease, afflicting mostly younger individuals from the Middle East. Almost all patients present with a diffuse abdominal lymphoma and malabsorption syndrome. The abdominal nodes and lamina propria of the gastrointestinal tract are massively infiltrated with lymphocytes, plasma cells, and reticuloendothelial cells. This infiltration is often accompanied by villous atrophy. The clinical course of the disease is usually progressive, but remissions have been reported with the use of cyclophosphamide, corticosteroids, and antibiotics.

**Mu Chain Disease.** This disease is the rarest of all the heavy chain disorders. It is also a chronic lymphocytic leukemia "look-alike." Visceral organs primarily are involved, in particular the spleen, liver, and abdominal lymph nodes. The patients may also present with light chainuria, pathologic fractures, and amyloidosis. The serum protein electrophoresis shows hypogammaglobulinemia. Treatment is the same as is used for chronic lymphocytic leukemia (i.e., chlorambucil, corticosteroids, and radiation treatment).

In contrast to the light chain disorders associated with multiple myeloma, these disorders are generally lymphoproliferative and are associated with an uncontrolled and excessive production of heavy chains only. Occasionally, light chains may be synthesized in addition; however, there is an inability to produce a whole immunoglobulin.

# Monoclonal Gammopathy of Undetermined Significance (MGUS)

This category of disorders includes those patients who present with an incidental finding of a serum M spike on routine testing.[8,13] It occurs as a result of idiopathic elaboration of abnormal monoclonal immunoglobulins, which generally accumulates in the absence of any other clinical symptoms. Most often the patients are not aware of any abnormality, and the M spike is discovered as an incidental finding.

MGUS was formerly called "benign monoclonal gammopathy," but the term "monoclonal gammopathy of undetermined significance" is preferred, because in most instances the biologic behavior of the proliferating cell of origin cannot be determined. Most importantly, the prognostic significance of this abnormal M protein cannot be determined at initial presentation. Indeed, "benign" is a misnomer, as there is a 10 percent chance of progression to a hematologic malignancy. The M spike may result from uncontrolled synthesis of whole immunoglobulins, but occasionally it is caused by excessive production of light chains only. Patients with MGUS usually have less than 2 g/dl of monoclonal protein in the serum and have less than 5 percent plasma cells in the marrow. The other clinical parameters found in multiple myeloma are generally absent in these patients. MGUS is relatively frequent and has been found in approximately 3 percent of persons past the age of 70 years and in 1 percent of those past 50.[8,13]

In one large series of patients with MGUS followed from the Mayo Clinic, after five years of follow-up almost 60 percent of patients failed to progress or to show significant increases in the M protein.[8,13] Nine percent of patients showed a greater than 50 percent increase in their M protein, and only 11 percent of patients progressed to a malignant monoclonal gammopathy. The remaining 23 percent of patients died from other causes prior to the conclusion of the study. There did not appear to be any significant difference among those patients who presented with an IgG, an IgA, or an IgM protein (Table 22–8).

It is impossible to predict which patients are likely to evolve to a more malignant presentation. Therefore, periodic examination of patients with MGUS is the only definitive way of categorizing those patients who develop insipient myeloma or other malignant monoclonal gammopathies and those patients who have a truly benign disorder.

## Tumor-Associated Gammopathy

This occurrence is very rare. However, certain patients with tumors mount immune responses of a

Table 22–8. MONOCLONAL GAMMOPATHY OF UNCERTAIN SIGNIFICANCE: 5-YEAR FOLLOW-UP

| | |
|---|---|
| No significant progression in M spike | 57% |
| >50% increase in M spike | 9% |
| Progression to malignant monoclonal gammopathy | 11% |
| Death from other causes | 23% |

humoral nature against the proliferating tumor cells, and conceivably this antibody production may be uncontrolled, producing a monoclonal immunoglobulin (gammopathy). These include those disorders not associated with neoplasms of cell types known to produce monoclonal paraproteins, such as squamous cell carcinoma of the lung, colon carcinoma, bile duct malignancy, and breast cancer.

### Biclonal Gammopathy

In this disorder, two parental B cells or mature plasma cell sources give rise to uncontrolled synthesis of two M proteins. The clinical significance of these disorders is uncertain, and this condition is extremely uncommon.

### Monoclonal Gammopathies Associated With Other Miscellaneous Disorders

Occasionally, M proteins may be seen in other conditions, including Gaucher's disease (see Chapter 23).

## Amyloidosis

### Classification

This includes a heterogenous group of disorders that are characterized by the extracellular deposition of an amorphous material derived from various proteins by differing mechanisms. The term "amyloid" is originally derived from the waxy, starchlike property of the material. Under the light microscope, this material appears as an amorphous eosinophilic structure that, on electron microscopy, shows a fibrillar pattern. The accumulation of this material within tissues and organs leads to loss of function and organ enlargement **(see Color Figure 195)**.[21-23]

Amyloidosis may be classified according to the suspected nature of the pathogenetic process, the presence or absence of associated disease, and the protein composition (Table 22–9). Two main types of amyloid protein are recognized:[21]

1. A protein with the N-terminal sequence that demonstrates homology with the variable region of an immunoglobulin light chain. This protein is termed (A = amyloid, L = light chain).
2. A protein with the N-terminal sequence that demonstrates homology with a nonimmunoglobulin protein. This form of amyloid is termed AA (second A = acute phase protein).

Amyloidosis was also formerly classified according to the distribution of the material within the tissues and organs. In this regard, so-called primary amyloid is mostly deposited in the gastrointestinal

**Table 22–9. CLASSIFICATION OF AMYLOIDOSIS**

Primary Systemic Amyloidosis (Idiopathic and Plasma Cell Neoplasm–Associated Amyloid) (AL)
Amyloid Secondary to Chronic Suppurative or Granulomatous Infections (AA)
   Tuberculosis
   Rheumatoid arthritis
   Ulcerative colitis
   Bronchiectasis
   Osteomyelitis
Heredofamilial Amyloid (AF)
   Familial Mediterranean Fever (AA)
   Portuguese polyneuropathy (AFp)
Isolated Organ Amyloid*
   Diabetes (pancreatic islets)
   Amyloid cardiomyopathy (heart)
   Brain (senile amyloid)

*Nature of protein unknown

tract, skin, and nerves. Secondary amyloid that is associated with a chronic inflammatory process is deposited in the spleen, liver, and kidneys. This classification, however, is inaccurate. In any of the amyloid syndromes, deposition may occur in either the primary or the secondary distribution. The classification of the amyloid syndromes is listed in Table 22–9.

### Clinical Features

The major clinical features occur from organ enlargement and loss of function, examples of which are an enlarged tongue (macroglossia), skin thickening, enlargement of the liver and spleen, and joint involvement (carpal tunnel syndrome). Examples of loss of organ function include gastrointestinal malabsorption, renal failure, cardiac failure, and disturbances in sympathetic nervous system function —particularly orthostatic hypotension.[21-23] The coagulation protein factor X may also be deficient in amyloidosis owing to adsorption onto the amyloid material.[20]

### Diagnosis

Generally, diagnosis is made by biopsy of the involved organ. When this cannot be accomplished, a rectal biopsy or bone marrow biopsy may reveal the eosinophilic deposits in the tissues. Special stains such as Congo red and metachromatic stains will also demonstrate the presence of amyloid.

### Prognosis and Treatment

In general, amyloidosis progresses relentlessly and fails to respond to therapy. Some successes have been reported with colchicine, particularly in the familial Mediterranean fever type of amyloid.[24] Chemotherapy and immunosuppressive therapy have usually been unsuccessful.

## PRINCIPLES OF THE DIFFERENTIAL DIAGNOSIS OF MONOCLONAL GAMMOPATHIES

Evaluation of patients with suspected monoclonal gammopathies involves the following principles (Table 22–10):

1. *Establish the presence of a monoclonal gammopathy by documentation of an M spike.*
   a. Perform serum protein electrophoresis (see Fig. 22-4).
   b. Perform urine protein electrophoresis (see Fig. 22-5*D*).
   c. Perform immunoelectrophoresis to document the nature of the paraprotein.
2. *Establish the nature of the proliferating cell type.*
   a. A bone marrow aspirate and biopsy will determine whether increased levels of lymphocytes, plasmacytoid lymphocytes, or plasma cells are present.
   b. Perform a skeletal survey to determine whether the proliferating cells are focally aggregated or whether their activity is associated with bone lysis. Specifically, roentgenography is performed to determine whether there is demineralization of bone (i.e., diffuse osteoporosis) or whether there are multiple or single areas of bone lysis.
3. *Establish the presence of an entire or partial protein (immunoglobulin) and the activity of the protein.*
   a. Test for Bence-Jones proteinuria (urine light chains) (see Fig. 22-5*D*).
   b. Perform quantitative analysis of total immunoglobulins by radial immunodiffusion, as well as qualitative analysis by immunoelectrophoresis.
4. *Establish the degree of organ involvement.*
   a. Assess renal function (BUN, creatinine).
   b. Investigate the skeletal system thoroughly.
   c. Evaluate the hemopoietic system.

### Table 22–10. PRINCIPLES IN DIFFERENTIAL DIAGNOSIS OF MONOCLONAL GAMMOPATHIES

Establish presence of a monoclonal gammopathy by
    documentation of an M spike
    Serum protein electrophoresis
    Urine protein electrophoresis
    Serum Immunoelectrophoresis
Establish nature of proliferating cell type
    Bone marrow aspirate/biopsy
    Skeletal survey
Establish presence of entire or partial protein and activity of
    the protein
    Urine light chains
    Quantitative analysis by radial immunodiffusion
Establish the degree of organ system involvement

d. All vital organ systems should also be thoroughly investigated.

With this general background, an evaluation can be made concerning whether the patient has a benign monoclonal gammopathy or a malignant monoclonal immunoproliferative disorder.

## CASE HISTORIES
### Case 1

A 60-year-old black man presented for evaluation of low back pain. The pain was aggravated by walking, was described as dull and aching, and was associated with lower limb weakness. The patient denied any fever or urinary symptoms but complained of fatigue with mild effort occurring for the previous two weeks. This was accompanied by shortness of breath and palpitations. He denied any chest pain.

He gave a history of pneumonia treated at another hospital two months before, that resolved on antibiotic therapy. He denied having had any other recent infections or any bleeding tendency. The rest of the systematic history was unremarkable. He did not smoke or drink alcohol and was not taking any drugs or medications.

**Physical Examination.** He was a well-developed, well-nourished black man in some distress, walking with a shuffled gait. His pulse was 96 per minute and regular. Blood pressure was normal. Examination of his head and neck was unremarkable; there was no cervical lymphadenopathy or thyromegaly, and his trachea was central. Chest examination showed scattered rales over both bases, worse on the left. His heart sounds were normal, but there was a grade II/VI ejection systolic murmur present down the left parasternal border and radiating into the neck. There was no evidence of hepatomegaly or splenomegaly and no significant clinical lymphadenopathy. There was tenderness over the lower lumbar spine to percussion. His reflexes were brisk yet equal, and his plantar reflexes were flexor.

**Laboratory Data.** His hematocrit was 30 percent with normochromic indices and a mean cell volume of 106 fl. His reticulocyte count was 1 percent. His white cell count was 4000/$\mu$l with a normal differential. Platelet count was 245,000/$\mu$l with normal platelet morphology. The peripheral smear showed marked rouleaux formation. His Westergren sedimentation rate was greater than 100 mm in the first hour. His blood urea nitrogen was 25 mg/dl, and creatinine was 1.8 mg/dl. Electrolytes were normal. His uric acid was 12 mg/dl, and calcium was 11 mg/dl. A serum protein was 9.5 mg/dl, with an albumin of 2.5 g/dl and globulin of 7.0 g/dl. A serum protein electrophoresis revealed a M spike in the gamma region. Immunoelectrophoresis showed a monoclonal IgG lambda paraprotein. Urinalysis showed 1+ protein, and 24-hour urine protein revealed 3 g/24 hours.

A skeletal survey showed multiple lytic bone lesions in the skull and pelvis with vertebral collapse over L4 and L5. There was general demineralization. A bone marrow showed a hypercellular marrow with 80 to 90 percent plasma cells. Many of the plasma cells showed binucleate and trinucleate morphology with prominent "punched out" nucleoli.

**Clinical Course.** The patient was initially given radiation therapy to the lower spinal region, which was followed up by melphalan and prednisone given daily for four days, cycled every one month. Despite an initial symptomatic response and alleviation of his low back pain, he developed additional painful areas over his ribs and upper throacic vertebrae. These were irradiated. Chemotherapy was continued. However, 10 months after the onset of treatment he developed a fulminant pneumonia and died.

**Comment.** This man had a fairly typical presentation of multiple myeloma, since bone pain constitutes one of the most common symptoms. A normochromic anemia, often with macrocytic indices is another common presenting feature. His history of pneumonia two months previously may have been the initial presentation of multiple myeloma—many patients do present with infections, particularly pneumonia. The diagnosis of multiple myeloma in this patient was not difficult, as he presented with the three classic presentations: a monoclonal M spike, marrow plasmacytosis, and skeletal lytic lesions. The weakness of his lower limbs and increased reflexes suggested early compression signs that responded well to initial radiation therapy. Radiation therapy or decompressive surgery or both are used in the initial treatment of cord compression.

His uric acid was also elevated, attesting to the increased turnover of cells and warranted the use of allopurinol treatment prophylactically prior to chemotherapy. His urinalysis showed a significant proteinuria that, on urine immunoelectrophoresis, revealed the presence of light chains. Light chains are not uncommonly found in the urine even in patients with a complete immunoglobulin M spike reflective of excess production. The moderate anemia and extensive lytic bone lesions are sufficient to categorize this patient's disease as stage III. The prognosis for patients with stage III is less than the median survival of two years, and in-

deed, his course was death in 10 months following diagnosis. Fulminant infection is probably the most common cause of death in these patients.

Figures 22-7 to 22-10 illustrate areas where lytic lesions occur in patients with multiple myeloma.

## Case 2

A 59-year-old white man presented with recurrent epistaxis and easy bruising. He also complained of swelling of his ankles, shortness of breath with mild effort, and fatigue. He noted that his vision had recently deteriorated, and he was troubled by continuous buzzing in his ears and by frequent headaches. He was taking atenolol (a beta blocker) and denied any alcohol consumption but had smoked one pack of cigarettes per day for 20 years, a habit he had stopped 10 years ago. His past history was significant for hypertension and a history of myocardial infarction.

**Physical Examination.** This showed a well-developed, well-nourished white man with mild shortness of breath. His pulse rate was 76 per minute. Blood pressure was 140/95. He was afebrile. He had evidence of ankle edema and

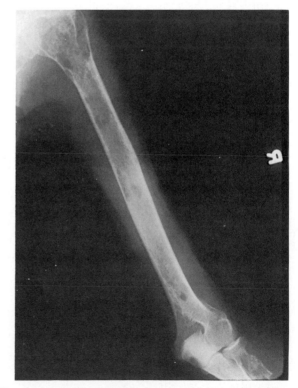

**Figure 22-9.** Radiograph of a humerus showing multiple lytic lesions, which, in the setting of multiple myeloma, are pathognomonic.

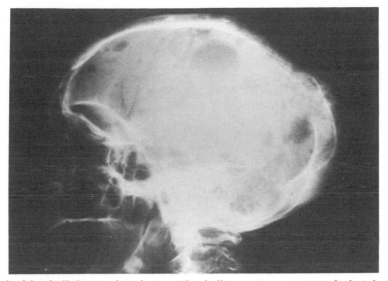

**Figure 22-10.** Radiograph of the skull showing lytic lesions. The skull is a very common site for lytic lesions and should be included in every skeletal series observing for these lesions.

jugular venous distention. Pupils were equal and reacted to light and accommodation, but fundoscopy showed venous engorgement with "sausage-linked" venous channels. There were no fundal hemorrhages. His gums and nose were normal. Examination of his chest revealed bibasilar rales, and heart sounds showed a normal S1, S2 with an S3 and S4 present. He had a grade I/VI ejection systolic murmur radiating into the neck. Examination of his abdomen showed enlargement of his liver to 3 cm below the right costal margin with a 13 cm span. His spleen was palpable 2 cm below the left costal margin. There was cervical and axillary lymphadenopathy with small firm, rubbery nodes, the largest measuring 2 × 1 cm. Examination of his skin showed scattered ecchymoses.

**Laboratory Data.** His hematocrit was 32 percent with normochromic, normocytic indices. His white cell count was 3500/$\mu$l with reversal of the normal neutrophil:lymphocyte ratio. Differential count showed 65 percent lymphocytes, many of which showed plasmacytoid features. His platelet count was 110,000/$\mu$l. His reticulocyte count was 1 percent. The sedimentation rate was 25 mm in the first hour and peripheral blood morphology showed rouleaux formation. A urinalysis showed trace protein with hyaline casts. Chemistry evaluation showed an elevated uric acid at 8 mg/dl and a total protein of 10.4 g/dl. The albumin was 4.0 g/dl, and globulins were 5.4 g/dl. A serum protein electrophoresis showed a monoclonal M spike of 3.5 g/dl. His serum viscosity was 5.1 (normal, 1.4 to 1.8). Bone marrow examination

revealed a hypercellular marrow with normal megakaryocytes and normal erythroid and myeloid differentiation. There was an increase marrow lymphocytosis with plasmacytoid lymphocytes constituting 20 percent of the marrow differential. His total serum IgM level was elevated.

Initial treatment with plasmapheresis was performed by a 1½ volume plasma exchange weekly, for three treatments every two weeks. His headaches improved and hemostatic problems abated. He was additionally given chemotherapy consisting of chlorambucil daily. This was associated with a significant improvement in his M spike and a decrease in the IgM level. His hematocrit improved and lymphadenopathy and splenomegaly resolved.

**Comment.** This man exhibits a typical clinical presentation of Waldenström's macroglobulinemia with hyperviscosity syndrome. The hemostatic abnormalities are a result of increasing plasma volume particularly affecting the unsupported vessels of the nose and easy bruisability. Interference in platelet function is also not uncommon. A mild pancytopenia is seen in patients who manifest marrow infiltration as did this patient. The finding of plasmacytoid lymphocytes in the peripheral smear with the presence of rouleaux can alert one to the diagnosis of Waldenström's macroglobulinemia. In addition, this patient exhibited the clinical features of congestive cardiac failure, another feature seen in patients with the hyperviscosity syndrome. His ocular findings are also typical. The diagnosis is ultimately established by the finding of the monoclonal protein and the documentation that the monoclonal protein is the macroglobulin IgM. Plasmacytoid lymphocytes in the bone marrow confirm the diagnosis.

Immediate treatment in symptomatic patients consists of plasmapheresis, and the fact that IgM is distributed mostly intravascularly is associated with a dramatic response to treatment. Plasmapheresis, however, is only a symptomatic treatment and must be followed by chemotherapy.

The clinical course of this disease is more benign than that of multiple myeloma, and many of the patients live as long as 5 to 10 years with this disease.

## References

1. Alexanian, R: Monoclonal gammopathy in lymphoma. Arch Int Med 135:62, 1975.
2. Bergsagel, DC: Plasma cell neoplasms and acute leukemia. Clin Haematol 11:221, 1982.
3. Cutler, SJ and Young, JL: Third National Cancer Survey Incidence Data. National Cancer Institute Monograph 41, 1975.
4. Durie, BGM: Staging and kinetics of multiple myeloma. In Salmon, SE (ed): Clinics in Haematology, Vol II(1) WB Saunders, London, 1982, pp 3–18.
5. Durie, BGM, Salmon, SE, and Mundy, GR: Relation of osteoclast activating factor production to extent of bone disease in multiple myeloma. Br J Haematol 47:21, 1981.
6. Hoogstraten, B: Multiple myeloma: A therapeutic enigma. Am J Clin Oncol 5:13, 1982.
7. Kapadia, SB: Multiple Myeloma. A clinico-pathologic study of 62 consecutive autopsied cases. Medicine (Balt) 59:380, 1980.
8. Kyle, RA: Monoclonal gammopathy of undetermined significance: Natural history of 241 cases. Am J Med 64:814, 1978.
9. Kyle, RA: Multiple myeloma: Review of 869 cases. Mayo Clin Proc 50:29, 1975.
10. Kyle, RA: Second malignancies associated with chemotherapeutic agents. Semin Oncol 9:131, 1982.
11. Kyle, RA: Treatment of multiple myeloma. A small step forward? N Engl J Med 310:1382, 1984.
12. Kyle, RA and Greipp, PR: Smouldering multiple myeloma. N Engl J Med 302:1347, 1980.
13. MacKenzie, MR, McIntyre, OR, and Durie, B: Monoclonal Gammopathies. Education Program, American Society of Hematology, 1983, p 33.
14. McIntyre, OR: Current concepts in cancer. Multiple myeloma. N Engl J Med 301:193, 1979.
15. Rosner, F and Grunwald, HW: Simultaneous occurrence of multiple myeloma and acute myeloblastic leukemia. Fact or myth. Am J Med 76:891, 1984.
16. MacKenzie, MR and Fudenberg, HH: Macroglobulinemia: An analysis of forty patients. Blood 39, 874, 1972.
17. Rywlin, AM, Civantos, F, Ortega, RS, et al: Bone marrow histology in monoclonal macroglobulinemia. Am J Clin Pathol 63:767, 1975.
18. Tursz, T, Brouet, JC, Flandrin, G, et al: Clinical and pathologic features of Waldenström's macroglobulinemia in seven patients with serum monoclonal IgG or IgA. Am J Med 63:499, 1977.
19. Waldenström, J: Incipient myelomatosis or "essential" hyperglobulinemia: New syndrome? Acta Med Scand 117:216, 1944.
20. Furie, B, Voo, L, McAdam, KPWJ, et al: Mechanisms of factor X deficiency in systemic amyloidosis. N Engl J Med 304:827, 1981.
21. Glenner, GG: Amyloid deposits and amyloidosis. N Engl J Med 302:1283, 1333, 1980.
22. Kyle, RA and Bayrd, ED: Amyloidosis: Review of 236 cases. Medicine 54:271, 1975.
23. Symmers, WStC: Primary amyloidosis: A review. J Clin Pathol 9:187, 1956.
24. Zemer, D, Pras, M, Shemer, J, et al: Daily prophylactic colchicine in familial Mediterranean fever. In Glenner, GG, Costa, PP, and Freitas, A (eds): Amyloid and Amyloidosis. Excerpta Medica, Amsterdam, 1980, p 580.
25. Rambaud, JC and Seligmann, M: Alpha chain disease. Clin Gastroenterol 5:341, 1976.
26. Seligmann, M, Mihaesco, E, Preud'homme, JL, et al: Heavy chain diseases: Current findings and concepts. Immunol Rev 48:145, 1979.

# CHAPTER 23

CATHERINE M. SPIER, M.D.

# Lipid (Lysosomal) Storage Diseases and Histiocytoses

## LIPID (LYSOSOMAL) STORAGE DISEASES

The lipid storage diseases, also known as lysosomal storage diseases because of the subcellular accumulation of unmetabolized material in lysosomes, are rare, autosomally inherited disorders. They are due to various enzyme defects (in-born errors) in lipid metabolism (Fig. 23-1). Although many different types have been documented, the most widely known and well-established are those described subsequently. Certain ethnic groups, most notably the Ashkenazi Jews, have an increased incidence of some lipid storage diseases, especially Gaucher's and Tay-Sachs, but all ethnic groups are known to be affected. This group of disorders has wide clinical expression, ranging from essentially asymptomatic to severe and incapacitating with early death. None has an effective therapy. The aim of control in these disorders has been directed at prenatal detection. However, newer techniques, such as enzyme replacement and gene manipulation are now being attempted. The results of these manipulations have shown variable degrees of success, and continued research is in progress. This chapter is devoted to a description of the clinical and pathologic features, as well as the prognosis and treatment, of the lipid storage diseases.

### Gaucher's Disease

This disorder was first described in 1882 by Philippe C. Gaucher in a 32-year-old woman with an enlarged spleen. Gaucher believed the abnormal cells found in her spleen at autopsy were part of a primary splenic tumor. His observations were studied further and the entity we call "Gaucher's disease"

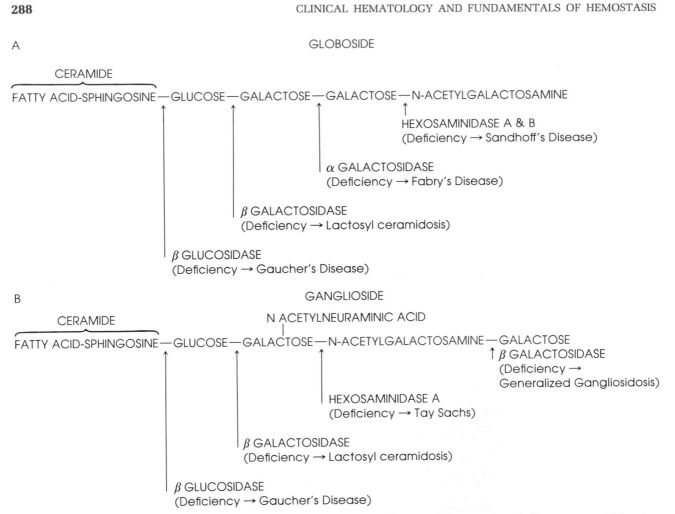

**Figure 23-1.** Schematic structure of globoside and ganglioside to show site of action of the several catabolic enzymes, which, when defective, result in one of the storage diseases. (From Wintrobe,[3] p 1341, with permission.)

was coined at the turn of the century by Dr. Nathan E. Brill of New York.[1]

Gaucher's disease has three clinically recognizable types, but all are due to a deficiency of the enzyme B-glucocerebrosidase with an accumulation of the unmetabolized glucocerebroside in cells, especially of the reticuloendothelial system (RES). The three types are the adult, or non-neuronopathic form (type I); the infantile, acute, or malignant neuronopathic form (type II); and the juvenile or subacute neuronopathic form (type III). All have in common the triad of hepatosplenomegaly **(see color Figure 198)**, Gaucher's cells in the bone marrow and an increase in serum acid phosphatase. The severity of the disease and the patient's age when the disease is first manifested are related to the magnitude of the enzyme deficiency. Each type will be described in detail subsequently. Table 23–1 briefly summarizes the features of each type.

## Clinical Features

**Type I (Adult Gaucher's Disease).** This is the most common type of Gaucher's and is also the most common of the lipidoses.[2] It is seen most frequently in Ashkenazi Jews. The clinical onset of the disease is variable, with most patients being discovered in childhood or early adulthood. It is not unheard of, however, for the diagnosis to be made in an older adult who comes to medical attention for other reasons, and is incidentally noted to have splenomegaly, anemia, or thrombocytopenia. On physical examination, these patients are often noted to have a yellow to yellow-brown pigmentation of the skin, and pingueculae, a yellowish discoloration near the corneal-scleral junction of the eye. Enlargement of the spleen, usually accompanied by an enlarged liver, is almost always present and is due to the accumulation of Gaucher's cells. Lymphadenopathy (enlargement of the lymph nodes), however, is uncommon. Bleeding episodes, most frequently of the nose or gums, are often described; normocytic anemia is common. Neurologic manifestations are rarely seen. Bony changes, noted especially in the femur, occur in from 50 to 75 percent of patients[3,4] and are due to the accumulation of Gaucher's cells in the marrow cavity, which expands and thins the

**Table 23–1. GAUCHER'S DISEASE—CLINICAL SUBTYPES**

| Clinical Features | Type 1: Non-neuronopathic | Type 2: Acute Neuronopathic | Type 3 Subacute Neuronopathic |
|---|---|---|---|
| Clinical onset | Childhood Adulthood | Infancy | Childhood |
| Hepatosplenomegaly | + | + | + |
| Hematologic complications secondary to hypersplenism | + | + | + |
| Skeletal deterioration | + | – | + |
| Neurodegenerative course | – | +++ | ++ |
| Death | Variable | By 2 yr | 2nd–4th decade |
| Ethnic predilection | Ashkenazi Jews | Panethnic | Swedish |

(From Desnick,[1] p. 445, with permission.)

overlying bone. This gives rise to the so-called flask-shaped deformity of the distal femur often seen on roentgenogram. Bone pain is common.[5] Survival of these patients is variable, and many have normal lifespans.

**Type II (Infantile, Acute, or Malignant Neuronopathic Gaucher's Disease).** This form of Gaucher's disease is not common and is seen in all ethnic groups, although uncommonly in Jews. Familial intermarriage is frequently found in the infant's family history. The onset of multiple neurologic signs including difficulty swallowing, opisthotonos (extreme arching of the spine), and other manifestations of brain stem involvement are noted early in infancy. Enlargement of the liver and spleen is also present. The infant has great difficulty in feeding and fails to grow. Usually death intervenes before the age of 2 years.

**Type III (Juvenile or Subacute Neuronopathic Gaucher's Disease).** This type has physical findings and survival intermediate between the first two forms. It has been noted especially in a group of 12 children from northern Sweden, the offspring of several related intermarriages.[2] These children have neurologic disease, with the onset between 6 months and 1 year of age. Their clinical course is more prolonged than in type II disease, with survival to late childhood or adolescence. The more severe the neurologic disease, the shorter the survival.

## Laboratory Diagnosis

Peripheral blood, bone marrow, and spleen are the sites most frequently examined in Gaucher's patients. The peripheral blood nearly always demonstrates a moderate normocytic anemia without active signs of replacement, such as polychromatophilic cells or nucleated red blood cells. There is pooling of blood in the enlarged spleen and some degree of ineffective erythropoiesis, with decreased incorporation of iron in erythroid precursors in the bone marrow. Leukocytes are commonly decreased in number. Platelets are also usually decreased in number as a result of splenic sequestra-

tion. These patients may have a bleeding tendency, with nosebleeds especially common. Gaucher's cells are noted only rarely in the peripheral blood.

Aspirates of bone marrow are often the first tissue in which Gaucher's cells are detected; these cells are required for the diagnosis **(see Color Figure 198)**. They are histiocytes, 20 to 80 $\mu$ in diameter, found in moderate numbers and as clumps of cells in the thickest areas of the smear. One or more round to oval nuclei are present in each cell. The cytoplasm is faintly blue with Wright's stain and has a "crumpled tissue paper" or finely folded appearance **(see Color Figure 198)**. Electron microscopy has demonstrated that this appearance is due to lamellar bodies stacked inside secondary phagolysosomes.[5] These cells have the following staining characteristics: positive with periodic acid–Schiff (PAS), acid phosphatase, Giemsa, iron, Sudan black B, and oil red O—all due to the accumulation of the unmetabolized glucocerebroside.

The spleen is enlarged to variable degrees owing to the accumulation of masses of Gaucher's cells. This enlargement is commonly up to 10 times normal splenic weight and can cause considerable discomfort to the patient.

Other organs and systems commonly affected include the liver and, in type II, the nervous system, pituitary gland, kidneys, lung, and ovaries.[6] All contain massive deposits of Gaucher's cells.

The serum acid phosphatase is increased, but proper detection requires the use of the substrate phenyl phosphate.[2] The isozyme measurement of this enzyme has shown that the tartrate-resistant fraction is what is increased in patients with Gaucher's disease.

Although the Gaucher's cell is pathognomonic of the disease in the proper clinical setting, so-called pseudo-Gaucher's cells have also been described. They are seen in disease states with increased cellular turnover, especially chronic myelogenous leukemia (CML), in which the phenomenon was first described. In theory, the increased cell turnover presents so much glycosyl ceramide to the reticuloendothelial system (RES) that its enzyme system is overwhelmed and cannot adequately metabolize all of the material. The excess is therefore stored in histiocytes, with their end morphologic expression identical to that of true Gaucher's cells. This phenomenon is also seen in a variety of other disorders, including acute myeloblastic leukemia (AML), chronic lymphocytic leukemia (CLL), plasma cell myeloma, aplastic anemia, idiopathic thrombocytopenic purpura (ITP), thalassemia major, and rheumatoid arthritis.[6] The presence of Gaucher-like cells in patients with these diseases has no known prognostic significance. It should be stressed that in each of these diseases there is no deficiency of the B-glucocerebrosidase, as there is in Gaucher's disease, but rather an overtaxation of a normal system.

## Prognosis

As previously stated, the length of survival in patients affected with Gaucher's disease is variable and depends on the type. The adult form has the longest survival, with patients surviving commonly into adulthood. Survival beyond 2 years of age in the infantile form is rare. As with its clinical features, the survival in the juvenile form is intermediate between the first two, but these individuals usually live into adolescence.

# Niemann-Pick Disease

Niemann-Pick disease is due to the deficiency of the enzyme sphingomyelinase with a secondary accumulation of the unmetabolized lipid sphingomyelin as well as cholesterol. Sphingomyelin is a common constituent of cell membranes as well as cellular organelles; thus, a deficiency of sphingomyelinase is most serious. There is an increased incidence of Niemann-Pick disease in Jews, especially in consanguinous populations. Because of the very different clinical manifestations the disease may take, it has been divided into five types—A through E. Only the first two types will be described, since they account for more than 85 percent of all cases.[7]

## Clinical Features

**Type A.** This form is also known as infantile or classic Niemann-Pick disease. This is the most common form of Niemann-Pick disease, accounting for up to 85 percent of all cases.[3,7] The onset is early in infancy, with failure to thrive, difficulty in feeding, and retarded physical and mental development. The skin has a waxy consistency. There is often jaundice at birth and usually hepatosplenomegaly, with a distended abdomen. The lymph nodes are enlarged as well. A "cherry-red spot" in the macula of the eye is found in approximately one half of the affected infants.[7] The neurologic symptoms are more pronounced in this type of Niemann-Pick dis-

ease than in any of the others. Deterioration is relentless and survival past the age of 1 or 2 years is rare.

**Type B.** Also called the chronic, or adult form, this type is seen much less frequently than type A, with only 13 reported cases in the literature.[2] Clinical onset consisting of hepatosplenomegaly is usually found in infancy, but the central nervous system is not involved. Individuals with this type of disease may have longer survival than those with type A, but they do not survive beyond childhood or early adolescence.

## Laboratory Diagnosis

There is a distinct pattern to the histiocytes in Niemann-Pick disease. These cells are most commonly seen in the bone marrow and spleeen, although they accumulate throughout the body and in the nervous system in patients with type A. They are large cells, 20 to 90 $\mu$ in diameter, with an inconspicuous nucleus. The cytoplasm is filled with and distended by round, uniformly sized droplets of accumulated lipid, giving the cell a very pale or light blue color when Wright-stained **(see Color Figure 199)**. Stains giving a positive reaction with Niemann-Pick cells are the lipid stains oil red O, Sudan black, and luxol fast blue; and acid phosphatase and nonspecific esterase. The PAS staining is weak, and the myeloperoxidase is negative.

Some adult patients with certain varieties of Niemann-Pick disease contain, in the bone marrow, a mixture of Niemann-Pick cells and sea-blue histiocytes, which are histiocytes distended with blue-staining ceroid on Wright's stain. It is believed that the sphingomyelin is gradually metabolized to the ceroid, thus generating the sea-blue histiocytes.[6] A marrow specimen with these findings would then need to be distinguished from the entity of sea-blue histiocytosis (see further on).

Other disorders that may cause Niemann-Pick–like cells to be contained in the bone marrow are $GM_1$ gangliosidosis, lactosyl ceramidosis, and Fabry's disease.[6]

The peripheral blood is most remarkable for the vacuoles that may be found in lymphocytes and monocytes of a routine peripheral blood smear. These vacuoles are round and from two to 20 may be found within one cell.[3] Anemia and leukopenia may be present but do not usually pose any threat to the patient.[3] Serum lipids are not usually increased.[3]

## Prognosis

There may be a slight increase in survival with the other types, but type A patients have a very short lifespan. Survival past the age of 2 years is uncommon. Type E is very rare and has been found only in adults who have a mild chronic course without any neurologic manifestations.[2]

## Tay-Sachs Disease

Also known as amaurotic infantile idiocy or $GM_2$ gangliosidosis, Tay-Sachs disease was first described in 1881 by the British ophthalmologist Warren Tay, and in 1886 by the New York neurologist Bernard Sachs. It has a particularly high incidence in the Ashkenazi Jewish population (those Jews who trace their origin to the Baltic Sea region) that is 100 times greater than the incidence in the non-Jewish population.[8] It is estimated that this high-risk group has a one in 30 carrier rate.[9] This autosomal recessive sphingolipidosis is due to a deficiency of the enzyme hexosaminidase A, with an increase of the other isoenzyme, hexosaminidase B. The unmetabolized $GM_2$ ganglioside accumulates in almost all tissues and has its most devastating effects within the central nervous system and eye.

### Clinical Features

Although affected infants appear normal at birth, by 6 months of age both physical and mental deterioration are notable. They have an exaggerated physical response to noise–the "startle reflex." In addition, a cherry-red spot in the macula of each eye is found. The infants eventually go blind. Along with the continual deterioration, there is enlargement of the head (macrocephaly), seizures, and paralysis. The neurons are greatly enlarged by accumulation of the unmetabolized ganglioside in vacuoles in the cytoplasm. In contrast to many other lipid storage diseases, the spleen, liver, and lymph nodes are not enlarged.[2] Feeding is poor, and death eventuates by 4 years of age.

### Laboratory Diagnosis

The major site of pathology is in the central nervous system, and examination of other tissues is less instructive. The peripheral blood contains vacuolated lymphocytes. The number and size of the vacuoles are related to the duration of the disease; it is postulated, but not definitely proven, that they contain the unmetabolized lipid (see Color Figure 200).[10] Vacuolated lymphocytes, however, are not pathognomonic for Tay-Sachs disease, as they are also seen in Niemann-Pick disease and in certain types of leukemias. Foam cells, or vacuolated histiocytes, are found in the bone marrow. Again, these cells are helpful but not diagnostic.

Because of the high frequency of disease in certain populations, prenatal detection has taken on greater importance. Culture of fetal fibroblasts from the amniotic fluid can be undertaken to detect hexosaminidase A levels in the fetus. Mass screening programs of adults at possible risk for transmitting

the disease have been undertaken, with variable success.[8]

### Prognosis

This disease is uniformly fatal before the age of 4 years. Attempts at enzyme replacement are just being undertaken, and the final results of the potential therapy are not yet known.

## Mucopolysaccharidoses (MPS)

The original descriptions of children affected with different forms of the mucopolysaccharidoses (MPS) were published within a relatively short time span at the turn of the century. Dr. John Thompson first described three young brothers with the characteristics now called Hurler's syndrome, in London in 1900; Gertrud Hurler elaborated on his description, describing two unrelated boys in Munich in 1919 with very similar characteristics. In 1917, Hunter described two brothers with a constellation of abnormalities now recognized as Hunter's syndrome.

Like the previously described disorders, the mucopolysaccharidoses show accumulations of unmetabolized material within lysosomes (see Color Figure 201). However, it is mucopolysaccharides, not sphingolipids, that accumulate. The clinical severity of these disorders varies widely. Products are found in the reticuloendothelial system (spleen, bone marrow, liver), lymph nodes, blood vessels, brain, heart, connective tissue, and urine.

### Categories

The mucopolysaccharidoses have been arranged into seven types (Table 23–2 gives an abbreviated classification scheme), but there are only four possible unmetabolized products: keratan sulfate, dermatan sulfate, heparan sulfate, or chondroitin sulfate. With the exception of Hunter's syndrome, which is X-linked recessive, these disorders have an autosomal recessive mode of inheritance. There does not appear to be a significant increase of affected individuals within any one ethnic group. The final classification of MPS is still somewhat unclear because of the interrelationships with cystic fibrosis and glycolipid storage diseases.[4]

### Clinical Features

There are many clinical abnormalities found within each type of MPS, and there are seven types of MPS; therefore, a detailed description of each is not possible here. The findings in Hurler's syndrome will be given in the most detail, because it is considered the prototype of the mucopolysaccharidoses.

In Hurler's syndrome (MPS I), there may be a short period of apparently normal development, but this is only temporary. These individuals are abnor-

## Table 23–2. MUCOPOLYSACCHARIDOSES (MPS)

| Name | Genetics | Accumulated Product | Enzyme Deficiency | Life Expectancy | Intelligence | Clinical Features |
|---|---|---|---|---|---|---|
| MPS I H (Hurler's) | AR | Heparan sulfate<br>Dermatan sulfate | α-L-iduronidase | 6–10 yr | Retarded | 1. Onset 6–8 mo<br>2. Dwarfism<br>3. Large, long head<br>4. Flat, broad nose with upturned nostrils<br>5. Corneal clouding<br>6. Hepatosplenomegaly<br>7. Valvular lesions<br>8. Coronary artery lesions<br>9. Skeletal deformities<br>10. Joint stiffness |
| MPS I S (Scheie's) | AR | Heparan sulfate<br>Dermatan sulfate | α-L-iduronidase | Normal | Normal | 1. Onset after 5 yr<br>2. Near normal height<br>3. Corneal clouding<br>4. Valvular lesions<br>5. Coronary artery lesions<br>6. Finger stiffness |
| MPS I H–S (Hurler-Scheie) | AR | Heparan sulfate<br>Dermatan sulfate | α-L-iduronidase | 3rd decade | Mild retardation (may be normal) | 1. Onset infancy<br>2. Dwarfism<br>3. Facial and bony lesions of Hurler's syndrome<br>4. Cardiac lesions |
| MPS II (Hunter) (wide range of severity) | X–R | Heparan sulfate<br>Dermatan sulfate | L-iduronosulfate sulfatase | 2nd decade to normal | Mild retardation to normal | 1. Similar to Hurler's syndrome, *but*<br>  a. No corneal clouding<br>  b. Retinal degeneration<br>  c. Deafness<br>  d. Nodular skin infiltrates |
| MPS III Sanfilippo's A Sanfilippo's B Sanfilippo's C (range of severity) | AR | Heparan sulfate<br>Heparan sulfate<br>Heparan sulfate | Sulfaminidase<br>α-N-acetylglucosaminidase<br>α-Glucosaminidase | 2nd–3rd decade | Retarded | 1. Onset after 3 yr<br>2. Normal growth<br>3. Hurler facies<br>4. No corneal clouding<br>5. No heart disease<br>6. No hepatosplenomegaly<br>7. Mild skeletal changes |
| MPS IV (Morquio's) (wide range of severity) | AR | Keratan sulfate<br>Chondroitin sulfate | N-acetylhexosaminidase Sulfatase | 3rd–6th decade | Normal | 1. Dwarfism<br>2. Thoracolumbar gibbus<br>3. Kyphoscoliosis<br>4. Facies similar to Hurler's syndrome<br>5. Corneal clouding<br>6. Valvular and coronary artery lesions<br>7. Joint hypermobility<br>8. Genu valgum |
| MPS VI (Maroteaux-Lamy) | AR | Dermatan sulfate | N-acetylhexosaminidase 4-SO$_4$ sulfatase | 2nd decade | Normal | 1. Similar to Hurler's syndrome, *but*<br>  a. Preservation of intelligence<br>  b. Longer survival |
| MPS VII (Glucuronidase deficiency disease) | AR | Dermatan sulfate<br>Heparan sulfate<br>Chondroitin sulfate | β-Glucuronidase | (?) Some restriction | (?) Retarded | Variable |

AR = Autosomal recessive; X–R = X-linked recessive. (From Robbins and Cotran,[9] p. 250, with permission.)

mally short and have coarse facial features, with a broad, flat nose, widely spaced eyes, and thickened tongue and lips. Some authors have described their appearance as similar to that of a gargoyle (the carved heads sometimes found on older European churches). The amount of body hair is increased, dark, and especially prominent on the forehead. The skin is thickened. Patients are mentally retarded. Clouding of the corneas in the eyes is present. These individuals may have hearing loss or be completely deaf. The heart is damaged, owing to the accumulation of mucopolysaccharide in the valves and blood vessels. There is a hump-back and prominent abdomen, with enlarged liver and spleen. The arms and legs are abnormal, with contractures of many joints. In addition, the hands are very wide and the fingers shortened.

In Hunter's syndrome (MPS II), the changes are similar, although not as severe. Corneal clouding is much less common. Patients affected with Sanfilippo's syndrome (MPS III) have a more normal stature but unfortunately many more severe neurologic problems and decreased survival. Compared with Hurler's syndrome, patients with Scheie's syndrome have more prominent corneal clouding but less abnormality in stature, facial appearance, or mental development. Patients with MPS VI (Maroteaux-Lamy syndrome) have growth and skeletal abnormalities, but mental retardation is not present. In Morquio's syndrome (MPS IV) patients have numerous skeletal changes, giving a markedly abnormal physical appearance; there is no mental retardation, however.

### Laboratory Diagnosis and Prognosis

In contrast to the other lysosomal storage diseases, nonmetabolized products may be detected in the urine of patients with MPS. Using the toluidine blue spot test or the turbidity test to detect acid mucopolysaccharides is the initial screening test. The spot test may be unreliable, however, and up to 32 percent false-negative test results in patients with Hurler's syndrome have been reported.[11] Also of note is that the urine of normal healthy newborns may give false-positive results, a phenomenon that disappears by 2 weeks of age.[11] Any positive screening test should be confirmed by column chromotography.

An interesting, but somewhat inconsistent, finding in the MPS in the peripheral blood is the presence of large granules in leukocytes, especially lymphocytes. These are known as Alder-Reilly bodies **(see Color Figure 141)**. In polymorphonuclear leukocytes (PMN), this needs to be distinguished from toxic granulation, but the large size of the granules in MPS usually leaves little doubt. A metachromatic stain, such as toluidine blue, will aid in confirmation. These granules are found with much greater

regularity, however, in histiocytes and lymphocytes in the bone marrow.[3]

The prognosis of the MPS varies somewhat with the type. Patients with Hurler's syndrome may live into their teens, while those affected with Hunter's syndrome may live into their twenties. Individuals who have Sanfilippo's syndrome do not usually survive to their teens. The theoretical aid of enzyme replacement therapy has yet to be translated into practical results.

## HISTIOCYTOSES
### Sea-Blue Histiocyte Syndrome

Although initially described in isolated case reports of young adults with an enlarged spleen, the syndrome of the sea-blue histiocyte is a genetic disorder with a benign course. The striking blue color of the histiocytes after staining with Wright's or May-Grünwald-Giemsa stain gives the syndrome its name.

The mode of transmission has not been clearly established, but autosomal recessive inheritance, with a variable degree of expression, appears most likely. Most patients are diagnosed before they reach 40 years of age. The earlier in life the disease is found, the more severe it is likely to be. Major findings on physical examination are splenomegaly and usually hepatomegaly. Also described, but occurring less consistently, are abnormalities of the eye, skin, and nervous system. Involvement of the lung may be noted on roentgenographic examination. Involvement of the lymph nodes is not seen.

Significant laboratory findings are usually confined to the blood. In the peripheral blood, thrombocytopenia is found with great frequency. Consequently clinical manifestations such as epistaxis, gastrointestinal tract bleeding, and purpura may be expected. However, there is no correlation of the degree of thrombocytopenia with the size of the spleen.[12] Blood lipids are normal. Abnormal liver function studies are only rarely seen.

The bone marrow aspirate is usually the site of diagnosis. Histiocytes of variable size (20 to 60 $\mu$) are present in greatly increased numbers. They contain the blue- to green-staining granules that vary in size, shape, and ability to take up the stain **(see Color Figure 202)**. Thus, not all cells will have the same staining intensity. It is not at present known why the granules stain blue with these stains. The cells will also react with the PAS, Sudan black B, and acid fast stains, but not with toluidine blue or iron stains.[12,13] Tissue sections stained with hematoxylin and eosin show some of the cells with pale-yellow pigmentation but without cytoplasmic staining. Both histochemical stains and tissue lipid analysis have shown the cells to contain largely glycolipid, phospholipid, and sphingolipid.

**Table 23–3. MAJOR FINDINGS IN HISTIOCYTIC DISORDERS**

| Disease | Age at Onset | Main Site(s) of Involvement | Course and Prognosis |
|---|---|---|---|
| Eosinophilic granuloma | Especially in males Children and young adults Often no symptoms until bone fracture | Unifocal: skull, rib, femur most common | Rare spontaneous healing; most require surgical removal; occasionally patients have recurrences |
| Hand-Schüller-Christian disease | Usually <5 yr old | Multifocal: bones, skin, lymphoid tissue; triad of pituitary, eye and skull involvement are characteristic but uncommon | 50%: spontaneous recovery 50%: recover with chemotherapy |
| Letterer-Siwe disease | Usually <3 yr old | Generalized: skin, lymphoid tissue, bones, ± bone marrow; more severe and extensive than H-S-C disease | Chemotherapy has improved prognosis, which was previously considered poor |

The great majority of patients with this syndrome do well and have normal lifespans. Splenectomy is not inevitable; many patients never require removal of the spleen. As previously mentioned, manifestations of the disease at an early age may imply more severe symptomatology.

Brief mention is made here of acquired, or secondary, sea-blue histiocyte syndrome. Cells identical in appearance to those in the primary disorder are found but in lesser numbers than in the primary syndrome. They are present in both the spleen and the bone marrow of patients with other, unrelated disorders. These disorders include ITP, CML, sickle cell anemia, thalassemia, polycythemia vera, sarcoidosis, and many other diseases.[3,13] The finding of these cells has led to the consideration that they may occur in individuals with a partial enzyme deficiency who are under stress from another disease.[12]

## Other Histiocytic Disorders (Eosinophilic Granuloma, Hand-Schüller-Christian Disease, Letterer-Siwe Disease)

The group of histiocytic disorders described here may be thought of as an abnormal proliferation and accumulation of mature histiocytes, or Langerhans' cells. These cells are normally found in small numbers in the skin and RES. Most patients are either children or young adults. A favorable outcome may be expected in most cases, with the exception of some patients with Letterer-Siwe disease, which may be fatal. These disorders may actually represent a continuum, from the unifocal and benign eosinophilic granuloma to the generalized and sometimes fatal Letterer-Siwe disease.[9] The term "histiocytosis X" is used generally to describe these

disorders. Table 23–3 summarizes their major findings. The malignant histiocytic disorders are discussed elsewhere in this book.

The clinical presentation of these disorders may consist of a myriad of findings, a solitary lesion, or anything between these two extremes. Removal of tissue for pathologic examination is necessary for the diagnosis. Microscopically, the different entities all have in common an accumulation of histiocytes with a distinctive appearance and a variable admixture of eosinophils, neutrophils, lymphocytes, plasma cells, giant cells, and foam cells in a fibrotic background. These histiocytes also have characteristic organelles—Langerhans' (Birbeck) granules—which may be seen only with the aid of the electron microscope.

There are no diagnostic findings in examination of the peripheral blood. In Letterer-Siwe disease, however, the presence of anemia or thrombocytopenia has been associated with a poor prognosis. This usually reflects involvement of the bone marrow by the disease.

## References

1. Desnick, RJ: Gaucher disease (1882–1982): Centennial perspectives on the most prevalent Jewish genetic disease. Mt Sinai J Med 49:443, 1982.
2. Kolodny, EH: Clinical and biochemical genetics of the lipidoses. Semin Hematol 9:251, 1972.
3. Wintrobe, MM: Clinical Hematology. Lea & Febiger, Philadelphia, 1981.
4. Stanbury, JB, Wyngaarden, JB, and Fredrickson, DS: The Metabolic Basis of Inherited Disease. McGraw-Hill, New York, 1972.
5. Lee, RE: The pathology of Gaucher disease. In Desnick, RJ, Gatt, S, and Grabowski, GA (eds): Gaucher Disease: A Century of Delineation and Research. Progress in Clinical and Biological Research. Vol 95. Alan R. Liss, New York, 1982, p 193.

6. Savage, RA: Specific and not-so-specific histiocytes in bone marrow. Lab Med 15:467, 1984.

7. Volk, BW, Adachi, M, and Schneck, L: The pathology of sphingolipidoses. Semin Hematol 9:317, 1972.

8. Goodman, MJ and Goodman, LE: The overselling of genetic anxiety. Hastings Cent Rep 12:20, 1982.

9. Robbins, SL and Cotran, RS: Pathologic Basis of Disease. WB Saunders, Philadelphia, 1979.

10. Brunning, RD: Morphologic alterations in nucleated blood and marrow cells in genetic disorders. Human Pathol 1:99, 1970.

11. Henry, JB: Todd, Sanford, Davidsohn. Clinical Diagnosis and Management by Laboratory Methods. WB Saunders, Philadelphia, 1984, p 454.

12. Sawitsky, A, Rosner, F, and Chodsky, S: The sea-blue histiocyte syndrome, a review: Genetic and biochemical studies. Sem Hematol 9:285, 1972.

13. Silverstein, MN and Ellefson, RD: The syndrome of the sea-blue histiocyte. Sem Hematol 9:299, 1972.

# CHAPTER 24

THOMAS J. FORLENZA, M.D., AND
D. HARMENING PITTIGLIO, Ph.D., M.T.(ASCP)

# The Lymphomas

Lymphomas represent an autonomous neoplastic growth of cellular elements of lymphoid tissue. Therefore, the lymph nodes and organs containing lymphoid tissue are usually primary sites of this type of malignancy.

Lymphomas are generally considered one of the lymphoproliferative diseases. This commonly used, broad term ("lymphoproliferative disorders" is also used) applies to a variety of localized or systemic proliferative disorders involving cell types indigenous to the lymphoreticular system. Cells of the lymphoreticular system include lymphocytes, plasma cells, histiocytes, and their precursors or derivatives. Table 24–1 lists diseases generally categorized as lymphoproliferative.

The term "lymphoma" refers to the asymmetrical enlargement of a group of lymph nodes, which destroys the normal histologic lymph node architecture. It is often this asymptomatic mass that usually forces the person to seek medical attention. Using this definition, lymphomas can be divided into Hodgkin's lymphoma, non-Hodgkin's lymphoma (malignant lymphoma usually of B-cell origin), and rare lymphomas such as T-cell lymphomas (lymphomas of the skin).

Since there is still some question regarding the pathogenesis of Hodgkin's lymphoma, as to whether it is a neoplastic disorder or is inflammatory in origin, the term "Hodgkin's disease" is more commonly used than "Hodgkin's lymphoma." Hodgkin's disease is regarded as a separate autonomous disorder, because there is a morphologic common denominator present among all forms, a distinctive giant cell known as the Reed-Sternberg cell **(see Color Figure 204)**. The Reed-Sternberg cell of Hodgkin's disease may not readily resemble the malignant transformation of a normal nodal element. However, the disturbed nodal architecture and the

**Table 24–1. LYMPHOPROLIFERATIVE DISORDERS**

1. Hodgkin's disease
2. Malignant non-Hodgkin's lymphomas
3. Lymphocytic and lymphoblastic leukemia
4. Plasma cell dyscrasias* (see Chapter 22)
5. Histiocytoses (see Chapter 23)

*Usually subcategorized as an immunoproliferative disorder.

consistent finding of this distinctive cell type make Hodgkin's disease the prototype lymphoma. Characteristically, various components of lymphocytes or histiocytes or both can be found in patients with Hodgkin's disease.

It is believed that the non-Hodgkin's lymphomas (NHL) result from a block in B-cell development with subsequent uncontrolled clonal proliferation of the neoplastic cell (Fig. 24-1). The massive B-cell proliferation replaces the normal architecture and invades the lymph node capsule, and the disease process ensues. These malignant lymphomas represent tumorous lesions composed mainly of lymphocytes or transformed lymphocytes and rarely of true histiocytic origin that arise in lymphoid tissue anywhere in the body. Most commonly these cohesive tumorous lesions develop within the lymph nodes and less frequently within the extranodal lymphatic tissue.

Hodgkin's lymphomas follow a step-wise and relatively consistent pattern of spread from one chain of nodes to adjacent groups. Advancement of the disease tends to involve contiguous areas in a progressive fashion. The non-Hodgkin's lymphomas may also follow a step-wise metastatic pattern, but this occurs less reliably than in Hodgkin's disease.

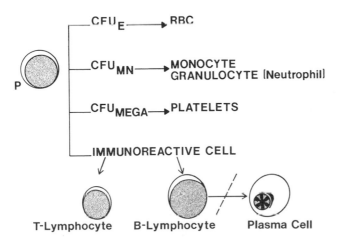

**Figure 24-1.** Schematic representation of differentiation of the various cell lines. The *dotted line* indicates the block in B-cell development, which may explain the clonal origins of some lymphomas. P = pluripotential cell; $CFU_E$ = colony-forming unit–erythroid; $CFU_{MN}$ = colony-forming unit–monocyte; neutrophil; $CFU_{MEGA}$ = colony-forming unit–megakaryocyte; T = T lymphocyte; B = B lymphocyte.

In the late stages of these disorders, widespread systemic metastases and visceral organ involvement may occur **(see Color Figure 203)**. Death may result from serious infiltration of vital organs, infection, severe malnutrition, or markedly reduced hematopoietic cell elements. The nature of nodal involvement is determined by a lymph node biopsy and histologic examination for determination of the histologic type. Clinical and radiologic evaluation will determine the clinical stage. Prognosis is dependent on both pathologic subtype and clinical stage of the disease, and will be discussed later.

In the terminal phases of the disease, patients with the non-Hodgkin's lymphomas can develop a leukemic phase, in contrast to those with Hodgkin's lymphomas, in whom there is virtually never a leukemic component.

## HODGKIN'S DISEASE
### History and Presentation

In 1832, Thomas Hodgkin of Guy's Hospital, London, described lymph node enlargement in seven patients, six of whom he had examined. He believed that the glandular enlargements were not reactive but represented a primary problem. Ninety-seven years later, subsequent examination of the tissue preserved from three of the cases in the Guy's Hospital Museum confirmed the diagnosis of Hodgkin's disease using present-day criteria.

Carl Sternberg in 1898 and Dorothy Reed in 1902 described the histologically characteristic giant cells as the common denominator among all forms of Hodgkin's disease. At that time, neither investigator, however, believed the disease to be malignant.

Even today there is still some question as to whether Hodgkin's disease is a neoplastic disorder or an inflammatory process. Almost invariably, Hodgkin's disease originates in the lymph nodes. Nodal involvement is contiguous, spreading from one chain of nodes to adjacent ones in a regular progression.

The diagnosis of Hodgkin's disease cannot be made unless the characteristic Reed-Sternberg cell is found in the appropriate histologic milieu **(see Color Figure 204)**. Cells resembling Reed-Sternberg cells may be found in patients with other malignant diseases (e.g., carcinoma of the breast and multiple myeloma) and in those with benign diseases (e.g., infectious mononucleosis, rubella, and toxoplasmosis). It is therefore imperative that the appropriate clinical and pathologic setting be present before a lymph node biopsy is performed and a diagnosis of Hodgkin's disease "established."

The origin of the Reed-Sternberg cell remains unresolved, but the macrophage seems to be a good candidate. In any event, the cell has very distinctive features and is readily recognized once found. Classically, Reed-Sternberg cells are giant cells that often are binucleated or bilobed. Their nuclei are often mirror images of each other with prominent large, "owl-eyed" nucleoli that generally are surrounded by a clear halo (see Color Figure 204).

## Classification

The Rye classification is almost unanimously accepted as the classification of Hodgkin's disease. Four distinctive, characteristic patterns have been recognized in this classification (Table 24 – 2), correlating with the general rule, the more abundant the lymphocytes, the more favorable the prognosis for the disease (see Color Figures 204 through 207).

## Incidence

Hodgkin's disease has a bimodal incidence. It is found in patients in their late twenties, and then again with increasing frequency after the age of 40 to 45, with a peak incidence between 50 and 60 years of age. Men are affected more frequently than women; the frequency recorded for men is 3.6/100,000 persons per year, compared with 2.6/100,000 persons per year for women. Although no specific etiology is known, an increased risk seems to exist if there is no early exposure to infection, a higher socioeconomic class, a one-sibling family, single-family housing, and few playmates.

There are studies supporting and disavowing the Epstein-Barr virus as the causative agent in Hodgkin's disease. However, there does seem to be a more frequent history of infectious mononucleosis in patients with Hodgkin's disease. An association with white cell antigens HLA-B5 and B18 has been suggested, but again, data seem to be inconsistent. Hodgkin's disease usually never has a leukemic component.

## Clinical Manifestations

Since the disease is initially confined to the lymph nodes, painless swelling — usually in the cervical area — is the most common presenting feature. Constitutional symptoms of low-grade fever, night sweats that usually drench the bed clothing, and weight loss of more than 10 percent of baseline body weight during the six months preceding the diagnosis comprise what are called "B symptoms." Their absence is designated by "A" after each stage. The classic Pel-Ebstein fever, with febrile periods of one to two weeks alternating with afebrile periods, is usually not seen. Lymph node size may vary with fever.

Other symptomology includes pruritis. Even though this is no longer considered one of the B symptoms, it may be the only symptom in someone with malaise and should alert the clinician to the possibility of a diagnosis of Hodgkin's disease. It is interesting to note that patients with Hodgkin's disease may complain of pain in the lymph node a few minutes after drinking alcoholic beverages. As with pruritis, the mechanism of this nonspecific symptom is unknown.

Although probably not an overt symptom, testicular dysfunction has been found in persons with untreated Hodgkin's disease. The complex etiology involves not only primary testicular failure but also both pituitary and gonadal abnormalities. These abnormalities are not present in men with other malignancies.

## Signs

The lymph node examination will be abnormal, with left cervical and supraclavicular nodes being swollen in 71 percent of patients and with these as the only sites of involvement in 43 percent. Right cervical or supraclavicular nodes (or both) and mediastinal nodes follow in frequency as sites of involvement in 59 percent and 62 percent of patients, respectively, as areas of sole involvement in 22 percent and 9 percent, respectively. The majority of patients with supraclavicular and mediastinal involvement have the nodular sclerosing variety (Kaplan). Waldeyer's ring is only rarely involved in patients with Hodgkin's disease.

Splenomegaly is present in about 65 percent of patients. Hodgkin's disease limited to the spleen is reported in about 25 percent (12 of 48) of cases of isolated splenomegaly. As the disease progresses, virtually every organ can be affected. Even the skin may be involved, via retrograde flow from involved nodes.

## Laboratory Features

The common laboratory profile at the onset of the disease is a normocytic normochromic anemia with a transitory increase in circulating lymphocytes, an absolute increase in monocytes and eosinophils, and often an increase in blood platelets. Large atypical lymphoid cells, almost totally lacking cytoplasm and demonstrating abnormal, irregular nuclear chromatin, may be present on the peripheral smear. During the advanced stages of the disease leukocytosis predominates, with an increase in the granulocytic series and a decrease in lymphocytes. The differential usually demonstrates prominent toxic granulation, with the presence of large, bizarre platelets. Occasionally, the Coombs test may be positive, and patients may present with an autoimmune hemolytic anemia or thrombocytopenia or both (see Chapter 12).

The Westergren sedimentation rate is commonly increased and serves as a useful nonspecific marker of disease activity. Disease infiltration of visceral organs may be reflected on the respective chemical test results (e.g., liver involvement, elevated alkaline phosphatase, and so forth).

Table 24–2. RYE CLASSIFICATION FOR HODGKIN'S LYMPHOMAS

| Pattern | General Age Group | Description | Presence of Reed-Sternberg (RS) cells | Frequency (% of Cases) | Prognosis | Color Figure |
|---------|-------------------|-------------|----------------------------------------|------------------------|-----------|--------------|
| 1. LP (lymphocyte predominant) | Young individuals | Characterized by a diffuse infiltrate of mature lymphocytes mixed with variable numbers of histiocytes. | Few in number | 5–10 | Best | 205 |
| 2. NS (nodular sclerosis) | Young individuals | Represents a distinct entity with a different epidemiology and biologic significance from the other three patterns. Unique to this pattern are two characteristics: (1) biopsy specimen characterized by birefringent bands of collagen, which traverse the lymph node, enclosing nodules of normal and abnormal lymphoid tissue; and (2) presence of a Reed-Sternberg cell variant called a lacunar cell, which looks like a Langhans' giant cell that sits in a lacunar space. | RS variant (lacunar cells present) | 35–60 | Second best | 207 |
| tx3. MC (mixed cellularity) | Middle age (30 yr old) | Characterized by a diffuse infiltrate of lymphocytes, histiocytes, eosinophils, and plasma cells, which obliterate the underlying nodal architecture. | Usually plentiful | 30–50 | Third best | 204 |
| 4. LD (lymphocyte-depletion) | Middle age | Characterized by a paucity of lymphocytes and diffuse fibrosis. | Few in number | 1–5 | Worst | 206 |

There appears to be a T-cell abnormality before and after treatment with chemotherapy in patients with Hodgkin's disease, with reduction in the percentage of E rosettes and mitogen-induced lymphocyte proliferation. Cutaneous anergy is a consistent finding, with depressed skin reactivity to common antigens such as Candida, mumps, streptokinase, and dermatophyton.

## Staging and Prognosis

The same staging system is used, regardless of whether the patient is staged clinically by physical examination or clinically and pathologically by staging laparotomy and lymph node biopsy. Hodgkin's disease is divided into four distinct clinical stages depending on which lymph node areas are involved (Table 24–3).

As described earlier, if constitutional symptoms of fever, night sweats, or weight loss are present, a "B" is appended to the staging categories; if these are absent, an "A" is appended. An "E" category has been described, to indicate extension from a lymph node group into adjacent organs except for the lung (e.g., into the thyroid gland). An "S" is used to describe isolated splenic involvement, which does not appear to have as grave a prognosis as does extranodal organ involvement.

The subdivision of stage IIIA into $III_1A$ (involvement of spleen, splenic, celiac, or portal nodes or any combination of these) and $III_2A$ (involvement of para-aortic, iliac, or mesenteric nodes, with or without upper abdominal involvement) has implications for treatment. The five-year survival rates in stage $III_1A$ were similar for those receiving chemotherapy and radiotherapy and those receiving radiotherapy alone; however, the disease-free survival was better in those receiving combined-modality treatment. Since there is no difference in five-year survival, it seems reasonable to save chemotherapy for patients who have relapses, rather than to expose the entire group to the increased risk of leukemia associated with combined-

modality treatment (5 percent + 1 percent per year after five years).

The different histologic types may carry different prognoses. Lymphocytic-predominant Hodgkin's disease is a relatively indolent disease and carries the best prognosis; this is followed by nodular sclerosis, mixed cellularity, and lymphocyte-depletion Hodgkin's disease. Among the last three subtypes, once remission is induced, relapse-free survival is best for lymphocyte depletion. This implies that nodular sclerosing histology has an adverse effect on survival, but this only seems to apply for the group of patients with nodular sclerosing type who have a depletion of lymphocytes. At the time of presentation, approximately 60 percent of cases will be nodular sclerosis, 30 percent mixed cellularity, 5 to 9 percent lymphocyte-predominant, and 1 to 2 percent lymphocyte-depletion Hodgkin's disease.

## Treatment

Pusey in 1902 and Senn in 1903 first reported impressive responses of patients with Hodgkin's disease to kilovoltage radiation. Alkylating agents were the first chemotherapeutic agents used. Subsequently, chemotherapeutic agents that happened to be effective in Hodgkin's disease were developed in 1949 and 1962. In 1963, de Vita and colleagues at the National Cancer Institute introduced MOMP, nitrogen mustard (mustargen), oncovin (vincristine), methotrexate, and prednisone. Procarbazine was shown to be more effective than methotrexate and was therefore substituted in the MOMP regimen in 1964; and it became MOPP therapy. This still serves as the mainstay of treatment for patients with Hodgkin's disease.

Today, treatment is usually determined by the clinical and pathologic staging and by whether there are A or B symptoms present.

Untreated Hodgkin's disease is almost universally fatal. Craft in the 1940s reported on all stages in an untreated population and found a median survival of less than one year and an 8 percent survival at five years. It is not possible to cure all stages of Hodgkin's disease. Survival curves in stages IA and IIA approach 80 to 90 percent cure rate, with radiation used as a single modality. Concurrent chemotherapy is not indicated, because it is possible to salvage the 10 to 20 percent of those patients with recurring disease with chemotherapy, and still achieve cure.

As already mentioned, subdividing Hodgkin's disease stage IIIA into $III_1A$ and $III_2A$ may have therapeutic implications. For reasons discussed under the section on prognosis, chemotherapy may be reserved for relapses in patients with stage $III_1A$ disease, and radiotherapy can be used as a primary modality. Combination chemotherapy has been shown to be far superior to single-agent treatment

**Table 24–3. STAGING OF HODGKIN'S DISEASE***

| | |
|---|---|
| I | One group of lymph nodes involved with disease, either above or below diaphragm |
| II | Two different groups of lymph nodes involved with disease, both being either above or below diaphragm |
| III† | Two different groups of lymph nodes involved with disease, on each side of diaphragm |
| IV | Extranodal involvement in areas not contiguous with lymph nodes.‡ |

*The A and B subdivisions can be affixed to each clinical stage depending on the clinical symptomology (see text).

†Stage IIIA is subdivided into 1 and 2 (see text).

‡E classification indicates extension from a lymph node area (see text).

for patients with stage III and IV disease and for those patients with B symptoms. Consolidation treatment with radiation is used, because the relapse rate in sites of initially bulky disease is high, despite effective and apparently curative doses of systemic multiagent chemotherapy. Patients who have stage IA and IIA disease have traditionally been treated with radiotherapy. There are groups studying combined-modality treatment in this group in an attempt to salvage the 10 percent of patients who have relapses. With improvement in radiation therapy and the ability to salvage radiation failures with combination chemotherapy, this approach should be attempted only in an investigational setting. Patients with stage II disease and with bulky mediastinal involvement and extension into lung or bone represent a special subset that may benefit from combined-modality treatment.

The advanced Hodgkin's disease stages IIIB and IV pose a different management problem, and aggressive eight-drug combinations have been used with very encouraging results, although MOPP therapy is still the first-line treatment in most cases.

The availability of effective salvage regimens, a good probability of salvage with MOPP therapy given a second time, and advances in supportive treatment modalities have made the management of Hodgkin's disease very favorable. The scheduling of chemotherapy and combination approach has served as a model for treating other malignancies.

## CASE HISTORY

A.D., a 24-year-old white male counselor, presented with the chief complaint of a small mass in the left supraclavicular region for two weeks.

Three weeks prior to admission, he noted soreness only at night in the upper part of the sternum, radiating to the supraclavicular regions bilaterally. The soreness woke him from sleep. Two weeks prior to admission, he developed a sore throat and noticed a small mass in the left supraclavicular area and in the right axilla and sought medical attention. He noted fever and weight loss but could not quantitate how much weight he had lost.

**Past History.** The patient's history was remarkable for German measles in 1980. He denied tobacco abuse and admitted to drinking a six-pack of beer per day. There were no known allergies.

**Family History.** The patient's father had hypertension; his mother, diverticulitis and hypertension; and his sister, a history of spontaneous pneumothorax.

**Review of Systems.** This was unremarkable, except as noted earlier.

**Physical Examination.** The patient was a pleasant white male in no acute distress. Blood pressure was 132/66; pulse 100, regular; respiratory rate 18, unlabored; temperature 100°F. There were no ecchymoses or petechiae. Lymph nodes were examined, and two firm nodes were revealed, one in the right supraclavicular area approximately 2 × 2 cm, the other in the left supraclavicular area 2 × 2 cm node. In the right axilla, nontender nodes were found. The remainder of the lymph node areas were unremarkable. Further examination revealed the following. Chest and lungs: clear to auscultation and percussion. Heart: regular rhythm; no murmurs, gallops, rubs, or clicks. Pulse: 3/4 to dorsalis pedis. Abdomen: no palpable hepatomegaly, splenomegaly, or masses. Neurologic examination: reflexes 5/5, symmetrical; no Babinski sign. Cranial nerves II through XII within normal limits.

**Laboratory Data.** Hb 14.6 g/dl, HCT 44.9 percent, MCV 81.5 $\mu^3$, MCH 26.5 $\mu\mu$g, MCHC 32.5 percent, WBC 14.5 × 10³, platelet count 509,000. Differential 80 percent neutrophils, 1 percent bands, 11 percent lymphs, 7 percent monocytes, and 1 percent eosinophils. A chemistry profile was within normal limits. A lymph node biopsy was obtained, and the diagnosis of

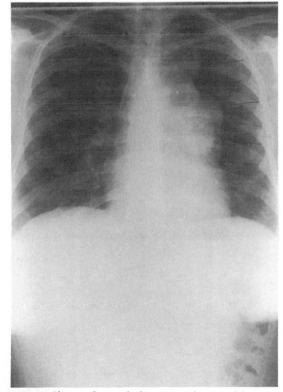

**Figure 24-2.** Chest radiograph showing widening of the mediastinum. This finding is strongly suggestive of lymphatic enlargement of any nature and in the setting of suspected lymphoma would warrant a mediastinal biopsy.

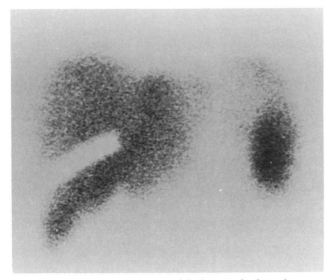

**Figure 24-3.** A radionucleotide scan of the liver and spleen showing a nonspecific pattern of heterogeneous uptake characteristic of the lymphomas.

mixed cellular type Hodgkin's disease with fibrosis was made.

Staging workup showed the following. On chest roentgenogram (Fig. 24–2), there was markedly widened mediastinum, with slight tracheal deviation to the right, suggesting parahilar and paratracheal lymphadenopathy. The lungs were clear. The heart was normal, and no pleural effusion or pneumothorax was present. Bilateral bone marrow biopsies and unilateral aspiration were negative. A liver-spleen scan (Fig. 24–3) showed hepatomegaly with minimal augmented splenic labeling. An abdominal

CT scan (Fig. 24–4) showed no gross adenopathy.

Because the patient's disease was clinically stage IIB and chemotherapy was to be given, no further staging via lymphangiography or staging laparotomy was done, as it would not have changed the management. Sperm deposits were made, and the patient was begun on chemotherapy as an outpatient.

**Treatment.** The patient was started on MOPP, and after the second complete cycle there was no clinical or roentgenologic evidence of Hodgkin's disease. The patient was given two more full cycles of MOPP, and it was then elected to give 2000 rads to the initial area of bulk masses in the mediastinum. During the radiation, there was a relapse in the right axilla. The patient was restarted on MOPP with prompt resolution of the adenopathy. Because of the recurrence of axillary adenopathy, it was elected to continue with six full cycles of MOPP chemotherapy. The patient at present is finishing his eighth cycle of MOPP, and there is no sign of recurrence.

## NON-HODGKIN'S LYMPHOMAS (MALIGNANT LYMPHOMAS)

As the process of lymphocyte differentiation into B and T cells has become appreciated, the non-Hodgkin's lymphomas have taken on an identity separate from Hodgkin's disease. Unfortunately, unlike the Hodgkin's lymphomas, there are as many classifications as there are experts! Figure 24-5 represents a classification of the non-Hodgkin's lymphomas ac-

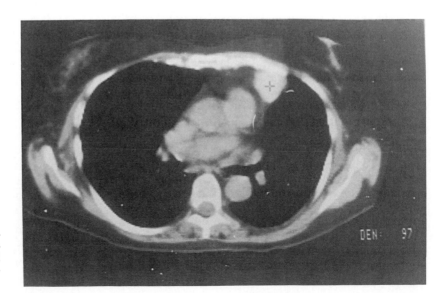

**Figure 24-4.** An abdominal CT scan of the retroperitoneal lymph nodes showing enlargement, which in the setting of documented lymphoma can serve as evidence of retroperitoneal involvement.

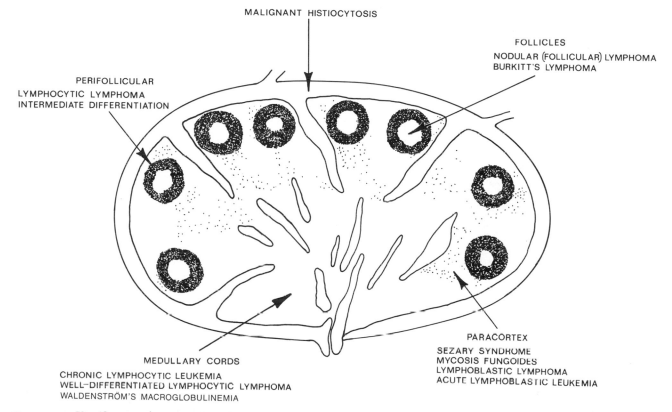

**Figure 24-5.** Classification of non-Hodgkin's lymphomas according to functional anatomy. (From Mann, RB, Jaffe, ES, and Berard, C: Am J Pathol 94:103,1979, with permission.)

cording to functional anatomy. Rapid advances in the appreciation of immunologic mechanisms have facilitated better "immunologic classifications." Traditionally, the staging and treatment approaches are very similar to those of the Hodgkin's lymphomas. Figure 24-6 describes the process of lymphocyte transformation and theoretical sites for development of non-Hodgkin's lymphoma.

A useful distinction is to divide the lymphomas on the basis of histologic appearance. The better-differentiated lymphomas tend to have a nodular appearance **(see Color Figure 209)** and have been termed grade I "favorable histology" because of the average six- to eight-year survival these patients experience. Less well differentiated tumors, referred to as grade II "poor histology" type, are more aggressive and are associated with a poorer prognosis **(see Color Figure 208)**.

Lymphomas, therefore, may be described according to the pattern of infiltration (nodular or diffuse), according to the cell type that is proliferating (lymphocytic, histiocytic, mixed), or on the basis of cell differentiation (well or poorly differentiated). These are the criteria used in the traditional Rappaport classification. There are two patterns of infiltration:

1. Diffuse lymphoma: infiltrating cells are spread throughout the lymph node, overshadowing the underlying architecture, which is replaced by a monotonous cell population **(see Color Figure 208)**.
2. Follicular or nodular lymphoma: tumor cells emanate from germinal center within the node, forming identifiable nodules within the lymph nodes; however, the infiltrating cells still exhibit a monotonous appearance **(see Color Figure 209)**.

The following cell types characterize the lymphomatous cell that is proliferating in a particular malignant lymphoma:

Well-differentiated lymphocyte
Poorly differentiated lymphocyte
Histiocytic cell
Mixed histiocytic-lymphocytic (both present)
Reticulum cell

Classifications other than the Rappaport have arisen with better understanding of the lymphocyte, its differentiation, and its function. Recent advances have shown that the Rappaport classifica-

## Follicular Center Cell Transformation

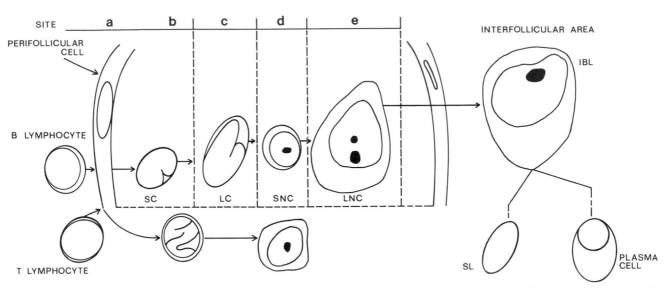

**Figure 24-6.** Process of lymphocyte transformation and potential sides for development of non-Hodgkin's lymphoma. SNC = small noncleaved cell; LNC = large noncleaved cell; SC = small cleaved cell; LC = large cleaved cell; IBL = immunoblast; SL = small lymphocyte—often with plasmacytoid features. (From Follicular center cell formation. JAMA 253(10):1432, 1985, with permission.)

tion does not take into account the immunologic origin or cell size and DNA content of the non-Hodgkin's lymphomas. In particular, the histiocytic cell referred to in the Rappaport classification is not a true histiocyte but a B lymphocyte. These features have prognostic and therapeutic implications. Many therapeutic studies, however, have used the Rappaport classification, which still has fairly accurate prognostic predictability.

The National Cancer Institute devised an interim classification called a "working formulation," dividing the non-Hodgkin's lymphoma into low grade, intermediate grade, high grade, and others (Table 24–4). In 1982, in the study conducted by the National Cancer Institute, the six major classifications in use at the time were applied to 1175 cases of non-Hodgkin's lymphoma; and it was found that all systems are *equally* predictive of clinical behavior. The working formulation represents a compromise classification that reconciles the advantages of the various classifications (Table 24–4). In following the literature, one will quickly realize the need to be familiar with two or three classifications. However, for the purpose of this text, only the Rappaport classification will be presented in any depth.

## Rappaport Classification

### Well-Differentiated Lymphocytic Lymphoma (WDLL)

In this type of lymphomatous infiltrate, normal-appearing, mature, small lymphocytes destroy the architecture of the lymph node with a uniform cellu-

lar infiltrate **(see Color Figure 210)**. The pattern of infiltration is diffuse, and the nodal capsule may be intact. The leukemic counterpart to this type of lymphoma is chronic lymphocytic leukemia (CLL), and the nodal morphology in both may be identical. The difference between a diffuse WDLL and CLL is simply that in the former process, the major pathology is within the lymph nodes rather than within the circulation (see Chapter 20). Diffuse WDLL may occur without the involvement of the bone marrow and peripheral blood. However, it may, late in the course of the disease, seed the blood and evoke a CLL-like blood picture that is impossible to differentiate from true CLL.

### Table 24–4. INTERNATIONAL WORKING FORMULATIONS AND APPLICABLE RAPPAPORT TYPES

Low-Grade Malignant Lymphoma
A. Small, lymphocytic (CLL, WDL)
B. Follicular, predominantly small, cleaved (NPDL)
C. Follicular, mixed small, cleaved, and large cell (NML)
Intermediate-Grade Malignant Lymphoma
D. Follicular, predominantly large cell (NHL)
E. Diffuse, small, cleaved (DPDL)
F. Diffuse, mixed small and large cell (DML)
G. Diffuse large cell (DHL)
High-Grade Malignant Lymphoma
H. Large cell, immunoblastic (DHL)
I. Lymphoblastic (undifferentiated/lymphoblastic)
J. Small, noncleaved (Burkitt's)
K. Miscellaneous
   1. Composite
   2. Mycoses fungoides (+ Sézary)
   3. Histiocytic (malignant histiocytosis)

## Poorly Differentiated Lymphocytic Lymphoma (PDLL)

This type is made up of cells ranging from normal to intermediate-sized lymphocytes to lymphoblasts (see Color Figure 211). Generally, the lymphocytes are larger and more variable in morphology. The nuclei are round, sometimes with deep clefts and convolutions. Normal-appearing lymphocytes may be intermixed with the larger cells.

In the older literature, this type of lymphoma was referred to as lymphoblastic lymphosarcoma. PDLL occurs in both the nodular and diffuse patterns of infiltration, with the nodular form being somewhat more common. In one review of reported cases, as many as 90 percent of the nodular lymphomas were PDLL.

These lymphocytes frequently spread beyond the capsule of the lymph node and invade the surrounding tissue. Diffuse PDLL may spill over into the peripheral blood, displaying an acute lymphocytic leukemia (ALL)–like hematologic picture, or exhibiting what has been termed "lymphosarcoma cell leukemia."

## Histiocytic Lymphoma (HL)

This type consists of larger cells and is a classification clouded by considerable controversy. In the new National Institute of Health Classification, the term "immunoblastic" is used to describe the cells that are of B-cell origin and not of histiocytic origin. Indeed, a great number of "histiocytic" lymphomas diagnosed in the past have not been revealed to be of B-cell origin. The malignant cells are generally larger than those found in poorly differentiated lymphoma, have a vesicular nucleus, prominent nucleoli, and abundant amphophilic cytoplasm (see Color Figure 212).

There are various subclassifications of histiocytic lymphoma, often applying the Rappaport classification inappropriately.

Various morphologic types of malignant cells have been described in the so-called histiocytic lymphoma, and nuclear pleomorphism is characteristic. The differentiated form of histiocytic lymphoma described is a large cell (up to 35 microns) with a primitive nucleus and open chromatin pattern. This cell often resembles the reticulum cell of the marrow, an undifferentiated cell that contains fibrils extending from the membrane into the surroundings. Multinucleated cells are common. This cell type constitutes a disease previously called reticulum cell sarcoma, which is an extranodal lymphoma morphologically indistinguishable from histiocytic lymphoma. It may represent a primary lesion in the bone, gastrointestinal tract, or the brain.

Another form of histiocytic lymphoma reported shows a more highly differentiated cell that is larger than the lymphoblast but smaller than the undifferentiated histiocyte mentioned previously. This cell is phagocytic, motile, and has an eosinophilic cytoplasm with a nucleus resembling a monocyte. The leukemic counterpart to this cell type may be acute monocytic leukemia.

Histiocytic lymphoma is often diffuse but can occur in the nodular form. Needless to say, subclassifications with surface markers and cell size identify another group of lymphomas with T-cell and null cell characteristics, adding more confusion to the complex classification of histiocytic lymphoma.

## Mixed Cell Type

This lymphoma is characterized by a mixture of both small and large lymphocytes (see Color Figure 213). Mixed cell lymphomas are most commonly nodular in the pattern of infiltration. However, normal-appearing small lymphocytes are uncommon in the follicles but common in the intervening tissue. This may lead to confusion with reactive hyperplasia. Extensive intranodular reticulum formation may be present.

## Lymphoblastic Lymphoma

The newest addition to the Rappaport classification consists of large immature lymphoid forms, lymphoblasts. Two variants with separate histologic patterns have been described, with similar clinical features and diffuse patterns of infiltration. Not uncommonly, this type may produce anterior mediastinal enlargement and may exhibit T-cell surface markers. Children and adolescents represent the major patient population and there is progressive involvement of the bone marrow and peripheral blood as an end stage of the disease. The leukemic counterpart to this lymphoma is acute lymphocytic leukemia. To subcategorize this type, surface markers should be performed.

## Undifferentiated Lymphoma (UL)

This lymphoma is characterized by the infiltration of undifferentiated cells having no signs of maturation toward lymphocytes or "histiocytes." These morphologically unidentifiable cells form a syncytial pattern of growth in the node. One form of undifferentiated lymphoma common in African blacks is Burkitt's lymphoma. This type frequently affects children, and the malignant cells destroy the normal bone formation of the jaw (see Fig. 24-7).

Characteristically, the lymphocytes in Burkitt's lymphoma, which are fairly uniform in size, form a diffuse sea of closely packed cells with round to oval nuclei that frequently demonstrate prominent nucleoli. Mitotic figures are usually apparent. Contrasting this darker background is the presence of larger pale-staining histiocytes that produce small clear spaces that appear similar to the "stars in the sky" (see Color Figure 214). This characteristic

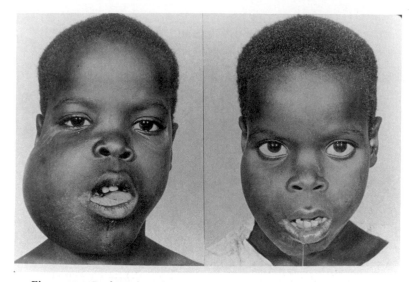

**Figure 24-7.** Burkitt's lymphoma before (*left*) and after treatment (*right*).

"starry sky" pattern is typical for Burkitt's lymphoma but not pathognomonic, since it has been described in other forms of lymphoma. This tumor is derived from B lymphocytes and consequently shows the appropriate B-surface characteristics.

The Epstein-Barr virus has been consistently isolated from these tumor cells, and the patients all show a high titer of antibody against this virus. The leukemic counterpart of this disorder called stem cell leukemia occurs when these malignant lymphocytes appear in the peripheral blood and bone marrow late in the course of the disease.

Burkitt's lymphoma fortunately is sensitive to chemotherapy and is associated with a good prognosis in early cases. Advanced cases, however, are rapidly fatal.

The second variant of undifferentiated lymphoma is referred to as non-Burkitt's or pleomorphic UL. As the name implies, these lymphocytes vary in size with pleomorphic nuclei containing prominent nucleoli. These cells are usually larger than Burkitt's lymphocytes and mitotic figures are numerous. However, the "starry sky" pattern characteristic of Burkitt's lymphoma is not apparent in this form of UL.

Table 24–5 summarizes the Rappaport classification of malignant lymphomas.

## Pathogenesis

The trigger mechanism for the lymphomas is not known. Localization to the B cell in the majority of non-Hodgkin's lymphomas is certain but again gives no insight into what makes the B cell malignant. Viruses have been implicated, but there has been no real isolation of virus particles. Recent work by Robert Gallo and his colleagues has shown that a normal complement of genetic material when transposed may become oncogenic. This transposition has been shown in human T-cell lymphoma.

Table 24–5. RAPPAPORT CLASSIFICATION OF NON-HODGKIN'S (MALIGNANT) LYMPHOMAS

| Abbreviation | Leukemic Counterpart | Pattern of Infiltration | Old Terminology |
|---|---|---|---|
| Well-differentiated lymphocytic lymphoma (WDLL) | CLL (chronic lymphocytic leukemia) | Diffuse | Lymphosarcoma |
| Poorly differentiated lymphocytic lymphoma (PDLL) | ALL (acute lymphocytic leukemia) | Diffuse or nodular | Lymphoblastic lymphosarcoma |
| Histiocytic lymphoma (HL) | AMonoL (acute monocytic leukemia) | Diffuse or nodular | Reticulum cell sarcoma |
| Mixed cellularity lymphoma (none) | None | Nodular | None |
| Undifferentiated lymphoma (UL) | Stem cell leukemia | Diffuse | Burkitt's lymphoma |
| Lymphoblastic lymphoma (none) | ALL (acute lymphocytic leukemia) | Diffuse | Newest addition to the Rappaport Classification |

Why the genetic material is transposed in some people leading to lymphoma and not in others is not known. DNA subsegment rearrangements have been shown in B-cell neoplasms and serve as a marker for monoclonal B-lymphocyte proliferation. Surface markers have allowed a better subclassification of lymphomas. A specific, seemingly unique antigen can be identified on the surface of tumor cells from some patients with non-Hodgkin's lymphoma by specific monoclonal antibody called BI antigen. It is present in tumors of B-cell origin, CLL, normal B cells, B and pre-B ALL, but is not found in T cells or in nonlymphoid tissue.

Certain immunodeficiency syndromes are complicated by concomitant lymphomas (e.g., ataxia telangiectasia, Wiskott-Aldrich syndrome, congenital sex-linked agammaglobulinemia, and the Chédiak-Higashi syndrome). Some acquired disorders including acquired hypogammaglobulinemia and Sjögren's syndrome are associated with a higher incidence of lymphoma. Also, patients on long-term immunosuppressive therapy may continue with long-term immunodeficiency when the therapy is discontinued and may also have a greater likelihood of developing lymphomas.

The non-Hodgkin's lymphomas can strike any age group, and the frequency increases with age. There is a high incidence of Burkitt's tumor among Central African children. In the Middle East, intestinal lymphoma is associated with immunoglobulin abnormalities. Sex appears not to have any influence on response to treatment or survival.

## Clinical Manifestations

The majority of patients will have painless lymphadenopathy for up to six months duration before consulting a physician. According to Rosenberg, fatigue, malaise, weight loss, or fever were noted in 2 to 14 percent of patients in his series. Bone pain is more specifically a symptom in the pediatric age group.

Unlike Hodgkin's disease, non-Hodgkin's lymphoma can present in extranodal sites as the primary clinical manifestation in 21, 24, and 37 percent of cases in three large studies (Desai, Rudders, and Rosenberg). The stomach and small intestine are involved with approximately equal frequency. Gastric lymphoma has the clinical appearance of gastric carcinoma. Small intestinal lymphoma is usually associated with malabsorption and appears to be particularly frequent in the Middle East. The spleen is rarely the only site of involvement. It occurred in approximately 1 percent of patients seen with lymphoma at the Mayo Clinic. However, isolated splenomegaly for no apparent reason is caused by lymphomatous infiltration in one third of cases. Solitary bone involvement is unusual and is difficult to distinguish from acute lymphoblastic leukemia and primary lymphosarcoma of the marrow.

## Laboratory Evaluation

Laboratory values are of little help in the diagnosis of non-Hodgkin's lymphoma. Usually there is not marked leukopenia or thrombocytopenia. Severe anemia may ensue if the marrow is the only site of disease; peripheral lymphocytes may carry monoclonal protein in 30 to 40 percent of patients in whom all lymphocytes appear normal.

Autoimmune hemolytic anemia or thrombocytopenia or both may be seen occasionally. In general, the subtypes have similar hematologic findings; however, thrombocytopenia is less common in nodular poorly differentiated and diffuse histiocytic lymphomas than in other subtypes. Thrombocytosis is less common in diffuse well-differentiated and nodular poorly differentiated lymphomas than in other subtypes.

Bone marrow biopsy and aspiration is a useful diagnostic tool. Forty of 108 patients (38 percent) had bone marrow involvement at the time of diagnosis. Fifty-seven percent of nodular poorly differentiated lymphocytic lymphomas and 27 percent of diffuse poorly differentiated lymphocytic lymphomas will have bone marrow involvement at the time of diagnosis. Additionally, 50 percent of the cases with bone marrow involvement show some degree of peripheral blood signs. Involvement of blood and bone marrow in histiocytic lymphoma is infrequent. Although when marrow involvement occurs, there is a greater association of central nervous system involvement as well. Since marrow involvement may be patchy, bilateral biopsies and biopsies of areas of increased uptake on bone scan have been reported to increase yield by 10 to 20 percent.

## Staging and Prognosis

The non-Hodgkin's lymphomas are staged from I to IV, as are the Hodgkin's lymphomas, and similarly are designated A and B according to symptoms. Evaluation must include a lymph node biopsy for tissue diagnosis, after other causes of nodal enlargement have been eliminated; abdominal CT scan; bilateral bone marrow biopsies and aspirations; evaluation of liver function; chest roentgenography; and occasionally lymphangiography. Figure 24-8 is a lymphangiogram showing characteristic enlargement of the pelvic lymph nodes in lymphoma. Staging laparotomy does not appear to improve the accuracy of staging. Once histologic material is obtained, diagnosis, prognosis, and staging may be ascertained and management planned.

The lymph node is usually replaced by neoplastic lymphocytes that destroy the normal architecture of the lymph node and invade the capsule, pulp, and sinuses. The disease may be patchy and there may be reactive areas in the lymph node. If the specimen is not properly evaluated, a malignant diagnosis

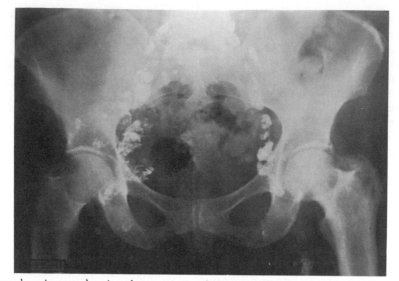

**Figure 24-8.** A lymphangiogram showing characteristic enlargement of the pelvic lymph nodes in lymphoma.

may be missed. Touch preparations should be made on freshly submitted tissue.

## Survival

Various factors affect prognosis and survival (Table 24–6), but histologic type, clinical stage, and the presence of A or B symptomatology seem to be the overriding factors. Survival is about the same in men and women in most reports, and children seem to do more poorly. Patients with nodular histology live longer than those with diffuse histologies, although the diffuse histology varieties are more amenable to cure. It has also been reported that serum lactic dehydrogenase seems to be a good predictor of survival. The level of this enzyme is inversely proportional to the length of survival.

There may be a leukemic phase to the non-Hodgkin's lymphomas. Lymphosarcoma cell leukemia is found in 13 percent of children and in 7 percent of adults. Incidences as high as 50 percent in children have been reported. In addition, acute myelogenous leukemia may develop as a complication of radiotherapy and chemotherapy, as already mentioned, in 5 percent of cases.

## Treatment

Most studies have used the Rappaport classification to report the disease-free interval and response to

**Table 24–6. FACTORS ADVERSELY INFLUENCING PROGNOSIS IN NON-HODGKIN'S LYMPHOMAS**

1. Bone marrow involvement
2. Increaased serum lactic dehydrogenase (LDH)
3. Presence of B symptoms
4. Liver involvement
5. Presence of gastrointestinal mass disease
6. Hematocrit <36%; hemoglobin <12 g/dl

chemotherapy or radiotherapy. Traditionally, the histologic groups have been divided into favorable and unfavorable and nodular and diffuse histologies. As in Hodgkin's disease, radiotherapy appears to have a role in stage I and II malignant lymphomas. Stages I and II had a 75 percent six-year disease-free survival. Total nodal radiation has been advocated, but only a 72 percent response rate has been obtained in stage III poorly differentiated lymphocytic and mixed cellular non-Hodgkin's lymphoma. The disease-free survival rates of patients randomized to total nodal radiation or COPP (cyclophosphamide, Oncovin, procarbazine, prednisone) showed no advantage to chemotherapy or radiotherapy, each being about equally effective. Complete responses have been reported with diffuse histologies — namely, diffuse poorly differentiated or diffuse mixed cell lymphomas with combination chemotherapy — but not for the nodular histologies, which tend to relapse within five years of complete remission.

An exception to the refractoriness of the nodular lymphomas was reported in a rare subtype of the nodular histiocytic lymphomas in the nodular mixed cellularity subtype.

In diffuse histiocytic lymphoma, pathologically staged patients with stage I or IE supradiaphragmatic lymph node involvement have a median survival of 72.5 months and a median disease-free survival of 69.5 months. Stage II and IIE patients have a median survival of 33 months and adjuvant chemotherapy or chemotherapy alone is recommended. Twenty to 30 percent of patients will present with pathologic stage I or II involvement. If pathologic staging is performed, radiation therapy in this group can be used as the treatment modality.

Recently, combination chemotherapy protocols employing the principle of (1) rapid chemotherapeutic cycling, (2) high dosage, and (3) non–cross-resistant regimens have achieved complete remission rates over 75 percent in aggressive histology lymphomas (intermediate and high grade). Most of these regimens employ five empiric drugs; cyclophosphamide, adriamycin, vincristine, prednisone, and methotrexate, with additional supplemental drugs such as bleomycin, cytosine arabinoside, procarbazine, and others. These regimens constitute a "new generation" of chemotherapeutic programs aimed at curing the aggressive non-Hodgkin's lymphomas.

If complete remission is achieved, there is a greater chance of survival. As mentioned, the chance for cure in the nodular lymphomas is very much less than that of the diffuse histology lymphomas.

Staging evaluation and treatment approaches for non-Hodgkin's lymphomas are not as standardized as they are for Hodgkin's disease. Individualization of approach is very important for the optimal management.

## RARE LYMPHOMAS

### Mycosis Fungoides: Sezary Syndrome

The T-cell non-Hodgkin's lymphomas have characterization very different from B-cell non-Hodgkin's lymphomas. They constitute a small percentage of the non-Hodgkin's lymphomas and so are listed in the rare category.

Mycosis fungoides is a T-cell type of non-Hodgkin's lymphoma with a predilection, in the initial stages, for the skin **(see Color Figure 216)**. Since any lymphoma may involve the skin as a sign of systemic spread, the specific characteristics of mycosis fungoides must be sought. Characteristic clinical manifestations of this disorder include plaque-like lesions of the skin, generalized erythroderma, intense pruritis, lymphadenopathy, and large abnormal T lymphocytes in the peripheral blood.

The Mycosis Fungoides Cooperative Group has defined a staging system for the cutaneous T-cell lymphomas, which uses clinical information readily obtained from physical examination. The depth of penetration of the skin and the number of lymph node groups involved have prognostic significance.

The course is variable, but approximately 40 percent of patients in stage IV have a survival of four years. The time from the development of skin rash to the development of plaques may be 0.1 to 48 years, the average being 6.1 years.

"Mycosis fungoides" is a term that describes the characteristic appearance of the tumor; it has no relation to a fungal disease. Sézary described characteristic large mononuclear cells with convoluted-cerebriform-nuclei in the blood **(see Color Figure 215)**, and most investigators believe that these represent the leukemic phase of the disease. Both the abnormal skin cells and the cells in the blood are helper T cells. In contradistinction to dermal involvement in B lymphoma, the epidermis is involved in mycosis fungoides, and characteristic Darier-Pautrier abscesses (the appearance of the Sézary cells clustered in the epidermis) are described.

Evaluation and staging is done as for any other lymphoma. A lymph node or liver biopsy may be delayed. However, in the early stages of disease, electron microscopy (EM) is very helpful in identifying the Sézary cell in mycosis fungoides. The presence of abnormal lymphocytes by light microscopy is highly predictive of finding abnormal lymphocytes by EM and cytogenetics. The absence of light microscopic findings does not rule out lymphocyte abnormalities.

Survival decreases with increasing stage of the disease. Involvement of blood, degree of lymph node involvement, and visceral involvement all have an unfavorable influence on prognosis. As with other lymphomas, infection is a major cause of death. It usually spreads from skin ulcers that become infected in the later stages of the disease.

### Treatment

There are two treatment approaches used, depending on the stage of the disease: topical and systemic. Early-stage disease is treated with topical preparations (e.g., nitrogen mustard, electron beam, and ultraviolet light, or PUVA, treatments). Later-stage disease is treated with systemic chemotherapy, extracorporeal treatment of blood with ultraviolet light and cis-retinoic acid. Remission ranges from 4 to 12 months. Late-stage treatment modalities are less effective in inducing a remission than are early-stage modalities. No treatment is curative.

### Lennert's Lymphoma

This lymphoma is considered a variant of diffuse mixed cell non-Hodgkin's lymphoma but with T-lymphocyte surface markers. It is characterized by a diffuse increase in epithelioid histiocytes within the lymph node. Clinical features include presentation in older individuals, generalized lymphadenopathy, and hepatosplenomegaly, with a high occurrence of constitutional B symptoms and advanced clinical stage.

### BENIGN LYMPHADENOPATHY SIMULATING LYMPHOMA

A review of the conditions classified under this category is beyond the scope of this text. These conditions have all been individually reported and have been reviewed by Dorfman and Warnke. The conditions are outlined in Table 24–7.

**Table 24-7. LYMPHADENOPATHY SIMULATING MALIGNANT LYMPHOMA**

Follicular (nodular) pattern
  Nonspecific reactive follicular hyperplasia
  Secondary syphilis
  Rheumatoid arthritis
    (Felty's syndrome and Still's disease)
  Giant lymph node hyperplasia
    (hyaline-vascular and plasma cell types)
Sinus pattern
  Histiocytosis X
  Sinus histiocytosis with massive lymphadenopathy
  "Lymphoma-like" Kaposi's sarcoma
  Vascular transformation of sinuses
  Lymphangiogram effect
  Metastatic carcinoma and melanoma
Diffuse pattern
  Postvaccinial lymphadenitis
  Hydantoin (Dilantin) hypersensitivity
  Viral (herpes zoster) lymphadenitis
  Immunoblastic lymphadenopathy
  Dermatopathic lymphadenopathy
  Lupus erythematosus
  Metastic carcinoma and melanoma
Mixed patterns
  Infectious mononucleosis
  Toxoplasmosis
  Cat scratch disease
  Lymphogranuloma inguinale
  Metastic carcinoma and melanoma

## Angio-Immunoblastic Lymphadenopathy (AIL)

This unusual disorder is characterized by a syndrome of (1) hyperimmunity (polyclonal proliferation of immunoblasts — transformed lymphocytes with excess polyclonal immunoglobin production), (2) cellular deficiency, and (3) propensity to behave like or evolve into a lymphoma. The pathologic features of AIL are diffuse effacement of the follicular and sinusoidal architecture, a prominence of blood vessels (hence the "angio"), and evidence of extensive "antigenic" stimulation with a prominence of immunoblasts and plasmacytoid lymphocytes. The condition usually presents in patients over the age of 50 years and is associated with constitutional symptoms (fever, weight loss, malaise, night sweats) lymphadenopathy, hepatosplenomegaly, and a skin rash with pruritis. The hematologic manifestations include normochromic normocytic anemia, leukocytosis, circulating atypical mononuclear cells, eosinophilia, and a positive Coombs test result (50 percent of cases). The overall prognosis is poor with a 50 percent one-year survival; 10 percent of cases undergo spontaneous remission. There is histologic evidence of transformation to immunoblastic sarcoma (lymphomas) in 43 percent of cases. For those cases that transform, the prognosis is dismal.

## MALIGNANT HISTIOCYTOSIS

Malignant histiocytosis, or histiocytic medullary reticulosis, is a true malignant disorder of histiocytes and represents uncontrolled histiocytic proliferation. As previously mentioned, the disorders classified as histiocytic lymphomas in the Rappaport classification are really clonal B lymphocytic, not histiocytic diseases. Malignant histiocytosis may be classified under the category of "histiocytic disorders"; however, because it represents a reticuloendothelial neoplasm, it may be discussed in the lymphoma category, even though it does not represent a true lymphoma.

The clinical features are characterized by a progressive wasting disease, with fever, generalized lymphodenopathy, hepatosplenomegaly, cutaneous nodular infiltrates, and often widespread tissue involvement. The pathologic features emphasize the invasive nature of the histiocytes, showing progressive systemic infiltration of morphologically atypical, malignant histiocytes.

Hematologic findings include normochromic normocytic anemia and leukopenia; however, the majority of patients are pancytopenic. The reticulocyte count is usually low. The peripheral blood may indicate abnormal mononuclear cells that usually constitute less than 10 to 30 percent of the differential leukocyte count. Marrow involvement is common, and bone marrow aspirates may suggest the diagnosis when the atypical mononuclear cells showing hemophagocytosis are found. The hemophagocytosis in conjunction with splenomegaly and marrow infiltration may explain the high incidence of pancytopenia. The indirect bilirubin is also occasionally elevated. The Coombs test result is invariably negative.

Malignant histiocytosis may be misdiagnosed as acute monocytic leukemia or other "lymphohemopoietic malignancy," and occasionally has been misdiagnosed as infectious mononucleosis.

The disorder is usually progressive within three to six months, although durable remissions have been reported with combination chemotherapy.

## Bibliography

### Hodgkin's Disease

Aisenberg, A: The changing face of Hodgkin's disease. Am J Med 67:921, 1979.
Andrieu, JM, Montagnon, B, Asselain, B, et al: Chemotherapy-radiotherapy association in Hodgkin's disease, clinical stage I A, II A: Results of a prospective clinical trial with 166 patients. Cancer 46:2126, 1980.
deVita, V: The consequences of the chemotherapy of Hodgkin's disease: The 10th David A. Karnofsky Memorial Lecture. Cancer 47:1, 1981.
Fisher, R, deVita, V, Bostick, F, et al: Persistent immunologic abnormalities in long-term survivors of advanced Hodgkin's disease. Ann Intern Med 92:595, 1980.

Gutensohn, N and Cole, P: Epidemiology of Hodgkin's disease. Semin Oncol 7:92, 1980.

Santoro, A and Bonadonna, G: Alternating drug combinations in the treatment of advanced Hodgkin's disease. N Engl J Med 306:770, 1982.

Smith, JL and Butler, JJ: Skin Involvement in Hodgkin's disease. Cancer 45:354, 1980.

Stein, R, Golomb, H, Diggs, CH, et al: Anatomic substage of stage III A Hodgkin's disease. Ann Intern Med 92:159, 1980.

Vigersky, R., Chapman, R, Berenberg, J, et al: Testicular dysfunction in untreated Hodgkin's disease. Am J Med 73:482, 1982.

## Non-Hodgkin's Lymphoma

Anderson, T, deVita, V, Simon, RM, et al: Malignant lymphoma. Cancer 50:2708, 1982.

Ault, KA: Monoclonal B lymphocytes in the blood of patients with lymphoma. N Engl J Med 300:1401, 1979.

Bitran, J, Golumb, H, Ultmann, J, et al: Non-Hodgkin's lymphoma, poorly differentiated lymphocytic and mixed cell types. Cancer 42:88, 1978.

Bloomfield, C, McKenna, RW, and Brunning, RD: Significance of haematological parameters in the non-Hodgkin's malignant lymphomas. Br J Haematol 32:41, 1976.

Chabner, B, Johnson, R, et al: Sequential non-surgical and surgical staging of non-Hodgkin's lymphoma. Ann Intern Med 85:149, 1976.

Dick, F, Bloomfield, C, and Brunning, R: Incidence, cytology, and histopathology of non-Hodgkin's lymphoma in the bone marrow. Cancer 33:1382, 1974.

Ferraris, AM, Giuntini, P, and Gaetani, GF: Serum lactic dehydrogenase as a prognostic tool for non-Hodgkin's lymphomas. Blood 54(4):928, 1979.

Glick, J, McFadden, E, Costello, W, et al: Nodular histiocytic lymphoma: Factors influencing prognosis and implications for aggressive chemotherapy. Cancer 49:840, 1982.

Lee, Yeu-Tsu N, Terry, R, and Lukes, R: Biopsy of peripheral lymph nodes. Am Surg 48(10):536, 1982.

Miller, DG: The association of immune disease and malignant lymphoma. Ann Intern Med 66:507, 1967.

Osborne, CK, Norton, L, Young, RC, et al: Nodular histiocytic lymphoma: An aggressive nodular lymphoma with a potential for prolonged disease free survival. Blood 56(1):98, 1980.

Rosenberg, SA, Berard, CW, Brown, BW, Jr, et al: National Cancer Institute Sponsored Study of Classification of Non-Hodgkin's Lymphomas. Summary and description of working formulation for clinical usage. Cancer 49:2112, 1982.

Rosenberg, SA, Diamond, H, Iaslowitz, B, et al: Lymphosarcoma: A review of 1,269 cases. Medicine 40:31, 1961.

Rudders, R, Kaddis, M, deLellis, RA, et al: Nodular non-Hodgkin's lymphomas (NHL). Cancer 43:1643, 1979.

Stein, R and Cousar, J: Malignant lymphomas of follicular center cell origin in man. Cancer 44:2236, 1979.

Straus, D, Filippa, D, Lieberman, PH, et al: The non-Hodgkin's lymphomas. Cancer 51:101, 1983.

Warnke, R and Levy, R: Immunopathology of follicular lymphomas. N Engl J Med 298:481, 1978.

Warnke, R and Miller, R: Immunologic phenotype in 30 patients with diffuse large-cell lymphoma. N Engl J Med 303:293, 1980.

Zulman, J, Jaffe, R, and Talal, N: Evidence that the malignant lymphoma of Sjogren's syndrome is a monoclonal B-cell neoplasm. N Engl J Med 299:1215, 1978.

## Mycosis Fungoides and Malignant Histiocytosis

Bunn, PA, Huberman, MS, Whang-Peng, J, et al: Prospective staging evaluation of patients with cutaneous T-cell lymphomas. Ann Intern Med 93:223, 1980.

Bunn, R and Lamberg, SI: Report of the committee on staging and classification of cutaneous T-cell lymphomas. Cancer Treat Rep 63(4):725, 1979.

Dorfman, RF and Warnke, R: Lymphadenopathy simulating lymphomas. Human Pathol 5:519, 1974.

Epstein, E, Levin, DL, Croft, JD, Jr, et al: Mycosis fungoides: Survival, prognostic features, response to therapy and autopsy findings. Medicine 15:61, 1972.

Lambert, IA, Catovsky, D, and Bergler, N: Malignant histiocytosis—a clinico-pathological study of 12 cases. Br J Haematol 40:65, 1978.

# CHAPTER 25

MILKA MUKHOLVA MONTEIL, M.D.

# Bone Marrow

## DEVELOPMENT OF HEMATOPOIETIC SYSTEM

Hematopoiesis originates from mesenchymal tissue and passes three stages of prenatal development. The first stage, the mesenchymal period, begins during the first month of embryonic development, in the yolk sac. It consists of intravascular erythropoietic islands in the yolk sac outside the embryo. The circulating red cells are nucleated and megaloblastic in character. Soon thereafter, and paralleling the yolk sac hematopoiesis, the second, hepatic, stage of red cell production starts. By the end of the 11th gestational week, the liver becomes the major hematopoietic organ. During this hepatic phase, the lymph nodes and the spleen also participate in hematopoiesis, but their contribution is less significant than that of the liver. In the liver, extravascular definitive erythroblasts are produced, which mature to enucleated macrocytic erythrocytes. Some megakaryocytes are produced in the yolk sac, but the actual megakaryocytic production begins mainly during the liver phase at about the sixth gestational week. In the same embryonic period granulopoiesis begins. The liver remains the main hematopoietic organ of the fetus up to the sixth gestational month. The bone marrow development starts early and simultaneously with the liver. Erythrocytes are produced in the bone marrow as early as 10th fetal week. The bone marrow grows and expands rapidly taking over erythropoiesis, thrombocytopoiesis, and finally granulopoiesis. After the sixth month of fetal life, the third and final stage, medullary hematopoiesis takes over. Marrow replaces the liver as the main hematopoietic organ and remains active throughout the person's entire life.[1] Lymphocyte production first starts in the liver and lymph nodes about the ninth week,[2] and lymphocytopoiesis remains a function of the bone marrow, thymus, lymph nodes, and spleen thereafter.

About the time of birth, the cavities of all bones contain hematopoietic marrow. During intrauterine life fetal erythropoiesis is partially megaloblastic; hence, the blood of a full-term newborn normally has high MCV and MCH, and the erythrocytes on blood film show marked anisocytocysis and macrocytosis. In full-term newborns, the foci of extramedullary hematopoiesis persist only occasionally. All bone cavities are filled with active, blood-forming elements. There is no reserve of marrow space, and if the hematopoiesis needs to expand at that early age, the extramedullary hematopoiesis in the liver, spleen, and even in the lymph nodes becomes active and immature cells spill over readily into the blood. For this reason, extramedullary hematopoiesis and immature cells in the blood of infants and young children do not have the same serious pathologic implication as in adults. After birth, the bones and their cavities grow and expand faster than the hematopoietic tissue. The extra space in the bones not occupied by marrow cells is filled by fat. In addition, a gradual replacement of the bone marrow by fat starts in the bones of the hands and feet and creeps centripetally toward the flat bone of the trunk. In adults, active hematopoietic tissue occupies about 40 to 50 percent of the cavities of the pelvic bones, ribs, sternum, the bodies of the vertebrae of spinal column, and the proximal end of the humerus and femur. The rest is replaced by fat. The mechanism that regulates this process of obliteration and fat replacement is poorly understood. The low body temperature and poor vascularization of the marrow spaces of the extremities have been thought to be determining factors, but locally inherited factors may also be important.

The bone marrow is one of the largest organs and represents 3.4 to 4.6 percent of the total body weight averaging about 1500 grams.[3] A discernible amount of fat is noticed by 3 to 4 years of age and increases very gradually thereafter. Small variations exist according to the site of the skeleton and according to the age of a person, but usually between the ages of 25 and 60 years the ratio of fat to hematopoietic marrow in the posterior iliac crest is about 1:1, with cellularity 50 percent.[4,5] After 60 years of age, the marrow cellularity decreases insignificantly and does not drop below 30 percent.

The bone marrow is a dynamic organ adapted to provide the environment for hematopoietic differentiation and maturation of stem cells. Such differentiation is influenced by distant humoral and local factors. It is well known that erythropoietin stimulates differentiation and maturation of erythrocytes; but under similar and less well known humoral influences, granulocytic, monocytic, and megakaryocytic differentiation and maturation also take place.

In addition, the bone marrow is also the source of immune stem cells, which mature to T for "thymic" and B for "bursa" lymphocytes, following the respective "conditioning." These stem cells are programmed to carry tissue and humoral immune functions correspondingly. The progenitor cells produced in the marrow mature immunologically in the thymus as T lymphocytes. The site of maturation of the B lymphocytes in humans is uncertain, but there is strong evidence that it most likely occurs in the bone marrow.[6] Therefore, the bone marrow and thymus are *primary* lymphoid organs of the antigen-independent process of division and differentiation, which give rise to new lymphocytes. Then these "new lymphocytes" populate the *secondary* lymphoid organs, where antigen-dependent effector cells proliferate and antibody production takes place.

## INDICATIONS FOR BONE MARROW STUDIES

Obtaining bone marrow for examination carries little procedural risk for the patient, but the procedure is quite painful and costly; therefore, bone marrow studies should be done only when clearly indicated. Hematologic conditions with a decrease or increase of any blood element are among the most common indications:

1. Anemias, erythrocytosis, polycythemia
2. Leukopenia and unexplained leukocytosis with appearance of immature or abnormal cells in the circulation
3. Thrombocytopenia and thrombocytosis

It is not rare for more than one blood element to be increased or decreased, as occurs in leukemias and some refractory anemias. In these situation, bone marrow study is essential and it precedes any other diagnostic procedure.

Bone marrow studies are also indicated in the diagnosis of diseases not primarily affecting the blood system, among which are the following:

1. Malignant tumors such as lymphomas, carcinomas, and sarcomas may metastasize to the bone marrow. Patients having any one of these types of solid malignant tumors have bone marrow studies done when the initial diagnosis is established for clinical staging of disease. Additional studies are performed periodically for monitoring the status of tumor spread and its therapeutic response.
2. Infections manifested clinically as "fever of unknown origin" may exhibit granulomas, focal necrosis, or histiocytic proliferation with intracytoplasmic organisms. Bone marrow for morphologic studies and bacterial cultures is obtained simultaneously during a single pro-

cedure. The diagnoses of disseminated tuberculosis, fungal infections (particularly histoplasmosis), and some protozoan infections are frequently confirmed through such procedures.

3. The histiocytes of the bone marrow can be involved in some hereditary or acquired storage diseases, such as Gaucher's disease, sea-blue histiocytosis, and others. A simple procedure such as bone marrow aspiration or biopsy or both may establish diagnosis.

Finally, whenever the physician expects a beneficial diagnostic result for his or her patient, bone marrow studies may be done.

## METHODS OF OBTAINING AND PREPARING BONE MARROW FOR HEMATOLOGIC STUDIES

During a bone marrow procedure hematopoietic tissue is obtained and processed in such a manner that maximum information can be obtained for diagnosis of a particular clinical problem.

The most common skeletal sites for hematologic studies in adults are the posterior superior iliac crest, sternum, anterior superior iliac crest, and very rarely spinal processes or vertebral bodies (Fig. 25-1). Occasionally, when a localized bone lesion is visualized on roentgenogram or computed tomographic (CT) scan, an "open" bone marrow-biopsy performed by a surgeon may need to be done in an operating room with the patient under anesthesia. In newborns and infants, marrow for studies can be obtained from the upper end of the tibial bone.

Before the procedure is performed, the patient (if adult) or the parent or guardian (if patient is a child) should be informed about the procedure, its risks, and its benefits for the diagnostic process. An authorized permission form, the so-called informed consent form, is signed, which allows the physician to perform the procedure. Signature of the permission form is witnessed by a second person, frequently the patient's nurse. The actual procedure is performed in the presence of and with the assistance of a medical technologist. While the physician performing the procedure and the nurse are attending the patient, the medical technologist gives full attention to the processing of the specimen. It is the responsibility also of the technologist to see that the samples are adequate. If not, the physician is informed immediately so that the procedure can be repeated before the patient is released. Samples are preserved appropriately for histologic, electron microscopic, cytogenetic, immunologic, microbiologic, and other studies as they may be requested in a particular case.

Bone marrow study in the diagnosis of hematopoietic disorders was first introduced by Arinkin.[7]

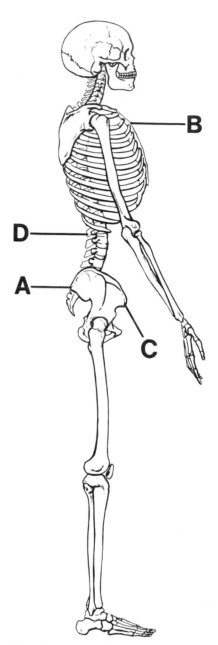

**Figure 25-1.** Posterior superior iliac crest (A), sternum (B), anterior superior iliac crest (C), and spinal processes (D) indicate the site of the skeleton in descending order of frequency from which bone marrow tissue is obtained for studies.

Although in earlier clinical practices it was a formidable procedure, with modern improved techniques, obtaining bone marrow tissue is a common everyday practice with insignificant patient discomfort or risk. Several techniques have been devised, each having its own merit and limitations. It is currently a common practice for bone marrow aspiration and bone marrow biopsy to be performed concurrently.

## Equipment

The tray used for assisting a bone marrow procedure should contain equipment to perform the procedure and to handle the preparation of the obtained tissues (Table 25–1). There are several different styles of aspiration needles and trephine bone biopsy needles. The most commonly used styles are the University of Illinois sternal needle with an adjustable guard for aspiration and various modification of the Vim-Silverman trephine needle for bone biopsy (Fig. 25-2). Examples of such modified trephine needles are the Westerman-Jensen, Jamshidi, and others. There are also smaller needles designed for use with infants and children.

Modifications of these original aspiration and trephine needles have been adapted by different companies and are manufactured as disposable equipment. Whole bone marrow trays are also sold as disposable equipment, which may be convenient for some laboratories with a low volume of bone marrow procedures. The disadvantages of the disposable trays include cost and loss of versatility.

A hematology laboratory that is involved in the assistance of bone marrow procedures should always have in readiness at least two bone marrow trays with a minimal inventory of equipment and reagents to handle routine bone marrow samples.

## Procedure

As a rule, very apprehensive patients and children receive a mild sedative beforehand. The site of the procedure is shaved, if hairy, and washed with soap. Then an antiseptic is applied and the area draped with sterile towels. A local anesthetic such as 2 percent lidocaine (Xylocaine) is infiltrated in the skin in the intervening tissues between the skin and bone and in the periosteum of the bone from which the marrow is to be obtained.

## Aspiration

The physician penetrates the bone cavity with an aspiration needle. A syringe is then attached to the free end of the needle, and the plunger is pulled to create a vacuum into which 1.0 to 1.5 ml of marrow particles and sinusoidal blood are drawn. The vacuum in the syringe is important for rapid and efficient detachment of cells and particles by suction. The syringe should be 5 ml or larger with a well-fitting plunger. The first aspirated material is used immediately for preparation of smears. More aspirate is obtained in additional syringes if it is needed for chromosome studies, bacterial cultures, and others. Despite the use of local anesthesia the patient normally experiences discomfort during the aspiration process (aspiration pain). Accomplishing the aspiration with a quick and continuous pull on the plunger diminishes the patient's discomfort and decreases the chance for clotting the specimen. A

### Table 25–1. INVENTORY TRAY FOR BONE MARROW ASPIRATION AND BIOPSY

**Required Materials**

1. 30 cc syringes
2. 20 cc syringes
3. 10 cc syringes
4. 5 cc syringes
5. 2% lidocaine
6. Prepodyne prep
7. Alcohol (70%) or prep
8. 23-gauge needles
9. 21-gauge needles
10. Filter papers
11. Buffered formalin 10% or other fixative for histologic processing of bone biopsy and marrow particles
12. Tube containing liquid EDTA anticoagulant
13. One box slides
14. One slide folder
15. One rubber bulb
16. Pasteur pipette
17. Petri dish
18. Sterile blades
19. Gloves (several pairs of different sizes)
20. Sterile gauze and cotton balls
21. Sterile bone marrow aspiration and trephine biopsy needles
22. Applicator sticks
23. Bandage
24. One culture bottle (*not* biphasic) for bacterial culture (Note: Save some bone marrow specimen in syringe for TB and fungal cultures, when indicated)
25. Pencil to label slides

clotted specimen is useless for smear preparation, because the fibrin threads strip the cytoplasm of the cell on smearing and hamper its spreading. Once an adequate aspirate is obtained, the quality of the smear depends entirely on the technologist's skill and speed in preparing and preserving the morphology of the marrow cells. Part of the first aspirate is used for the preparation of direct and marrow particle smears. The other part is placed in an EDTA anticoagulant-containing tube for use later in the laboratory. If some aspirate still remains, it can be left to clot. The clot is fixed in buffered formalin and processed for histologic sections.

## Preparation of Marrow Aspirate for Examination

To avoid any delay, all necessary materials, preservatives, and slides should be meticulously clean and in readiness. The aspirated material in the first syringe contains mostly marrow cells and particles and should be used for smears. Several *direct smears* can be prepared immediately, using the technique for blood film preparation. A small drop is placed on a glass slide, and the blood and the particles are dragged behind a spreading slide. Although this method of preparation preserves well the cell morphology, it is inadequate for evaluation of the cells in relationship to each other and does not offer ade-

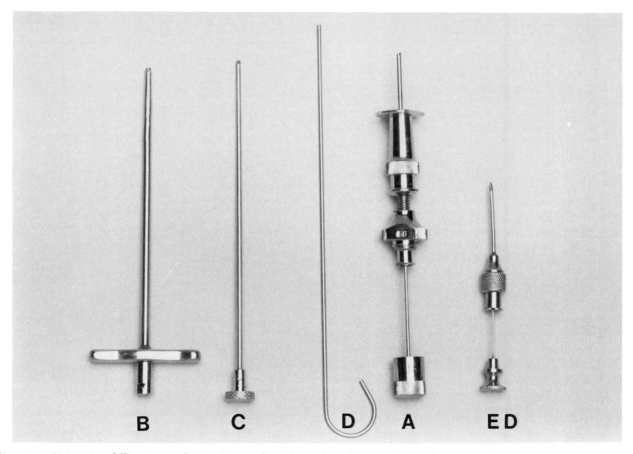

**Figure 25-2.** University of Illinois sternal aspiration needle with an adjustable guard and stylet (A); Jamshidi trephine needle biopsy (B) includes a stylet (C) and probe (D). A smaller-sized pediatric aspiration needle and trephine biopsy (ED) are also shown.

quate smears for estimation of marrow cellularity.

*Smears of marrow particles* are prepared by pouring a small amount of the aspirate on a glass slide. The marrow tissue is seen as gray particles floating in blood and fat droplets. The particles are aspirated selectively with a plastic dropper or Oxford pipette and transferred to a clean glass slide. These are covered gently with another slide. The two slides are pulled in opposite and parallel directions to smear the particles without crushing the cells. Some techniques recommend using two cover glasses instead.[8] The marrow particle is squashed between two coverslips, which are gently pulled apart so that particle smears are prepared on the two cover glasses.

Techniques for preparing particle smears vary from person to person and from laboratory to laboratory. The aspirate can be transferred in a watch glass and the particles can be fished out with a capillary pipette or broken end of a wooden stick applicator. With experience, technologists usually adapt a technique that best suits themselves, to produce high-quality slides.

Marrow particle smears are good for evaluation of the cellularity and the relationship of the cells to each other. In well-prepared smears there is the added advantage of excellent cell morphology so that subtle changes in cell maturation and cytoplasmic inclusions can be easily recognized.

All direct and particle smears should be labeled with the patient's name, number, and date at the bedside. Then the smears are quickly air dried by blowing on them or by exposing them to an air flow from a fan.

## Quantitative Measurement of Bone Marrow Aspirate

The EDTA-anticoagulated aspirate can be used for quantitative studies.[9] About 1 ml of this aspirate is transferred to a Wintrobe tube and is centrifuged at 2800 rpm (at 850 g) for 8 minutes. The fluid is separated into four layers representing fat and perivascular cells, plasma, buffy coat or myeloid-erythroid, and erythrocytes, respectively. Each layer is measured and read as a percentage directly from the Wintrobe tube, its volume correlates with a given basic element of the marrow. Smears can be prepared from each layer and can be used accordingly to study iron from the top layer and hematopoietic cell and myeloid-to-erythroid (M : E) cell ratio from the buffy coat layer. Such quantitative studies may be useful in estimating cellularity (fat versus buffy coat) when no histologic sections of bone biopsy and marrow particles are available.

## Staining of Bone Marrow Smears

Dried bone marrow smears are stained with Romanovsky's polychromic stains such as Wright's, Wright-Giemsa, or May-Grünwald-Giemsa stain. Before staining, the hematopoietic cells have to be fixed in absolute methyl alcohol for 3 to 5 minutes. Some commercially sold dyes are dissolved in methyl alcohol, which may eliminate the step of fixation, but most of the methanol solutions of these stains are standardized for blood films. The thick cellular particle smear of the bone marrow may not be adequately fixed during the staining procedure. A smear with a washed-out appearance of nuclei and loss of cytoplasmic details indicates underfixation, which can be corrected by prefixation for 2 to 3 minutes in absolute methyl alcohol. For best results the aspirate smears are stained as soon as they are dried. If the staining is to be done later, the smears should be fixed and stored in a dust-free box.

## Equipment and Reagents

1. Stain. Wright's stain or any of the preferred polychromatic stains can be used for staining hematopoietic cells. It is highly recommended to follow the manufacturer's directions, which are enclosed with the staining solutions.
2. Buffer solution. A distilled water solution of monobasic potassium phosphate and dibasic sodium phosphate with a pH of about 6.4 is also supplied commercially with the stain.
3. Staining rack and rack dish.

## Procedure

A staining rack with its draining dish is preferably situated close to a sink to facilitate the draining of the fluids and washing. The slides are placed on the rack horizontally with the dried smear facing upward and are well spaced so that the fluid from one slide does not overflow onto the other slides. With a dropper or bottle stopper the smears on the slides are covered with stain, but the stain from one slide must not spill over to another slide. After a proper time period, usually 3 to 6 minutes, an equal amount of buffer solution is added on the surface of each slide. Stain and buffer solution are mixed by gently blowing on several points of the slides. A metallic sheen appears on the surface of the dye-buffer solution within 6 to 8 minutes. While still on the rack the stain is floated off with tap water and then the slides are washed more vigorously for an additional 20 to 30 seconds. The excess dye is cleaned from the back and margin of the slides with the rack moistened in alcohol, and the slides are then air dried. For best results with different

batches of stain, some experimentation is needed to determine the correct timing. Technicians in busy laboratories with a large volume of bone marrow specimens may prefer to use some semiautomated or automated staining equipment, which is available commercially.

The stained bone marrow slides are preserved better if covered with coverglasses. Stained and well-dried slides are dipped in a Coplin jar with xylene for a few seconds. A small drop of a commercially available synthetic media is applied along the long margin on the slide, and then the cover glass is pressed from that margin toward the opposite side to expel the air before the cover slide is rested on the marrow smear. After drying, the glass-covered slide can be kept for years and reviewed numerous times without damage to the smear.

## Bone Biopsy

Bone biopsy is performed customarily in conjunction with marrow aspirate and has an advantage when the aspirate yields a "dry" tap owing to unaspirable marrow. Trephine bone biopsy is also indicated for diagnosis of neoplastic and granulomatous diseases. For clinical staging of lymphomas and carcinomas, bilateral posterior superior iliac crest biopsies are recommended, which increase the chance to diagnose a focal process. In adults, an 11-gauge Jamshidi biopsy needle is used, whereas in children a 13-gauge needle is preferred. An adequate biopsy is at least 15 mm in length.[8,10] The aspirate is performed after the biopsy by changing the direction of the needle to avoid aspiration of the biopsy site. It is better yet for the aspiration of the marrow to be done through a new puncture site in the anesthetized area.

### Preparation of Trephine Biopsy for Examination

**Touch Preparation.** The bone core is supported lightly without pressure between the blades of a forceps and touched several times on two or three clean slide surfaces. The biopsy core should not be rubbed on the slide, because rubbing destroys the cells. The slides are air dried rapidly. The touch preparations are fixed in absolute methanol and stained with Wright-Giemsa stain.

**Histologic Tissue Preparation.** The biopsy specimen is immersed without delay in B-5 or 5 percent buffered formalin fixative. Histology laboratories may have a choice of other preferred fixatives such as Zenker's solution, Carnoy's solution, and others.[11] After fixation the biopsy undergoes standard histologic processing of decalcification, dehydration, embedding in paraffin blocks, and sectioning on 2 to 3 $\mu$ thick sections for staining. The advantage of bone marrow biopsy is that it represents marrow structures in their natural relationship. A variety of different stains can be used to demonstrate marrow iron, reticulum, collagen, acid-fast organisms, and fungi in granulomatous diseases. This offers great advantages in diagnosing bacterial and fungal infections. The bacterial cultures may require long periods of incubation to show growth of organisms. While on tissue sections, the histologic and etiologic diagnosis may be made within 10 to 12 hours. At present, when metastatic tumors and lymphomas are found in the bone marrow, monoclonal hybridoma antibodies can be used on histologic material to demonstrate specific receptors. Thus, a very precise diagnosis of the origin of a tumor can be made.

A disadvantage of the bone biopsy is that fine cellular details are lost in the processing; therefore, it is of little value in the diagnosis of leukemias and of some refractory anemias. In these situations, the touch preparation from the biopsy may supply the missing morphologic details.

## BONE MARROW STRUCTURE

The hematopoietic marrow is organized around the bone vasculature.[12,13] A nutrient artery enters the bone and gives out branches, which run toward the periphery leading to specialized vascular spaces — sinuses. Several sinuses may combine in a collecting sinus, which leads to a central vein. The central vein runs parallel to the nutrient artery. Outside of the sinuses and in intimate relationship with them are the hematopoietic cords. The development of the hematopoietic cells is extravascular in the cords and highly compartmentalized. The two major compartments are the sinuses and cords. Upon maturation in the cords, the hematopoietic cells traverse the walls of the sinuses and enter the blood.[14-16] There is also hemopoietic compartmentalization in the cords. The erythropoiesis takes place in distinct anatomic units; a macrophage surrounded by a cluster of maturing erythroblasts is known as an erythropoietic island.[17] The granulopoiesis is less conspicuously oriented toward a distinct reticular cell but still is recognizable as an entity.[18] The megakaryopoiesis is located subjacent to the sinus endothelium. The megakaryocytes protrude with small cytoplasmic processes through the wall delivering the platelets straight in the sinusoidal blood (Fig. 25-3).[19] Marrow immunocytes consist of lymphocytes and plasma cells. The lymhocytes are compartmentalized in lymphocytic nodules and random diffuse dispersion of lymphocytes occurs throughout the cords. The lymphocytic nodules are unevenly distributed and tend to influence the lymphocyte count in bone marrow samples **(see Color Figure 217)**. Plasma cells are oriented around blood vessels.

The meshwork of stromal cells in which the he-matopoietic cells are suspended is in a delicate semifluid state and is composed of reticulum cells, histiocytes, fat cells, and endothelial cells. The reticulum cells are associated with fibers that can be visualized after silver staining. They are adjacent to the sinus endothelial cells forming the outer part of the walls as an adventitial reticular cell. Their fine cytoplasmic projections are extended deep into the cords, which make contact with similar projections of other cells. Occasionally the nuclear region of these cells can be seen deep in the cords associated with granulopoiesis **(see Color Figure 218)**. Cytochemically these cells are alkaline-phosphatase positive. The histiocyte-macrophage is seen as a perisinusoidal cell related to the bone marrow–blood barrier and as a central macrophage part of the erythropoietic islands. In the role of a nutrient cell delivering iron to the growing immature erythroblasts, the central macrophage sends out long, slender sytoplasmic processes that envelope the erythroid precursors **(see Color Figure 219)**. This extensive and intimate contact with the maturing erythropoietic cells is necessary in the transferring of iron from the macrophage to the red cell precursors. Histochemically, the macrophages are acid-phosphatase positive.

The fat cells vary in amount according to the age of the patient and the location whence the marrow is obtained. In children only a few fat cells are seen, whereas in adults fat cells average about 50 percent of the total marrow volume. The marrow fat and the ground mucopolysaccharide substance are dynamic tissues similar to the hematopoietic marrow, and these are altered rapidly in disease.

In marrow aspirates, cells are occasionally seen originating from bone tissue. Osteoblasts are found usually in groups. They resemble plasma cells but are slightly larger. The nucleus of osteoblast has a fine chromatin pattern with a prominent nucleolus. A perinuclear halo, detached from the nuclear membrane with a cytoplasmic bridge, represents the Golgi apparatus area **(see Color Figure 220)**. The osteoblast, a bone matrix synthesizing cell, is alkaline-phosphatase positive. Osteoblasts are seen usually in children and patients having metabolic bone diseases.

Osteoclasts are multinucleated giant cells resembling megakaryocytes. The nuclei of the osteoclasts are separated from each other and may have nucleoli (compared with the megakaryocyte nucleus, which is lobated). The acidophilic or basophilic cytoplasm is granular and well delineated **(see Color Figures 221 and 222)**.

The bone marrow is a highly vascularized tissue from which endothelial cells can occasionally be aspirated. Endothelial cells are more visible in hypoplastic marrows and should not be mistaken for metastatic tumors **(see Color Figure 223)**.

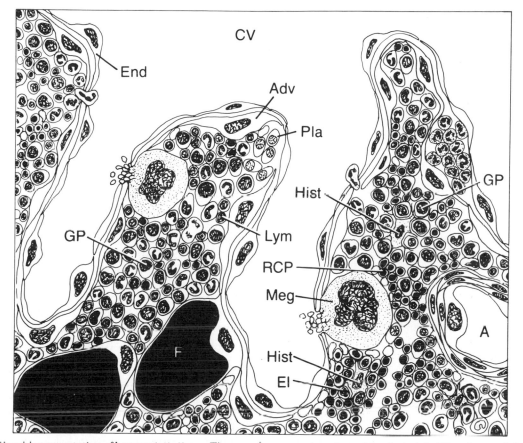

**Figure 25-3.** Graphic presentation of hemopoietic tissue. The vascular compartment consists of arteriole (A) and central sinus (CV). The venous sinusoids are lined by endothelial cells (End), and their wall outside is supported by adventitial-reticulum cells (Adv). Fat tissue (F) is part of the marrow. The compartmentalization of the hemopoiesis is represented by areas of granulopoiesis (GP), areas of erythropoiesis (RCP), and erythropoietic islands (EI) with its nutrient histiocyte (Hist). The megakaryocytes protrude with small cytoplasmic projections through the vascular wall (meg). Lymphocytes (lym) are randomly scattered among the hemopoietic cells while plasma cells are usually situated along the vascular wall (Pla).

## BONE MARROW EXAMINATION

The examination of the bone marrow slides starts with low magnification with a dry objective of ×10. A scan over the slide permits selection of a suitable area for examination and differential count. "Bare nuclei" due to destruction of the marrow cells by squashing them or stripping their cytoplasm by fibrin thread should be avoided. An area is selected where the cells are well spread, intact, and not diluted by sinusoidal blood. When marrow particles are examined, such areas are found at the periphery of the particles. On this low magnification, marrow cellularity is also evaluated. The number and the distribution of the megakaryocytes is noted (usually about three per low-power field adjacent to spicule). Under this power, nonhematopoietic tumor cells infiltrating to the bone marrow are also observed for, which are usually larger than the granulocytic or erythropoietic precursors, and which can be seen in clusters **(see Color Figure 224)**.

After the initial scan, immersion oil is applied on the slide and the examination continues on high magnification (oil immersion objective ×63 or ×100). The high magnification provides details of the nuclear and cytoplasmic maturation process. The iron in histiocytes is visualized as brown-blue granules. Cytoplasmic inclusions of a diagnostic nature can be seen in histiocytes and granulocytes. Differential counts of bone marrow are also done with the oil immersion objective.

## ESTIMATION OF MARROW CELLULARITY

The cellularity is reflected in the ratio of hemopoietic to fat cells. The bone marrow in infancy and early childhood has no fat. After 2 to 3 years of age, fat tissue gradually permeates the hemopoietic marrow, and by age 20 years, half of the marrow in the posterior iliac crest is replaced by fat. In the sternum at that age the marrow has about 60 percent cellularity. There follows a gradual and insignificant decrease in the marrow cellularity, so that by the age of 60 to 65 years the marrow cellularity is about 35 to 40 percent.

Overall marrow cellularity of adults is about 50 percent (±10 percent). The bone biopsy is the most reliable assessment of cellularity, because it offers a large amount of tissue for evaluation. However, the evaluation of the cellularity can be done also on good aspirate smears. The best areas for examination of cellularity in smears is the areas between two uncrushed particles. The ratio of cells to fat is evaluated on low magnification (objective ×10), so that larger areas are included in the field of observation. Usually the ratio of fat to packed cells should be 1:1. The empty spaces that result from the spreading of the cells but are not occupied by fat cells are disregarded and treated as an artifact. The term "decreased" or "increased" cellularity is implied when less or more than the expected normal amount of cells is seen. Precise evaluation can be achieved with experience, and good reproducibility can be attained among several observers. The marrow cellularity is variable, and random samples may not be representative of the cellular status throughout the bone marrow. On the other hand, a random sample is a fairly good representation of the differential count. Therefore, the judgment of marrow hypoplasia and aplasia cannot be done on a single hypocellular bone marrow aspirate or biopsy. Even in the presence of blood cytopenia (anemia, granulocytopenia, and thrombocytopenia) more than one marrow sample should be obtained from different sites of the skeleton to diagnose marrow aplasia. Marrow cellularity has its diagnostic value when it is related to the M:E ratio, which is calculated after a differential count is performed. The M:E ratio is obtained by determining the number of granulocytes and their precursor cells to the number of nucleated red cells.

## BONE MARROW DIFFERENTIAL COUNT

A bone marrow differential count has limited diagnostic value and is not necessary or useful in most nonhemopoietic diseases. However, a differential count is an excellent tool for training a novice in bone marrow morphology and is widely used in diagnosing and following up patients with leukemias, refractory anemias, and myelodysplastic syndromes. Because of the compartmentalization of the hemopoietic cells, at least 500 to 1000 nucleated cells need to be classified for a correct differential count. During the first month after birth, dramatic alteration occurs in the distribution of the different marrow compartments. At birth there is a predominance of granulocyte precursors, which switches

within a month to a predominance of lymphoid elements. In early infancy many lymphocytes have fine chromatin, high nucleus cytoplasmic ratio, and distinct nucleoli. They can be misinterpreted as blasts if the observer is unfamiliar with these characteristics. Suggestion has been made that these lymphoid cells may represent stem cells in the infant marrow.[20] In children up to 3 years old, one third or more of the marrow cellularity is made up of lymphocytes. The lymphocyte number gradually declines to the normal adult level thereafter. In adult marrow the lymphocytes are distributed both at random among the hemopoietic cells and in lymphocytic nodules. This can introduce great variation in the differential count from sample to sample in the same patient. The great mass of the marrow is composed of granulopoietic and erythropoietic precursors. For the purpose of the differential count these are enumerated in their different categories according to their stage of maturation. When adequate numbers of cells are tabulated, the percentage of each category is calculated. Some hematologists prefer to exclude the segmented neutrophils from the differential count as being part of the neutrophil storage pool of the marrow. The normal M:E ratio in this case is between 1.5 and 3. However, pathologists and hematologists who interpret the bone marrow histologic sections of particle and biopsies in conjunction with marrow smears include the segmented neutrophils in the differential counts, because these cannot be excluded in the evaluation of histologic specimens. The normal M:E ratio then is slightly higher and ranges between 3 and 4. The granulopoietic tissue occupies two to four times greater marrow space than the erythropoietic precursor, owing to the shorter survival of the granulocytes in the circulation (neutrophils 2 to 5 hours versus erythrocytes 120 days). Megakaryocytes are unevenly distributed, and a differential count is a poor means for their evaluation. Usually 5 to 10 megakaryocytes are seen per microscopic field on low magnification (objective ×10). When clusters of megakaryocytes and promegakaryocytes are seen, it is an indication of megakaryocytic hyperplasia. In a normal cellular marrow, finding two or less megakaryocytes per field on screening may indicate megakaryocytic hypoplasia. Decreased and increased numbers of megakaryocytes are better evaluated on histologic sections of biopsy and particle specimens.

Bone marrow differential counts may show great variability because of compartmentalization of the hematopoiesis.[8,21,22] Table 25–2 represents the data of normal reference ranges used by the computer resources of the Medical Center Hospital and University of Texas Health Service Center at San Antonio.

Table 25-2. DIFFERENTIAL CELL COUNT OF BONE MARROW IN PERCENT OF TOTAL NUCLEATED CELLS*

| | At Birth | Up to 1 Mo | Children | Adults |
|---|---|---|---|---|
| Undifferentiated cells | 0-2 | 0-2 | 0-1 | 0-1 |
| Myeloblast | 0-2 | 0-2 | 0-2 | 0-2 |
| Promyelocyte | 0-4 | 0-4 | 0-4 | 0-4 |
| Myelocytes | | | | |
|   Neutrophilic | 2-8 | 2-4 | 5-15 | 5-20 |
|   Eosinophilic | 0-5 | 0-3 | 0-6 | 0-3 |
|   Basophilic | 0-1 | 0-1 | 0-1 | 0-1 |
| Metamyelocytes and bands | | | | |
|   Neutrophilic | 15-25 | 5-10 | 5-15 | 5-35 |
|   Eosinophilic | 0-5 | 1-5 | 1-8 | 0-5 |
|   Basophilic | 0-1 | 0-1 | 0-1 | 0-1 |
| Segmented neutrophils | 5-15 | 3-10 | 5-15 | 5-15 |
| Pronormoblast | 0-3 | 0-1 | 0-2 | 0-1.5 |
| Basophilic normoblast | 0-5 | 0-3 | 0-5 | 0-5 |
| Polychromatophilic normoblast | 6-20 | 5-20 | 5-11 | 5-30 |
| Orthochromatic normoblast | 0-5 | 0-2 | 0-8 | 5-10 |
| Lymphocytes | 5-15 | 5-50 | 5-35 | 10-20 |
| Plasma cells | 0-2 | 0-2 | 0-2 | 0-2 |
| Monocytes | 0-5 | 0-2 | 0-4 | 0-5 |
| M:E ratio based on 500 cell count | 3-4.5 | 3-4.5 | 1.5-4 | 2-4 |

*Normal reference range from the Laboratory Computing Resources of The University of Texas Health Science Center and Medical Center Hospital, San Antonio, TX.

## BONE MARROW AND BLOOD INTERPRETATION BASED ON CELLULARITY AND M:E RATIO CHANGES

A bone marrow sample represents a minute part of a very large organ. The bone marrow activity and responses are reflected in blood changes; therefore, evaluation of the bone marrow should be done always in conjunction with evaluation of the peripheral blood. In adult humans with 50 percent marrow cellularity, about 30 to 40 percent represents granulopoiesis and 10 to 15 percent erythropoiesis with an average M:E ratio of 4:1 **(see Color Figure 225)**. When marrow cellularity increases or decreases preserving the normal M:E ratio, this is indicative of a balanced granulocytic and erythrocytic hyperplasia or hypoplasia correspondingly. However, if the cellularity change occurs simultaneously with M:E ratio changes, the interpretation requires a broader understanding of hemopoietic tissue physiology and reactions, as well as experience, and cannot be translated in simple terms.

Table 25-3 is included to be used only as a simple guide and to give some basic information to the reader, but it cannot and should not be used as a diagnostic tool without the patient's clinical history and physical evaluation of the disease. Also, the problems frequently presented by different patients with the same disease will not fit in such a simplistic concept.

## CORRELATIONS OF SMEARS AND HISTOLOGIC SECTIONS OF BONE MARROW SPECIMENS

Bone marrow smears represent a very limited sample of a huge and very dynamic tissue, but the cell morphology and the M:E ratio are well depicted in random specimens. The variations are not significant even when samples are compared from sternal and iliac crest aspirates.[23] On the other hand, marrow cellularity is poorly represented in random smears; thus, the interpretation should be with some degree of reservation. Even large biopsy specimens may have a great degree of cellular variations.[4] For this reason, in diseases when marrow cellularity is crucial for the diagnosis, more than one sample of bone biopsies may need to be obtained.

### Bone Marrow Iron Stores

The evaluation of marrow iron stores is essential in diagnosis of some anemias and especially in refractory and dyserythropoietic anemias. When the morphologic characteristic of the iron particles in the storage nutrient histiocyte and erythroblastic precursors is an important diagnostic clue, an iron stain is done on particle smear. If the overall distribution of the amount of iron is of clinical importance, then histologic sections of bone marrow biopsy and marrow particles stained for iron are a more reliable

**Table 25-3. MARROW AND BLOOD INTERPRETATION BASED ON CELLULARITY AND M:E RATIO**

| Complete Blood Count | Bone Marrow Cellularity | M:E Ratio | Bone Marrow Interpretation |
|---|---|---|---|
| Normal | Increased or decreased* | Normal range | Normal |
| Pancytopenia | Decreased | Normal range | Marrow hypoplasia |
| Neutropenia | Decreased | Decreased | Granulocytic hypoplasia |
| Anemia | Normal or decreased | Increased | Red cell hypoplasia |
| Neutrophilia | Normal or increased | Increased | Granulocytic hyperplasia |
| Erythrocytosis (polycythemia) | Normal or increased | Decreased | Erythrocytic hyperplasia |
| Anemia | Normal or increased | Decreased | Erythrocytic hyperplasia or ineffective erythropoiesis† |
| Neutropenia | Normal or increased | Increased | Decreased neutrophilic survival or ineffective granulopoiesis |
| Pancytopenia | Increased | Normal, increased, or decreased | Ineffective myelopoiesis or hypersplenism |

*Because of poor presentation of cellularity in random specimen.
†Reticulocyte count is necessary to differentiate between erythrocytic hyperplasia and ineffective erythropoiesis.

source of information, because they represent a large sample of hematopoietic tissue. Bone biopsy for iron studies should be decalcified by the EDTA chelating method, which does not affect the storage iron.[12] Acid decalcifying solutions extract iron and must not be used in these cases. The storage iron of the bone marrow is in the form of hemosiderin. The iron content of hemosiderin is higher than it is in the ferritin. Other components of hemosiderin are protein, ferritin, some lipids, and membranes of cellular organelles. Hemosiderin can be seen on unstained smears as golden-yellow granules. On Wright-Giemsa–stained smears, it appears as brownish-blue granules. However, for more precise evaluation Prussian blue reaction is used to demonstrate intracytoplasmic iron of histiocyte and red cell precursors.

### Iron Staining of Aspirate Smear[24]

Two smears with good marrow particles are selected. Particles are used, because they contain storage histiocytes.

### Reagents

Reagents commonly used include potassium ferrocyanide 2 percent, hydrochloric acid (HCl) 1 percent, and nuclear fast red. For a working solution of nuclear fast red, 5 percent anhydrous aluminum sulfate is prepared by heating to dissolve the aluminum sulfate. After cooling the solution is filtered and a crystal of thymol is added as a preservative. Nuclear fast red 0.1 g is dissolved in this 5 percent aluminum sulfate solution. The mixture can be kept indefinitely in an air-tight bottle.

### Procedure

First, air-dried smears of marrow particles are fixed for 10 minutes in formalin vapor by moistening gauze or filter paper with a few drops of 10 percent formalin and placing it together with the slides in a Coplin jar. Second, fresh-staining solution is prepared for each batch of slides. The procedure is as follows:

1. 12 ml of 2 percent potassium ferrocyanide is mixed with 36 ml of 1 percent HCl.
2. The slides are immersed in the solution for 10 minutes.

Next, the slides are rinsed with distilled water, air dried, and counterstained with nuclear fast red for another 10 minutes. Finally, the counterstained slides are rinsed with tap water, dried, and coverslipped.

Modification of Prussian blue reaction is used also to stain iron in histologic sections of bone biopsies and marrow particles. Hemosiderin and some ferritin aggregates are seen after staining, as bright-blue specks and granules **(see Color Figure 226)**. Hemoglobin iron does not stain. The storage iron may be reported verbally as "absent," "decreased," "adequate," "moderately increased," and "markedly increased," or it can be given corresponding numerical values from 0 to 5, where 2 represents the normal or adequate iron stored in an adult.

## BONE MARROW REPORT

The bone marrow report consists usually of seven parts:

1. Patient's addressograph data, including age and relevant clinical summary
2. Description of material received for studies, such as smears of aspirate, marrow particles, and/or bone biopsy(ies).
3. Data of the CBC, WBC, differential count, and a description of the blood smear usually on the day on which the bone marrow specimen is obtained. Platelet count and reticulocyte count should be included.
4. Bone marrow differential count.
5. Description of cellularity, M:E ratio, granulo-

poiesis, erythropoiesis, and megakaryopoiesis. Any change of the nonhematopoietic elements of marrow or metastatic tumor cells are included in this section of the report. The status of iron stores is reported.

6. Description of histologic sections of bone marrow biopsy and particles if available.

7. Diagnostic conclusion.

The technologist's contribution in this phase is limited to performing the blood and bone marrow differential count when needed. The actual examination of the blood and the bone marrow, as well as the diagnostic conclusions on each specimen, is the responsibility of a physician who has adequate preparation and experience to integrate all available clinical and laboratory information in reaching the correct diagnosis.

## References

1. Gilmour, JR: Normal hematopoiesis in intrauterine and neonatal life. J Pathol 52:25, 1941.

2. Gupta, S, Pahwa, R, O'Reilly, R, et al: Ontogeny of lymphocyte subpopulations in human fetal liver. Proc Natl Acad Sci 73(3):919, 1976.

3. Mechanik, N: Untersuchung uber das Gewicht des Knochenmarkes des Menshen. Z Gesamte Anat 79:58, 1926.

4. Hartsock, RJ, Smith, EB, and Petty, CS: Normal variations with aging of the amount of hematopoietic tissue in bone marrow from anterior iliac crest. Am J Clin Pathol 43:326, 1965.

5. Custer, RP: An Atlas of the Blood and Bone Marrow. WB Saunders, Philadelphia, 1974, p 33.

6. Claman, HN, Chaperon, EA, and Triplett, RF: Immunocompetence of transferred thymus — marrow cell combinations. J Immunol 97:828, 1966.

7. Arinkin, MJ: Intravitale Untersuchungsmethodik der Knochenmarks. Folia Haematol (Leipz) 38:233, 1929.

8. Wintrobe, MM: Clinical Hematology. Lea & Febiger, Philadelphia, 1981, p 58.

9. Nelson, DA: Hematopoiesis. In Henry, JB (ed): Clinical Diagnosis and Management by Laboratory Methods. WB Saunders, Philadelphia, 1979, p 956.

10. Brynes, RK, McKenna, RW, and Sunberg, RD: Bone marrow aspiration and trephine biopsy, an approach to a thorough study. Am J Clin Pathol 70:753, 1978.

11. Sheeham, DC and Hrapchak, BB: Theory and Practice of Histotechnology. CV Mosby, St Louis, 1980, pp 46, 94.

12. Tavassoli, M and Jossey, JM: Bone marrow, structure and function. Alan R. Liss, New York, 1978, p 43.

13. Lichtman, MA: The ultrastructure of the hemopoietic environment of the marrow: A review. Exp Hematol 9:391, 1981.

14. Tavassoli, M and Shaklai, M: Absence of tight junctions in endothelium of marrow sinuses: Possible significance for marrow cell egress. Erythropoiesis in BM. Br J Haematol 41:303, 1979.

15. Aoki, M and Tavassoli, M: Dynamics of red cell egress from bone marrow after blood letting. Br J Haematol 49:337, 1981.

16. Aoki, M and Tavassoli, M: Red cell egress from bone marrow in state of transfusion plethora. Exp Hematol 9:231, 1981.

17. Bessis, M: L'ilot erythroblastique, unite fonctionelle de la moelle osseuse. Rev Hematol 13:8, 1958.

18. Western, H and Bainton, DF: Association of alkaline-phosphatase-positive reticulum cells in bone marrow with granulocytic precursors. J Exp Med 150:919, 1979.

19. Lichtman, MA, Chamberlain, JK, Simon W, et al: Parasinusoidal location of megakaryoctes in marrow. A determinant of platelet release. Am J Hematol 4:303, 1978.

20. Rosse, C, Kraemer, MJ, Dillon, TL, et al: Bone marrow cell population of normal infants: The predominance of lymphocytes. J Lab Clin Med 89:1225, 1977.

21. Mauer, AM: Pediatric Hematology. McGraw-Hill, New York, 1969, p 17.

22. Oski, FA and Naiman, LJ: Hematologic Problems of the Newborn. WB Saunders, Philadelphia, 1982, p 21.

23. Rubinstein, MA: Aspiration of bone marrow from iliac crest comparison of iliac crest and sternal bone marrow studies. JAMA 137:1821, 1948.

24. Nelson, DA and Davey, IR: Hematopoiesis. In Henry, JB (ed): Clinical Diagnosis and Management by Laboratory Methods. WB Saunders, Philadelphia, 1984, p 646.

# CHAPTER 26

D. HARMENING PITTIGLIO, Ph.D., M.T.(ASCP)

# Introduction to Hemostasis: An Overview of Hemostatic Mechanism, Platelet Structure and Function, and Extrinsic and Intrinsic Systems

## PLATELETS AND HEMOSTATIC MECHANISMS

Hemostasis is the process by which the body spontaneously stops bleeding and maintains blood in the fluid state within the vascular compartment. Four major systems are involved in maintaining hemostasis:

1. Vascular system
2. Platelets
3. Fibrin-forming (coagulation) system
4. Fibrin-lysing (fibrinolytic) system

Three additional minor systems are also related to hemostasis:

1. Kinin system
2. Serine protease inhibitors
3. Complement system

The hemostatic mechanisms are designed to rapidly repair any vascular breaks and maintain blood flow within the vessels. However, there are potential risks associated with this rapid localized hemostasis: imbalance in one direction leads to excessive bleeding, and in the other to thrombosis. There are also limits to the degree of vascular injury that may be controlled since the process of hemostasis involves consumption of platelets and coagulation factors. The relative importance of the hemostatic mechanisms varies with vessel size. For example, breaks in capillaries seal directly and immediately with little dependence on hemostasis. However, arterioles and venules, once ruptured, become quickly occluded with a mass of fused platelets. Hemostasis in veins depends on vascular contraction as well as on perivascular and intravascular activation of hemostatic factors, as these vessels rupture easily with increased hydrostatic pressure due to trauma. Arterial hemorrhage is the most severe test of hemostasis, even though arteries are the most resistant of all vessels to bleeding because of their thick, muscular walls. The process of vasoconstriction is crucial to successful thrombus formation in arteries. Generally, the larger the area of bleeding, the larger the vessel involved.

Bleeding from arterioles and venules results in pinpoint petechial hemorrhages. Hemorrhaging from veins results in large, ill-defined, soft tissue bleeding termed "ecchymoses." Bleeding from arteries manifests in rapidly expanding "blowout" hemorrhage. Each major and minor hemostatic system will be considered separately and then interrelated into the entire sequence of events in the maintenance of hemostasis.

## Vascular System

The vascular system acts to prevent bleeding by (1) contraction of vessels (vasoconstriction) and reflex stimulation of adjacent vessels, (2) diversion of blood flow around damaged vasculature, (3) initiation of contact-activation of platelets with subsequent aggregation, and (4) contact-activation of the coagulation system (both extrinsic and intrinsic) leading to fibrin formation. Vascular integrity, which is influenced by vitamin C intake, is important in maintaining the fluidity of the blood. The blood vessel, with its smooth and continuous endothelial lining and fibrous coat, is designed to facilitate blood flow as well as participate in the process of hemostasis. The endothelial surface of the blood vessel is usually inert to coagulation factors and platelets. It is termed a "nonwettable" surface in that the physical and chemical characteristics of the endothelium allow a minimum of interaction between blood and the endothelial surface. However, when the endothelial lining is disrupted, underlying collagen and basement membrane are exposed, activating platelets and the plasma coagulation factors. This break in endothelium leads to platelet adhesion and thrombus formation, because the endothelial cells contain ADP, which is important in inducing aggregation of platelets. In addition, released tissue thromboplastin initiates fibrin formation through the extrinsic pathway of the coagulation system. The vascular response involved in the hemostatic mechanism usually lasts less than one minute.

## Metabolic Functions of the Endothelium

One of the most important functions of the endothelial surface is its multiple antithrombotic properties. Glycocalyx, a mucopolysaccharide, coats the luminal surface of the endothelium and possesses the ability to stimulate weakly the physiologic anticoagulant antithrombin III (AT-III) through one of its constituents known as heparin sulfate. In addition, the vascular endothelial membrane also contains thrombin receptor sites, termed "thrombomodulin," that neutralize the active enzyme thrombin, which is necessary in producing a fibrin clot with the coagulation cascade (see section on fibrin-forming system). This thrombomodulin-thrombin complex activates another important plasma protein called protein C, which is a potent and specific anticoagulant as well as an effective fibrinolytic agent important in maintaining the endothelium in a nonthrombogenic state (see section on protease inhibitors).

Other nonthrombogenic properties of the vascular endothelium include the enzyme ADPase, which degrades ADP, and synthesis of prostacyclin ($PGI_2$), which functions as a potent vasodilator and inhibitor of the platelet response. The endothelium is also rich in an activator of fibrinolysis called tissue plasminogen activator (TPA). With an appropriate stimulus, this substance is released and activates the plasma protein plasminogen to the enzyme plasmin, which ensures rapid lysis of the forming fibrin clot.

The endothelium plays a major role in the delicate balance between halting the bleeding (procoagulant activity, formation of a clot) and prevention of excessive pathologic thrombus formation by initiation of fibrinolysis and release of anticoagulant factors. The endothelium is also intimately involved in the metabolism and clearance of several small molecules such as angiotensin, serotonin, and bradykinin. These substances affect the regulation of blood pressure, the egress of fluid across the endothelium, and inflammation.

The vascular endothelial cells also synthesize a number of substances such as type IV collagen and fibronectin (a noncollagen glycoprotein) that are important for normal hemostasis and vascular integrity. Von Willebrand's factor, a part of the plasma factor VIII molecule, is also produced by the vascular endothelial cells as well as by megakaryocytes. A glycoprotein receptor for this factor is present on the surface of activated platelets and mediates platelet adhesion to a foreign surface such as collagen (see next section).

## PLATELET STRUCTURE AND FUNCTION

Platelets are intimately involved in "primary hemostasis," which is the interaction of platelets and the vascular endothelium in halting bleeding following vascular injury. As discussed in Chapter 1, platelets are cellular fragments derived from the cytoplasm of megakaryocytes present in the bone marrow. Platelets are released and circulate approximately 9 to 12 days as small, disc-shaped cells with an average diameter of 2 to 4 microns. On a Wright-stained peripheral smear, platelets appear as round or oval, granular purple dots. The platelet's typical stained morphology consists of a clear zone of cytoplasm, termed "hyalomere," which surrounds a highly stained granulomere (Fig. 26-1). The normal platelet count ranges from 150,000 to 350,000, depending on the methodology employed. In the peripheral blood, approximately 30 percent of the platelets are sequestered in the microvasculature or in the spleen as functional reserves after their release from the bone marrow. Aged or nonviable platelets are removed by both the spleen and the liver. These anuclear cytoplasmic fragments (platelets) contain a number of interesting organelles, which are listed in Figure 26-2.

## Structure

The platelet structure is quite distinct, leading to the subdivision into three defined zones that possess unique functional capabilities. These include (1) the peripheral zone (the stimulus receptor/transmitter region), (2) the sol-gel zone (the cytoskeletal/contractile region), and (3) the organelle zone (the metabolic/organellar region). Table 26-1 summarizes the three described zones and their contents. These zones are prominently delineated by the circumferential band of microtubules found in the platelet (Fig. 26-3).

## Peripheral Zone

The peripheral zone is a complex region of the platelet consisting of the glycocalyx (an amorphous exterior coat), plasma membrane, numerous deeply penetrating surface-connecting channels known as the open canalicular system (OCS), and a submembranous area of specialized microfilaments.

The glycocalyx intimately surrounds the platelet and is considered an important component of the platelet membrane. A number of glycoproteins present in this area are responsible for blood group specificity (ABO), tissue compatibility (HLA), and platelet unique immunologic antigenicity. In addition, glycoproteins also serve as receptors and facilitate transmission of stimuli across the platelet membrane. For example, platelet membrane glycoprotein Ib is the receptor for the plasma coagulation protein called von Willebrand's factor, and glycoproteins IIb and IIIa are involved with fibrinogen binding. In addition to these, the platelet membrane includes receptors for the following substances: adenosine diphosphate (ADP), thrombin, epinephrine, and serotonin. Various enzymes have also been isolated in the plasma membrane of platelets.

The platelet membrane, similar to other plasma membranes, represents a fluid lipid bilayer composed of glycoproteins, glycolipids, and lipoproteins. The membrane phospholipid portion of the activated platelet serves as a surface for the interaction of the plasma proteins involved in blood coagulation, which assemble in complexes on the platelet's surface. Coagulation factors V and VIII also are present on the surface of the platelet membrane, as are various platelet factors that participate in the formation of fibrin (i.e., PF3, PF4). In addition to containing receptors for various stimuli, the periph-

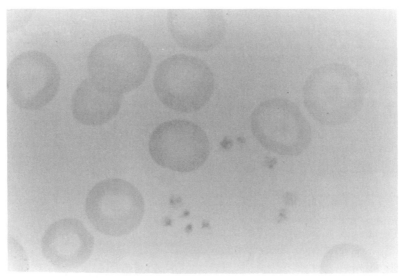

**Figure 26-1.** Normal platelets; Wright-stained blood smear.

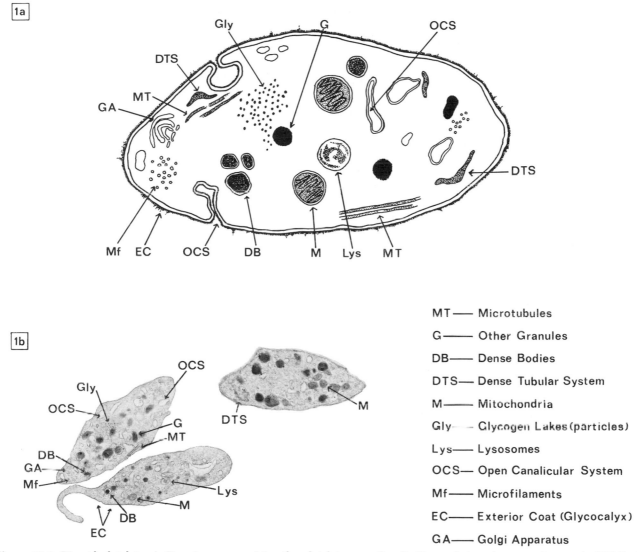

**Figure 26-2.** Discoid platelets. *A*, Drawing summarizing the platelet organelles. *B*, Transmission electron micrograph (TEM) of cross-sectioned platelets illustrating basic ultrastructure.

MT —— Microtubules

G —— Other Granules

DB —— Dense Bodies

DTS —— Dense Tubular System

M —— Mitochondria

Gly —— Glycogen Lakes (particles)

Lys —— Lysosomes

OCS —— Open Canalicular System

Mf —— Microfilaments

EC —— Exterior Coat (Glycocalyx)

GA —— Golgi Apparatus

## TABLE 26–1. PLATELET ULTRASTRUCTURAL ZONES

**I. Peripheral Zone (Stimulus Receptor/Transmitter Region)**
   A. Glycocalyx
   B. Plasma membrane
   C. Open canalicular system (OCS)
   D. Submembranous region
**II. Sol-Gel Zone (Cytoskeletal/Contractile Region)**
   A. Circumferential microtubules
   B. Microfilaments
   C. Thrombosthenin
**III. Organelle Zone (Metabolic/Organellar Region)**
   A. Granules
      1. Alpha granules
      2. Dense granules
      3. Glycogen granules
   B. Mitochondria
   C. Dense tubular system (DTS)
   D. Lysosomes and peroxisomes

eral zone of the platelet also contains the mechanism for the development of "stickiness," which is essential for the platelet functions of adhesion and aggregation.

The membranous surface connecting system referred to as the open canalicular system (OCS) consists of tubular invaginations of the plasma membrane that articulate throughout the platelet, even though it is part of the peripheral zone. Platelet stored products are released to the exterior through the OCS. The OCS also facilitates collection of plasma procoagulants that aid in fibrin formation by providing increased surface absorptive area.

### Sol-Gel Zone

The aqueous sol-gel zone contains microtubules and microfilaments. Microfilaments are interwo-

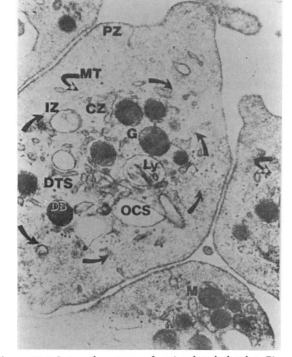

**Figure 26-3.** Internal anatomy of a stimulated platelet. Circumferential band of microtubules (MT) leads to reorganization of the internal structure of the platelet into three zones. The peripheral zone (PZ) is the region external to a circumferential band of microtubules (MT with * on *curved arrows*). The intermediate zone (IZ), designated by the *encircling arrows*, includes the microtubules and the closely adjacent cytoplasmic material. The central zone (CZ) is internal to the microtubule band and contains many organelles such as granules (G), dense bodies (DB), dense tubular system (DTS), lysosomes (Ly), mitochondria (M), and many profiles of the open canalicular system (OCS). Magnification ×49,700. (From Barnhart, MI: Platelet responses in health and disease. Mol Cell Biochem 22:115, 1978, with permission.)

ven throughout the cytoplasm of the platelet and are composed of thrombosthenin, a microfibrillar "contractile" protein similar to the actinomyosin protein involved in muscle tissue contraction. Thrombosthenin comprises approximately 15 percent of the total platelet protein. Although some of this protein is unorganized, the majority is aligned into a bundle of circumferential microtubules. This circumferential band of hollow tubular structures, similar to the microtubules of other cells, lies immediately beneath the platelet membrane. This structure, together with microfilaments actin and myosin, forms the platelet's cytoskeleton, which contracts as the platelet's shape changes.

The cytoskeleton is responsible for maintaining its normal discoid shape. In the stimulated platelet (Fig. 26-3), contraction of the circumferential band of microtubules is postulated to be responsible for the centripetal movement and reorganization of organelles, pseudopod formation, and the so-called release reactions of platelets.

## Organelle Zone

The organelle region is responsible for the metabolic activities of the platelet. Generally, the most numerous organelles are the platelet granules, which are heterogeneous in size, electron density, and chemical contents. Two types of granules are considered unique to platelets: alpha granules and dense bodies. The alpha granules are more numerous (20 to 200 per platelet) and contain a number of different proteins which are summarized in Table 26-2. The physiologic role of these proteins present in the alpha granules of platelets has not been clearly defined. However, it is known that platelet factor 4 does neutralize the anticoagulant heparin.

Dense bodies are fewer in number (2 to 10 per platelet) and represent densely opaque granules in transmission electron microscope (TEM) preparations. Table 26-3 lists the contents of the dense body granules in the platelet. The intragranular concentration of ADP and ATP found in the dense bodies of the platelets is called the "storage pool" of adenine nucleotides. This contrasts with the "metabolic pool" of ATP and ADP that is found in the platelet cytoplasm.

Acquired abnormalities of platelet alpha or dense granules have been reported in patients who have undergone coronary bypass surgery. Congenital abnormalities of alpha granules have also been reported, such as the "gray platelet syndrome" (see Chapter 27). These patients usually experience a mild clinical bleeding. The contents of both the alpha granules and dense bodies are released during the process called the "release reaction," which is energy dependent. As a result of ADP released from dense bodies during the "release reaction," additional platelets are drawn to the site of the vascular injury resulting in the formation of platelet aggregates. Both acquired and hereditary disorders have been described, resulting in decreased storage pool adenine nucleotides. For example, patients with antibodies to platelets that induce platelet release in conditions of compensated autoimmune thrombocytopenia represent one type of *acquired* storage pool disease. In contrast, a group of rare heterogeneous *hereditary* storage pool disorders also exist,

## TABLE 26-2. PROTEINS PRESENT IN PLATELET'S ALPHA GRANULES

| Platelet-Specific Proteins | Plasma Proteins |
|---|---|
| 1. Platelet factor 4 | 1. Fibrinogen |
| 2. B-thromboglobulin (BTG) | 2. Factor VIII vWF |
| 3. Platelet-derived growth factor | 3. Factor V |
| 4. Thrombospondin (TSP) | 4. Albumin |
| 5. Chemotactic factor | 5. Fibronectin |
| 6. Permeability factor | |
| 7. Bactericidal factor | |
| 8. Acid hydrolases | |

## TABLE 26–3. CONTENTS OF PLATELET DENSE BODY GRANULES

| | |
|---|---|
| ADP | ATP |
| Calcium | Serotonin |
| Catecholamines (epinephrine, Norepinephrine) | Pyrophosphate |

which include Chédiak-Higashi syndrome, Hermansky-Pudlak syndrome, and Wiskott-Aldrich syndrome (see Chapter 27 for more details on these disorders). Other granules, which can be found in the platelet as well as in other cells, include lysosomes, peroxisomes, and glycogen granules.

The dense tubular system (DTS) is another important structure present in the cytoplasm of the organelle zone of platelets. This complex of dense tubules is analogous to the sarcotubules in skeletal muscle. It is derived from the smooth endoplasmic reticulum (ER) of immature megakaryocytes. The DTS is the site of prostaglandin synthesis and sequestration of calcium. It is primarily the release of calcium from the DTS that triggers contraction of thrombosthenin and subsequent internal activation of platelets. It is also postulated that the DTS is involved in limited protein synthesis and serves as a reservoir for microtubular elements and submembranous and other microfilaments. Platelet activation is an energy-dependent process that relies on the metabolic function of mitochondria. Approximately 10 to 60 mitochondria per platelet are present, which require glycogen as their source of energy for metabolism. It is estimated in the "resting" platelet that ATP (energy) production is generated by 50 percent glycolysis and 50 percent oxidative Krebs cycle. In the "activated state," 80 percent of the ATP production in platelets occurs through the glycolytic pathway.

## Function

Platelets have specific roles in the hemostatic process, which are critically dependent on an adequate number of circulating thrombocytes as well as on normal platelet function. The role of platelets in hemostasis includes (1) maintenance of vascular integrity, (2) initial arrest of bleeding by platelet plug formation, and (3) stabilization of the hemostatic plug by contributing to the process of fibrin formation.

Numerous stimuli can trigger a platelet response termed "activation," which may be transient, reversible, or irreversible. Activation refers to several separate responses of platelet function, which include "stickiness," adhesion, shape change, aggregation, and release. Platelets respond in a graded fashion, depending on the strength of stimuli, duration, and physiologic or pathologic state.

The reader should refer to Figure 26-2, to review the structure of the platelet before proceeding, in order to visualize and understand subsequent events that occur in the platelet at the ultrastructural level during hemostasis.

### Maintenance of Vascular Integrity

Platelets are involved in the nurturing of endothelial cells lining the vascular system. When a platelet adheres to the endothelial cell, the amount of cytoplasm between platelet and cell is reduced and the platelet may eventually become incorporated into the endothelial cell. This process has an effect of "nurturing" or "feeding" the tissue cells by releasing endothelial growth factor. In addition, through the release of this mitogen (platelet derived growth factor) vascular healing is promoted, by stimulating endothelial cell migration and medial smooth muscle cell migration in the vessel wall. Figure 26-4 shows a scanning electron micrograph (SEM) demonstrating platelet adherence at the site of endothelial loss compared with the normal smooth contour of the endothelial cell. In the absence of platelets

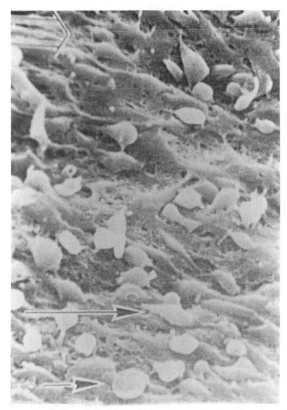

**Figure 26-4.** SEM of platelet adherence at the site of endothelial loss. *Short arrow* points to a discoid intact platelet with a single pseudopod. *Long arrow* points to an elongated adherent platelet. *Double arrow* marks densely adherent platelets appearing as elongated humps fused to the subendothelial layer. (From Robbins and Cotran: Pathologic Basis of Disease, ed 1. WB Saunders, Philadelphia, 1979, p. 120, with permission.)

from the circulation, red cells migrate through the vessel walls in large numbers and enter the lymphatic drainage or appear as petechiae or purpura in the skin or mucous membranes. This process of maintenance of normal vascular integrity, involving "nourishment" of the endothelium by the platelet, or actual incorporation of platelets into the vessel wall, requires less than 10 percent of the platelets in the circulation but is nevertheless an important function.

## Platelet Plug Formation

Various steps or processes are involved in the initial formation of a platelet plug: platelet adhesion, platelet aggregation, and platelet release reaction.

**Adhesion.** Exposure to subendothelial connective tissue, such as collagen fibers, initiates platelet adhesion. Adhesion is a reversible process whereby platelets stick to foreign surfaces. This process of platelet adhesion involves the interaction of platelet surface glycoproteins with the connective tissue elements of the subendothelium.

Adhesion of platelets to subendothelial fibers is dependent on a plasma protein called von Willebrand's factor, abbreviated VIII vWF, denoting that this factor is a component of factor VIII complex (see section on coagulation system). Evidence indicates that VIII vWF is synthesized by endothelial cells and megakaryocytes (precursors of platelets). Absorption of VIII vWF occurs both on exposed subendothelial fibers and on the surface of circulating platelets as it attaches to the appropriate membrane surface glycoprotein (Ib). In certain hereditary disorders, no platelet adhesion occurs and abnormal bleeding results because of the absence either of this plasma factor (von Willebrand's disease) or of the appropriate platelet membrane glycoprotein Ib (Bernard-Soulier syndrome). Platelets thus adhere to the area of injury at the endothelial lining or to each other when injured, acting to arrest the initial episode of bleeding. In Figure 26-5, a transmission electron micrograph (TEM) demonstrates platelet adherence to subendothelial connective tissue at the focus of endothelial loss. A decrease in platelet number, therefore, leads to failure to block the site of injury, resulting in increased bleeding. Other platelets may adhere to the original contact platelets (adhering to the site of injury), producing the phenomenon of aggregation and resulting in thrombus formation in order to stop bleeding. It is interesting to note that platelet adhesion consumes little energy as measured by ATP use.

**Aggregation.** During platelet aggregation, the injured platelet changes shape from discoid to spherical, with pseudopod formation (Fig. 26-6). Initial aggregation of platelets is caused by ADP, which is released from adherent platelets or endothelial cells. ADP is a potent initiator of aggregation resulting in the transformation of ambient discoid plate-

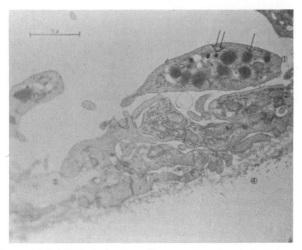

**Figure 26-5.** TEM of platelet adherence to subendothelial connective tissue at the focus of endothelial loss. *1*, Intact platelet with pseudopod (*thin arrow* is alpha granule; *thick arrow* is dense body); *2*, partially degranulated platelet; *3*, degranulated platelet "ghost"; *4*, internal elastic lamina. (From Robbins and Cotran: Pathologic Basis of Disease, ed 1. WB Saunders, Philadelphia, 1979, p. 116, with permission.)

lets to reactive spiny spheres. These spheres react with one another to form a mass of aggregated platelets (see Fig. 26-5). By binding specific membrane receptors, ADP induces further shape change of nearby circulating platelets, promoting additional aggregation. Both calcium and the plasma protein fibrinogen (coagulation factor I) are necessary for platelet aggregation. The interaction of ADP with its platelet membrane receptor mobilizes specific fibrinogen-binding sites consisting of two membrane glycoproteins.

The platelet-to-platelet interaction (initial aggregation) is a process of $Ca^{++}$-dependent ligand formation between membrane-bound fibrinogen molecules. Platelets will not aggregate in the absence of membrane glycoprotein, fibrinogen-binding sites, fibrinogen, or calcium. Binding of ADP to the platelet membrane activates phospholipase, which cleaves the phospholipids present in the platelet membrane, freeing such fatty acids as arachidonic acid. This released arachidonic acid is converted in the cytoplasm of the platelet into the cyclic endoperoxides, PGG2 and PGH2 by prostaglandin synthetase. This enzyme is commonly known as cyclooxygenase. PGG2 and PGH2 are unstable compounds that are converted to thromboxane A2 (TxA2) by the enzyme thromboxane synthetase (Fig. 26-7). Thromboxane A2, a potent aggregating agent of platelets, mediates the platelet release reaction as well as vasoconstriction. With its in vivo half-life of 30 seconds, thromboxane A2 activity is limited in time, because it hydrolyzes spontaneously within the platelet to an inactive form (TxB2). As TxA2 is generated with subsequent aggregating effects on platelets, calcium, sequestered in the dense tubular system of the platelet, is extruded in

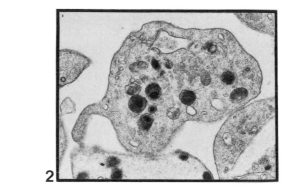

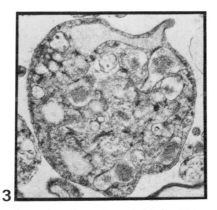

**Figure 26-6.** TEM showing disk-to-sphere transformation of an activated platelet. Note progression from (1) disk shape to (2) pseudopod formation to (3) degranulated ballooned sphere.

the sol-gel zone. This process activates the $Ca^{++}$-dependent microfilament, thrombosthenin. Activation of thrombosthenin results in a contractile wave centralizing organelles, which leads to the release of dense granules and activation of platelet factor 3 (PF3). Receptor sites of PF3 now become exposed on the surface of the platelet membrane. PF3 facilitates thrombin formation by the intrinsic coagulation system (see section on fibrin formation). Thrombin, also a potent platelet aggregator, can induce the release reaction of both types of granules (dense and alpha).

In vitro platelet aggregation can be initiated by a variety of agents, listed in Table 26–4. In vitro aggregation may be visualized as a two-phase process that may be reversible, biphasic, or irreversible, depending on the strength of the activation stimulus. Early aggregation, the primary (initial or first) wave of aggregation, involves contraction of the circumferential microtubular band and reorganization and centralization of platelet organelles. This contraction and centralization of organelles results in decreased absorbance as measured by an instrument called a platelet aggregometer. (For a review of the laboratory procedure for aggregation, see Chapter 31.) This first wave of aggregation is a reversible

process, as platelets form loosely attached aggregates under such conditions as low concentrations of aggregating reagents or pathologically diminished platelet response.

The secondary wave of aggregation is dependent on the activation stimulus being strong enough to evoke the release of platelet granules as a consequence of stronger, more complete contraction. Ultrastructurally, the internal reorganization of organelles is more severe and degranulation is evident by the lack of density of the granules with transmission electron microscopy (see Fig. 26-6). Biochemical studies have confirmed the release of substances such as ADP, serotonin, and epinephrine; these are

**TABLE 26–4. IN VITRO PLATELET AGGREGATORS**

| | |
|---|---|
| ADP Collagen Epinephrine Thrombin Ristocetin | Common Laboratory Aggregating Reagents |
| Arachidonic acid Immune products Snake venoms | Other Aggregators |

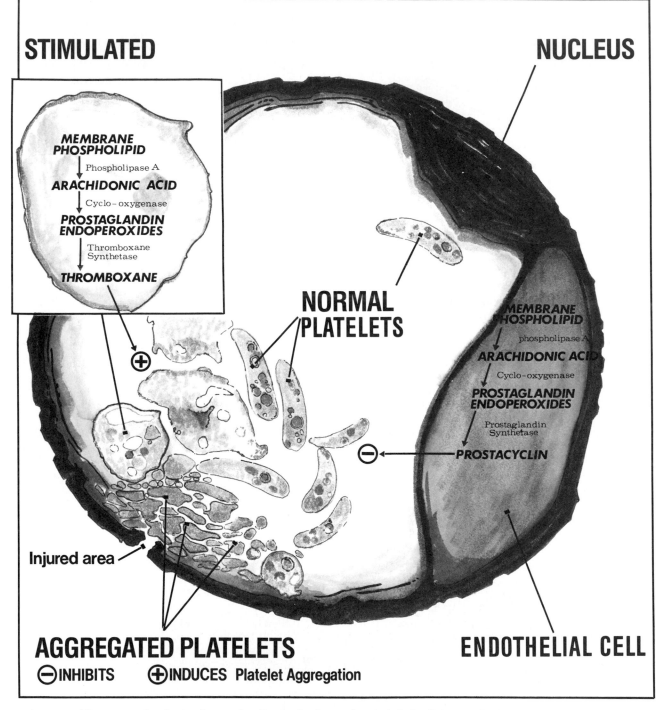

**Figure 26-7.** Synthesis of prostaglandins in platelets and endothelial cell during platelet plug formation.

responsible for the secondary wave of aggregation, which is usually irreversible. Figure 26-8 depicts a typical biphasic response of in vitro platelet aggregation to ADP as recorded by an aggregometer. It should be noted that aggregation is an energy-dependent process that greatly exhausts the platelet energy resources.

**Release Reaction.** The release reaction from dense granules involves the secretion of ADP, serotonin (a vasoactive amine), and calcium. ADP is responsible for further aggregation of more platelets serving to amplify the process previously described. Elevation of intracellular $Ca^{++}$ also amplifies the process by activating more calcium-sensitive phos-

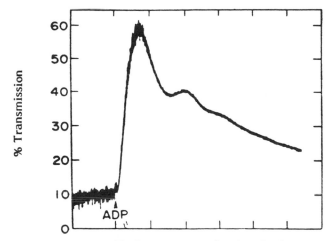
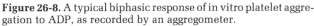

**Figure 26-8.** A typical biphasic response of in vitro platelet aggregation to ADP, as recorded by an aggregometer.

pholipases, leading to further formation of thromboxane A2, as previously described. Thus, amplification of the initial aggregation of platelets (a reversible phenomenon) results in secondary aggregation of many other platelets into an irreversible aggregation of a mass of degenerative platelet material without membranes. This mass is termed "viscous metamorphasis" (Fig. 26-9). Different substances are released at different rates, suggesting a heterogenicity of granules. The release of substances such as fibrinogen, catecholamines, and acid hydrolases confirms the degranulation of alpha granules. The release reaction is an energy-dependent secretion process that occurs only after internal reorganization and transformation have oc-

curred, given a sufficiently strong platelet stimulus that results in an irreversible process (Fig. 26-10).

## Effect of Aspirin on Platelet Plug Formation

Aspirin inhibits the enzyme cyclooxygenase, which blocks the formation of prostaglandins, thus preventing aggregation. Prostaglandins are present in many different tissues, including endothelium. In endothelium, there is a pathway similar to the one described in platelets (see Fig. 26-7). Arachidonic acid in endothelium is converted to PGG2 by cyclooxygenase, but thromboxane is not formed. Instead prostacyclin, PGI2, is formed from the cyclic endoperoxides by the enzyme prostacyclin synthetase. PGI2, produced in the endothelium, has an effect opposite to that of thromboxane on the platelet. PGI2 is a potent inhibitor of platelet aggregation and a vasodilator. Therefore, as long as the endothelium is intact and PGI2 is made and secreted, platelet aggregation is limited in time. Aspirin, which has previously been stated to inhibit cyclooxygenase activity, is more inhibitory for the platelet enzyme cyclooxygenase than endothelial cyclooxygenase. However, if very high doses of aspirin are taken, both the endothelial and platelet cyclooxygenase will be affected, and the effect will cancel out. Thus, a potential for thrombosis may occur.

## Stabilization of Hemostatic Plug

The last stage involved in arresting bleeding after vessel damage is the formation of a stable platelet plug. This stabilization is achieved through the formation and deposition of fibrin, the end product of coagulation. Fibrin is formed as a result of a series of

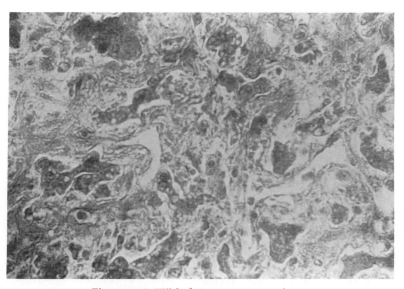

**Figure 26-9.** TEM of viscous metamorphasis.

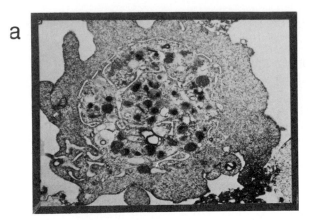
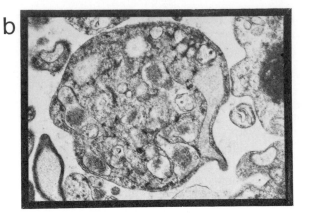

**Figure 26-10.** TEM of an activated and a degranulated platelet. A, Early aggregation of activated platelet (the primary wave of aggregation, a reversible process). B, Degranulated platelet (the secondary wave of aggregation, an irreversible process). (From Barnhart, MI: Platelet responses in health and disease. Mol Cell Biochem 22:117, 1978, with permission.)

reactions that involve not only platelets but also various blood proteins, lipids, and ions (see section on fibrin-forming system).

As mentioned previously, platelets provide an

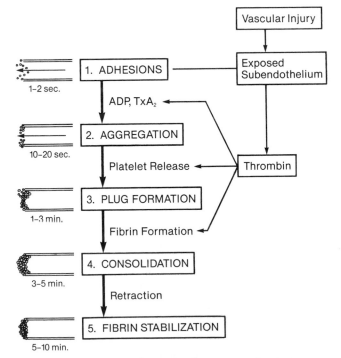

**Figure 26-11.** Sequence of events in hemostatic plug formation. *1*, Platelet adhesion to exposed subendothelial connective tissue structures. *2*, Platelet aggregation by ADP, thromboxane A2, and thrombin recruitment through transformation of discoid platelets into reactive spiny spheres that interact with one another through calcium-dependent fibrinogen bridges. *3*, Contribution of platelet coagulant activity to the coagulation process, which stabilizes the plug with a fibrin mesh. *4*, Retraction of the platelet mass to provide a dense thrombus. *5*, Fibrin polymerization and fibrin stabilization factor XIII. (From Thompson and Harker: Manual of Hemostasis and Thrombosis. FA Davis, Philadelphia, 1983, with permission.)

optimal environment for fibrin formation by exposing certain phospholipids (PF3) on the platelet membrane surface during aggregation. These membrane phospholipids provide a catalytic surface for the activation of various clotting enzymes or factors, such as factor X. In addition, certain coagulation factors (V and VIII) are present on the platelet membrane. All of these factors, in addition to others, are involved in the coagulation system, which leads to the generation of large quantities of thrombin on the aggregated platelet's surface. Thrombin, then, converts fibrinogen to fibrin (see section on fibrin-forming system). This allows stabilization of both adherent and aggregating platelets by the fibrin strands that form around them. These fibrin strands trap and enmesh all the activated platelets resulting in the formation of a stable hemostatic plug. Figure 26-11 provides a review of the sequence of events involved in platelet plug formation and the approximate time involved in each stage.

## FIBRIN-FORMING (COAGULATION) SYSTEM

This system is mediated by many coagulation proteins normally present in the blood in an inactive state (coagulation factors). "Secondary hemostasis" is used to define the coagulation factor's role in the hemostatic mechanism (see Tables 26–5 and 26–8, for a review of the appropriate nomenclature and characteristics of these factors).

It should be noted that the coagulation factors are designated by Roman numerals. The numerical system adopted assigns the number to the factors according to the sequence of discovery and *not* to the point of interaction in the cascade. Table 26–5 lists the coagulation factors and their most commonly used designations. All the coagulation proteins are produced in the liver, with the possible exception of factor VIII.

**TABLE 26–5. NOMENCLATURE OF COAGULATION FACTORS**

| | |
|---|---|
| Factor I | Fibrinogen |
| Factor II | Prothrombin |
| Factor III | Tissue thromboplastin (tissue factor) |
| Factor IV | Calcium |
| Factor V | Labile factor (proaccelerin) |
| Factor VI | Not assigned |
| Factor VII | Stable factor (serum prothrombin conversion accelerator, or SPCA) |
| Factor VIII | AHF (antihemophilic factor) |
| Factor IX | Christmas factor (plasma thromboplastin component, or PTC) |
| Factor X | Stuart-Prower factor |
| Factor XI | PTA (plasma thromboplastin antecedent) |
| Factor XII | Hageman factor (contact factor) |
| Factor XIII | FSF (fibrin-stabilizing factor) |
| Fitzgerald factor | HMWK (high molecular weight kininogen) |
| Fletcher factor | Pre-kallikrein |

## Hemostatic Function

In terms of hemostatic function, the coagulation factors can be divided into three categories: substrate, cofactors, and enzymes. Factor I, fibrinogen, is regarded as the substrate of the blood coagulation system, since the formation of a fibrin clot from fibrinogen is the ultimate goal. Cofactors are proteins that accelerate the enzymatic reactions involved in the coagulation process. Factors III (tissue factor), V (labile factor), and VIII (antihemophilic factor, or AHF) and Fitzgerald factor (high molecular weight kininogen, or HMWK) are the cofactors of the blood coagulation system. All the rest of the coagulation factors are categorized as enzymes. These enzymes involved in coagulation can be divided into two groups: serine proteases and a transamidase. Factor XIII (fibrin-stabilizing factor) is the only transamidase of the coagulation proteins that functions to create covalent bonds between the fibrin monomers formed during the coagulation process to produce a stable fibrin clot. All the other factors that function as enzymes in coagulation are serine proteases. These proteases have serine as a portion of their active enzymatic site and function to cleave peptide bonds.

## Physical Properties

On the basis of their physical properties, the coagulation proteins may also be conveniently divided into three other groups: (1) the contact proteins, (2) the prothrombin proteins, and (3) the fibrinogen or thrombin-sensitive proteins.

The contact group includes factors XII (Hageman factor), XI, prekallikrein (Fletcher factor), and high molecular weight kininogen (Fitzgerald factor). This group is involved in the initial phase of the intrinsic activation of coagulation; its factors are not consumed during coagulation, and therefore are present in both plasma and serum. The contact group of coagulation factors is fairly stable, is not absorbed by the reagent barium sulfate ($BaSO_4$), and is not dependent on vitamin K for synthesis. Although deficiencies of these coagulation proteins are associated with markedly abnormal laboratory tests, an isolated factor XI deficiency is associated with a mild bleeding disorder. Ironically, problems with thrombosis have been reported in patients with factor XII and Fletcher factor deficiencies.

The prothrombin proteins are generally low molecular weight proteins that include factors II, VII, IX, and X. This group is also known as the vitamin K–dependent coagulation proteins. Each member of this group contains a unique amino acid— gamma carboxyglutamic acid—that is necessary for attraction of these coagulation factors to the surface of activated platelets, where the formation of a fibrin clot occurs. The active participation of these proteins in blood coagulation is dependent on vitamin K, which is necessary for the conversion of glutamic acid to gamma carboxyglutamic acid. Drugs that act as antagonists to vitamin K inhibit this vitamin K–dependent reaction, which is required for functionally active coagulation factors of the prothrombin group. Patients who are vitamin K deficient exhibit decreased production of functional prothrombin proteins. Acquired deficiencies of the vitamin K–dependent coagulation factors are relatively common, as the body does not contain appreciable stores of vitamin K. Characteristic prototypes for developing a vitamin K deficiency include patients who have just had surgery and are receiving parenteral feeding, patients who are receiving high doses of intravenous antibiotics, and patients suffering from liver disease. The factors of the prothrombin group, except for factor II (prothrombin), are not consumed during coagulation. These factors are absorbed by the reagent $BaSO_4$ and are, therefore, not present in adsorbed plasma. However, they are present in fresh and stored plasma as well as in serum.

The fibrinogen group consists generally of high molecular weight proteins that include factors I (fibrinogen), V (labile factor), VIII (AHF), and XIII (fibrin-stabilizing factor). During coagulation, generated thrombin acts on all the factors in the fibrinogen group. Thrombin enhances the activity of factors V and VIII by converting these proteins to active cofactors, which are involved in the assembly of macromolecular complexes on the surface of activated platelets. Thrombin also activates factor XIII and converts fibrinogen (factor I) to fibrin. The fibrinogen group of coagulation factors is consumed during the coagulation process; therefore, these factors are not present in serum. These factors are not absorbed by the reagent $BaSO_4$ and are present in adsorbed plasma. Factors V and VIII are the least stable factors, since their activity is relatively labile to degradation and denaturation. These factors are therefore not present in stored plasma. In addition to the presence of the fibrinogen group in plasma, these factors are also found within platelets. The fibrinogen group of coagulation factors have been reported to increase during conditions of inflammation, in pregnancy, and with the use of oral contraceptives.

## Blood Coagulation: the "Cascade" Theory

The process of blood coagulation involves a series of biochemical reactions that transforms circulating blood into an insoluble gel through conversion of soluble fibrinogen to fibrin. This process requires plasma proteins (coagulation factors), as well as phospholipids and calcium.

Blood coagulation leading to fibrin formation can be separated into two pathways; the extrinsic and intrinsic, both of which share specific common coagulation factors with the common pathway (Fig. 26-12). Both pathways require initiation, which leads to subsequent activation of various coagulation factors in a "cascading," "waterfall," or "domino" effect. According to the cascade theory, each coagulation factor is converted to its active form by the preceding factor, in a series of biochemical chain reactions. Each reaction is promoted by the preceding reaction, and if there is a deficiency of any one of the factors, the following consequences result:

1. Coagulation cannot proceed at a normal rate
2. Initiation of the next subsequent reaction is delayed
3. The time required for the clot to form is prolonged
4. Bleeding from the injured vessel continues for a longer time

Eventually, both the extrinsic and intrinsic systems lead to generation of the enzyme thrombin which converts fibrinogen to fibrin (Fig. 26-12).

The term "extrinsic" is used because this pathway is initiated when factor III (tissue thromboplastin), a substance not found in blood, enters the vascular system. The tissue factor includes a phospholipid component that is the source of required phospholipid in the extrinsic system. Phospholipid provides a surface for interaction of various factors. The phospholipids required in the intrinsic pathway are provided by the platelet membrane. In the intrinsic pathway, all the factors necessary for clot formation are "intrinsic" to the vascular compartment, as they are all found within the circulating blood (Fig. 26-12).

### Extrinsic Pathway

In the extrinsic pathway, factor VII is activated to VIIa in the presence of calcium (IV) and the tissue factor (III), which is released from the injured vessel wall. In the extrinsic coagulation system, it is important to realize that this pathway bypasses the activation of factors XII, XI, IX, and VIII, requiring only activated factor VII, $Ca^{++}$, and factor III (a lipoprotein) to activate factor X to Xa. In Figure 26-12, one can see that the extrinsic pathway provides a means for quickly producing small amounts of thrombin, leading to fibrin formation. In addition, the thrombin generated by this pathway can accelerate the intrinsic pathway by enhancing the activity of factors V and VIII. In the laboratory, the prothrombin time (PT test) is used to monitor the extrinsic pathway (for a review of the procedure, see Chapter 31).

### Intrinsic Pathway

Following exposure to foreign substances such as subendothelial collagen, activation of factor XII to XIIa initiates clotting through the intrinsic pathway. It should be noted that factor XII is only partially activated by this contact with a foreign substance. Fletcher and Fitzgerald factors are additionally needed to enhance or amplify the contact factors involved in the intrinsic system (Fig. 26-13). The activation of factor XII acts as the common link between many aspects of the hemostatic mechanism, including the fibrinolytic system, the kinin system, and the complement system. (Fig. 26-13; also see section on fibrin lysing). Contact activation occurs in the absence of calcium and also refers to the activation of factor XI to factor XIa by factor XIIa.

The next reaction in the intrinsic pathway is the activation of factor IX to factor IXa by factor XIa, in the presence of calcium. Activated factor IX (IXa) participates along with the essential cofactor VIII in the presence of calcium and platelet factor 3 (PF3), a source of phospholipid, to activate factor X, which leads to the generation of thrombin and formation of fibrin. The macromolecular complex of IXa, VIII, X, and $Ca^{++}$ assembles on the surface of the activated platelet during the intrinsic pathway of blood coagulation. This surface provides a protective environment that facilitates the enzymatic reactions of the coagulation cascade without interference from the physiologic anticoagulants normally present in plasma.

In regard to the intrinsic pathway, it is also important to be familiar with the properties of the factor VIII complex (Table 26-6). Factor VIII, which consists of several components, is the largest protein involved in the clotting cascade. The major portion of this protein is considered to be a carrier protein called von Willebrand's factor (VIII vWF). A smaller

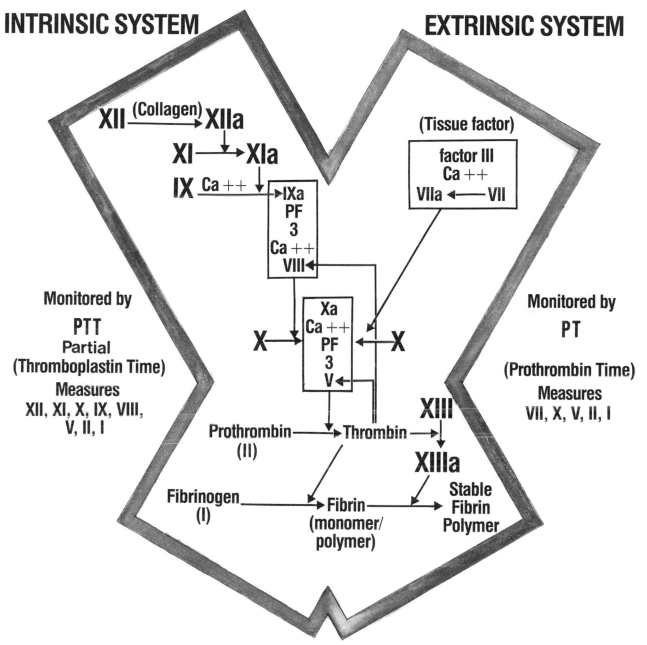

**Figure 26-12.** Formation of the "cascade" theory of coagulation.

subunit or protein that is tightly associated (VIIIc) is responsible for the clotting or procoagulant activity. Two other subunits have also been defined (Table 26-6). It should be noted that factor VIII requires enhancement by the generated enzyme thrombin to amplify its activity. In the laboratory, the activated partial thromboplastin time (APTT) test is used to evaluate the intrinsic pathway (for a review of this procedure, see Chapter 31).

## Common Pathway

The common pathway begins with the activation of factor X either by factor VIIa in the presence of co-factor, tissue thromboplastin (factor III), and calcium; or by factor IXa in the presence of the cofactor, factor VIII, calcium, and PF3. After the formation of factor Xa, this activated factor along with another cofactor, V, in the presence of calcium and PF3, converts factor II, prothrombin, to the active enzyme thrombin. This additional macromolecular complex of Xa, V, Ca++, and II also assembles on the surface of activated platelets.

Activation of thrombin is slow, but once generated it further amplifies coagulation. Thrombin functions to:

1. Convert fibrinogen to fibrin

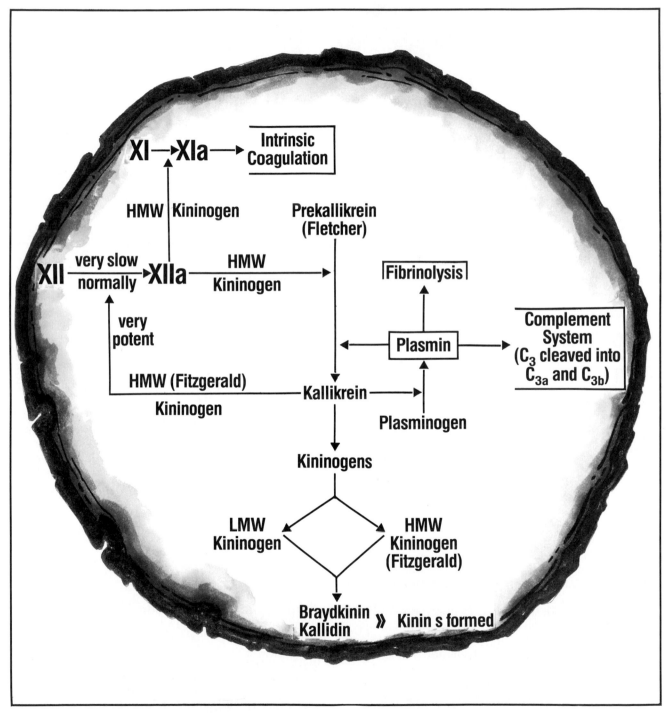

**Figure 26-13.** Interrelationship of coagulation, fibrinolytic, kinin, and complement systems.

## TABLE 26 – 6. FACTOR VIII COMPLEX

I. Smaller Protein Subunit
   **Nomenclature**
   VIII:C (the factor VIII procoagulant protein or
   VIII:AHF (the antihemophilic factor)
   **Components**
   a. VIII:CAg—antigen determinant of VIII:C, measured by immunoassays with human antibodies to VIII:C
   b. VIII:C—procoagulant property of normal plasma measured in the APTT test as procoagulant activity
   **Characteristics**
   1. Inherited recessive, sex-linked
   2. Acts as a cofactor in a complex with factor IXa, $Ca^{++}$, and PF3 to activate X to Xa.
II. Major Protein Portion
   **Nomenclature**
   VIII:vWF (von Willebrand's factor) or
   VIII:R (factor VIII–related protein)
   **Components**
   a. VIIIR:Ag—antigen determinant on VIII-related protein which is detected by using heterologous antibodies to von Willebrand's factor
   b. VIIIR:RC$_o$ (VIIIR:vW)—the property of normal plasma VIIIR that supports ristocetin-induced agglutination of washed normal platelets
   **Characteristics**
   1. Inherited autosomal dominant
   2. Responsible for platelet adhesion
   3. Responsible for ristocetin induced aggregation of platelets
   4. Plays a role in regulating VIII:C synthesis; therefore, affects the plasma concentration of VIII:C as well as release of VIII from the site of production into circulation
   5. Stabilizes VIII:C when bound to VIII:R during circulation, and functions in prevention or protection of VIII:C from inactivation

---

2. Activate factor XIII
3. Enhance factor V and VIII activity
4. Initiate plasminogen to plasmin
5. Aggregate more platelets

Thrombin acts on fibrinogen to form fibrin monomers. Fibrinogen is composed of three pairs of polypeptide chains (two alpha, two beta, and two gamma). Thrombin cleaves a portion of each of the alpha and beta polypeptides to form fibrinopeptides A and B. After this cleavage, the fibrinogen molecule is converted to a fibrin monomer (Fig. 26-14). Fibrin monomers quickly polymerize to form fibrin. Weak hydrogen-bonding holds together the fibrin monomers in this initial clot, which can be dissolved by certain substances such as mild acid and urea. Activated factor XIII, a transamidase, converts hydrogen bonding to covalent bonding (S-S), resulting in a stronger, more stable clot.

By using the PT and PTT test results in the laboratory, one can identify defects or deficiencies as occurring in the intrinsic, extrinsic, or common pathways of blood coagulation. Table 26-7 allows the reader to practice interpretation of these tests in identifying possible factor deficiencies. Table 26 8 summarizes the properties of the coagulation factors.

### Current Concepts of the Coagulation System

Division of the coagulation process into strictly defined extrinsic and intrinsic pathways has been abandoned, because the cascade theory has been extensively modified. It has been reported that factor VIIa of the extrinsic pathway can directly activate factor IX of the intrinsic pathway. Additionally, it is reported that factor VII can be activated by factors XIIa, IXa, Xa, and thrombin. It has therefore been hypothesized that factor VII may be the key regulatory protein that initiates blood coagulation. Until more information is generated, and for the simplicity of presentation, the reader should still be able to assimilate the classic "cascade" presentation of fibrin formation.

## FIBRIN-LYSING (FIBRINOLYTIC) SYSTEM

The fibrin-forming and fibrin-lysing systems are intimately related. Activation of coagulation also activates fibrin lysis. Fibrinolysis, the physiologic process of removing unwanted fibrin deposits, represents a gradual, progressive enzymatic cleavage of fibrin to soluble fragments. These fragments are then removed from the circulation by the fixed macrophages of the reticuloendothelial system (RES). This action of the fibrinolytic system re-establishes blood flow in vessels occluded by a thrombus and facilitates the healing process following injury. The fibrinolytic system is mediated mainly by the enzyme plasmin, which acts primarily on fibrin to produce lysis of the clot. Plasmin is generated from the circulating inactive zymogen called plasminogen. Plasminogen is activated to plasmin by various substances:

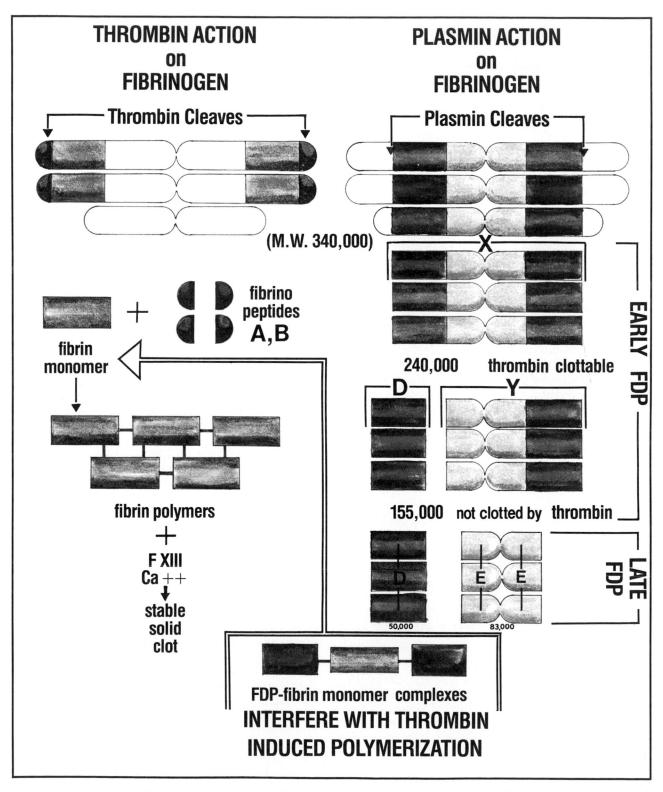

**Figure 26-14.** Comparison of thrombin and plasmin activity of fibrinogen.

**TABLE 26–7. USE OF PT AND PTT FOR IDENTIFICATION OF FACTOR DEFICIENCIES IN COAGULATION STUDIES**

| | | Correction Studies | | | | |
| | | PT | | PTT | | |
| Patient PT | Results PTT | Adsorbed Plasma Reagent | Serum Reagent | Adsorbed Plasma Reagent | Serum Reagent | Deficiency |
|---|---|---|---|---|---|---|
| N | Ab | — | — | C | NC | VIII |
| N | Ab | — | — | C | C | XI, XII* |
| N | Ab | — | — | NC | C | IX |
| Ab | Ab | C | NC | C | NC | V |
| Ab | Ab | NC | C | NC | C | X |
| Ab | Ab | NC | NC | NC | NC | II |
| Ab | N | NC | C | — | — | VII |

N = normal time; Ab = abnormal time; C = time corrected to normal; — = not applicable; NC = time not corrected to normal.
*No associated bleeding occurs in this deficiency.

1. Tissue plasminogen activator (tissue kinase released from injured tissue or endothelium)
2. Thrombin
3. Kallikrein
4. Other substances: urokinase, streptokinase, and staphylokinase

In addition to plasmin, plasminogen, and plasminogen activators, inhibitors of plasmin are also a part of the fibrinolytic system.

Again, it is important to realize that some of the same substances that initiate or enhance clot formation also initiate clot degradation. For example, in tissue, both tissue thromboplastin (initiator of extrinsic pathway of fibrin formation) and tissue plasminogen activator (which activates plasminogen) are released with endothelial damage. Tissue plasminogen activator (TPA) is produced by vascular endothelial cells and selectively binds to fibrin as it activates fibrin-bound plasminogen. Because circulating plasminogen is not activated by TPA, this biologic substance is efficient in dissolving a clot without causing systemic fibrinolysis and serves as an ideal therapeutic fibrinolytic agent. Biologic TPA has been successfully produced by recombinant DNA technology and is currently in clinical trials. It is also important to note that thrombin generates fibrin and plasmin formation. In addition, prekallikrein (Fletcher factor) and high molecular weight kininogen (Fitzgerald factor) indirectly initiate clotting (via factor XIIa) as well as plasmin formation (see Fig. 26-13).

## Action of Plasmin

Plasmin is a broad-spectrum endopeptidase (proteolytic enzyme) that acts nonspecifically, with a strong affinity for fibrin. Plasmin, however, cannot distinguish between the protein fibrin and fibrinogen. The action of plasmin begins by splitting off pieces of each of the alpha and beta polypeptides (a larger portion than that cleaved by thrombin) and a smaller piece of each of the two gamma polypeptides from fibrinogen. The remaining molecule is called the X monomer (which is still thrombin clottable). As plasmin continues its action, it further splits the X monomer into a Y fragment (not clottable by thrombin) and a smaller D fragment. Further action of plasmin cleaves the Y fragment into D and E fragments. Therefore, the final fibrin-split products are 2D and 1E fragments generated from one molecule of fibrinogen (Fig. 26-14). These products are collectively known as either fibrin degradation products (FDP) or fibrin-split products (FSP). Early FDPs include X monomer and Y fragments. Late FDPs include D and E fragments. These fragments are important clinically, because they can increase vascular permeability and interfere with thrombin induced fibrin formation. In patients with certain disease conditions, when plasmin is activated, FDP are measured.

In addition to its action on fibrin and fibrinogen, plasmin also destroys factors V, VIII, and other coagulation factors.

Thus, plasmin acts to:

1. Destroy fibrin and fibrinogen
2. Produce FDP, which increases vascular permeability and interferes with thrombin-induced fibrin formation (Fig. 26-14)
3. Destroy factors V, VIII, and other coagulation factors
4. Indirectly enhance or amplify XII to XIIa (see Fig. 26-13)
5. Enhance or amplify prekallikrein conversion to kallekrein, liberating kinins from kininogen
6. Cleave C3 into fragments (see section on complement)

Enhanced fibrinolysis may be observed not only in various coagulopathies but also in traumatic inju-

# TABLE 26–8. COAGULATION FACTOR NOMENCLATURE AT A GLANCE

| Factor | Synonym | Clotting Pathway | Molecular Weight | Site of Production | Plasma Concentration μg/ml | Half-life Disappearance | Minimum Hemostatic Level | Storage Stability | Active Form | Other Characteristics (all factors are present in normal fresh plasma) |
|---|---|---|---|---|---|---|---|---|---|---|
| I | Fibrinogen | Both intrinsic, extrinsic, common pathway | 340,000 | Liver | 2500 (250 mg%) | 120 hr | 50–100 mg% | Stable | Protein | Activity destroyed during coagulation process/present in absorbed plasma |
| II | Prothrombin | Both intrinsic, extrinsic, common pathway | 70,000 | Liver—Vitamin K dependent | 100 | 100 hr | 40% concentration | Stable | Serine protease | Consumed during coagulation process |
| III | Tissue thromboplastin | Extrinsic system only | 45,000 | Thromboplastic activity present in most tissues | 0 | | | | Cofactor | |
| V | Labile factor proaccelerin | Both intrinsic, extrinsic, common pathway | 330,000 | Liver | 5–12 | 25 hr | 5–10% concentration | Labile | Cofactor | Activity destroyed during coagulation process/present in absorbed plasma |
| VII | Stable factor proconvertin | Extrinsic system only | 55,000 | Liver—Vitamin K dependent | 1 | 5 hr | 5–10% concentration | Stable | Glycoprotein | Present in serum |
| VIII/vWF | Antihemophilic factor (AHF)/von Willebrand factor | Intrinsic system only | 1–2 million | Possibly endothelial cells & megakaryocytes | 7 | 10 hr | 30% concentration | Labile | Cofactor | Activity destroyed during coagulation process/present in absorbed plasma |
| IX | Christmas factor, plasma (PTC), thromboplastin component | Intrinsic only | 57,000 | Liver—Vitamin K dependent | 4 | 20 hr | 30% concentration | Stable | Serine protease | Present in serum |
| X | Stuart Prower factor | Both intrinsic, extrinsic, common pathway | 59,000 | Liver—Vitamin K dependent | 5 | 65 hr | 8–10% concentration | Stable | Serine protease | Present in serum |
| XI | Plasma thromboplastin antecedent (PTA) | Intrinsic only | 160,000 | Liver | 4 | 65 hr | 20–30% concentration | Stable | Serine protease | Present in serum and absorbed plasma |
| XII | Hageman factor/contract factor | Intrinsic only | 80,000 | Liver | 29 | 60 hr | 0% | Stable | Serine protease | Present in serum and absorbed plasma |
| XIII | Fibrin stabilizing factor (FSF) | Both intrinsic, extrinsic, common pathway | 300,000 | Liver or platelets | 10 | 150 hr | 1% concentration | Stable | Transglutaminase | Actively destroyed during coagulation process/present in absorbed plasma |
| Prekallikrein | Fletcher factor | Intrinsic only | 80,000 | Liver | 50 | ? | ? | ? Stable | Serine protease | |
| High molecular weight kininogen | Fitzgerald factor | Intrinsic only | 120,000 | Liver | 70 | ? | ? | ? Stable | Cofactor | |

**Note:** Although not a coagulation protein or factor calcium is sometimes denoted as factor IV.

ries, major surgery, liver cirrhosis, and other pathologic states.

## KININ SYSTEM

The kinin system, important in inflammation, vascular permeability, and chemotaxis, is activated by
both the coagulation and fibrinolytic systems. In
this system, prekallikrein (Fletcher factor) is activated to kallikrein by factor XIIa (Hageman factor)
and plasmin. Kallikrein is an enzyme that can act on
kininogens—low molecular weight (LMW) and
high molecular weight (HMW, or Fitzgerald factor)
—and converts them to kinins. The kinins generated may include kallidin and bradykinin. Bradykinin functions to:

1. Increase vascular permeability
2. Contract smooth muscle
3. Dilate small blood vessels
4. Induce inflammation and pain
5. Cause release of prostaglandins from tissues

The kinin system is also involved in the contact
activation phase of the intrinsic pathway of coagulation. Activation of factor XII to XIIa does not occur
without kallikrein or HMW kininogen. Kallikrein
amplifies the generation of XII; and HMW kininogen
is an essential factor in the activation of XI to XIa.
Fitzgerald factor (HMW) is necessary in both the
fibrin-forming and fibrin-lysing systems (see Fig.
26-13).

## PROTEASE INHIBITORS

Because the fibrinolytic system is activated when
coagulation is activated, extra fibrin is degraded
and eliminated along with some of the coagulation
factors. However, enzymes such as plasmin and
kallikrein still circulate until they are eliminated by
(1) liver hepatocytes (which have an affinity for activated enzymes), (2) reticuloendothelial system
(which picks up particulate matter), or (3) serine
protease inhibitors present in plasma. Serine protease inhibitors attach to various enzymes and inactivate them. Important serine protease inhibitors
include the following.

*Antithrombin III (AT-III)*, also termed "heparin
cofactor" or "factor Xa inhibitor," is the major inactivator of thrombin and Xa. It is considered the most
important physiologic anticoagulant, as 80 percent
of the antithrombin activity of normal human
plasma is due to AT-III. In addition, AT-III inhibits
factors XIIa, XIa, IXa, and VIIIa. AT-III is also capable of inhibiting kallikrein and plasmin. In its natural state, AT-III is a slow progressive inhibitor. However, in the presence of heparin, it becomes a very
potent inhibitor of coagulation. Therefore, the efficacy of heparin therapy depends on the level of AT-
III. Individuals who lack this inhibitor fail to re-

spond to heparin therapy. Heparin forms a complex
with AT-III. This combination exposes further sites
on the AT-III molecule, increasing its ability to
combine with sites on either thrombin or Xa, rendering the factor inactive. This complex is 100 times
more potent as an anticoagulant than AT-III alone.
The hemostatic result is an increase in the coagulation time. (Antithrombin III deficiency, also known
as "hereditary thrombophilia," is an autosomal
dominant disorder in which there is an increased
tendency toward thrombosis. It is suggested that
this inherited reduction in AT-III may account for as
many as 2 percent of the cases of clinical pulmonary
thromboembolism.)

*Alpha-2 macroglobulin* is a nonspecific inhibitor
that works on many coagulation factors. *Alpha-2
antiplasmin* is the major blood inhibitor of plasmin.
*Alpha-1 antitrypsin* inhibits coagulation factors as
well as fibrinolysis. *C1 esterase inhibitor* inhibits
plasmin, kallikrein, and thrombin.

All of these protease inhibitors have broad spec-
trums of inhibition, even though specificity for one
factor or more may be exhibited. Both kallikrein
and plasmin are inhibited by all of these serine protease inhibitors.

Also included in this group is a vitamin K–
dependent protein inhibitor known as protein C
(autoprothrombin II-A). Protein C is a serine protease inhibitor that (1) inactivates factors V and VIII,
(2) competitively inhibits factor Xa by the platelet-
bound factor V mechanism, and (3) promotes fibrinolysis by stimulating the release of TPA from endothelial cells.

Another vitamin K–dependent protein, protein
S, has been proposed as a necessary cofactor for activated protein C in its role of inactivation of factor
V. Deficiencies of protein C are associated with a
predisposition for thrombosis.

Finally, it should be mentioned that the generation of activated protein C is believed to be regulated by its own specific inhibitor. It has been postulated that a deficiency of this inhibitor to inhibit
activated protein C is responsible for the inherited
combined deficiencies of factors V and VIII.

## COMPLEMENT SYSTEM

The complement system is composed of approximately 22 serum proteins, which, working together
with antibodies and clotting factors, play an important role as a mediator of both the immune and
allergic reactions. The reactions in which complement participates take place in the blood or in other
body fluids. The most important biologic role of
complement is the production of cell membrane
lysis of antibody-coated target cells. Two independent pathways of activation of the complement cascade may occur along with a common cytolytic
pathway. These are designated the classic and the

alternate pathways of complement activation (see Chapter 11 for a review of the complement system).

Both the coagulation system and the fibrinolytic system are interrelated with complement. Plasmin is an important activator of complement, possessing the ability to cleave directly C3 into C3a and C3b. C3a is an anaphylotoxin causing increased vascular permeability via degranulation of mast cells releasing histamine. C3b is an opsonin causing immune adherence. C5a is not only an anaphylotoxin but is also a potent aggregator of platelets and a chemotactic agent for white blood cells. In addition, C1-esterase inhibitor is an inactivator of the complement sequence as well as thrombin and plasmin.

The interrelationship of the coagulation, complement, and fibrinolytic systems is clinically demonstrated in the condition known as hereditary angioneurotic edema. In this disease, there is no inhibition of C1 enzyme activity. The allergic-type symptoms are increased in stressful conditions. Stress results in increased blood levels of plasmin and therefore, complement activation. In the absence of adequate C1 inactivation, the body cannot rid itself of the complement products.

## LABORATORY EVALUATION OF HEMOSTASIS

The diagnosis of any hemostatic disorder is made by the systematic evaluation of information obtained in the history and physical examination, along with the appropriate laboratory testing. Diagnostically, the most valuable data from a patient's history include:

1. Documentation of the physical appearance, site, severity, and frequency of bleeding episodes
2. A family history of bleeding disorders
3. An accurate drug history
4. Other contributing or underlying illnesses

Bleeding disorders present themselves differently depending on the causative problem. Patients with platelet disorders usually exhibit petechiae and mucous membrane bleeding. Patients with coagulation defects usually develop deep spreading hematomas and bleeding into the joints with evident hematuria.

Alteration of any aspect of the hemostatic mechanism may cause abnormal bleeding in a wide variety of familial and acquired clinical disorders. These defects may be classified into three broad categories that can be diagnostically approached by a systematic laboratory evaluation. These include (1) vascular and platelet disorders, (2) coagulation factor deficiencies, and (3) fibrinolytic disorders.

Although many laboratories differ in their approach to a bleeding disorder, a general profile of laboratory tests is usually established. This profile can often be used as a means of differentiation of various hemostatic problems. Laboratory screening tests routinely ordered usually include platelet count and peripheral smear examination, prothrombin time (PT), partial thromboplastin time (PTT), and template bleeding time (TBT). Several laboratories also include the thrombin time as a part of their initial coagulation workup.

As mentioned previously, the PT test measures the factors of the extrinsic pathway of coagulation (factors VII, X, V, II, and I). Factor VII is the only factor listed that is restricted to the extrinsic system, since factors X, V, II, and I are part of the common pathway (see Fig. 26-12). The PT test is ideally used to detect early vitamin K deficiencies, as factor VII has the shortest half-life of the coagulation factors and is vitamin K dependent. The PT test is also used to monitor oral anticoagulant therapy. Any abnormalities of these factors, a vitamin K defect, liver disease, or the presence of inhibitors will result in an abnormally prolonged PT time.

The APTT, or PTT, test measures factors of the intrinsic pathway of blood coagulation (XII, Fletcher, Fitzgerald, XI, IX, VIII, X, V, II and I). It should be noted that factors XII, XI, IX, VIII, Fletcher, and Fitzgerald are limited to the intrinsic system. Deficiencies or inhibitors of any of these factors will result in an abnormally prolonged APTT time. Both the PT and APTT tests will show prolonged results with an abnormality of the shared factors of the common pathway (X, V, II, I). A factor abnormality refers to a deficiency of that factor in plasma owing to any one of the following reasons:

**TABLE 26-9. INTERPRETATION OF COAGULATION TEST RESULTS**

| Test | Test Result | | Possible Defect(s) |
|---|---|---|---|
| APTT and PT: TT: | Abnormal Normal | Multiple: | 1. Vitamin K defect<br>2. Liver Disease<br>3. Inhibitor present<br>4. Factors in common pathway (II, V, X) |
| APTT: | Abnormal | Factor: | 1. VIII, IX, XI, XII, Fletcher, Fitzgerald |
| PT: | Normal | | 2. Lupus anticoagulant |
| PT: APTT: | Abnormal Normal | Factor: | 1. VII |
| APTT, PT, TT: | Abnormal | Multiple: | 1. Factor deficiencies (I)<br>2. Severe liver disease<br>3. DIC<br>4. Potent inhibitor<br>5. Hypo- or dysfibrinogenemia |

**TABLE 26–10. CLASSIFICATION OF BLEEDING DISORDERS BY SCREENING TESTS**

| Test | Vascular Disorder | Quantitative Platelet Disorder | Qualitative Platelet Disorder | Factor Deficiency | Fibrinolytic Disorder (Acquired) |
|---|---|---|---|---|---|
| Platelet count | N | AbN | N | N | AbN |
| PT | N | N | N | AbN* | AbN |
| PTT | N | N | N | AbN* | AbN |
| TBT | AbN | AbN | AbN | N | AbN |

N = normal; AbN = abnormal; PT = prothrombin time; PTT = partial thromboplastin time; TBT = template bleeding time.
*Dependent on the factor deficiency.

1. Decreased synthesis
2. Synthesis of an abnormal functioning factor molecule
3. Excessive destruction of factors through acquired disorders
4. Inactivation of factors through circulating inhibitors

Table 26–9 summarizes the interpretation of the PT and APTT test results.

The thrombin time is a measure of the ability of thrombin to convert fibrinogen to fibrin and is particularly useful in the evaluation of circulating anticoagulants (pathologic inhibitors). The thrombin time is prolonged in the following conditions:

1. Hypofibrinogenemia and dysfibrinogenemia
2. Treatment with heparin
3. Circulating FDPs
4. Pathologic circulating inhibitors

Table 26–10 may be used as a general guide toward categorizing bleeding disorders into the groups previously listed using the suggested screening tests. Additional laboratory testing is designed to narrow down the abnormality to one of these specific areas. As a result, laboratory testing can be divided into the following categories:

1. Screening tests for vascular or platelet dysfunction (e.g., platelet aggregation, PF3 assay)
2. Tests for coagulation (e.g., factor assays)
3. Special tests (e.g., for fibrinolytic disorders; such as tests for determination of FDPs, and protamine sulfate and ethanol gel tests for detection of fibrin monomers)

The reader may refer to subsequent chapters for a detailed discussion of the previously listed hemostatic disorders.

## Bibliography

Barnhart, MI and Baechler, CA: Endothelial cell physiology, perturbations and responses. Sem Thromb Hemost 5(2):50, 1978.
Barnhart, MI: Platelet responses in health and disease. Mol Cell Biochem 22:113, 1978.
Baugh, RF and Hougie, C: Structure and function in blood coagulation. In Poller, L (ed): Recent Advances in Blood Coagulation. Churchill Livingstone, Edinburgh, p 81, 1981.
Booth, NA, Bennett, B, Wijngaards, G, et al: A new life-long hemorrhagic disorder due to excess plasminogen activators. Blood 61:267, 1983.
Collen, D: On the regulation and control of fibrinolysis. Thromb Haemost 42:77, 1980.
Evans, VJ: Looking at platelets. J Med Tech 1:9, 1984.
Evans, VJ: Platelet morphology and the blood smear. J Med Tech 1:9, 1984.
Farced, J, Messmore, HL, Fenton, JW II, et al: Perspectives in Hemostasis. Pergamon Press, NY, 1981.
Fritsma, G, Engelmann, G, and Yousuf, M: A review of platelet function and testing. J Med Tech 47(9):723, 1981.
Gastpar, H, Kuhn, K, and Marx, R: Collagen-Platelet Interaction. F. K. Shattauer Verlag, Munich, pp 1 36, 1979.
Kisiel, W and Davie, EW: Protein C (a review). Meth Enzymol 80:320, 1981.
Knaer, TVM, Stel, HV, Voorman, ECI, et al: Localization of VIII CAg using different monoclonal antibodies against VIII C. Thromb Haemost 50:17, 1983.
La Croix, KA and Davis, GL: A review of protein C and its role in hemostasis. J Med Tech 2:2, 1985.
Long, MW: Current concepts in the development and regulation of the bone marrow megakaryocyte. J Med Tech 1:9, 1984.
Marlar, RA, Kleiss, AJ, and Griffin, JH: Human protein C: inactivation of factors V and VIII in plasma by the activated molecule. Ann NY Acad Sci 370:303, 1981.
Mason, RG, Sharp, D, Chuang, HYK, et al: The endothelium: Roles in thrombosis and hemostasis. Arch Pathol Lab Med 101:61, 1977.
McGann, MA and Triplett, DA: Laboratory evaluation of the fibrinolytic system. Lab Med 14:18, 1983.
Murano, G: The "Hageman" connection: Interrelationships of blood coagulation, fibrino(geno)lysis, kinin generation, and complement activation. Am J Hematol 4:409, 1978.
Nemerson, Y and Bach, R: Tissue factor revisited. Prog Hemost Thromb 6:237, 1982.
Nichols, WL, Gerrard, JM, and Didisheim, P: Platelet structure, biochemistry and physiology. In Poller, L (ed): Recent Advances in Blood Coagulation. Churchill Livingstone, Edinburgh, p 1, 1981.
Owen, WG and Esmon, CT: Functional properties of an endothelial cell cofactor for thrombin-catalyzed activation of protein C. J Biol Chem 256:5532, 1981.
Pennica, D, Holmes, WE, Kohr, WJ, et al: Cloning and expression of human tissue-type plasminogen activator with DNA in E. coli. Nature 301:214, 1983.
Stemerman, MB: Anatomy of the blood vessel wall. In Coleman, RW, Hirsh, JW, Marder, VJ, et al (eds): Hemostasis and Thrombosis. JB Lippincott, Philadelphia, p 525, 1982.
Thaler, E and Lechner, K: Antithrombin III deficiency and thromboembolism. Clin Haematol 10:369, 1981.
Triplett, DA and Harms, CS: Procedures for the coagulation laboratory. ASCP Press, Chicago, 1981.

# CHAPTER 27

ROBERT M. SILGALS, M.D., AND
RONALD A. SACHER, M.D., F.R.C.P.(C)

# Quantitative and Qualitative Vascular and Platelet Disorders, Both Congenital and Acquired

Platelets play a very important role in normal hemostasis. Following vascular injury, a series of prompt sequential and interrelated responses occur, with the resultant formation of a platelet plug and cessation of bleeding.[1] Initially the platelets undergo a change in shape from the normal discoid appearance to a sphere. This is followed by adhesion to the site of vascular disruption, primary aggregation (recruitment) of additional platelets, an energy-dependent release of platelet granules, and recruitment of other thrombocytes with secondary (irreversible) aggregation. Subsequent involvement of coagulation factors and the fibrinolytic system results in clot stabilization, in clot retraction, and eventually in resorption of the thrombus with recanalization of the vascular channel.

A large number of abnormalities may result in platelet dysfunction. Although platelet disorders are most commonly associated with an increased risk of bleeding complications, in some instances thromboembolic events may occur instead of or in addition to hemorrhagic tendencies. Obviously, the absolute number of platelets is important. In severe thrombocytopenia, there may simply not be enough platelets present for normal hemostasis to occur. The risk of bleeding is then increased. In addition, the qualitative function of platelets is important for normal hemostasis. An abnormality in the platelet function just outlined, whether it be congenital or acquired, can place the patient at risk for hemorrhage or thrombosis even if the platelet count is normal. In some conditions, when the platelet count is elevated, bleeding may occur. Last, blood vessels themselves are important in normal hemostasis. Vascular abnormalities may predispose to bleeding, which clinically may be confused with disorders of platelet function.

As a general rule, the hemorrhagic manifestation of platelet disorders differs from bleeding in patients with coagulation system abnormalities.[7] Superficial surface areas such as the skin and mucous membranes are more likely sites of bleeding in individuals with platelet disorders. Patients may present with petechial bleeding (**see Color Figure 227**), epistaxis, abnormal menstrual bleeding, or gastrointestinal hemorrhage. Intra-articular and deep muscle bleeds that can be seen in hemophiliacs are unusual events in patients with platelet abnormalities. Postsurgical bleeding can be seen in those with disorders of either platelets or the coagulation system. However, the risk of hemorrhage in patients with platelet abnormalities can vary greatly, depending on the specific disorder and the individual patient.

## QUANTITATIVE PLATELET ABNORMALITIES: THROMBOCYTOPENIA

The causes of thrombocytopenia may be classified into two major categories: (1) failure of the bone marrow to produce an adequate number of platelets and (2) increased peripheral destruction or loss of platelets.

The diagnosis of thrombocytopenia is usually made using automated platelet counters. In all cases of suspected thrombocytopenia, it is essential that the patient's peripheral blood smear be evaluated. Not only may the peripheral smear suggest an etiol-ogy for the thrombocytopenia, but also it may reveal artifactual thrombocytopenia (pseudothrombocytopenia), which must be excluded.[3] For several reasons, platelet clumping may occur after collection of the blood sample, particularly if blood is collected in an ethylenediaminotetraacetic acid (EDTA) tube. An automated platelet count may interpret this phenomenon as an actual decrease in the platelet number. Preview of the peripheral smear to document true thrombocytopenia and to rule out the presence of platelet clumps is necessary before embarking on costly and potentially morbid evaluation or therapy. Once the diagnosis of thrombocytopenia is confirmed, the appearance of the peripheral smear may provide clues as to the cause of the disorder. For example, fragmented red blood cells would suggest a microangiopathic hemolytic anemia with platelet consumption. The presence of altered red cell and white cell morphology might lead to consideration of vitamin deficiencies, myelophthisis, leukemia, or a dysmyelopoietic syndrome. However, an evaluation of the bone marrow is essential in most cases of thrombocytopenia.

The presence of abundant megakaryocytes and normal maturation of the other cell lines will lead to a suspicion of peripheral destruction of platelets. Absence of megakaryocytes, abnormal hematopoiesis, or the presence of fibrosis, foreign cells, or leukemia will suggest a primary failure of platelet production. Last, a thorough physical examination and a careful medical history with emphasis on symptoms, other illnesses, family history, and drug history are essential.

## Thrombocytopenia Secondary to Decreased Platelet Production

### Causes of Decreased Platelet Production

In general, disorders that directly affect bone marrow maturation often cause thrombocytopenia as one of several hematologic manifestations. Anemia and leukopenia often coexist in many patients. The particular cell line that is decreased and the degree of the cytopenia can vary markedly from patient to patient and may change in the same patient as the underlying disorder progresses. Occasionally, thrombocytopenia may antedate the other hematologic findings. Last, a few conditions appear to affect thrombopoiesis primarily, with little effect on the erythroid and myeloid cell lines. Table 27-1 lists causes of thrombocytopenia secondary to decreased platelet production.

The hematologic conditions that include thrombocytopenia as a manifestation of marrow dysfunction are fairly distinct entities, which are fully described in other chapters of this book. They will be mentioned only briefly here. Aplastic anemia results from an often undefined insult to a pluripoten-

**Table 27–1. ACQUIRED THROMBOCYTOPENIA SECONDARY TO DECREASED PLATELET PRODUCTION**

Aplastic anemia
Paroxysmal nocturnal hemoglobinuria
Leukemia (acute, chronic, hairy cell)
Preleukemic syndromes (myelodysplasia)
Metastastic lymphoma or carcinoma
Myelofibrosis (primary or secondary)
Folate and vitamin $B_{12}$ deficiencies
Cytotoxic and immunosuppressive chemotherapy
Viral infections*
Drugs*
Idiopathic*

*Conditions in which thrombocytopenia is often the predominant hematologic finding.

tial stem cell with resultant failure of the stem cell to populate the erythroid, myeloid, and megakaryocytic lines. Pancytopenia with a hypocellular marrow subsequently occurs. Paroxysmal nocturnal hemoglobinuria (PNH) and the myelodysplastic (preleukemic) syndromes are clonal disorders in which stem cells are also damaged. Although anemia often is the initial finding, abnormalities in other cell lines are common and many patients either present with or develop thrombocytopenia. In the setting of the leukemias, myelofibrosis, lymphoma, or carcinoma metastatic to the bone marrow, the architecture of the bone marrow is damaged with a resultant myelophthisic anemia. It is also common for thrombocytopenia to occur. Folate and vitamin $B_{12}$ are necessary for normal maturation and development of all rapidly dividing cells. Although usually considered to be causes of anemia, deficiencies in these vitamins actually result in pancytopenia in many cases. The majority of cancer chemotherapeutic agents are also marrow suppressants. However, certain agents, such as mitomycin C and the nitrosoureas including BCNU and CCNU, are particularly prone to the production of severe, long-lasting thrombocytopenia.[4]

Obviously, these disorders are often associated with specific findings on history, physical examination, and laboratory evaluation. However, in most cases examination of the bone marrow aspirate and biopsy is necessary to confirm the correct diagnosis. (See specific chapters for a more detailed discussion of these conditions.)

Many viral infections are associated with the development of thrombocytopenia. Although pancytopenia, leukopenia, and even aplastic anemia have been reported to occur, thrombocytopenia is the most important hematologic result of several viral infections.[5] In some instances, viral inclusions have actually been identified in marrow megakaryocytes. However, it is often difficult to differentiate the role of direct suppression of platelet production from the role of peripheral destruction of platelets by either immune or nonimmune mechanisms. As discussed later in this chapter, many patients with autoimmune thrombocytopenia give a history of previous viral infection. In addition, bone marrow aspirates during viral infections often show the presence of a normal number of megakaryocytes. Consequently, viral inhibition of thrombopoiesis is often a diagnosis of exclusion.

Certain drugs have the ability to cause thrombocytopenia through direct suppression of thrombopoiesis. Alcohol may cause severe thrombocytopenia in certain predisposed patients.[6,7] Although ethanol (and the lifestyle of the alcoholic) may have profound and variable effects on bone marrow function (direct suppression of erythropoiesis, folate and other nutritional deficiencies, blood loss and iron deficiency from gastrointestinal bleeding, hypersplenism secondary to cirrhosis of the liver), a subset of alcoholics seem to develop thrombocytopenia even in the absence of these complicating factors. The thrombocytopenia may be severe with consequent bleeding. Anemia and a mild leukopenia may or may not be present. Recovery of the platelet count usually occurs after alcohol withdrawal, often in a matter of a few days. This disorder has been seen both in chronic alcoholics and in binge drinkers. Repeated episodes of thrombocytopenia in the same patient are well documented. The commonly used diuretic and antihypertensive agent hydrochlorothiazide has also been associated with thrombocytopenia.[8] The fall in platelet count is usually only mild to moderate and most often transient.

Occasionally, patients present with thrombocytopenia, reduced megakaryocytes in the bone marrow, minimal abnormalities in other hematologic cell lines, and no evidence of any underlying disease.[9] The thrombocytopenia appears to be secondary to an isolated failure of thrombopoiesis. The course of these patients seems to be varied. Some remain clinically stable for a significant period of time, whereas others have subsequently developed aplastic anemia or a preleukemic syndrome. Additionally, systemic lupus erythematosus should be considered in all such cases.

## Management

**Definitive.** The management of patients with thrombocytopenia secondary to decreased platelet production depends on the underlying cause of the problem and the clinical situation. Therapy is primarily directed at the etiology of the thrombocytopenia. This might entail the withdrawal of offending drugs—alcohol or cytotoxic chemotherapy—or the initiation of appropriate vitamin therapy (vitamin $B_{12}$ or folate), specific immunotherapy (steroids in the case of lupus erythematosus) or chemotherapy (leukemia, lymphoma).

**Supportive: Platelet Transfusions.** In most cases

of thrombocytopenia secondary to decreased platelet production, platelet transfusions will be successful in raising the peripheral count and in controlling abnormal bleeding. However, platelet transfusions are not without hazard. Fever and other transfusion reactions may occur. The risk of transmission of hepatitis is always present. Repeated platelet transfusions may also lead to the development of alloantibodies in the recipients directed toward donor platelet antigens. Over time, repeated platelet transfusions may not be effective in raising the count, as the donor platelets will be rapidly destroyed because of these antibodies. Subsequently, the use of platelet transfusions requires a clinical decision based on the individual patient. Factors to consider include the severity of the thrombocytopenia, the presence or absence of abnormal bleeding, the nature of the etiology of the disorder, and the expected duration of the thrombocytopenia. Rough guidelines for platelet transfusions can be suggested based on the risk of bleeding for various degrees of thrombocytopenia. For example, in patients with acute leukemia, severe spontaneous bleeding is unusual (although it certainly can occur) when the platelet count is greater than 20,000/mm³.[10] The risk for bleeding after trauma or surgery rises significantly when the platelet count falls below 50,000/mm³.

With these figures in mind, the following guidelines can be used. In patients in whom the platelet count is greater than 20,000/mm³ and who do not have bleeding complications, the risks of platelet transfusions probably outweigh the benefits. Careful observation alone is appropriate. On the other hand, the thrombocytopenic patient with significant bleeding (gastrointestinal, genitourinary, or intracerebral) should receive therapeutic platelet transfusions even if the platelet count is greater than 20,000/mm³. At times it may be necessary to maintain the platelet count as high as 100,000/mm³ in order to treat appropriately the bleeding complications, particularly if intrinsic platelet function is abnormal. The management of patients with severe thrombocytopenia (less than 20,000/mm³) but without bleeding is more controversial.[11,12] Some physicians would recommend careful follow-up and would perform platelet transfusions only if bleeding developed. Others would use platelet transfusion prophylactically if the duration of thrombocytopenia was likely to be brief (less than two weeks), especially in patients with acute leukemia during aggressive chemotherapy. Patients with severe refractory thrombocytopenia present an even more difficult clinical problem, as they are very likely to develop platelet antibodies if repeated transfusions are given. In this case, transfusions are usually held unless bleeding occurs or surgery is required, even if the platelet count is less than 20,000/mm³.

## Thrombocytopenia Secondary to Increased Peripheral Destruction or Sequestration of Platelets

Thrombocytopenia in the face of normal marrow function indicates that the lifespan of platelets is significantly reduced. Compared with thrombocytopenia from decreased platelet production, evaluation of the bone marrow in these instances shows the presence of abundant megakaryocytes (**see Color Figure 228**). Platelet transfusions are usually unsuccessful in raising the platelet count and controlling abnormal bleeding as the transfused platelets will also be destroyed by the underlying disease process that caused the thrombocytopenia. These disorders of platelet survival may be classified according to the mechanism of platelet destruction — whether it is immune mediated or not. In several conditions, however, the pathophysiology of platelet destruction has not been well elucidated, and in others an immune mechanism has been postulated but not proven.

### Immune Thrombocytopenia

The immune thrombocytopenias are a heterogenous group of disorders characterized by the production of specific antibodies directed against the platelets. Subsequently, the antibody coated thrombocytes are removed by the reticuloendothelial system.[10] As compensatory marrow thrombopoiesis is insufficient to overcome the peripheral destruction of platelets, thrombocytopenia and the possibility of a hemorrhagic complication develops. The immune thrombocytopenias may occur in association with an underlying disease or may have no discernible etiology. When no underlying condition can be documented, the disorder is referred to as idiopathic thrombocytopenic purpura (ITP).

**Idiopathic Thrombocytopenic Purpura (ITP).** ITP can be broadly classified into three groups.[13] Chronic ITP generally occurs in adults.[14,15] Women predominate over men in this disorder, with a history of petechiae (**see Color Figures 227 and 230**), epistaxis, or abnormal menstrual bleeding that has preceded the diagnosis for several weeks to months. A history of a recent viral infection may be present. Spontaneous remission is unusual. Therapy with corticosteroids or splenectomy is usually undertaken and will be discussed more fully subsequently.

Acute ITP, on the other hand, occurs predominantly in children, is usually of abrupt onset, and generally resolves spontaneously.[14,16] Approximately 50 percent of cases occur after viral infection; acute ITP shows a predilection for the winter and spring seasons. The male and female incidence is equal. Approximately 85 percent of children spontaneously recover, one half in the first month after onset of the disease. The remainder develop the chronic form of the disease. Serious complications are unusual. Therapy generally consists of bed rest and symptomatic management. Although controversy over interventional therapy exists, most authors suggest reserving steroids for patients with severe thrombocytopenia (less than 10,000 to 20,000/m³) or significant hemorrhage manifested by widespread petechiae and ecchymoses or gastrointestinal, genitourinary, or intracerebral bleeding.[17,18] Steroid therapy has not been shown to shorten the duration of the disease or prevent the development of the chronic type. Splenectomy is undertaken only in patients who develop chronic ITP and in whom the platelet counts cannot be maintained on steroids.

Last, an intermittent, relapsing variety of ITP, in which intervals of thrombocytopenia are interspersed with periods when the platelet count is normal, can be seen in both children and adults.

The diagnosis of ITP is usually one of exclusion. Standard criteria include the presence of thrombocytopenia or shortened platelet survival, the finding of abundant megakaryocytes on bone marrow examination (**see Color Figure 228**), and the absence of an underlying condition (including medications) that could account for the clinical picture (see further on, secondary immune thrombocytopenias).[13] The physical examination of these patients may be normal or may reveal petechiae (**see Color Figure 227**) or other sites of bleeding (**see Color Figure 230**). The finding of lymphadenopathy or splenomegaly should raise the suspicion of thrombocytopenia secondary to lymphoma or viral infection.[13,15] Serositis or joint findings would suggest systemic lupus erythematosus. Collagen vascular serologic tests — particularly those for antinuclear antibodies (ANA) —should be done routinely. Serologic tests for infectious mononucleosis or cytomegalovirus (CMV) are indicated if the clinical picture suggests a specific viral syndrome.

Since platelet destruction in ITP is mediated by IgG autoantibodies, there has been much interest in the development of specific diagnostic tests to identify these antibodies. Antibody bound to platelets (platelet-associated immunoglobulin, or PAIg) has been shown to be increased in patients with ITP and to correlate with the severity of the disease.[13] Several institutions have reported various methods of determining PAIg.[19-21] However, the reliability, specificity, and pathophysiologic significance of the so-called platelet Coombs' test has been questioned.[22] Although progress has been made, no specific reliable serologic test for ITP is generally available.

As previously discussed, treatment of acute ITP is usually conservative, with therapeutic intervention reserved for the most serious cases. Initial therapy for chronic ITP usually entails the use of corticosteroids (for example, prednisone 1 mg/kg body weight/day). Most patients will respond to steroid therapy with an increase in platelet counts. However, complete responses, with platelet counts rising to greater than 150,000, occur in less than half of all patients.[13,23] Additionally, many patients relapse when steroids are discontinued, and only a small percentage have long-lasting remissions.[23] In situations when steroids fail or platelet counts can only be maintained with moderate to high steroid doses, splenectomy is usually undertaken. The rationale for splenectomy is twofold: both a major source of antibody production and the primary site for platelet destruction are eliminated when the spleen is removed. The majority of patients will respond to splenectomy. A minority will not benefit from splenectomy, and relapse can occur after an initial response.[23]

An impressively large number of therapeutic regimens have been suggested for patients with disease that is refractory to or that relapses after splenectomy. Vinca alkaloids, given intermittently[24] or by continuous infusion,[25] as well as the transfusion of platelets labeled in vitro with vinca alkaloids,[26] have been successfully used. Immunosuppressive therapy with cyclophosphamide[27] and azothiaprine,[28] high-dose intravenous gamma globulin,[29] and the androgen danazol[30] also have been suggested as possible therapies. These measures cannot be expected to be curative, and as some have potentially serious side effects. Karpatkin[13] has emphasized the important point, that the goal of therapy is to keep the patient free of bleeding complications. Raising the platelet count to normal levels is not necessary, and the physician must avoid "treating the number" in a patient with moderate thrombocytopenia and no evidence of bleeding. In fact, patients with refractory disease often seem to do quite well, and spontaneous late recoveries of adequate platelet counts have been reported.[31] Although some patients will most certainly be candidates for the newer therapies, these patients should be carefully chosen.

**Secondary Immune Thrombocytopenia.** Immune-mediated thrombocytopenias may occur as a manifestation of several disorders (Table 27–2). These underlying conditions must be ruled out before a diagnosis of ITP can be established. The relationship between immune thrombocytopenias and viral infections is interesting. As mentioned previously, approximately 50 percent of patients with ITP give a history of a recent viral-like illness, often an upper respiratory tract infection, at the time of presentation. A role for viral infection in the initiation of the disease process is a tempting theory. There have been occasional reports of "ITP" associated with specific viral infections and one instance of acute infectious mononucleosis presenting as an ITP.[32] ITP may be a coexistent feature of human immune virus (HTLV III) infection.

**Table 27–2. THROMBOCYTOPENIA SECONDARY TO INCREASED PERIPHERAL DESTRUCTION OF PLATELETS**

I. Immune-mediated thrombocytopenia
  A. Idiopathic thrombocytopenic purpura (ITP)
    1. Acute ITP
    2. Chronic ITP
    3. Intermittent/recurrent ITP
  B. Secondary immune thrombocytopenias
    1. Viral infections
    2. Collagen vascular diseases
    3. Lymphoproliferative malignancies
    4. Carcinomas
    5. Drugs
    6. After blood transfusions
II. Nonimmune-mediated thrombocytopenias
  A. Thrombotic thrombocytopenic purpura
  B. Hemolytic uremic syndrome
  C. Disseminated intravascular coagulation
  D. Heparin administration
  E. Complications of pregnancy
  F. Infections

Collagen vascular diseases, particularly systemic lupus erythematosus (SLE), may cause an immune-mediated thrombocytopenia. Although thrombocytopenia may occur at any time in the natural history of SLE, thrombocytopenic purpura may occasionally be the presenting sign of the disease. In fact, it has been reported that between 3 and 16 percent of patients with ITP later develop other signs of SLE.[13,23] Immune thrombocytopenias may also occur in the setting of malignancy. Although most commonly associated with chronic lymphocytic leukemia, cases have also been reported in patients with lymphomas and solid tumors. Steroid therapy and splenectomy appear to be beneficial.[33] Elevated levels of PAIg have been noted.[34] Recently, immune thrombocytopenia has been reported in a group of homosexual men who did not meet the criteria for having the acquired immune deficiency syndrome (AIDS).[35] It was suggested that a basic abnormality of immune regulation might be present in this population, resulting in autoimmune phenomena in some and opportunistic infections in others.

Immune thrombocytopenias have been described as occurring secondary to an almost endless list of drugs.[36] The most common and best described drug-induced immune thrombocytopenia has been associated with the cardiac antiarrhythmic quinidine.[37,38] In this disorder, the onset is usually explosive, with severe thrombocytopenia, petechial bleeding, and, occasionally, life-threatening hemorrhage. Thrombocytopenia may occur early in the course of treatment with quinidine, after the patient has been taking the drug for many months, or when the drug has been given intermittently. Platelet destruction in quinidine purpura appears to occur through an "innocent bystander" immune mechanism. Antibodies to the drug are produced; the drug,

the antibody, and the platelet then form a complex. Platelet destruction by the reticuloendothelial system follows. As the presence of the drug is necessary for antibody binding to occur, the disorder is usually self-limited. The platelet count will quickly return to normal once the drug has been cleared from the body.[14] This usually occurs within several days. Therapy is usually supportive. Steroids are often administered in the hope that capillary fragility will be improved and bleeding lessened. Capillary fragility may be monitored by the tourniquet test (**see Color Figure 229**). Steroids, however, have little effect on the underlying disease process or the duration of thrombocytopenia. Quinidine should never be readministered to a patient suspected of having had quinidine thrombocytopenia. A single dose may result in a significant thrombocytopenia, with potentially serious bleeding complications.[14]

Last, in rare cases, patients may lack a specific platelet antigen (Pl^A1) and may develop thrombocytopenia following blood transfusions.[39] Although the mechanism is not entirely clear, it is thought that in these patients the few platelets present in transfused packed cells are positive for Pl^A1. An antibody-mediated immune response is generated in the recipient against Pl^A1 that somehow results in destruction of the patient's own platelets.[40] The disorder is usually self-limited and is known as post-transfusion purpura (PTP) (**see Color Figure 231**). In severe cases plasmapheresis through removal of the antibodies may be effective.[39] Recently, steroids have been reported to be beneficial in an isolated case despite previous reports to the contrary.[41]

**Role of Platelet Transfusion in Immune-Mediated Thrombocytopenia.** Platelet transfusions are of limited benefit in patients with immune thrombocytopenias. The survival of transfused platelets will be short in most cases as the antibodies directed against the patient's own platelets can destroy the transfused platelets as well. Subsequently, prophylactic platelet transfusions are not indicated. In patients with severe hemorrhage, however, platelet transfusions are usually given in an attempt to control bleeding. Therapy of the underlying condition is essential when such a disorder exists.

**Immune Thrombocytopenias in Pregnancy.** The presence of immune thrombocytopenia in a pregnant patient presents a difficult clinical problem. As the autoantibodies of ITP are of the IgG class, they are able to cross the placenta. The fetus is then at risk for the development of thrombocytopenia. The trauma of passage through the birth canal could result in significant complication to the infant with a low platelet count. On the other hand, a normal platelet count in the child should exclude any increased risk of morbidity.

Unfortunately, the management of ITP in pregnancy is controversial. Approximately 50 percent of infants born to mothers with ITP will be thrombocytopenic.[42] Platelet counts may actually fall in the baby after birth.[43] Predicting which infant will have a low platelet count is difficult. There is little correlation between platelet levels in the mother and those in the infant.[42] In addition, the amount of PAIg in the mother is of little predictive value.[44] Women in remission after splenectomy may actually have babies that are thrombocytopenic. Several strategies of management have been suggested. The performance of cesarean section in all mothers with ITP has been advocated by some. Others recommend checking the baby's platelet count from a scalp vein sample early in delivery.[42] If the platelet count is normal, vaginal delivery is allowed to take place. More recently, steroid therapy for the mother has also been suggested to be beneficial to both the infant and the mother.[45] The presence of circulating (not platelet-bound) antiplatelet antibody has been strongly correlated with the platelet count in the infant.[44] Although tests for platelet antibodies are not widely available, this technique may in the future help identify patients who require cesarean section. The impact of cesarean section on infant mortality in this situation has not been elucidated.[42]

### Nonimmune Thrombocytopenia Secondary to Destruction of Platelets

**Thrombotic Thrombocytopenic Purpura (TTP).** Thrombotic thrombocytopenic purpura (TTP) is a poorly understood syndrome with prominent hematologic and systemic manifestations. Diagnosis is based on the presence of five clinical criteria in the absence of an underlying explanation for the illness: (1) thrombocytopenia, (2) microangiopathic hemolytic anemia, (3) fever, (4) neurologic abnormalities, and (5) renal dysfunction.[46] Initially TTP was recognized as an acute, severe condition in which short-term prognosis was dismal. A compilation of early case reports showed a long-term survival rate of less than 10 percent.[46] More recently, a wider spectrum of presentations has been noted, and the prognosis may not always be as poor as previously appreciated.[47]

TTP usually occurs in young adults.[46] A history of a viral-like illness can often be illicited. Petechiae and abnormal bleeding are almost always present. The peripheral blood smear shows thrombocytopenia and fragmented red blood cells consistent with a microangiopathic hemolytic anemia (**see Color Figure 121**). Neurologic manifestations include headache, altered mental status, seizures, paresis, cranial nerve abnormalities, and coma. Renal findings include proteinuria, hematuria, and acute renal failure (**see Color Figure 232**). Almost any organ system can be involved, and damage to the cardiac conduction system with resultant arrhythmias is not unusual.[48] Abnormal laboratory studies are secondary to the hemolytic anemia (increased reticulocyte count, elevated bilirubin, and lactate dehydrogenase [LDH]) and the renal failure. Al-

though fibrin-split products may be elevated, other coagulation studies are usually normal and there is little evidence of disseminated intravascular coagulation.[49] Death may occur secondary to bleeding, renal failure, or CNS or cardiac complications.

The pathophysiology of the disease is unclear. It has been suggested that uncontrolled platelet aggregation is a major underlying mechanism[49] with resultant thrombocytopenia, shearing of red cells by the intravascular platelet aggregates, and damage to organs secondary to vascular occlusion (**see Color Figure 232**). Certain investigators have suggested that a normal plasma substance that inhibits platelet aggregation is absent in this disorder.[50] Pathologically, hyaline-like deposits are frequently noted in the luminae and subendothelial areas of capillaries and small arterioles without the presence of perivascular inflammation. Gingival biopsy has been used as a diagnostic test.[51]

At this point there is no standard therapy for TTP. Although many treatments have been reported to produce remissions, the variable nature and natural history of the disorder make evaluations of these therapies difficult. Steroid administration and splenectomy have occasionally resulted in remission but are generally considered to be ineffective in reversing the course of the disease.[49,51] Antiplatelet agents such as aspirin and dipyridamole are often employed,[52] but their effectiveness has been questioned.[47] The infusion of large amounts of plasma[53] and the performance of plasma exchange[49] have been advocated; the latter is currently in vogue as the treatment of choice in many centers. Dextran infusion in association with splenectomy and steroid therapy has also been said to be beneficial.[54] More recently, vincristine[55] and intravenous prostacycline[56] have both been reported to induce remissions. The multitude of suggested therapies are consistent with our poor understanding of this disorder, and delineation of the most effective treatment awaits further trials. The use of platelet transfusions has been criticized for fear of actually worsening the clinical situation.[57]

**Hemolytic Uremic Syndrome (HUS).** The hemolytic uremic syndrome (HUS) is another poorly understood disorder that in many ways resembles TTP. The cardinal manifestations are thrombocytopenia, microangiopathic hemolytic anemia (**see Color Figure 127**), and renal failure.[58,59] As opposed to TTP, the primary pathologic findings in HUS are limited to the kidneys, with involvement of small vessels and glomeruli.[59] Hemolytic anemia and thrombocytopenia appear to be secondary to the local renal abnormalities. Although fever is a common sign and neurologic manifestations have been reported, the presence of severe neurologic dysfunction or the pathologic evidence of widespread vessel disease would suggest the diagnosis of TTP.

The disorder has most frequently been noted in children between the ages of 2 and 4 years. Previous viral and bacterial infections are commonly reported. Proteinuria, hematuria, oliguria, or anuria is usually present. Prognosis in children seems to depend on the degree and reversibility of renal dysfunction.[58] Although management is usually conservative, therapeutic intervention with anticoagulants, antiplatelet agents, steroids, and fibrinolytic agents has been attempted.

The disorder may also occur in adults and has been related to pregnancy, obstetric complications, and the use of oral contraceptives.[58,60] The prognosis in adults is generally felt to be worse than in children, with mortality rates and permanent renal dysfunction being more common. Treatment with heparin and antiplatelet agents has been recommended.[58]

**Disseminated Intravascular Coagulation (DIC).** Disseminated intravascular coagulation (DIC) is classically associated with thrombocytopenia secondary to intravascular consumption of platelets in addition to clotting factors. The severity, chronicity, and natural history of this disorder are extremely variable. DIC is usually a manifestation of an underlying condition rather than an independent disease entity, and the prognosis often depends more on the cause of DIC than on the presence of DIC itself.[61] This topic is covered more fully in Chapter 29.

**Heparin Administration.** Thrombocytopenia may also be seen during the therapeutic use of heparin.[62,63] Although the incidence of heparin-induced thrombocytopenia varies in different reports, a recent review suggests an overall occurrence rate of approximately 5 percent.[62] The incidence seems to be higher in patients receiving bovine, as compared with porcine, heparin. Thrombocytopenia usually occurs 6 to 12 days after initiation of therapy but may occur sooner in patients who have previously received the drug. The degree of thrombocytopenia is often mild to moderate, and bleeding complications are fairly unusual. However, in some instances, heparin-induced thrombocytopenia has been associated with arterial or venous thrombosis, occasionally with disastrous complications.[62] The mechanism of heparin-induced thrombocytopenia is not clear. An immune mechanism has been suggested, and elevated levels of platelet IgG and complement have been reported.[63]

Management is dependent on the findings in a specific case. If thrombocytopenia is mild and if bleeding or thrombotic complications are absent, then heparin can be continued and oral anticoagulation with Coumadin immediately started. In some cases, platelet counts will rise despite continued heparin therapy. Obviously, careful follow up assessment of platelet count is mandatory if this course of therapy is undertaken. However, if the thrombocytopenia is severe or results in hemorrhage or if thrombotic events occur, then the heparin must be discontinued. Depending on the specific situation, oral anticoagulation,

fibrinolytic therapy, or vena caval interruption may be appropriate.[62]

**Nonimmune Thrombocytopenia in Pregnancy.** Pregnancy may be associated with a number of conditions in which thrombocytopenia occurs.[65] For example, pre-eclampsia has been associated with low platelet counts in the absence of DIC. However, when faced with a pregnant patient with a low platelet count, one must also consider the possibilities of DIC secondary to obstetric complications, TTP, HUS, and ITP.

**Miscellaneous Causes of Thrombocytopenia.** Thrombocytopenia has also been associated with infections due to bacterial, viral, and protozoal agents. Several mechanisms can be involved, including direct marrow suppression (see previous section on viral thrombocytopenia), autoimmunity, and DIC. However, several infectious agents have been reported to cause thrombocytopenia due to peripheral destruction of platelets. Bacterial septicemia, for example, can result in falling platelet counts in the absence of DIC.[36] Thrombocytopenia has also been reported as a complication of severe burns, the adult respiratory distress syndrome, and certain snake bites.[36]

## Platelet Sequestration and Washout

Two additional mechanisms of thrombocytopenia bear brief mention. Normally one third of the circulating platelet mass is present in the spleen. Sequestration of platelets with variable thrombocytopenia may occur in patients with splenomegaly. As much as 90 percent of the total platelet mass may be sequestered in large spleens.[66] The degree of thrombocytopenia is often mild to moderate but occasionally may be severe. Leukopenia and a normocytic anemia commonly occur in addition to the low platelet count. The severity of the hematologic abnormalities depends greatly on the underlying condition causing the splenomegaly.

Last, patients who require massive blood transfusions for severe hemorrhage may develop a mild to moderate thrombocytopenia.[67] This can occur with the administration of whole banked blood or packed red cells. The condition has been termed a "washout" effect, as whole blood (including normal platelets) is lost during hemorrhage and replaced by packed red cells (with few platelets) or banked whole blood (with nonusable old platelets). Thrombocytopenia is usually mild, and therapy is seldom indicated.

## QUANTITATIVE PLATELET ABNORMALITIES: THROMBOCYTOSIS

Elevated platelet counts are encountered relatively commonly in clinical medicine (Table 27–3).[68] In some instances, thrombocytosis presents as a manifestation of an underlying hematologic disease, usually one of the myeloproliferative syndromes.

Table 27-3. CAUSES OF THROMBOCYTOSIS

I. Myeloproliferative syndromes
  A. Essential thrombocythemia
  B. Polycythemia vera
  C. Myelofibrosis with agnogenic myeloid metaplasia
  D. Chronic myelogenous leukemia
II. Secondary (reactive) thrombocytosis
  A. Mobilization of pooled platelets
    1. Postsplenectomy
    2. After epinephrine administration
  B. Rebound thrombocytosis
    1. After blood loss (including surgery)
    2. Accompanying bone marrow recovery
      a. After cytotoxic chemotherapy
      b. After treatment of vitamin $B_{12}$ or folate deficiency
  C. Iron Deficiency
  D. Malignancy
  E. Chronic inflammatory conditions
    1. Collagen vascular diseases
    2. Inflammatory bowel diseases
  F. Chronic infections
    1. Tuberculosis
    2. Osteomyelitis

More commonly, however, high platelet counts are found in the absence of any intrinsic hematologic abnormality. A large number of underlying conditions may be associated with such a reactive or secondary thrombocytosis. The distinction between reactive thrombocytosis and the elevated platelet count seen in primary hematologic conditions are important. Not only will therapy and prognosis differ but also the risk of complications will vary depending on the cause of high platelet count. Patients with a myeloproliferative syndrome are at an increased risk for both thrombotic and hemorrhagic events.[69,70] In reactive thrombocytosis, however, platelet function is normal, and complications secondary to the high platelet counts are unusual.[68,71]

## Thrombocytosis in Primary Disorders

The myeloproliferative syndromes are a group of disorders that have in common loss of control of normal hematopoiesis. In a sense, they are neoplastic conditions arising from the progeny of an abnormal pluripotential stem cell in the marrow and peripheral blood.[69] The myeloid, erythroid, and megakaryocytic lines are all involved in the process. The clinical manifestations depend on which element tends to predominate. In essential thrombocythemia a high platelet count (often greater than 1 million/mm³) is the predominant finding.[72] However, polycythemia vera (PV), chronic myelogenous leukemia (CML), and myelofibrosis with agnogenic myeloid metaplasia (MF) often result in thrombocytosis as well. The incidence has been stated to be 60 percent for PV and 29 percent for MF.[70] Specific characteristics of these disorders are covered in detail in Chapters 15, 20, and 21.

As mentioned earlier, patients with a myeloproliferative syndrome have an increased risk of both hemorrhagic and thrombotic complications. Resultant morbidity and mortality may be quite significant.[71] Bleeding manifestations can involve the skin (easy bruising) or mucous membranes (epistaxis, gastrointestinal tract bleeding), or may present as abnormal bleeding after surgery.[69,70] Thromboembolic complications can include deep vein thrombosis, pulmonary embolus, stroke, or thrombosis of portal or mesenteric veins.[69] The underlying reasons for the hemostatic abnormalities are not entirely clear. Several factors are probably involved. It has been suggested that the degree of thrombocytosis is important and that patients with very high platelet counts are more likely to suffer complications. Control of platelet counts with chemotherapy has been suggested to lessen the risk of neurologic manifestations of essential thrombocytothemia.[72] The risk of bleeding may also be decreased if the platelet count is lowered. However, patients with reactive thrombocytosis do not seem prone to develop hemostatic complications even if the platelet count is very high (see further on). In addition, complications have been noted in patients with myeloproliferative syndromes at times when platelet counts were normal.[69] Consequently, attributing the bleeding and thrombotic complications solely to the level of thrombocytosis is not a satisfactory explanation.

As the megakaryocytic line is involved in the neoplastic process in the myeloproliferative disorders, it is not surprising that abnormalities in platelet morphology and function are commonly found. Giant platelets are often seen on the peripheral smear (**see Color Figure 233**), and electron microscopy frequently reveals ultrastructural abnormalities.[70] The bleeding time is frequently prolonged except in the case of CML.[70] Platelet aggregation studies are often abnormal, although results with specific agents can vary from patient to patient.[70,73] The loss of the secondary wave of epinephrine induced aggregation has been suggested to be particularly common but not universal.[69,74] It thus seems reasonable to assume that the hemostatic complications of the myeloproliferative syndrome are due in part to intrinsic platelet abnormalities that arise through the neoplastic process.

Factors not directly related to platelet function may also contribute to the thrombotic and hemorrhagic manifestations of the myeloproliferative syndrome. For example, the frequency of complication varies greatly among the specific disorders.[71] Both thrombotic and hemorrhagic events are unusual in patients with CML, in the absence of thrombocytopenia. Myelofibrosis is more likely associated with bleeding than with thrombotic complications. Both bleeding and thrombosis may occur in patients with polycythemia vera or with idiopathic thrombocythemia. In addition, the bleeding time seems to have little correlation with the frequency of complications.[70] In polycythemia vera, the erythrocytosis and resultant increase in blood viscosity may actually interfere with normal clotting. Phlebotomy to control the red cell count may be more important than treating the elevated platelet count, and in preventing complications.[69]

Because therapy of the myeloproliferative syndromes is discussed in the respective chapters, it will only be briefly mentioned here. When thrombotic or hemorrhagic complications occur in the face of significant thrombocytosis, platelet pheresis can rapidly lower the platelet count.[72] However, the effects are very transient and this technique is not suitable for long-term management. Chemotherapeutic agents such as busulfan and hydroxyurea, as well as radioactive phosphorus, are preferred for the long-term control of thrombocytosis.[69,72] Other measures to consider include phlebotomy when erythrocytosis is present and anticoagulation when thrombotic manifestations predominate. The role of antiplatelet agents is controversial.[69,72] Although their administration theoretically could lessen thrombotic complications, it could conceivably increase the risk of bleeding.

## Secondary (Reactive) Thrombocytosis

Even though secondary thrombocytosis may occur in a large number of underlying conditions and diseases,[68,75] a reasonable pathophysiologic mechanism can only be suggested in a minority of cases. Usually the degree of thrombocytosis is mild to moderate; however, platelet counts greater than 1 million/mm³ are sometimes seen.

Thrombocytosis may occur when peripheral platelet pools are mobilized. Normally, the spleen contains approximately one third of the total number of circulating platelets. In addition, the spleen is a major site for removal of platelets. Splenectomy will result in an immediate increase in the platelet count. The thrombocytosis in this case is usually transient, and the platelet count will return to normal over one to two months.[68] The administration of epinephrine can cause release of platelets from the spleen, with a resultant thrombocytosis.[68] High platelet counts can also occur when the bone marrow is stimulated by blood loss, particularly in the presence of acute, brisk hemorrhage. In addition, when a damaged or suppressed marrow begins to show recovery function, a transient rebound thrombocytosis is often seen. This may occur after treatment of a vitamin deficiency (vitamin $B_{12}$ or folate) or in the recovery phase after cytotoxic chemotherapy. The mechanism by which thrombocytosis develops in patients with malignancy,

iron deficiency, or chronic inflammatory or infectious disease is poorly understood.

In patients with reactive thrombocytosis, platelet morphology is normal, platelet function tests are usually normal, and bleeding or thrombotic complications are rare.[71,73] Therapy is indicated only as dictated by the underlying disease, whereas specific therapy of the high platelet count is not warranted in the absence of complications. The major concern in patients with high platelet counts is the differentiation of secondary thrombocytosis from one of the myeloproliferative syndromes. In many cases this may be accomplished fairly easily. The medical history, physical examination, and routine studies often are suggestive of the etiology. Careful abdominal examination is important, as the presence of an enlarged spleen could suggest a myeloproliferative disorder. Similarly, an elevated hematocrit could lead to the consideration of polycythemia vera; a high white cell count might suggest CML; and the presence of teardrop red cells would raise the possibility of myelofibrosis. In some cases, however, the diagnosis is not clear at the time of presentation, and the patient must be followed over time before a firm etiology of the thrombocytosis can be established.

## QUALITATIVE PLATELET ABNORMALITIES

As discussed in Chapter 26, platelet response to vascular injury is complex. Various abnormalities in the platelet function may predispose to abnormal bleeding even in the face of a normal platelet count. Hemostatic disorders secondary to platelet dysfunction are often referred to as thrombocytopathies and may occur as congenital or acquired conditions. In addition, abnormalities in thrombocyte function may be due to intrinsic defects in the platelets themselves or to the presence or absence of extrinsic factors in the plasma. For example, abnormalities in platelet membrane structure may adversely affect the initial steps in the formation of a platelet plug: change in platelet shape and adhesion to the site of vascular injury. Absence of platelet granules or dysfunction in the release of these granules may result in failure of recruitment and aggregation. On the other hand, the absence of factor VIII complex (von Willebrand's factor) will result in bleeding tendencies produced by abnormal platelet plug formation. Similarly, drugs such as aspirin and abnormal plasma components such as paraproteins may interfere with normal platelet function. Table 27-4 presents a classification of platelet disorders.

The clinical manifestations of qualitative platelet abnormalities may be quite variable. Many patients are prone to development of abnormal bleeding. This may take the form of superficial skin and mucous membrane bleeding (petechiae or epi-

**Table 27–4. QUALITATIVE PLATELET ABNORMALITIES**

I. Inherited platelet abnormalities
  A. Intrinsic platelet defects
    1. Bernard-Soulier syndrome
    2. Glanzmann's thrombasthenia
    3. Storage pool disorders
  B. Extrinsic platelet abnormalities
    1. Von Willebrand's disease
    2. Congenital afibrinogenemia
II. Acquired platelet abnormalities
  A. Intrinsic platelet abnormalities
    1. Preleukemic and acute nonlymphocytic leukemia
    2. Myeloproliferative syndromes*
    3. Paroxysmal nocturnal hemoglobinemia*
  B. Drug-related platelet abnormalities
    1. Aspirin and other nonsteroidal anti-inflammatory agents
    2. Sulfinpyrazone
    3. Dipyridamole
    4. Dextran
    5. Heparin*
    6. Penicillins
  C. Extrinsic platelet abnormalities
    1. Uremia
    2. Paraproteins (multiple myeloma, Waldenström's macroglobulinemia

*Associated with increased risk of thromboembolic events

staxis), abnormal menstrual bleeding, or abnormal bleeding after surgery.[2] A history of prolonged hemorrhage after dental extractions is often obtained. As previously mentioned, joint and deep muscle bleeding are unusual. However, specific manifestations may vary, and in some qualitative disorders, platelet dysfunction is actually associated with an increased risk of thrombotic events.

The importance of the medical history as a first step in evaluation of thrombocytopathies has been previously stressed. A careful and complete family history and a thorough physical examination are essential. A meticulous history of drug use must be obtained. Initial laboratory tests should include a complete blood count and an evaluation of the peripheral blood smear. The number and morphology of platelets should be noted. Several laboratory tests are available to aid in the evaluation of thrombocytopathies. The individual procedures are discussed in greater detail in Chapter 31. Assessment of bleeding time is the most commonly used screening test, and bleeding time is prolonged in patients with most disorders associated with significant platelet dysfunction. The bleeding time, however, may be prolonged in other conditions not directly affecting platelets and is an unreliable measure of platelet function in patients with moderate to severe thrombocytopenia. In addition, it gives little information regarding the specific abnormality accounting for platelet dysfunction. Other laboratory techniques sometimes used include retention of platelets by a column of glass beads (to test adhesion) and platelet interaction with rabbit aorta endothelium (to test adhesion and aggregation). Last, the ability of several substances such as ADP, collagen, epinephrine, and ristocetin to directly cause platelet aggregation can be measured. Although the patterns of aggregation seen when a battery of such agents is used may be suggestive or even diagnostic of certain conditions, in many instances the results are less specific.

## Hereditary Disorders of Platelet Function

### Intrinsic Platelet Abnormalities

The *Bernard-Soulier syndrome* is a rare familial disorder inherited as an autosomal recessive trait. Clinical manifestations may be quite variable but are often severe and in some instances fatal.[76,77] Sites of bleeding are those typical for platelet disorders (petechiae, epistaxis, gastrointestinal bleeding, menstrual bleeding). Intracranial hemorrhage has been reported. The platelet count may be normal or low. On bone marrow examination, megakaryocytes are quantitatively normal. Platelets on the peripheral blood smear are often large and show a clustering of granules in the center. The bleeding time is usually prolonged, and platelet interaction with rabbit endothelium is decreased. Platelet aggregation studies show a characteristic pattern—normal responses to collagen and ADP and an absent response to ristocetin.[78] As compared with the response found in patients with von Willebrand's disease, ristocetin aggregation in patients with this syndrome is not corrected by the addition of factor VIII. The disorder is believed to be secondary to a membrane defect with resultant abnormal platelet adhesion. A decrease in a specific membrane component, glycoprotein I-B, has been reported.[76] Interestingly, this is the proposed binding site for von Willebrand's factor. Iron replacement and blood and platelet transfusions for bleeding episodes are the mainstays of therapy. Steroid administration and splenectomy are ineffective.

*Glanzmann's thrombasthenia* is also a congenital thrombocytopathy of autosomal recessive inheritance.[76,77] Clinical manifestations are similar to those of the Bernard-Soulier syndrome. Symptoms may be quite variable, but fatalities have been reported. As opposed to the Bernard-Soulier syndrome, however, platelet counts and platelet morphology in this disease are normal.[79] The bleeding time is prolonged, glass bead retention is decreased, but platelets do adhere to subendothelium.[76,79] Clot retraction has been reported to be decreased. Platelet aggregation studies are a mirror image of those found in Bernard-Soulier syndrome—aggregation to ristocetin is normal; aggregation to collagen, ADP, and epinephrine is absent.[79] The failure of these platelets to aggregate in response to ADP is the hallmark of this abnormality. A membrane defect (decreased glycoprotein III-A and II-B) has been noted.[80] Platelet antigen A-1 is decreased.[81] It has been suggested that the functional defect in thrombasthenia is one of platelet aggregation rather than of adhesion or release.[80,82] Treatment is supportive.

The *inherited storage pool disorders* are a heterogeneous group of conditions that have in common an abnormality of the secretory phase of platelet response.[77,83] These conditions may occur as isolated phenomena involving platelet function only or may be associated with other congenital conditions. In some cases, platelet granules are absent; in others, granules are present but the release mechanism is impaired.[84] Clinically, bleeding manifestations tend to be mild to moderate. Postoperative bleeding, menorrhagia, and easy bruising often occur. The patient's platelet count and platelet morphology are usually but not invariably normal; the bleeding time may or may not be prolonged. Glass bead retention and adhesion to subendothelium are usually decreased. Platelet aggregation studies show a specific pattern. When ADP and epinephrine are employed, the first wave of aggregation is normal but the second wave does not occur. Aggregation with collagen is also impaired. As the same pattern can be seen in aspirin use, a careful drug history is required before the diagnosis can be made. Electron microscopy is helpful in further classifying the disorder. If normal platelet granules are present, a defect in platelet secretion is felt to be present. In the majority of cases, however, dense bodies or alpha granules, or both may be decreased or absent, and a true storage pool deficiency is present. Weiss and colleagues[84] have suggested a classification system based on the morphologic findings of platelet granules by electron microscopy. In addition to occurring as isolated phenomena, storage pool disorders have been described in a large number of conditions including the Hermansky-Pudlak, Chédiak-Higashi, and Wiskott-Aldrich syndromes.[76] If therapy is required, it is generally supportive. Patients should be instructed to avoid all aspirin-like products. The prognosis is usually excellent.

### Extrinsic Platelet Abnormalities

*Von Willebrand's disease* is in most cases an autosomal dominant inherited condition in which all elements of the factor VIII complex (VIII coagulant activity, VIII von Willebrand activity, and VIII antigen) are decreased.[85] The disorder is discussed more fully in Chapter 28 and will be covered only briefly here. In classic von Willebrand's disease, patients present with an abnormal partial thromboplastin time (PTT) secondary to the decreased coagulant activity of factor VIII and a prolonged bleeding time secondary to the decrease in von Willebrand's fac-

tor. However, both the presentation and the findings on laboratory evaluation may vary greatly among different patients and in the same patient over time.[85] Platelet function is defective because of the decrease in von Willebrand's factor. Glass bead retention is abnormal. Platelet aggregation studies are normal with collagen, ADP, and epinephrine; but no aggregation occurs with ristocetin. That this disorder is not due to an intrinsic platelet abnormality is shown by the ability of normal plasma (with normal von Willebrand's factor activity) to correct the platelet aggregation defect and the bleeding tendencies of the patient.[82] Von Willebrand's factor appears to be necessary for normal platelet adhesion to occur.[1,82]

*Congenital afibrinogenemia*[86] has been associated with several abnormalities in tests of platelet function: prolongation of the bleeding time, decrease in platelet aggregation, and decrease in glass bead retention. The abnormalities are corrected by the addition of fibrinogen, both in vivo and in vitro. Apparently small amounts of fibrinogen are necessary for normal platelet function to occur.

## Acquired Platelet Dysfunction Including Drug Therapy

### Intrinsic Platelet Abnormalities

*Primary disorders of the bone marrow*, including acute nonlymphocytic leukemia (ANLL) and the preleukemic syndromes, have been associated with both structural and functional abnormalities of platelets. Giant platelets, abnormalities in platelet granules, and acquired storage pool deficiencies have all been reported.[74,87] Both ANLL and the preleukemias are now felt to be clonal disorders in which the erythroid, megakaryocytic, and myeloid lines are involved in neoplastic transformation.[88] That platelet structure and function can be abnormal in these disorders is not surprising.

The *myeloproliferative syndromes* (essential thrombocythemia)—chronic myelogenous leukemia, polycythemia vera, and myelofibrosis with agnogenic myeloid metaplasia)—are all clonal marrow disorders. As discussed in the section on thrombocytosis, these disorders may be associated with elevated platelet counts. Thrombosis and hemorrhage may complicate the course of these diseases.

*Paroxysmal nocturnal hemoglobinuria* (PNH) has already been mentioned as a cause of thrombocytopenia. Abnormalities in platelet function have been noted in patients with PNH, and they are at an increased risk for thromboembolic phenomena.[89] Abnormal thrombosis may occur at unusual sites, including the hepatic, portal, splenic, and cerebral veins. These complications may be serious and in some instances fatal. The etiology of the tendency toward thrombosis in this disorder is unclear. PNH appears to be a clonal disorder in which erythroid, myeloid, and megakaryocytic cell lines are all involved. It is clear that complement deposition and activation occurs on red blood cells with resultant intravascular hemolysis. It has been suggested that complement activation on platelet surfaces may result in platelet aggregation with subsequent thrombotic complications.[89]

**Drug-Related Thrombocytopathies.** Several drugs may interfere with platelet function. Although in most cases platelet function is decreased and the risk of abnormal bleeding is increased, occasionally, as in the case of heparin use, the incidence of abnormal thromboembolic events is also increased. The risks to the individual patients can vary considerably. Individual differences in susceptibility to the effects of the drugs are great. In addition, patients with underlying hemostatic abnormalities are at an increased risk of complications when the so-called antiplatelet agents are used.

**Aspirin and Other Nonsteroidal Anti-inflammatory Agents.** The effects of the nonsteroidal anti-inflammatory agents (NSAIAs) on platelet function appear to be mediated through effects on prostaglandin synthesis.[90] NSAIAs inhibit the enzyme cyclooxygenase. Cyclooxygenase normally converts arachidonic acid to intermediates that are then converted to prostaglandins and related compounds such as thromboxane A-2 and prostacyclin.[90] Platelet thromboxane A-2 is a strong mediator of platelet aggregation and granule release, as well as local vasoconstriction. It may function by inhibiting the enzyme adenylcyclase and thus reduce cyclic AMP levels. The antiplatelet effects of aspirin and related drugs are felt to be secondary to this inhibition of thromboxane A-2 production. However, the NSAIAs also inhibit production of prostacyclin in blood vessel walls.[90] Prostacyclin normally increases cyclic AMP levels and is a potent platelet antiaggregating agent and vasodilator. Theoretically, aspirin may inhibit platelet function through its effects on platelet thromboxane A-2 production while at the same time enhancing the tendency to thrombosis by inhibiting prostacyclin production by the vessel wall. Clinically, however, the antiplatelet properties of these drugs appear to be more important.

Aspirin inhibits platelet cyclooxygenase by irreversibly acetylating the enzyme.[90] The subsequent inhibition of thromboxane A-2 lasts for the lifespan of the platelet, because mature platelets cannot produce additional cyclooxygenase. Inhibition of prostacyclin production by the vessel wall, however, is reversible, as more cyclooxygenase can be produced.[90] These observations may have significant clinical implications concerning the dose and frequency of administration of aspirin when antiplatelet effects are desired. Salicylates that do not carry acetyl groups do not affect platelet function.[91] Other NSAIAs such as indomethacin, phenylbutazone, and ibuprofen have transient antiplatelet effects because cyclooxygenase is reversibly inhibited.[92]

The laboratory findings produced by nonsteroidal anti-inflammatory agents resemble those in patients with storage pool disorders. Prolongation of the bleeding time is variable. Platelet aggregation studies show a loss of the second wave of aggregation upon testing with epinephrine and ADP. Collagen aggregation is significantly decreased.[93] Glass bead retention and subendothelial adhesion are not effected.[94]

The widespread use of aspirin over many years indicates that the antiplatelet effects of these drugs have little adverse clinical significance in most patients. However, individuals with underlying hemostatic abnormalities are at an increased risk of bleeding complications when given aspirin. Aspirin should never be used in patients with von Willebrand's disease, hemophilia, or significant underlying platelet abnormalities. On the other hand, it has been suggested that the antiplatelet effects of these drugs may actually be beneficial in certain clinical situations. The use of antiplatelet agents has been suggested in the treatment of ischemic heart disease, cerebral vascular disease, and thrombotic thrombocytopenic purpura, as well as several other conditions.[95]

*Sulfinpyrazone* is occasionally used as an antiplatelet agent. Its mechanism of action is unclear. It may reversibly inhibit cyclooxygenase, and it may also have effects on the vessel wall that inhibit thrombus formation.[91] Bleeding time is not prolonged in patients treated with this drug, and platelet aggregation studies are usually normal.[94]

*Dipyridamole* has been shown to increase platelet levels of cyclic AMP, inhibiting its breakdown by the enzyme phosphodiesterase.[91] Dipyridamole is often used in conjunction with aspirin when antiplatelet effects are desired. Although individual reports vary, the effects of dipyridamole on platelet function tests appear to be minimal.[94] In addition to its effect on cyclic AMP metabolism, the drug also can cause vasodilation, which theoretically could enhance the effect of prostaglandin inhibitors such as aspirin.[91]

*Dextran* may also significantly alter platelet function. In patients receiving dextran infusions, the bleeding time is commonly prolonged and glass bead retention decreased.[74] Effects appear to be greater with higher molecular weight dextran. Although the mechanism of action is unclear, effects on platelets' surface membranes may be involved, resulting in abnormal platelet adhesion to sites of vascular injury.[74,94]

*Heparin,* as previously mentioned, can cause both thrombocytopenia and abnormal thrombosis.[63]

The *penicillins* have also been shown to affect platelet function, particularly when the drugs are used in high doses. The effects have been best studied with carbenicillin.[96,97] The bleeding time is commonly prolonged, and platelet aggregation studies are often abnormal. Bleeding tendencies seem to be directly related to the dose of drug given. As these drugs are frequently used in patients with significant underlying illnesses, clinical bleeding may occasionally be problematic.

Several other drugs including alcohol, clofibrate, propranolol, and hydroxychloroquine have been reported to effect platelet function. The clinical significance of these findings is unclear.[74]

### Extrinsic Platelet Abnormalities

**Uremia.** Abnormal bleeding and abnormalities in platelet function may be seen in patients with renal failure. Prolonged bleeding times and decreased platelet adhesiveness have been reported.[98] The abnormalities are usually correctable by dialysis, suggesting that some as of yet unidentified antiplatelet factor accumulates in renal failure.

**Paraproteinemia.** As can occur with multiple myeloma or Waldenström's macroglobulinemia, paraproteinemia may also result in platelet dysfunction. Bleeding times are often prolonged and platelet adhesion is decreased. Factors associated with abnormal platelet function include the type of paraprotein (IgM and IgA have greater effects than IgG), the amount of the paraprotein in the blood, and the serum viscosity.[99] Effective therapy of the underlying conditions should improve the bleeding tendencies. Plasmapheresis may be effective in patients with very high levels of circulating paraproteins and the hyperviscosity syndrome. **Color Figure 237** demonstrates cryoglobulinemic purpura; amyloid purpura can be seen in **Color Figure 238,** showing the characteristic periorbital distribution.

Table 27–5 summarizes the profiles of the various platelet disorders.

## VASCULAR ABNORMALITIES ASSOCIATED WITH BLEEDING

Abnormal bleeding may occur in association with a wide variety of diseases that affect the vascular system either as a primary or secondary manifestation (Table 27–6). These disorders are characterized by easy bruising and spontaneous bleeding, particularly from small blood vessels. The underlying abnormality may affect the supporting connective tissue or the vessels themselves. The disorder may be inherited or acquired. Examination may show ec-

chymoses or petechiae in the skin, although in some cases mucosal bleeding may predominate. Laboratory investigation shows a normal platelet count and coagulation profile and occasionally a prolonged bleeding time.

## INHERITED VASCULAR DEFECTS

Von Willebrand's Disease (see also Chapter 28). As mentioned earlier in this chapter, this disorder manifests as a mixed coagulopathy and as a qualitative platelet defect due to a deficiency of elements of the factor VIII complex. It is believed that the autosomal dominant form of this disorder results from decreased or defective release of VIII:vWF multimers from the vascular endothelial cell.

**Hereditary Hemorrhagic Telangiectasia (Rendu-Weber-Osler Syndrome).** This disorder is characterized by capillary dilatations (telangiectasias), particularly in the skin and mucous membranes. The disorder is inherited as an autosomal dominant trait and may present clinically as an iron-deficient anemia. Examination may show the occurrence of the capillary telangiectasias, especially on the lips and oral cavity. Bleeding occurring from these sites results from the fragility of the abnormal vessels. Coagulation tests, platelet count, and bleeding times are normal. Treatment is directed to local bleeding sites and replacement of iron.

### Acquired Vascular Defects

**Easy Bruisability Syndrome.** This is a benign condition usually occurring in young women who present with cutaneous purpura. Clinical examination and laboratory data are otherwise normal. No treatment other than reassurance is necessary.

**Henoch-Schönlein Purpura.** Vascular damage occurs from immune complex deposition within the blood vessel walls following a viral or bacterial infection, usually in children. Characteristically, purpura develops symmetrically on the buttock and posterior thighs. **Color Figure 234** demonstrates this type of purpuric lesions located on the foot. The disorder is associated with other manifestations of immune complex injury such as arthritis, glomerulonephritis, and abdominal pain. Similarly, purpura may occur in association with other disorders producing "vasculitis" or in association with DIC.

**Decreased or Defective Vascular Supporting Tissue.** Disorders causing alterations in the vascular supporting connective tissue are often associated with ecchymoses or purpura.

In the elderly (senile purpura), in persons receiving prolonged corticosteroid therapy, or in those with Cushing's syndrome (excess endogenous corticosteroid production), purpura occurs commonly

Table 27–5. PLATELET DISORDERS

| Disorder | Pathogenesis | Clinical | Laboratory |
|---|---|---|---|
| Alport's syndrome | Hereditary nephritis and deafness. | Mild epistaxis. Occasionally fatal CNS bleeding. | Thrombocytopenia. Giant platelets. BT—abnormal. Platelet aggregation—may be abnormal, often normal. PF3 release—may be abnormal. |
| Bernard-Soulier syndrome (autosomal recessive) | Lack of glycoprotein Ib. Platelets do not bind factors V, XI. | Rather severe hemorrhagic diathesis. | Thrombocytopenia. Giant atypical platelets. Platelet retention—abnormal. Platelet adhesion—abnormal. Ristocetin agglutination—abnormal. Platelet aggregation—normal. |
| Chédiak-Higashi syndrome (autosomal recessive) | Storage pool deficiency. Large organelles, some with acid phosphatase. | Increased susceptibility to pyogenic infections. | BT—abnormal. Platelet adhesion—abnormal. Platelet aggregation—abnormal. |
| Cyclooxygenase deficiency (inheritance undetermined) | Inability to activate prostaglandin pathway. "Aspirin-like" defect. | Moderate bleeding tendency. Ecchymoses. | BT—abnormal. Platelet aggregation—abnormal. |
| Essential athrombia | | Mucosal bleeding. Easy bruising. | BT—abnormal. Platelet count—normal. Platelet aggregation—abnormal. |
| Fanconi's syndrome (autosomal recessive) | Inborn error of metabolism. Megakaryocytic hypoplasia. | Pancytopenia. Dwarfism. Microcephaly. Hypogenitalism. Strabismus. Mental retardation. Micro-ophthalmia. Splenic atrophy. Anomalies of thumbs, radial bones, kidneys. | Thrombocytopenia. |
| Glanzmann's thrombasthenia | Lack of glycoproteins IIb, IIIa. | Severe bleeding—purpuric with spontaneous mucosal and cutaneous bleeding aggravated by trauma. Occasional hemarthrosis. Severity decreases with age. | BT—abnormal. Clot retraction—none. Platelet adhesion—abnormal. Platelet count—generally normal. Platelet aggregation—abnormal. Ristocetin agglutination—normal. |
| Glycogen storage disease, type I (autosomal recessive?) | Storage pool deficiency. Glucose-6-phosphatase deficiency | Mild bleeding. Corrects with treatment for enzyme deficiency. | BT—abnormal. Platelet aggregation—abnormal. PF3 activity—abnormal. |
| Gray platelet syndrome (autosomal recessive?) | Storage pool deficiency. Absence of α-granules. Platelets appear amorphous. Large platelets. | | BT—abnormal. Platelet adhesion—abnormal. Platelet aggregation—abnormal. Thrombocytopenia. |

**Table 27–5. PLATELET DISORDERS** *(continued)*

| Disorder | Pathogenesis | Clinical | Laboratory |
|---|---|---|---|
| Hermansky-Pudlak syndrome (autosomal recessive) | Storage pool deficiency. Absence of dense bodies. | Oculocutaneous albinism. Ceroid-like pigment in macrophages. | BT—abnormal. Platelet aggregation—abnormal. Platelet adhesion—abnormal. |
| May-Hegglin (autosomal dominant) | Ineffective thrombopoiesis. | Giant platelets. Doehle bodies. Generally asymptomatic. Possible severe bleeding. | Thrombocytopenia. BT—abnormal. |
| Tar-baby syndrome (thrombocytopenia with absent radii) (autosomal recessive) | Storage pool deficiency. Megakaryocytic hypoplasia. | Skeletal, renal, and cardiac malformations. Decreased dense bodies. | BT—abnormal. Platelet aggregation—abnormal. |
| Thrombocythomia (essential/primary) | | Associated with myeloproliferative disorders—polycythemia rubra vera, myeloid metaplasia, CML. | Platelet count—high, may be > 1,000,000/$\mu$l. Large platelets. Platelet retention—abnormal. Platelet aggregation—abnormal. BT—abnormal. |
| Von Willebrand's syndrome (autosomal dominant) | Low levels of plasma co-factor (VIII:vWF). | Variable clinical symptoms—may bleed. Generally vascular and mucosal bleeding. Severity depends on VIII:C levels. | Lab-testing variable. BT—abnormal. Platelet retention—abnormal. Platelet aggregation—normal. Ristocetin agglutination—abnormal. VIII R:Ag—abnormal. VIII:C—abnormal. |
| Wiskott-Aldrich syndrome (sex-linked recessive) | Storage pool deficiency. Immunologic disorders—B & T cell dysfunction. Isohemagglutinins absent. | Recurrent pyogenic infection. Eczema. Increased lymphoreticular malignancies. Very small platelets. Decreased or absent dense bodies. Mild-moderate bleeding—mucocutaneous bleeding, epistaxis, easy bruising. | Thrombocytopenia—severe. Shortened survival. BT—abnormal. Platelet aggregation—abnormal. IgM—low. IgG, IgA—normal. |

From Pittiglio, DH: Treating hemostatic disorders. A problem-oriented approach. In Hemostasis Overview. American Association of Blood Banks, Arlington, VA, 1984, p 22.
BT = bleeding time.

**Table 27–6. VASCULAR ABNORMALITIES ASSOCIATED WITH BLEEDING**

I. Inherited vascular defects
  A. Von Willebrand's disease
  B. Hereditary hemorrhage telangiectasia
II. Acquired vascular disorders
  A. Easy bruisability syndrome
  B. Henoch-Schönlein purpura
  C. Senile purpura
  D. Steroid purpura
  E. Scurvy
  F. Toxins
  G. Nonsteroidal drugs

on the hands and forearms (**see Color Figures 235 and 236**). Vascular connective tissue may also be abnormal because of defective collagen synthesis found in patients with vitamin C deficiency (scurvy), or because of abnormal deposits in the connective tissue, as may occur in those with amyloid purpura, with hemorrhages occurring in the gums, periosteal-perifollicular distribution, and periorbital areas, respectively.

**Toxins and Drugs.** Toxic damage to the vasculature may occur during infections or with use of nonsteroidal anti-inflammatory drugs (NSHIDs), despite a normal platelet count and bleeding time.

Table 27–7 summarizes the profiles of the various vascular disorders.

Table 27-7. VASCULAR DISORDERS

| Disorder | Pathogenesis | Clinical | Laboratory |
|---|---|---|---|
| Hereditary hemorrhagic telangiectasia (Osler-Weber-Rendu) (autosomal dominant; most common vascular disorder associated with hemorrhagic diathesis) | Large capillaries. Elastic fibers possibly missing. Pinpoint, nodular, or spider-like telangiectatic lesions in adults. | Epistaxis in childhood. Mucocutaneous bleeding. Associated classic DIC-type syndrome. | BT—normal or abnormal. Tourniquet test—often abnormal. Normal platelet function test results. |
| Marfan's syndrome (autosomal dominant) | Collagen vascular disorder. Skeletal defects—long extremities, arachnodactylia, "Lincolnesque" features. Cardiovascular abnormalities—diffuse or descending aortic aneurysm. Ocular defects. | Easy bruising. | Large platelets. Platelet adhesion—abnormal. Platelet aggregation—abnormal. |
| Osteogenesis imperfecta (autosomal dominant) | Collagen vascular disorder. Brittle bone disease—lack of bone matrix. Blue sclera. | Skin and subcutaneous hemorrhages. Easy bruising. Epistaxis. | BT—abnormal. Tourniquet test—abnormal. Platelet adhesion—abnormal. Platelet aggregation—abnormal. |
| Pseudoxanthoma elasticum (autosomal recessive; rare) | Abnormal elastic fibers throughout arterial system. | Significant hemorrhage. Easy, spontaneous bruising. Petechiae. Purpura. Marked predisposition to thrombosis. | |
| Homocystinuria (autosomal recessive) | Cystathione synthetase deficiency. | Occasional mild bleeding. Generally have arterial and venous thrombosis. | Possibly short platelet survival. Unknown effect on platelet function. |
| Kasabach-Merritt syndrome | Giant cavernous hemangioma. | Mild bleeding at site of hemangioma. Diffuse bleeding in association with DIC. | Thrombocytopenia. Low fibrinogen. High plasma fibrinopeptide A and FDP. |

From Pittiglio, DH: Treating hemostatic disorders. A problem-oriented approach. In Hemostasis Overview. American Association of Blood Banks, Arlington, VA, 1984, p 19.
BT = bleeding time.

# References

1. Shattil, SJ and Bennett, JS: Platelets and their membranes in homeostasis: Physiology and pathophysiology. Ann Intern Med 94:108, 1980.
2. Williams, WJ: Clinical manifestations of disorders of homeostasis. In Williams, WJ, Beutler, E, Erslev, AJ, et al (eds): Hematology. McGraw-Hill, New York, 1983, p 69.
3. Payne, BA and Pierre, RV: Pseudothrombocytopenia: A laboratory artifact with potentially serious consequences. Mayo Clin Proc 59:123, 1984.
4. Chabner, BA and Myers, CE: Clinical pharmacology of cancer chemotherapy. In DeVita, VT, Hellman, S, and Rosenberg, SA (eds): Cancer: Principles and Practice of Oncology. JB Lippincott, Philadelphia, 1982, p 156.
5. Young, N and Mortimer, P: Viruses and bone marrow failure. Blood 63:729, 1984.
6. Lindenbaum, J and Hargrove, RL: Thrombocytopenia in alcoholics. Ann Intern Med 68:526, 1968.
7. Post, RM and Desforges, JF: Thrombocytopenia and alcoholism. Ann Intern Med 68:1230, 1968.
8. Dutti, J and Weinfeld, A: The frequency of thrombocytopenia in patients with heart disease treated with diuretics. Acta Med Scand 183:245, 1968.
9. Stoll, DB, Blum, S, Pasquale, D, et al: Thrombocytopenia with decreased megakaryocytes: Evaluation and prognosis. Ann Intern Med 94:170, 1981.
10. Gaydos, LA, Freirich, EJ, and Mantel, N: The quantitative relation between platelet count and hemorrhage in patients with acute leukemia. N Engl J Med 266:905, 1962.
11. Lister, TA and Yankee, RA: Blood component therapy. Clin Haematol 7:407, 1978.
12. Gardner, FH: Preservation and clinical use of platelets. In Williams, WJ, Beutler, E, Erslev, AJ, et al (eds): Hematology. McGraw-Hill, New York, 1983, p 1556.
13. Karpatkin, S: Autoimmune thrombocytopenic purpura. Blood 56:329, 1980.
14. Koller, CA: Immune thrombocytopenic purpura. Med Clin North Am 64:716, 1980.
15. McMillan, R: Chronic idiopathic thrombocytopenic purpura. N Engl J Med 304:1135, 1981.
16. McClure, PD: Idiopathic thrombocytopenic purpura in children: Diagnosis and management. Pediatrics 55:68, 1975.
17. McClure, PD: Idiopathic thrombocytopenic purpura: Should corticosteroids be given? Am J Dis Child 131:357, 1977.

18. McElfresh, AE: Idiopathic thrombocytopenic purpura: To treat or not to treat. J Pediatr 87:160, 1975.

19. Dixon, R, Rosse, W, and Ebbert, L: Quantitative determination of antibody in idiopathic thrombocytopenia purpura: Correlation of serum and platelet-bound antibody with clinical response. N Engl J Med 292:230, 1975.

20. Hedge, UM, Gordon-Smith, EC, and Worledge, S: Platelet antibodies in thrombocytopenic patients. Br J Haematol 35:113, 1977.

21. LoBuglio, AF, Court, WS, Vinocur, L, et al: Immune thrombocytopenic purpura: use of a $^{125}$I-labeled antihuman IgG monoclonal antibody to quantify platelet-bound IgG. N Engl J Med 309:459, 1983.

22. Murphy, S: In search of a platelet Coombs test. N Engl J Med 309:490, 1983.

23. DiFino, SM, Lachart, NA, Kirshner, JK, et al: Adult idiopathic thrombocytopenia: Clinical findings and response to therapy. Am J Med 69:430, 1980.

24. Ahn, YS, Harrington, WJ, Seelman, RC, et al: Vincristine therapy of idiopathic and secondary thrombocytopenias. N Engl J Med 291:376, 1974.

25. Ahn, YS, Harrington, WJ, Mylvaganam, R, et al: Slow infusion of vinca alkaloids in the treatment of idiopathic thrombocytopenic purpura. Ann Intern Med 100:192, 1984.

26. Ahn, YS, Byrnes, JJ, Harrington, WJ, et al: The treatment of idiopathic thrombocytopenia with vinblastine loaded platelets. N Engl J Med 298:1101, 1978.

27. Laros, RK and Penner, JA: "Refractory" thrombocytopenic purpura treated successfully with cyclophosphamide. JAMA 215:445, 1971.

28. Sussman, LN: Azathioprine in refractory idiopathic thrombocytopenic purpura. JAMA 202:259, 1967.

29. Fehr, J, Hofmann, V, and Kappeler, V: Transient reversal of thrombocytopenia in idiopathic thrombocytopenic purpura by high-dose intravenous gamma globulin. N Engl J Med 306:1254–8, 1982.

30. Ahn, YS, Harrington, WJ, Simon, SR, et al: Danazol for the treatment of idiopathic thrombocytopenic purpura. N Engl J Med 308:1396, 1983.

31. Picozz, VJ, Roeske, WR, and Cregor, WP: Fate of therapy failures in adult idiopathic thrombocytopenic purpura. Am J Med 69:690, 1980.

32. Ellman, L, Carvelho, A, Jacobson, BM, et al: Platelet autoantibodies in a case of infectious mononucleosis presenting as thrombocytopenic purpura. Am J Med 55:723, 1973.

33. Kim, HD and Boggs, DR: A syndrome resembling idiopathic thrombocytopenic purpura in 10 patients with diverse forms of cancer. Am J Med 67:371, 1979.

34. Bellone, JD, Kunicki, TJ, and Aster, RH: Immune thrombocytopenia associated with carcinoma. Ann Intern Med 79:470, 1983.

35. Morris, L, Distenfeld, A, Amorosi, E, et al: Autoimmune thrombocytopenic purpura in homosexual males. Ann Intern Med 96:714, 1982.

36. Aster, RH: Thrombocytopenia due to enhanced platelet destruction. In Williams, WJ, Beutler, E, Erslev, AJ, et al (eds): Hematology. McGraw-Hill, New York, 1983 p 1313.

37. Bolton, FG and Damesheck, W: Thrombocytopenia due to quinidine: I. Clinical studies. Blood 11:527, 1956.

38. Bolton, FG: Thrombocytopenic purpura due to quinidine: II. Serologic mechanisms. Blood 11:547, 1956.

39. Abramson, N, Eisenberg, PD, and Aster, RH: Post-transfusion purpura: immunologic aspects and therapy. N Engl J Med 291:1103, 1974.

40. Shulman, NR, Aster, RH, Leitner, A, et al: Immunoreactions involving platelets: V. Post-transfusion purpura due to a complement fixing antibody against a genetically controlled platelet antigen: a proposed mechanism for thrombocytopenia and its relevance in "autoimmunity." J Clin Invest 40:1597, 1961.

41. Weisberg, LJ and Linker, CA: Prednisone therapy and post-transfusion purpura. Ann Intern Med 100:76, 1984.

42. Kelton, JG: Management of the pregnant patient with idiopathic thrombocytopenic purpura. Ann Intern Med 99:796, 1983.

43. Kelton, JG, Inwood, MJ, Barr, RM, et al: The prenatal prediction of thrombocytopenia in infants of mothers with clinically diagnosed immune thrombocytopenia. Am J Obstet Gynecol 144:449, 1982.

44. Cines, DB, Dusak, B, Tomaski, A, et al: Immune thrombocytopenia purpura and pregnancy. N Engl J Med 306:826, 1982.

45. Karpatkin, M, Porges, RI, and Karpatkin, S: Platelet counts in infants of woman with autoimmune thrombocytopenia. N Engl J Med 305:936, 1981.

46. Amorosi, EC and Ultman, JE: Thrombotic thrombocytopenic purpura. Report of 16 cases and review of the literature. Medicine 45:135, 1966.

47. Rosove, MH, Ho, WG, and Goldfinger, D: Ineffectiveness of aspirin and dipyridamole in the treatment of thrombotic thrombocytopenic purpura. Ann Intern Med 96:27, 1982.

48. Rudolf, RL, Hutchins, GM, and Bell, WR: The heart and cardiac conduction system in thrombotic thrombocytopenic purpura. Ann Intern Med 91:357, 1979.

49. Myers, TJ, Wakem, CJ, Ball, EA, et al: Thrombotic thrombocytopenic purpura: Combined treatment with plasmapheresis and antiplatelet agents. Ann Intern Med 92:149, 1980.

50. Lian, EC-Y, Harkness, DR, Byrnes, JJ, et al: Presence of a platelet aggregating factor in the plasma of patients with thrombotic thrombocytopenic purpura (TTP) and its inhibition by normal plasma. Blood 53:333, 1979.

51. Goodman, A, Ramos, R, Petrolli, M, et al: Gingival biopsy in thrombotic thrombocytopenic purpura. Ann Intern Med 89:501, 1978.

52. Amorosi, EL and Karpatkin, S: Antiplatelet therapy of thrombotic thrombocytopenic purpura. Ann Intern Med 86:102, 1977.

53. Byrnes, JJ and Khurana M: Treatment of thrombotic thrombocytopenic purpura with plasma. N Engl J Med 297:1386, 1977.

54. Cuttner, J: Splenectomy, steroids, and dextran 70 in thrombotic thrombocytopenic purpura. JAMA 227:397, 1974.

55. Gutterman, LA and Stevenson, TD: Treatment of thrombotic thrombocytopenic purpura with vincristine. JAMA 247:1433, 1982.

56. Fitzgerald, GA, Maas, RL, Stein, R, et al: Intravenous prostacyclin in thrombotic thrombocytopenic purpura. Ann Intern Med 95:319, 1981.

57. Harkness, DR, Byrnes, JJ, Lian, EC-Y, et al: Hazard of platelet transfusion in thrombotic thrombocytopenic purpura. JAMA 246:1931, 1981.

58. Goldstein, MH, Churg, J, Strauss, L, et al: Hemolytic uremic syndrome. Nephron 23:263, 1979.

59. Musgrave, JE, Taluclken, YB, Puri, HC, et al: The hemolytic-uremic syndrome. Clin Pediatr 17:218, 1978.

60. Ponticelli, C, Rivolta, E, Imbasciati, E, et al: Hemolytic uremic syndrome in adults. Arch Intern Med 140:353, 1980.

61. Bick, RL: Disseminated intravascular coagulation and related syndromes: Etiology, pathophysiology, diagnosis, and management. Am J Hematol 5:205, 1978.

62. King, DJ and Kelton, JG: Heparin-associated thrombocytopenia. Ann Intern Med 100:535, 1984.

63. Bell, WR, Tomasulo, PA, Alving, BM, et al: Thrombocytopenia occurring during heparin administration. A prospective study in 52 patients. Ann Intern Med 85:155, 1976.

64. Cines, DB, Kaywin, P, Bina, M, et al: Heparin-associated thrombocytopenia. N Engl J Med 303:788, 1980.

65. Perkins, RP: Thrombocytopenia in obstetrical syndromes: V. A review. Obstet Gynecol Surv 34:101, 1979.

66. Wintrobe, MM, Lee, GR, Boggs, DR, et al (eds): Disorders primarily involving the spleen. In Clinical Hematology. Lea & Febiger, Philadelphia, 1981, p 1426.

67. Wintrobe, MM, Lee, GR, Boggs, DR, et al (eds): Thrombocytopenia following massive blood transfusions. In Clinical Hematology. Lea & Febiger, Philadelphia, 1981, p 1116.

68. Williams, WJ: Thrombocytosis. In Williams, WJ, Beutler, E, Erslev, AJ, et al (eds): Hematology. McGraw-Hill, New York, 1983, p 1342.

69. Murphy, S: Disorders of platelet production. In Colman, RW, Hirsh, J, Marder, VJ, et al (eds): Hemostasis and Thrombosis. JP Lippincott, Philadelphia, 1982, p 259.

70. Weinfeld, A, Branehog, I, and Kutl, J: Platelets in the myeloproliferative syndrome. Clin Haematol 4:373, 1975.

71. Walsh, PN, Murphy, S, and Barry, WE: The role of platelets in pathogenesis of thrombosis and hemorrhage in patients with thrombosis. Thromb Haemost 38:1085, 1977.

72. Jabaily, J, Ilard, HJ, Laszlo, J, et al: Neurologic manifestations of essential thrombocythemia. Ann Intern Med 99:513, 1983.

73. Ginsburg, AD: Platelet function in patients with high platelet counts. Ann Intern Med 82:506, 1975.

74. Malpacs, TW and Harker, LA: Acquired disorders of platelet function. Sem Hematol 17:242, 1980.

75. Wintrobe, MM, Lee, GR, Lee, GR, Boggs, DR, et al (eds): Thrombocytosis. In Clinical Hematology. Lea & Febiger, Philadelphia, 1981, p 1128.

76. Weiss, H: Congenital disorders of platelet function. Sem Hematol 17:228, 1980.

77. George, JN and Reimann, TA: Inherited disorders of the platelet membrane: Glanzmann's thrombasthenic and Bernard-Soulier disease. In Colman, RW, Hirsh, J, Marder, VJ, et al (eds): Hemostasis and Thrombosis. JP Lippincott, Philadelphia, 1982, p 496.

78. Howard, MA, Hilton, RA, and Hardisty, RM: Hereditary giant platelet syndrome: A disorder of a new aspect of platelet functions. Br Med J 2:586, 1973.

79. Caen, JP, Casteldi, PA, Leclerc, JC, et al: Congenital bleeding disorders with long bleeding times and normal platelet counts. I. Glanzmann's thrombasthenia. Am J Med 41:4, 1966.

80. Phillips, DR and Pom Agin, P: Platelet membrane defects in Glanzmann's thrombasthenia. J Clin Invest 60:535, 1977.

81. Kunichi, TJ and Aster, RH: Deletion of the platelet specific alloantigen P1^A1 from platelets with Glanzmann's thrombasthenia. J Clin Invest 61:1225, 1978.

82. Weiss, HJ: Platelet physiology and abnormalities of platelet function. N Engl J Med 293:531, 1975.

83. Weiss, HJ: Inherited disorders of platelet secretion. In Colman, RW, Hirsh, J, Marder, VJ, et al (eds): Hemostasis and Thrombosis. JP Lippincott, Philadelphia, 1982. p 507.

84. Weiss, HJ, Wittie, LD, Kaplan, KL, et al: Heterogeneity in storage pool deficiency: Studies on granule bound substances in 18 patients including variants deficiency in alpha granules, platelet factor 4, beta-thromboglobulin, and platelet derived growth factor. Blood 54:1293, 1979.

85. Bloom, AL: The Von Willebrand syndrome. Sem Hematol 17:215, 1980.

86. Weiss, HJ and Rogers, J: Fibrinogen and platelets in the primary arrest of bleeding: Studies in two patients with congenital afibrinogenemia. N Engl J Med 285:369, 1971.

87. Cowan, DH, Graham, RC, and Baunach, D: The platelet defect in leukemia. J Clin Invest 56:188, 1975.

88. Koeffler, HP and Golde, DW: Human preleukemia. Ann Intern Med 93:345, 1980.

89. Schreiber, AD: Paroxysmal nocturnal hemoglobinuria revisited. N Engl J Med 309:723, 1983.

90. Moncada, S and Vane JR: Arachidonic acid metabolites and the interaction between platelets and blood-vessel walls. N Engl J Med 300:1142, 1979.

91. Fuster, V and Chesboro, JH: Antithrombotic therapy: Role of platelet-inhibitor drugs. II. Pharmacologic effects of platelet inhibition drugs. Mayo Clin Proc 56:185, 1981.

92. O'Brien, JR, Finch, W, and Clark, E: A comparison of an effect of different anti-inflammatory drugs on human platelets. J Clin Pathol 23:522, 1970.

93. Wintrobe, MM, Lee, GR, Boggs, DR, et al (eds): Thrombosis and antithrombotic therapy. In Clinical Hematology. Lea & Febiger, Philadelphia, 1981, p 1262.

94. Weiss, HJ: Antiplatelet therapy. N Engl J Med 298:1344, 1978.

95. Weiss, HJ: Antiplatelet therapy. N Engl J Med 298:1403, 1978.

96. Brown, CH, Natelson, EA, Bradshaw, MW, et al: The hemostatic defect produced by carbenicillin. N Engl J Med 291:265, 1974.

97. Brown, CH, Bradshaw, MW, Natelson, EA, et al: Defective platelet function following the administration of penicillin compounds. Blood 47:949, 1976.

98. Eknoyan, G, Wacksman, SJ, Glueck, HI, et al: Platelet function in renal failure. N Engl J Med 280:677, 1969.

99. Perkins, HA, Mackenzie, MR, Fudenberg, HH: Hemostatic defects in dysproteinemia. Blood 35:695, 1970.

# CHAPTER 28

G. ROCK, M.D., Ph.D.

# Defects of Plasma Clotting Factors

The plasma clotting factors circulate as inactive precursors, known as zymogens. When coagulation is initiated, each zymogen and cofactor is converted to its active form, an enzyme, which then participates in the coagulation cascade leading to the formation of thrombin. Thrombin then converts the soluble plasma protein fibrinogen into an insoluble fibrin clot (see Chapter 26).

Impaired coagulation can result from a number of defects in the individual plasma clotting factors, which can alter both the rate of coagulation and the type of clot that is formed. These defects can be produced by:

1. Decreased synthesis of the factors
2. Synthesis of abnormal molecules
3. Loss or consumption of the factors
4. Inappropriate inactivation of these factors by inhibitors or antibodies

Such defects may be inherited or acquired, with their frequency ranging from extremely rare to relatively common and their occurrence ranging from causing little harm to life-threatening problems. The acquired coagulation disorders are seen in clinical practice more frequently than the hereditary disorders and are usually associated with multiple clotting factor deficiencies. They can be caused by vitamin K deficiency, liver disease, diffuse intravascular thrombosis, and fibrinolysis. Massive transfusion without fresh frozen plasma (FFP) replacement can also cause coagulation defects. The coagulation disorders will be discussed in sequence.

## FACTOR I—FIBRINOGEN

Fibrinogen, a protein with a molecular weight of 345,000, is synthesized in the liver and is the most abundant coagulation factor present in the circulation of normal individuals with plasma levels of 200 to 400 mg/dl. Fibrinogen is converted, by the action of thrombin, to insoluble fibrin, one of the main constituents of the clot. The formation of a stable clot is essential for achieving effective hemostasis. During clotting, thrombin cleaves a single peptide bond in each of the chains of fibrinopeptide A and B. The resulting fibrin monomers polymerize spontaneously to form insoluble fibrin polymers, which are strengthened by the action of factor XIIIa to produce a tough fibrin clot (see Chapter 26).

Fortunately, congenital afibrinogenemia, or absence of fibrinogen, is a rare disorder. About 60 cases of this inherited disease, in which there is an almost total lack of circulating fibrinogen, have been reported. It appears to result from a failure of synthesis of adequate amounts of fibrinogen, rather than an increased rate of destruction (i.e., fibrinogenolysis), or from loss through consumption. This disorder is transmitted by an autosomal recessive gene, with the disease occurring in both sexes, although more cases have been reported in men than in women. These patients have repeated episodes of bleeding throughout their lives, but they may have long periods without serious bleeding. Bleeding may occur from the umbilical cord at birth, although patients with congenital afibrinogenemia have less severe bleeding than the average patient with hemophilia A. Two patients with this disorder who have been treated by repeat infusions of fibrinogen have developed antibodies to fibrinogen.

Congenital hypofibrinogenemia has also been reported; this too is a rare disorder. These patients usually have mild hemorrhagic symptoms, and although their blood usually clots spontaneously, the fibrinogen levels are moderately low (20 to 100 mg/dl).

Congenital dysfibrinogenemia, on the other hand, is due to the presence of qualitatively abnormal and therefore functionally defective fibrinogen. The presence of the abnormal protein can result in problems at any stage of the conversion of fibrinogen to fibrin by thrombin, which can result in altered rates of clotting. In some patients, it has been determined that there is a defect in aggregation of the fibrin monomers, whereas in others there is a defect in the cleavage of fibrinopeptides A and B, or A and AP (a subclass of A), possibly as a result of molecular defects in the proteins themselves. Other biochemical abnormalities in the fibrinogen protein have also been reported and, again, result in defective formation of fibrin. This disorder appears to be autosomal dominant, with both sexes equally affected. The presence of abnormal fibrinogens has not been associated with any single clinical presentation: rather, there appears to be a wide variety of manifestations including mild bleeding tendencies, occurrence of thrombosis, and no symptomatic problems.

In most patients with congenital dysfibrinogenemia, a visible clot is spontaneously formed; this is in contrast to patients with congenital afibrinogenemia whose blood does not form clots. The clotting time of whole blood or recalcified plasma in patients with congenital afibrinogenemia may be normal or prolonged, but the appearance of the clot may be abnormal, appearing soft and friable.

Acquired dysfibrinogenemia has been demonstrated and, although it must be distinguished from the inherited form of the disorder, it presents clinically in much the same way. Acquired deficiencies of fibrinogen are distinguished from dysfibrinogenemia on the basis of comparable reduction of fibrinogen regardless of the techniques used to measure fibrinogen and the fact that there is no family history of the disorder.

## Laboratory Assessment

Diagnosis of congenital afibrinogenemia is relatively simple. Laboratory abnormalities are severe despite the mild clinical symptoms usually seen. The diagnostic laboratory tests for afibrinogenemia include an infinite prothrombin time (PT), partial thromboplastin time (PTT), thrombin time (TT), reptilase time, and the absence of clot formation. Assay of fibrinogen levels by clotting techniques involving the use of thrombin show markedly decreased to absent fibrinogen levels in congenital afibrinogenemia; however, trace levels may be found by immunologic methods. Other laboratory findings that may be associated with congenital afibrinogenemia include mild thrombocytopenia, normal to prolonged bleeding time, normal thromboplastin generation test, and an abnormal sedimentation rate.

Patients with hypofibrinogenemia present with laboratory findings less severe than in those with afibrinogenemia. This disorder might be suggested in patients with a previous history of mild bleeding and when coagulation studies reveal an abnormal clot retraction and a variable PT and PTT. The typical coagulation profile found in patients with hypofibrinogenemia would show a prolonged PT and PTT, abnormal clot retraction with increased red cell fallout, and slightly to moderately decreased fibrinogen levels.

Laboratory findings in patients with dysfibrinogenemia may demonstrate a wide variety of abnormalities. With the exception of fibrinogen Oslow (short thrombin time) and Oklahoma (normal thrombin time), all the dysfibrinogenemias are well characterized by a prolonged to infinite thrombin time and reptilase time. Also characteristic of the dysfibrinogenemias is a normal level of fibrinogen with immunologic or precipitation methods, but decreased levels of fibrinogen based on the measurement of thrombin clottable protein. Other laboratory findings associated with dysfibrinogenemia include normal to prolonged whole blood clotting time, a friable clot, clots insoluble in 5M urea, prolonged PT, prolonged Stypven time, normal to prolonged PTT, normal thromboplastin generation test, and a normal to prolonged bleeding time in the face of normal platelet numbers and morphology (see Chapter 31).

It should be noted that the thrombin time cannot be used as a means to assess the level of fibrinogen in patients on heparin therapy. The thrombin time will be prolonged in the presence of heparin. The snake venom (Bothrops atrox) known as reptilase R has a direct action on fibrinogen to convert it to fibrin, which is not inhibited by the presence of heparin. The use of reptilase R as an adjunct to the thrombin time is helpful in evaluating an abnormal thrombin time. A normal reptilase time and a prolonged thrombin time suggest the presence of heparin. A prolonged reptilase time and a prolonged thrombin time suggest a fibrinogen deficiency, dysfibrinogenemia, or high levels of circulating fibrin(ogen) degradation products (see Chapter 31).

## Half-Life and Treatment of Deficiency

The biologic half-life of fibrinogen in humans has been reported to be from 1.5 to 6.3 days.

Fibrinogen replacement therapy may be accomplished by infusing cryoprecipitate or purified fibrinogen. Each bag of cryoprecipitate contains approximately 250 mg of fibrinogen. The initial loading dose of cryoprecipitate is approximately 4 bags/10 kg or 100 mg/kg for the purified fibrinogen. Maintenance is carried out using 1 bag of cryoprecipitate/10 kg/48 hr or 20 mg purified fibrinogen/kg/48 hr. Although most factor VIII concentrates contain a high level of fibrinogen, they are not generally used to treat this deficiency, owing to the waste of factor VIII. Because of its stability, fibrinogen can be prepared from plasma separated from outdated blood. The supernatant from cryoprecipitate can also be used as a source of fibrinogen. Fibrinogen concentrates are seldom used because of the substantially high risk of hepatitis.

## FACTOR II — PROTHROMBIN

This glycoprotein, which is one of the vitamin K–dependent clotting factors, is the precursor substance of thrombin. Thrombin, the terminal proteolytic enzyme produced by the coagulation cascade, attacks not only fibrinogen but also fibrin and other proteins. The molecular weight of prothrombin appears to be between 52,000 and 70,000. Purified prothrombin contains 10 percent carbohydrate and migrates electrophoretically as an alpha globulin. No subunits have been demonstrated. The actual chemistry of prothrombin is closely related to that of factors VII, IX, and X. Plasma levels of prothrombin are calculated by the number of units of thrombin formation.

Congenital deficiency of prothrombin is extremely rare, and in general, hemorrhagic manifestations have been mild with bleeding from mucous membranes, excessive bruising, and menorrhagia.

Acquired defects of single vitamin K–dependent coagulant factors are rare, and deficiencies generally relate to all of the vitamin K–dependent factors (factors II, VII, IX, and X). The most common causes are liver dysfunction, abnormalities in the absorption of vitamin K from the intestinal tract, continued use of broad-spectrum antibiotics, and vitamin K intake depleting oral anticoagulant drugs (e.g., Coumadin).

## Laboratory Assessment

There is a prolonged one-stage prothrombin time that is not corrected by the addition of absorbed normal plasma or aged serum, or when using Russell's viper venom as the thromboplastin (see Chapter 31). There is a prolonged PTT but normal levels of factors I, V, VII, and X. Prothrombin measured by either the one- or the two-stage method is significantly decreased. The one-stage assay involves mixing adsorbed ox plasma (which supplies factor V and fibrinogen) and normal serum (which supplies factors VII and X) as substrate or using commercial factor II–depleted plasma. Care must be taken to adsorb the ox plasma twice so that it is absolutely free of prothrombin. The assay is performed using the PT method. The two-stage assay is more reliable and involves generating thrombin and adding fibrinogen. The amount of the thrombin formed is proportional to the amount of prothrombin present.

## Half-Life and Treatment of Deficiency

The half-life of prothrombin in the circulation is about eight hours, with approximately 30 to 40 percent of the total body prothrombin distributed in the extravascular compartment. Treatment of the deficiency involves administering prothrombin complex, which contains factors II, VII, IX, and X. Alternately, fresh frozen plasma may be administered. Approximately 40 percent of the normal level of prothrombin is required for hemostasis.

## FACTOR V (PROACCELERIN)

Factor V is one of the unstable labile coagulation factors, a property that has made its characterization very difficult. It has a molecular weight estimated to be greater than 200,000 and, when attacked by thrombin, is activated, producing both an increase in activity and a decrease in molecular size.

Hereditary deficiencies of factor V were first reported in 1947. The disorder is transmitted as an incompletely recessive autosomal disease and equally affects both sexes. The number of clinically affected individuals is relatively low; however, heterozygotes with factor V levels ranging from 20 to 60 percent of normal are encountered more frequently. In patients with this disorder bruising follows trivial injury and epistaxis may be severe, with bleeding from mucous membranes being the most frequent manifestation. Menorrhagia is a common complaint in female patients with this disorder; deep intramuscular hematoma or hemarthrosis rarely occurs.

A rare but well-documented autosomal inherited coagulation defect is a combined deficiency of factors V and VIII, which may result from a deficiency of protein C inhibitor. The laboratory findings are characteristic of both of these deficiencies.

Acquired deficiency of factor V occurs in patients with disseminated intravascular coagulation and those with severe liver disease.

## Laboratory Assessment

The PT and PTT (activated or unactivated) are prolonged. Despite a very long prothrombin time (which indicates a low level of factor V), some patients do not have severe manifestations of the disease.

When testing for this deficiency, it is important to remember that a phospholipid source other than normal platelets must be used, because factor V is present in normal platelets. It is not present in platelets of factor V–deficient patients; therefore, their platelets could be used.

## Half-Life and Treatment of Deficiency

Usual values for the half-life of factor V range from 12 to 15 hours, although values up to 36 hours have also been reported. There appears to be an extravascular pooling of factor V, and in addition, factor V is found adsorbed to the surface of platelets.

This deficiency is treated by the administration of fresh frozen plasma. The usual dose is 10 to 15 ml/kg, and the level required for hemostasis is approximately 10 to 15 percent of normal.

## FACTOR VII

Factor VII is a glycoprotein containing up to 50 percent carbohydrate. The molecular weight as estimated from gel filtration studies is 48,000 in serum and 63,000 in plasma. The concentration of factor VII in human serum has been estimated at about 8 to 16 $\mu$g/ml. Factor VII is said to be stable during storage in both plasma and in serum.

Hereditary deficiency of factor VII is transmitted

as a highly penetrant, incompletely recessive, autosomal trait. It is manifested as a hemorrhagic state characterized by a prolonged prothrombin time but a normal PTT or whole blood clotting time. This disease is very rare, with a variable presentation of bleeding, depending on the level of factor VII. Based on reactivity with rabbit antibody, it is possible to define at least two different types of hereditary factor VII deficiency. Some patients who have only a slight prolongation of the one-stage prothrombin time have very little clinical effect; however, when the PT is more prolonged, significant bleeding can occur.

Acquired defects relate to those of the other vitamin K–dependent factors.

## Laboratory Assessment

The PTT in these patients is completely normal, whereas the PT is prolonged. The PT is fully corrected by using a snake venom (Russell's viper venom) as the thromboplastin (see Chapter 31 for the reptilase time). All tests that do not use tissue factor have normal results. A definitive diagnosis is obtained by testing prothrombin time with a mixture of equal parts of patient's plasma and plasma from a patient with a previously established deficiency.

## Half-Life and Treatment of Deficiency

There are two phases to the disappearance curve of factor VII. The first phase has a half-disappearance time of 18 to 35 minutes and is thought to be due to equilibrium with extravascular sites. The second phase, which is believed to represent biologic degradation, has a half-disappearance time ranging from 100 to 300 minutes.

Treatment of factor VII deficiency is with the prothrombin complex, which contains factors II, VII, IX, and X. Fresh frozen plasma may also be administered. Approximately 5 to 10 percent of the normal level is required for hemostasis.

## FACTOR VIII (ANTIHEMOPHILIC FACTOR)

Factor VIII is a glycoprotein present in only trace quantities in the plasma of healthy individuals. One hundred percent factor VIII activity is defined as 1 unit of factor VIII/ml of plasma, although there is a wide range of normal, with values from 50 to 200 percent. The plasma levels of factor VIII are increased in a number of situations, including after exercise, during pregnancy, when taking oral contraceptives, and in renal disease. It has also been demonstrated that administration of adrenalin or 1-desamino-9-D-arginine vasopressin (DDAVP) can produce a marked transient rise in circulating levels of factor VIII clotting activity. Factor VIII is not stable in citrated plasma where 50 percent of the activity is lost following incubation at 22°C for 24 hours.[1] However, when physiologic levels of calcium are maintained, such as when heparin is used as the anticoagulant, 100 percent of the factor VIII activity is present after 24 hours.

Defects in factor VIII have been related to hemophilia A and von Willebrand's disease. To better understand these disorders, a knowledge of the factor VIII complex is required (see Chapter 26).

As shown in Table 28–1, there are two biologic functions of the factor VIII complex, with the designation VIII:C representing the procoagulant or clotting activity, and VIII:vWF, the von Willebrand activity.

The factor VIII:C activity is measured in a one- or two-stage clotting assay (see Chapter 31).[2,3] The VIII:C or procoagulant (or clotting) protein can be purified quite separately from the factor VIII complex, and, indeed, the gene for this protein has now been cloned and expressed independently of VIII:vWF. The VIII:C protein has an apparent native molecular weight of 270,000. The VIII:vWF activity is determined by the response of washed, normal platelets to aggregation in the presence of test plasma and the antibiotic ristocetin (Fig. 28–1). The activity is associated with the high molecular weight factor VIII glycoprotein complex.

The precise nature of the relationship between VIII:C and VIII:vWF is not yet clear. The VIII:C activity is known to be associated with von Willebrand's factor in the plasma and during early purification. Indeed, until very recently, it was thought that procoagulant activity and the von Willebrand activity were part of the same molecule having a combined molecular weight of greater than $1 \times 10^6$. It is now generally believed that these two proteins are separate, although in some circumstances they copurify.

In addition to the biologic activities, immunologic markers of factor VIII can also be measured. Antibodies directed toward various parts of the factor VIII complex recognize either the procoagulant antigen (VIII:Ag) or that of the higher molecular weight complex (vWF:Ag) (Table 28-1). The vWF:Ag

antibodies, originally developed in rabbits, were first used to demonstrate the coprecipitation of the vWF:Ag.[4] Subsequently, it has been possible to use the antibody to quantitate vWF:Ag using Laurell rocket electrophoresis techniques, as shown in Figure 28-2. More recent techniques involve the use of enzyme-linked immunoabsorbant assay (ELISA) to measure the vWF:Ag.[5]

The VIII:Ag antibodies, on the other hand, are generally IgG in nature and are nonprecipitating. A number of radioimmune and other assays have now been used to quantitate VIII:Ag.[6] Originally, only antibodies from hemophilia A patients were used; however, a number of monoclonal antibodies to factor VIII have been developed and are being used for the assay.

It should be pointed out that the immunologic markers of factor VIII do not necessarily measure the sites of biologic activity; therefore, care should be exercised in the interpretation of data obtained from immunologic measurements.[7]

Hemophilia A is a hereditary disorder characterized by a defect in factor VIII, or procoagulant activity. This is a sex-linked hemorrhagic disease of males that results from a mutation of the locus on the X chromosome. It is characterized by a lack of the procoagulant activity of factor VIII, as measured by a prolonged PTT. Although almost exclusively limited to men, there have been rare reports of female hemophiliacs. The daughters of patients with hemophilia A are obligatory carriers, and sons of patients with hemophilia A are normal; the female carriers then transmit the disorder to half their sons and the carrier state to half their daughters.

The incidence of the disease is estimated to be approximately 1/10,000 of the male population. Although the majority of cases are inherited, spontaneous mutations do occur. The patients are divided into three groups according to their factor VIII level: severe, less than 1 percent; moderate, 3 to 5 percent; and mild, 5 to 12 percent.

It was originally thought that because patients with hemophilia A lacked the biologic capability to achieve clotting, they were totally deficient in factor VIII. However, in 1965 Zimmerman and coworkers[4] developed the heterologous antibody (anti vWF:Ag) against the purified factor VIII complex from healthy individuals and demonstrated that this antibody would react with plasmas from all normal persons and from all persons with hemophilia, showing that the latter had at least a part of the factor VIII molecule.

Further immunologic study of hemophilia was possible using human antibodies to VIII:Ag, which develop spontaneously in approximately 10 percent of patients with hemophilia A. Plasma from these patients will neutralize the VIII:C activity of normal plasma. Using these antibodies it was determined that some hemophiliacs had material in their

**Table 28–1. NOMENCLATURE FOR PROPERTIES OF FACTOR VIII COMPLEX**

| Term | Description |
|---|---|
| VIII:C | Procoagulant activity specifically deficient in hemophilia A |
| VIII:Ag | Antigenic property of the factor VIII complex recognized by homologous antibodies |
| VIIIR:RC$_o$ | Ristocetin cofactor activity, the property of the factor VIII complex that supports the aggregation of platelets by ristocetin |
| vWF:Ag | Antigenic property of the factor VIII complex recognized by heterologous antibodies |

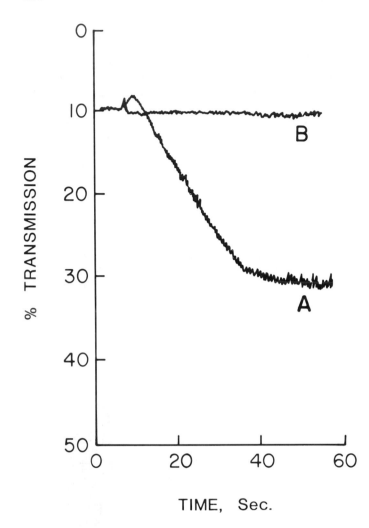

**Figure 28-1.** Factor VIII:vWF and platelet aggregation. Plasma is incubated with washed normal platelets and ristocetin. The aggregation slope is observed over 60 seconds after addition of (A) plasma containing a normal level of vWF and (B) plasma containing a low VIII:vWF level (patient with von Willebrand's disease).

plasma that would cross-react with this antibody.[8] Recently, data have indicated that VIII:C antibodies can be found that will react with plasmas of all patients with severe hemophilia, depending on the assay technique.[9] This suggested that a factor VIII:C–like protein is present in the plasma of the majority, if not all, persons with hemophilia. Subsequently, we have demonstrated a factor VIII:C material that is deficient in procoagulant activity but reactive when tested against the VIII:C antibody in four patients with severe hemophilia.[10] Polyacrylamide gel electrophoresis showed similar patterns for the unreduced factor VIII:C–like proteins, compared with normal individuals (Fig. 28-3); however, when the samples were reduced, different patterns were seen. Biochemical analysis showed that different amounts of carbohydrate were associated with the hemophilic VIII:C.[10] Thus, it is likely that the biochemical defect in hemophilia A is due to the presence of an abnormal glycoprotein. Recently, studies using factor VIII DNA probes showed that in seven out of 200 patients with hemophilia, the ge-

netic information for factor VIII protein was identified as abnormal.[11] The alterations in other patients with hemophilia remain to be defined.

Von Willebrand's disease is due to defects in both factor VIII and VIII:vWF. This disease affects both sexes, and patients exhibit prolonged bleeding. Two in vitro platelet assays are usually abnormal in von Willebrand's disease: ristocetin-induced platelet aggregation and retention of platelets in glass bead columns (platelet adhesion). Both of these deficiencies are corrected following infusion of plasma or cryoprecipitate.

In patients with von Willebrand's disease, ristocetin does not cause platelet aggregation as it does with normal platelets. The problem in using ristocetin-induced platelet aggregation for diagnosis is that, in patients with primary platelet disorders, false-positive results may occur. In addition, the reaction is not sufficiently understood to be certain that other factors are not involved.

The hemostatic disorder in von Willebrand's disease is transmitted by an autosomal locus that af-

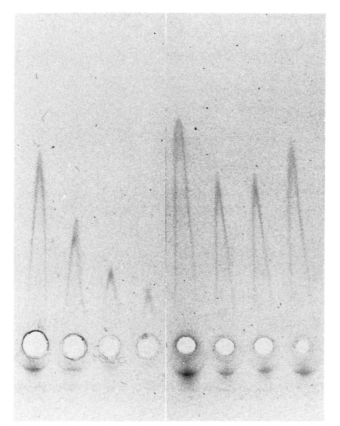

**Figure 28-2.** Quantitative immunoelectrophoresis of normal and hemophilic plasmas. Wells 1 through 4 contain serial dilutions of a standard plasma (Cutter Laboratories). Wells 5 and 8 contain plasmas from two patients with severe hemophilia; wells 6 and 7 contain normal plasmas.

fects both the structure and concentration of vWF:Ag. Using the heterologous antibody and two-dimensional electrophoresis, it has been possible to show both fast- and slow-moving forms of vWF:Ag (Fig. 28-4). This permitted definition of subtypes of von Willebrand's disease. Recently, far more sophisticated techniques have become available for measuring the presence of vWF:Ag multimers. These multimers are different-sized subunits or aggregates of the factor VIII:vWF complex, all of which are detected by their reactivity with heterologous antibody to vWF:Ag. As shown in Figure 28-3, one can define a large number of multimers of the factor VIII:vWF complex. Definition of certain of the subtypes of von Willebrand's disease depends on the presence or absence of different molecular weight forms or multimers of vWF:Ag in addition to determination of the amount of vWF:Ag present. Using these various techniques, different subtypes of von Willebrand's disease have been determined based on both quantitative and qualitative defects, as listed in Table 28-2.[12]

The most common form of von Willebrand's disease (type I) is a mild and moderate disorder, in which levels of all the components of the factor VIII complex are reduced and the bleeding time is prolonged. During the bleeding time test, platelets from patients with von Willebrand's disease do not adhere to the endothelial lip of the wound, although they do adhere normally to perivascular collagen. The plasma VIII:C and VIII:Ag activities are decreased although they may generally be slightly higher than the VIIIR:RC$_o$ and vWF:Ag. The increase in bleeding time is variable but it is usually correlated with the reduced ristocetin cofactor activity. The hemostatic effect may be quite inconsistent and, consequently, laboratory measurements may vary considerably. The platelet count is normal, and petechiae are rare. Epistaxis and easy bruising are common, as is excessive bleeding associated with surgery. This may be prevented or corrected with appropriate therapy. Hemarthrosis is rare, and permanent joint deformities are usually associated with trauma. This disease is relatively less common than hemophilia A.

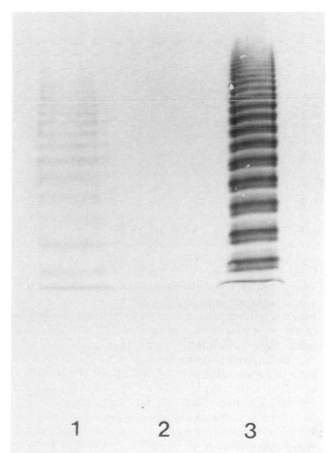

**Figure 28-3.** vWF:Ag multimers. Samples of (1) normal plasma, (2) von Willebrand plasma, and (3) cryoprecipitate underwent electrophoresis in SDS-agarose gel. A western blotting technique was performed. The gel on nitrocellulose paper was incubated first with a rabbit antihuman vWF:Ag antibody and then with goat antirabbit IgG; then it was stained.

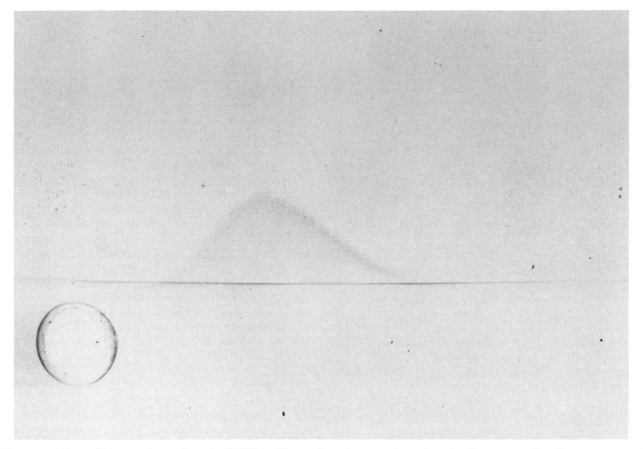

**Figure 28-4.** Crossed immunoelectrophoresis of vWF:Ag. Electrophoresis was performed on the plasma in the first dimension toward the anode. The agarose was then cut and the sample electrophoresed in the second dimension against rabbit antibody to vWF:Ag which was incorporated into the gel. The gels were stained with Coomassie blue to show the arc of immunoprecipitation.

Acquired deficiencies of factor VIII are rare and attributed to the development of antibodies or inhibitors. Patients with such acquired antibodies usually suffer from a disorder such as rheumatoid arthritis, asthma, ulcerative colitis, systemic lupus erythematosus (SLE), or allergic states, or are postpartum patients or elderly.

Antibodies to factor VIII also occur in 10 to 15 percent of patients with hemophilia A. These inhibitors are usually detected at the time of a systematic investigation. They are nonprecipitating and almost always IgG in nature. The antibodies are present in both plasma and serum, are stable at 56°C for 30 minutes, are not absorbed by barium sulphate or aluminum hydroxide, and will slowly neutralize factor VIII during incubation at 37°C. Replacement therapy with factor VIII usually leads to a rise in antibody titer. Recently, therapeutic use of activated prothrombin complex has been successful in these patients; however, the cost is quite high and it is not widely available and it is generally considered that this should be used only in extreme situations. Alternatively, factor IX concentrates can be used to correct the bleeding episodes. These concentrates generate factor Xa in the absence of VIII. Although the precise mechanism or mechanisms by which these concentrates "bypass" the inhibitors are uncertain, this therapy seems to be effective in certain types of bleeding as judged by clinical response.

Patients with von Willebrand's disease may also produce antibodies; these are precipitating in nature and directed against the vWF portion of the

### Table 28–2. CLASSIFICATION OF VON WILLEBRAND'S DISEASE

| Type | Description |
|------|-------------|
| Ia | All forms present with large multimers predominant |
| Ib | All forms present with relatively reduced content of large multimers |
| IIa | Large multimers absent; no ristocetin-induced platelet aggregation |
| IIb | Large multimers absent; greater than normal platelet aggregation with low concentrations of ristocetin |
| II (unclassified) | Large multimers absent; no data on ristocetin-induced aggregation in platelet-rich plasma |
| IIc | Increased concentration of smallest multimers |
| Severe | vWF:Ag too low for multimer analysis |

factor VIII complex. In some disease states (SLE, CLL, diabetes), acquired von Willebrand's syndrome has been described.

The clinical and laboratory presentations of classic hemophilia and von Willebrand's disease are shown in Table 28–3.

## Laboratory Assessment

In patients with hemophilia A, the PTT and whole blood clotting time are abnormal; the prothrombin and bleeding times are normal. The factor VIII level is approximately 1 to 15 percent of normal. Factor VIII:C assays are performed by a one- or two-stage technique. The one-stage assay involves the correction of the abnormal PTT of hemophilic plasma by the test plasma; the two-stage assay is based on the thromboplastin generation test, in which the only variable is the VIII:C content of the test plasma. The VIIIR:RC$_o$ and vWF:Ag are normal; the VIII:Ag usually parallels the low factor VIII:C value (Table 28–3).

In those with von Willebrand's disease, the PTT and the bleeding time are abnormal; the prothrombin and thrombin times are normal. In the classic form of the disease, the levels of all the factor VIII markers, that is, VIIIR:RC$_o$, vWF:Ag, VIII:C, and VIII·Ag, are decreased. The abnormal PTT is related to the low factor VIII:C level (Table 28–3).

Testing for factor VIII inhibitors in patients with hemophilia and nonhemophiliacs involves incubating the person's citrated serum at 37°C with a known amount of VIII:C and assaying for residual VIII:C after one to two hours. One unit of inhibitor is defined as the amount of antibody capable of neutralizing one half of a unit of factor VIII:C. The patient's serum rather than plasma must be used in this assay, because in some patients who do not have hemophilia the plasma may contain a measurable amount of VIII:C, which would interfere with the assay. In a patient with an inhibitor, the titer

usually increases two to four days following stimulation by the factor VIII received during replacement therapy.

## Half-life and Treatment of Deficiency

The survival of VIII:C in the circulation is six to 10 hours in patients with hemophilia;[13] some patients with von Willebrand's disease actually show a secondary rise in VIII:C two to four hours after infusion of cryoprecipitate, which is greater than expected from the amount of VIII:C in the infusate. The half-life of VIII:vWF, on the other hand, is less than VIII:C at three to four hours.

Hemophilia A patients are treated with factor-specific, concentrated or purified, factor VIII preparations. In 1965, Poole[14] discovered that factor VIII precipitated when plasma was thawed. This enriched plasma fraction, termed "cryoprecipitate," was used for many years to treat these patients. Cryoprecipitates contain, on average, 80 to 120 units of VIII:C, 0.5 g of protein, 250 mg of fibrinogen, and 45 mg of fibronectin. However, there are drawbacks to the use of cryoprecipitate; the absolute dose of factor VIII:C is not known, there are a number of other plasma contaminants, and the cryoprecipitates must be stored frozen at below −20°C to maintain activity.

Thus, more highly purified, lyophilized preparations of factor VIII concentrates have become widely used. Although concentrates made from porcine or bovine plasma have been used, most treatment is carried out using concentrates made from human plasma. These factor VIII concentrates contain approximately 25 units VIII:C, 100 units vWF:Ag, and 10 units VIIIR:RC$_o$/ml.

The effective hemostatic level is approximately 30 percent of normal. For major bleeds, 3.5 bags cryoprecipitate per 10 kg are administered as the loading dose, and the maintenance dose is 1.75 bags per 10 kg/8 hours for one to two days, and every 12

Table 28–3. COMPARISON OF HEMOPHILIA A AND CLASSIC VON WILLEBRAND'S DISEASE

|  | Hemophilia A | von Willebrand's |
|---|---|---|
| Deficiency | VIII:C, VIII:AHF | VIII:vWF, VIII:R |
| Inheritance | Recessive, X-linked | Dominant, autosomal |
| Clinical Bleeding | Hemarthrosis, muscle, soft tissue, visceral | Gums, GI tract, mucous membranes |
| Bleeding Disorder | Moderate to severe (60%—severe) | Mild to moderate |
| Laboratory Tests |  |  |
| Bleeding Time | N | A |
| Clot Retraction | N | N |
| Glass Bead Retraction | N | A |
| Platelet Count | N | N |
| Ristocetin Aggregation | N | A |
| PT | N | N |
| PTT | A | A |
| VIII | A | A |
| vWF:Ag | N | A |

N = normal; A = abnormal.

hours thereafter. The regimen when using purified concentrate is a loading dose of 30 units/kg, and 10 to 15 units/kg/8 hours for one to two days, and every 12 hours thereafter. The predicted response to therapy may be calculated by using this formula:

$$C_1 + \frac{C_2 \times V_2}{V_1 + V_2}$$

where $C_1$ = level in the patient before infusion (%/ml); $C_2$ = factor VIII:C level in the infusate (%/ml); $V_2$ = volume of the infusate (ml); and $V_1$ = plasma volume of the patient (ml).

Minor bleeds do not require a loading dose and maintenance is achieved by 1.25 to 1.75 bags of cryoprecipitate per 10 kg/12 hours for two to four days; concentrates are administered in doses of 10 to 15 units/kg /12 hours for two to four days.

Patients with von Willebrand's disease respond to treatment with either fresh frozen plasma or cryoprecipitate. Factor VIII concentrates do not provide effective treatment in von Willebrand's disease. It seems that the VIII:vWF is either destroyed or removed during purification of cryoprecipitate to make the concentrates. Efficacy of replacement therapy in von Willebrand's disease is measured by the correction of the abnormal bleeding time as well as an increase in factor VIII.

Several drugs (such as catecholamines, vasopressin derivatives, and insulin) are known to increase factor VIII levels, but unpleasant side effects limit potential clinical applications. 1-Desamino-8-D-arginine vasopressin (DDAVP), a synthetic analogue of the antidiuretic hormone 8-arginine vasopressin, is well tolerated when infused intravenously in healthy volunteers and produces a marked, rapid, transient increase in plasma factor VIII procoagulant activity, factor VIII–related antigen, and the factor needed for aggregation of washed platelets by the antibiotic ristocetin. This increase is observed both in patients with von Willebrand's disease and those with hemophilia A, although the drug is not effective in raising factor VIII levels in patients with the severe forms of either disease.

Because of this response, DDAVP has been given both intravenously and intranasally to patients with mild to moderate hemophilia and von Willebrand's disease. Using doses of 0.4 to 0.5 $\mu$g/kg in patients with 9 percent or more starting factor VIII levels, it was possible to achieve values of 100 percent of normal and to permit dental extraction and major surgery in six patients with mild hemophilia and in two with von Willebrand's disease.[15] Following this regimen the mean half-life of the autologous VIII:C was 9.4 hours.

## FACTOR IX (CHRISTMAS DISEASE)

Factor IX has not been highly purified; however, it appears to be a glycoprotein that migrates on electrophoresis as either alpha or beta globulin. The molecular weight has been estimated as between 56,000 and 110,000 with the molecular weight of the serum factor greater than that of plasma.

Hereditary deficiency of factor IX is also known as hemophilia B, Christmas disease, or hereditary plasma thromboplastin component (PTC) deficiency. This disorder closely resembles hemophilia A, having a sex-linked recessive mode of inheritance and similar clinical manifestations. The incidence of the disease is approximately 1/100,000 of the population.

Carriers of factor IX deficiency have a wide range of factor IX activity. The approximate hemostatic level of factor IX is 25 percent. There also appears to be considerable heterogeneity in the patient population. Factor IX inhibitors do occur but are very rare. They are present in both plasma and serum, are stable at 56°C for 30 minutes, act rapidly, and can be detected without an incubation period.

Patients with hemophilia B have been segregated into two groups on the basis of prothrombin time. In one group the prothrombin time is normal, while in the other group it is prolonged. This prolongation is due to an inhibitory substance that can be absorbed by barium sulfate and has been identified as an abnormal form of the factor IX protein.

The acquired deficiencies of factor IX are due to the same causes as the other vitamin K–dependent deficiencies. However, it should be noted that factor IX deficiency can develop without a significant decrease in the plasma levels of the other vitamin K–dependent clotting factors. Factor IX deficiency is also seen occasionally in patients whose urinary loss of protein exceeds 10 to 15 g/day, owing to the nephrotic syndrome.

## Laboratory Assessment

The PTT is abnormal in these patients; the prothrombin and the bleeding times are normal. A variant form has been described in which the one-stage prothrombin time is prolonged when ox brain is used as the thromboplastin, and returns to normal upon the addition of factor IX antibodies. These patients have a substance that is functionally inactive but antigenically similar to factor IX; their disorder is termed hemophilia B$^+$. The factor IX level is low in these patients.

## Half-life and Treatment of Deficiency

An in vivo half-life of 20 to 24 hours has been demonstrated with little difference in survival between factor IX derived from serum and that derived from plasma. The prothrombin complex concentrates contain factor IX and are used as replacement therapy. The in vivo recovery of factor IX is usually 50 percent of the expected value obtained with the formula for calculating factor VIII:C recovery.

In patients with factor IX deficiency, it is difficult to restore hemostatic levels of factor IX with fresh frozen plasma alone.

## FACTOR X (STUART-PROWER FACTOR)

This glycoprotein has a molecular weight between 50 and 100,000. It is generally stable during storage but can be activated by chemical interaction to produce factor Xa, which is an enzyme with esterolytic and anticoagulant activity and the ability to activate chymotrypsinogen.

Hereditary deficiencies of factor X (Stuart-Prower or Stuart factor) occur in less than 1/500,000 of the population, however, the heterozygous state occurs in roughly 1/500 of the population. Hereditary factor X deficiency exists in at least three different forms, with the patients representing a fairly heterogeneous group. The clinical manifestations of the disease depend on the level of factor X and may include easy bruising, bleeding from mucous membranes, or menorrhagia. Marked deficiency of factor X may lead to hemarthrosis or serious bleeding after injury.

Since this is one of the vitamin K–dependent coagulant factors, again, the acquired disorders are generally due to the same causes as for the others. In addition, several reports have been published on the occurrence of isolated factor X deficiency in association with amyloidosis.

## Laboratory Assessment

In these patients, the PT and PTT are prolonged, and the reptilase R time may be normal or prolonged.

## Half-life and Treatment of Deficiency

A biphasic survival curve has been obtained for factor X, with the first phase showing a half-life of 1.7 to 9 hours and the second a half-life of 32 to 48 hours. There appears to be an extravascular distribution of this factor.

In severe factor X deficiency it is necessary only to increase the circulating level of factor X to approximately 10 percent in order to achieve hemostasis. Therefore, fresh frozen plasma can be used for treatment. This disease does not respond to vitamin K therapy.

## FACTOR XI (PLASMA THROMBOPLASTIN ANTECEDENT)

Factor XI is a glycoprotein and, as one of the contact factors, is involved in the earliest phases of clotting. It is partially consumed during coagulation, but is also found in serum. The molecular weight of the precursor form or zymogen is 124,000. It is absorbed by kaolin but only partially absorbed by aluminum hydroxide and barium sulfate.

Hereditary factor XI deficiency is transmitted as a recessive autosomal trait and was first reported in 1953. This disease appears to occur mainly in those of Jewish ancestry. The majority of recorded cases have been found in New York and Los Angeles, where the disease is almost as common as classic hemophilia. The deficiency occurs with equal frequency in men and women. Heterozygotes have 10 to 20 percent of the normal mean level of factor XI. Factor XI levels are low in neonates (approximately 30 percent of adult values) and are also known to decline in women during pregnancy. The clinical manifestations of hereditary factor XI deficiency are mild; bruising, epistaxis, and menorrhagia are the most common manifestations. Hemarthroses are rarely seen.

Acquired deficiency of factor XI is sometimes seen in disseminated intravascular coagulation. This is due to consumption following activation.

## Laboratory Assessment

The PTT is prolonged in this disorder, and the PT is normal. Usually the bleeding time is normal. PTT can be corrected with normal plasma or normal serum.

## Half-life and Treatment of Deficiency

The half-life of factor XI in the circulation is 60 hours.

Treatment of the severe hereditary deficiency is generally carried out with plasma infusion, to which the patients usually respond well. On occasion, higher than expected in vivo results are obtained when the one-stage assay is used; this phenomenon is not observed with the two-stage assay. Inhibitors to factor XI are rare.

## FACTOR XII (HAGEMAN FACTOR)

Factor XII has been purified from both human and bovine sources, with the molecular weight of human factor XII given as approximately 20,000 when established by ultracentrifugation data and 100,000 when established by gel filtration, suggesting the possibility of subunits. Factor XII is stable on storage in plasma or serum and is activated by exposure to glass and a variety of other substances, including collagen and fatty acids. The mechanism of activation of factor XII by surfaces or chemicals is not known: there is disagreement regarding the enzymatic properties of factor XIIa, which has many characteristics of an enzyme during blood coagulation.

Hereditary deficiency of factor XII is also known as the Hageman trait. This deficiency is autosomal recessive. Usually it is not associated with any hemorrhagic manifestations, but patients may present with thromboembolic complications.

## Laboratory Assessment

Hageman factor exists as a proenzyme in plasma and is strongly adsorbed by a variety of "foreign surfaces" such as glass, celite, skin, collagen, and long-chain fatty acids; thus, it is necessary to collect blood with plastic equipment to maintain activity. Diagnosis of disorder is based on a low level of factor XII, which is adsorbed by aluminum hydroxide and barium sulfate. The PT is normal; the disorder is characterized by a prolonged PTT, abnormal whole blood clotting time, and prolonged clotting in siliconized tubes.

## Half-life and Treatment of Deficiency

On the very rare occasions when treatment is required, fresh frozen plasma or stored plasma is recommended.

The half-life of the infusate is 60 to 70 hours.

## FACTOR XIII (FIBRIN-STABILIZING FACTOR)

The final stage of the coagulation process involves the stabilization of the fibrin gel by the action of factor XIII, which is present in both plasma and platelets. Platelet fibrin-stabilizing factor is activated by thrombin and acts much sooner than does the plasma fibrin-stabilizing factor, which is activated through a process that requires calcium. The net result is the formation of covalent cross-links between the polypeptide chains of the fibrin subunit.

Inherited defects of this factor are extremely rare and appear to be autosomal recessive in nature. Prominent bleeding from the umbilical cord is frequently seen, as is poor wound healing following surgery or trauma. Initial hemostasis in factor XIII–deficient patients is usually normal but short-lived, with bleeding often occurring 36 hours or longer after the initial trauma. In patients with factor XIII deficiency, bleeding is often first noted when the umbilical cord separates; death occurs at this time more frequently than in patients with factor VIII or IX deficiency.

Acquired defects of this factor may occur in patients who have leukemia.

## Laboratory Assessment

All the routine clotting test results are normal in patients with this disorder. The first clue of a defect is that the clot appears friable. If factor XIII is completely absent, the clot will be soluble in 5M urea or 1 percent monochloroacetic acid. The presence of 1 to 2 percent factor XIII renders the clot insoluble.

## Half-life and Treatment of Deficiency

The half-life is long, at six days, and hemostasis can be achieved with very low levels of therapy (0.5 percent). The replacement therapy is fresh frozen plasma.

## OTHER COAGULATION FACTORS

There are a number of other defects of coagulation, which are determined mostly by reactions that occur in the laboratory. Most of these problems are not related to a specific absence of an identifiable plasma protein, but they do have importance in the investigation of bleeding disorders or of abnormal laboratory results, or both.

## Fletcher Trait (Prekallikrein)

Deficiency of Fletcher factor or prekallikrein is determined in the laboratory but manifests clinically as an asymptomatic coagulation disease. The PTT is prolonged and the PT is normal. The abnormal PTT is corrected by aluminum hydroxide adsorbed to fresh plasma and serum; plasma deficient in factors VIII, IX, XI, and XII will also correct the abnormality. The PTT will gradually return to normal levels with prolonged incubation in the test system or with prolonged contact with glass; however, this is not seen with the prothrombin time. The prekallikrein level is decreased, as is the kinin-generating capacity. Prekallikrein has been studied in the past for its role in inflammation and chemotaxis. It is also necessary for the optimal activation and fragmentation of factor XII in the early stages of coagulation.

## Fitzgerald Factor

Deficiency of the Fitzgerald factor is also an asymptomatic defect. In this situation, the PTT is prolonged and the PT is normal. The PTT can be corrected by the addition of plasma deficient in all the coagulation factors, including Fletcher factor and factor XII. This deficiency appears to be identical to the Flaujeac clotting defect.

## Passovoy Trait

Patients with this trait have a moderate bleeding diathesis, which is transmitted as an autosomal dominant disorder. The PTT is slightly prolonged, and the PT is normal. The trait is the result of an abnormality in the intrinsic pathway of coagulation. Levels of all the known clotting factors are normal.

## INHIBITORS

Normal human plasma contains protease inhibitors that regulate the activity of activated clotting factors and fibrinolytic enzymes. These have been referred to as naturally occurring inhibitors, to be differentiated from acquired inhibitors or circulating anticoagulants that arise from an underlying disease process or pathology. Some well-characterized naturally occurring inhibitors include antithrombin III, $\alpha_2$-macroglobulin, $\alpha_1$-antitrypsin, $\alpha_2$-antiplasmin, $C_1$-inactivator, and protein C. Recently, protein C has gained much attention as a regulator of hemostasis and thrombosis. The activation of protein C provides a direct link between coagulation and the formation of anticoagulant activity.

Circulating anticoagulants (inhibitors) are seen in a variety of pathologic processes, such as SLE, multiple myeloma, and hemophilia, as well as in postpartum women. These inhibitors present as acquired hemostatic defects and are usually immunoglobulins. They are recognized by unexplained bleeding or screening tests as a prolonged APTT that is not corrected by a 1:1 mix of patient's plasma with normal plasma. These pathologic inhibitors may be directed against a specific clotting factor or may have a less-defined mechanism, as in SLE. Specific factor inhibition most often involves antibodies directed against factor VIII:C and less commonly, against factors V, VII, IX, XI, and XIII. In the case of SLE, most evidence suggests that inhibition is directed against prothrombin or the prothrombin complex.

The presence of a circulating anticoagulant appears to be an increasing problem in clinical laboratories. The type of inhibitor most often determines the probability of bleeding complications and the approach to patient management.

## Lupus Anticoagulant

Inhibition of coagulation is often seen in association with collagen disorders such as SLE. In these patients, there is a prolonged PTT and a mild to moderately prolonged PT. The anticoagulant in lupus may affect various stages in the coagulation process in different patients. In general, bleeding is unusual; thrombosis is more common (see Chapter 31).

## Presence of Paraproteins Acting As Anticoagulants

A number of platelet and clotting functions are inhibited in myeloma and Waldenström's macroglobulinemia, both of which induce a complex hemostatic defect. The most common single abnormality is the prolongation of the thrombin time owing to the interference of the abnormal protein with orderly fibrin monomer polymerization. The correlation between laboratory findings and hemorrhagic manifestations is usually poor.

Table 28–4 summarizes the factor deficiencies, listing their clinical profile, and Table 28–5 summarizes their various test results.

## SUMMARY

Once a history of bleeding in the patient is ascertained, certain basic screening tests should be done, including:

1. Platelet count
2. Prothrombin time (PT)
3. Partial thromboplastin time (PTT)
4. Bleeding time (BT)
5. Thrombin time (TT)

When the platelet count is normal, the possible results of the PT and PTT are as follows:

1. Abnormal PT (this could be due to deficiencies in fibrinogen, prothrombin, factor V, VII, or X, or to an inhibitor to any of these factors or to thrombin)
2. Abnormal PTT (this could be due to deficiencies in factor VIII, IX, X, XI, XII, V, II, Fletcher, or Fitzgerald, or to inhibitors to these factors)
3. Normal PT, abnormal PTT (this could be due to defects in factors VIII, IX, XI, XII, Fletcher, or Fitzgerald, or to inhibitors to these factors)
4. Normal PTT, abnormal PT (this could be due to defects in factor VII)
5. Abnormal PT and PTT (this may be due to defects of fibrinogen, factor II, V, VIII, IX, X, XI, or XII; to a combined deficiency of factors V and VIII; or to the presence of inhibitors of the aforementioned factors)

The deficiencies of factors VIII, IX, XI, XII, Fitzgerald, and Fletcher should be differentiated by performing specific factor assays or by adding plasma (or serum) to the test plasma and observing for correction of PTT.

The thrombin time (TT) assesses thrombin-fibrinogen interaction and may be abnormal in patients who have hypofibrinogenemia or dysfibrinogenemia, and as a result of circulating inhibitors. In these cases, the PT and PTT both may be prolonged. Inhibitors such as fibrin-degradation products (FDPs) occurring in patients with disseminated intravascular coagulation (DIC) and following administration of heparin usually prolong the TT. The TT is the most sensitive index of heparin presence and of DIC.

## CASE STUDY

**History.** Ten-year-old male with frequent bruising; walks with a limp. Patient has two sisters, alive and well; both parents, alive and well; maternal grandfather died as a result of "bleeding" following a car accident.

**Physical Examination.** Patient has no lymphadenopathy or splenomegaly. Large bruises on left elbow; is unable to straighten both arms. Abdomen is rigid and tender; patient complains of acute abdominal pain.

## Table 28-4. FACTOR DEFICIENCIES

| Factor | Deficiency | Minimum for Hemostasis | Half-life | Laboratory | Clinical |
|---|---|---|---|---|---|
| I | Afibrinogenemia Autosomal recessive— homozygous Rare | 50–100 mg | 3.2–4.5 days | No clot formation <5 mg fibrinogen | Umbilical stump bleeding, easy bruising, ecchymosis, epistaxis, gingival oozing, hematuria, poor wound healing. |
|  | Hypofibrinogenemia Autosomal recessive— heterozygous Rare |  |  | Abn: PT APTT TCT Low fibrinogen | Mild bleeding, thrombotic episodes. |
|  | Dysfibrinogenemia Variable inheritance Uncommon—variants |  |  | Fibrinogen— Qualitative abnormal Quantitative normal | Possible hemorrhage, possible thrombosis, possible asymptomatic. |
| II | Hypoprothrombinemia Autosomal recessive Extremely rare | 30%–40% | 2.8–4.4 days | Abn: PT APTT | Postop bleeding, epistaxis, menorrhagia, easy bruising. |
| V | Parahemophilia Autosomal recessive 1/1,000,000– homozygote | 10%–25% | 20 hr | Abn: PT APTT BT | Epistaxis, easy bruising, menorrhagia. |
| VII | Hypopro- convertinemia Incomplete autosomal recessive—variable expression 1/500,000 | 10%–20% | 100–300 min | Abn: PT Norm: APTT | Epistaxis, menorrhagia, cerebral hemorrhage. |
| VIII | Hemophilia A (Classic hemophilia) Sex-linked recessive 1/100,000 | 10%–40% | 9–18 hr | Abn: APTT Norm: PT BT | May be severe, moderate or mild- spontaneous hemorrhage, hemarthroses, crippling, ecchymoses, muscle hemorrhage, post-traumatic and postsurgical bleeding. |
|  | von Willebrand's syndrome Variable inheritance —variants– autosomal dominant, variable penetrance; 1/80,000 | 20%–40% | 16–24 hr | Variable results: Platelet studies BT APTT | Mucous membrane bleeding, superficial wound bleeding— variable depending on VIII:C levels. |
| IX | Hemophilia B (Christmas disease) Sex-linked recessive 1/100,000 | 20%–50% | 18–30 hr | Abn: APTT Norm: PT | May be severe, moderate or mild— spontaneous hemorrhage, hemarthroses, crippling, ecchymoses, muscle hemorrhage, posttraumatic and postsurgical bleeding. |
| X | Stuart-Prower defect Autosomal recessive <1/500,000– homozygous 1/500–heterozygous | 15%–20% | 32–48 hr | Abn: PT APTT | Menorrhagia, ecchymoses, CNS bleeding, excessive bleeding after childbirth. |

Table 28–4. FACTOR DEFICIENCIES (continued)

| Factor | Deficiency | Minimum for Hemostasis | Half-life | Laboratory | Clinical |
|---|---|---|---|---|---|
| XI | Hemophilia C Incomplete autosomal recessive–pseudo–dominant Rare | 15%–25% | 40–84 hr | Abn: APTT Norm: PT | Mild bleeding, bruising, epistaxis, retinal hemorrhage, menorrhagia. |
| XII | Hageman trait Autosomal recessive Rare | ? | 48–52 hr | Abn: APTT Norm: PT | Asymptomatic— rarely bleed, may thrombose. |
| XIII | Factor XIII deficiency Autosomal recessive Rare | 1% | 12 days | Norm: PT APTT Clot soluble in 5 M urea | Umbilical cord bleeding, delayed wound healing, minor injuries cause prolonged bleeding, fetal wastage, excessive fibrinolysis, male sterility, intracranial hemorrhage. |
| PK | Fletcher trait Autosomal recessive Rare | ? | ? | Abn: APTT (normal after prolonged activation) | Asymptomatic. |
| HMWK | Fitzgerald deficiency Autosomal recessive Rare | ? | ? | Abn: APTT | Asymptomatic. |
| Plasminogen | Abnormal functional Plasminogen Autosomal Rare | ? | 2–2.5 days | Abnormal plasminogen function–normal clotting tests | Thrombosis. |
| Protein C | Protein C deficiency Autosomal dominant | ? | 6–8 hr | Normal clotting tests | Thrombosis— thrombophlebitis, recurring pulmonary emboli. |

From Pittiglio, DH, et al.: Treating hemostatic disorders. A problem-oriented approach. In Pittiglio, DH: Hemostasis Overview. American Association of Blood Banks, Arlington, VA, 1984, p. 28, with permission.)

Table 28–5. FACTOR DEFICIENCIES AND TEST RESULTS

| | BT | PT | APTT | Adsorbed Plasma | Aged Serum | Thrombin Time | Fibrinogen | Urea Solubility | Platelet Count | Protamine Sulfate | FDP |
|---|---|---|---|---|---|---|---|---|---|---|---|
| I | N | A | A | C | NC | A | A | N | N | — | — |
| II | N | A | A | NC | NC | N | N | N | N | — | — |
| V | A | A | A | C | NC | N | N | N | N | — | — |
| VII | N | A | N | NC | C | N | N | N | N | — | — |
| VIII:C | N | N | A | C | NC | N | N | N | N | — | — |
| VIII:vWF | A | N | A | C | C | N | N | N | N | — | — |
| IX | N | N | A | NC | C | N | N | N | N | — | — |
| X | N | A | A | NC | C | N | N | N | N | — | — |
| XI | N | N | A | C | C | N | N | N | N | — | — |
| XII | N | N | A | C | C | N | N | N | N | — | — |
| XIII | N | N | N | — | — | N | N | A | N | — | — |
| PK | N | N | A* | C | C | N | N | N | N | — | — |
| HMWK | N | N | A | C | C | N | N | N | N | — | — |
| Plasminogen | N | N | N | — | — | N | N | N | N | — | — |
| $\alpha_2$-AP | N | N | N | — | — | N | N | N | N | — | — |
| AT-III | N | N | N | — | — | N | N | N | N | — | — |
| DIC | — | A | A | — | — | A | A | N | A | A | A |
| Fibrinolysis | — | N | N | — | — | A | A | N | N | N | A |

N = normal; C = correction; A = abnormal; NC = no correction; BT = bleeding time; PT = prothrombin time; APTT = activated partial thromboplastin time; FDP = fibrin-degradation products.
*The APTT returns to normal after prolonged activation of the contact system.
From Pittiglio, DH, et al.: Treating hemostatic disorders. A problem-oriented approach. In Pittiglio, DH: Hemostasis Overview. American Association of Blood Banks, Arlington, VA, 1984, p. 31, with permission.)

**Provisional Diagnosis**

*Laboratory Findings.* PT 11 sec; PTT 90 sec; bleeding time 3 min; and platelet count 275,000/$\mu$l.

*Additional Laboratory Findings.* Factor VIII <1 percent activity; factor IX 105 percent activity; vWF:Ag 110 percent activity; factor VIII inhibitor 4 units.

**Diagnosis.** The patient has a factor VIII deficiency with an inhibitor.

# References

1. Rock, GA and Tittley, P: The effect of temperature variations on cryoprecipitate. Transfusion 19:86, 1979.
2. Hardisty, RM and Macpherson, JC: A one-stage Factor VIII (antihemophilic globulin) assay and its use on venous and capillary plasma. Thromb Diath Haemorr 7:215, 1962.
3. Pool, JG and Robinson, J: Assay of plasma antihemophilic globulin (AHG). Br Med J 5:17, 1959.
4. Zimmerman, TS, Ratnoff, OD, and Powell, AE: Immunologic differentiation of classic hemophilia (Factor VIII deficiency) and von Willebrand's disease. J Clin Invest 50:244, 1971.
5. Cejka, J: Enzyme immunoassay for Factor VIII-related antigen. Clin Chem 28:1356, 1982.
6. Lazarchick, J and Hoyer, LW: Immunoradiometric measurement of the Factor VIII procoagulant antigen. J Clin Invest 62:1048, 1978.
7. Rock, G, Ganz, P, and Tackaberry, E: The relationship of biological and immunological activities of Factor VIII. Biochem Biophys Res Comm 115:981, 1983.
8. Hoyer, LW and Breckenridge, RT: Immunologic studies of antihemophilic Factor (AHF, Factor VIII) II. Properties of cross-reacting material. Blood 35:809, 1970.
9. Poon, MC and Ratnoff, OD: Immunologic evidence that the antihemophilic factor (Factor VIII)-like material in hemophilic plasma possesses a non-functional low molecular weight subcomponent. Blood 50:367, 1977.
10. Rock, G, Cruickshank, WH, and Palmer, DS: Variant forms of procoagulant-like Factor VIII in hemophiliacs. Thromb Res 21:53, 1981.
11. Lawn, RM and Vehar, GA: The molecular genetics of hemophilia. Sci Am 254:48, 1986.
12. Hoyer, LW, Rizza, CR, and Tuddenham, EGD: Von Willebrand factor multimer patterns in von Willebrand's disease. J Haematol 55:493, 1983.
13. Rock, G, Smiley, RK, Tittley, P, et al: In vivo effectiveness of a high-yield Factor VIII concentrate prepared in a blood bank. N Engl J Med 311:310, 1984.
14. Pool, JG: Cryoprecipitate quality and supply. Transfusion 15:305, 1975.
15. Mannucci, PM, Ruggeriz, M, Pareti, FI, et al: 1-Deamino-8-D-Arginine Vasopressin: A new pharmacological approach to the management of haemophilia and von Willebrand's disease. Lancet 1:869, 1977.

# CHAPTER 29

JOHN LAZARCHICK, M.D., AND JOETTE KIZER, M.L.T.(ASCP)

# Interaction of Fibrinolytic, Coagulation, and Kinin Systems and Related Pathology

Normal hemostasis is the result of the balanced interaction of the vascular endothelium and platelets with four biochemical systems:[1,2] the coagulation, the fibrinolytic, the kinin, and to a lesser extent the complement systems. The interrelationship between these systems is illustrated in Figure 29–1. When a stimulus initiates activation of the coagulation system with resultant fibrin formation and the establishment of a hemostatic barrier, a series of enzymes comprising the fibrinolytic system are simultaneously activated to control local thrombus formation and subsequently to lyse the fibrin thrombus, re-establishing vessel lumen integrity and blood flow. This chapter deals with the biochemistry of the components of this fibrinolytic system, its associated pathophysiologic disorders, and laboratory tests available to evaluate individual components and overall function.

## MOLECULAR COMPONENTS: PHYSICOCHEMICAL AND FUNCTIONAL PROPERTIES

The molecular components of the fibrinolytic system consist of (1) the plasma protein plasminogen; (2) its active enzymatic form, plasmin; (3) a group of plasminogen activators, which convert plasminogen to plasmin; (4) plasmin inhibitors, most prominently $\alpha_2$-plasmin inhibitor; and (5) fibrin/fibrinogen, which serves as substrate for the active enzyme plasmin (Table 29–1).

### Plasminogen

Native plasminogen is a single-chain plasma zymogen of approximately 90,000 daltons molecular

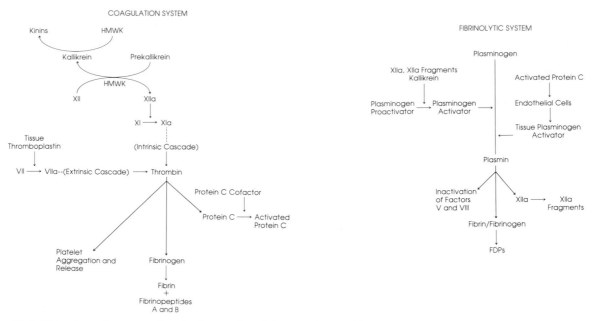

**Figure 29-1.** This schematic summarizes the interaction of the coagulation, fibrinolytic, and kinin systems. High molecular weight kininogen and prekallikrein catalyze the activation of factor XII to XIIa. Factor XIIa then promotes the conversion of prekallikrein to kallikrein. The latter liberates kinins from high molecular weight kininogen, thus completing the positive feedback loops of the contact phase of coagulation. Thrombin formed through the extrinsic or intrinsic cascade system then converts fibrinogen to fibrin and induces platelet aggregation release. Thrombin with protein C cofactor activates protein C, which promotes tissue plasminogen activator release from endothelial cells. A second point of interaction between these systems can also result in formation of plasminogen activator. Kallikrein, in association with factor XIIa and XIIa fragments, converts a plasmin proactivator to its activated state. Through either activating system, plasminogen can then be proteolytically cleaved to form plasmin. Plasmin not only lyses fibrin and inactivates factors V and VIII but also degrades factor XIIa to inactivate fragments that are a component of the second plasminogen activator system.

## Table 29-1. COMPONENTS OF THE FIBRINOLYTIC SYSTEM

|  | Comments |
|---|---|
| 1. Plasminogen | Circulating zymogen forms with molecular weight of 90,000 daltons. |
| 2. Plasminogen activators:<br>Tissue activator | Endogenous activator liberated from endothelial cells by the action of protein C. |
| Factor XIIa, kallikrein<br>Factor XIIa fragments<br>Factor XIa | Contact phase activator generated with the initiation of coagulation. |
| Urokinase | Proteases produced in the kidney and secreted in the urine. |
| Streptokinase | Bacterial cell product. Forms complex with plasminogen which has intrinsic activating activity. |
| 3. Plasmin | Active serine protease of 70–75,000 daltons. |
| 4. $\alpha_2$-Plasmin inhibitor | Primary inhibitor of plasmin. Forms irreversible complex with plasmin. |
| $\alpha_2$-Macroglobulin | Serves as a plasmin inhibitor only when $\alpha_2$-plasmin inhibitor binding sites are saturated. |
| 5. Fibrinogen, fibrin | Plasmin substrates. Proteolytic cleavage results in the generation of degradation products. |

weight, which circulates in two molecular forms, differing only in their carbohydrate content.[3] It is synthesized by the liver and has a half-life of two days. The plasma content is approximately 20 mg/dl. Each form of this molecule has an amino acid terminal glutamic acid (Glu-plasminogen) and is capable of undergoing limited proteolytic cleavage of this region to an incomplete molecule with lysine as the new terminal amino acid (Lys-plasminogen). This latter form is more readily converted to active plasmin by plasminogen activators than the Glu-plasminogen form and is probably of greater physiologic significance.

## Plasminogen Activators

The conversion of either form to active plasmin can be initiated through a variety of direct or indirect mechanisms.[4] This group of activating proteins is collectively known as plasminogen activators. Regardless of the initiating mechanism, activation of plasminogen to yield plasmin proceeds through the cleavage of the same arginine 560–valine 561 bond in the Glu and Lys forms of plasminogen. These activators are either endogenous or exogenous in origin.

Endogenous activators are serine proteases present in the blood and a variety of other tissues, particularly the vascular endothelium. With the initiation of the contact phase of coagulation (see Chapter 26), factor XIIa, XIIa fragments, XIa, kallikrein, and high molecular weight kininogen interact to yield plasminogen activating ability.[5] The exact biochemical steps involved in the formation of this intrinsic activator are not completely understood. The activator activity generated by this pathway slowly converts plasminogen to plasmin. A great deal of interest has been most recently directed toward the endogenous activator system because of its potential for pharmacologic manipulation and its greater efficiency in thrombolytic therapy. This mechanism is probably the major physiologic activator of plasminogen. Tissue plasminogen activator (TPA) is an endothelial cell product with a molecular weight of approximately 68,000 daltons.[6] The mechanism controlling its release from vascular endothelium is unsettled, but protein C, a vitamin K–dependent serine protease, is a likely candidate. Thrombin generated during the coagulation process causes the release of protein C cofactor from the vascular endothelium. Once complexed with thrombin this cofactor rapidly activates protein C. Activated protein C then promotes clot lysis by indirectly liberating TPA from endothelial cells, thus initiating endogenous fibrinolysis. At the same time, protein C exerts a negative feedback control on the coagulation process by inactivating coagulant factors V and VIII, thus limiting further clot formation.[7,8] TPA has a high affinity for fibrin and its adsorption to fibrin clots greatly enhances plasminogen conversion to plasmin. Because of a higher affinity of both the plasminogen activator and plasminogen for fibrin rather than fibrinogen, the effect of this reaction is accentuated on the surface of and within the clot. Release of TPA from the endothelium is also responsive to a variety of other stimuli including venous occlusion, strenuous exercise, and treatment with vasoactive drugs including the vasopressin derivative DDAVP. TPA activity is increased severalfold under these conditions.[9]

Exogenous activators have been available for clinical use for a number of years. One of these, urokinase, is synthesized by the kidney and excreted in the urine.[10] It can also be identified in vitro using kidney cell cultures and is a potent direct activator of plasminogen. Its major drawbacks are its expense and its relatively lower affinity for fibrin compared with TPA. A consequence of the latter property is that the plasmin generated will digest not only fibrin but also circulating fibrinogen, and, therefore, the development of severe hypofibrinogenemia is not uncommon with its use. The other exogenous activator, streptokinase, is a product of beta-hemolytic streptococci. It is not a serine protease and has no intrinsic proteolytic activity but is capable of forming a 1 : 1 stoichiometric complex with plasminogen. This interaction results in a conformational change of the plasminogen molecule and exposure of its active serine site.[11] The streptokinase-plasminogen complex can then undergo autocatalysis to yield other activators: SK-Glu-plasmin and SK-Lys-plasmin. Any of these forms will readily convert free plasminogen to plasmin. Since streptokinase is a bacterial protein, a major limitation with its use in thrombolytic therapy is the induction of an immune response with resulting antibody development and an inhibition of its activity.

## Plasmin

The pivotal serine protease generated through these complex biochemical processes is plasmin. This protein has a molecular weight of 77,000 to 85,000 daltons, depending on whether Lys-plasmin or Glu-plasmin is formed, and has a transient plasma half-life measured in seconds.[12] Plasmin has the ability to proteolytically degrade both fibrin in clots and native fibrinogen in the circulation into a series of well-characterized end products collectively known as fibrin/fibrinogen-degradation products (FDPs). This process results in an asymmetrical, progressive breakdown of fibrin and fibrinogen.[13] The earliest recognized component is fragment X, which is still capable of clotting. A recent finding has been the identification of a small peptide fragment from the B beta chain of fibrinogen, which is released simultaneously with the formation of the X fragment. Measurement by radioimmunoassay of this B beta 15-42 related peptide may prove of value in the documentation of early fibrinolytic states.[14,15] The X fragment undergoes further plasmin attack to yield unclottable Y and D fragments. The Y fragment is further digested to yield an additional D fragment and a single E fragment. It is now realized that the proteolytic cleavage of cross-linked fibrin (i.e., fibrin transamidated through the action of factor XIIIa and calcium) results in other intermediate degradation products (e.g., $D_2E$ without the generation of fragment D or E).

These breakdown products have specific inhibitory effects on the coagulation system and thereby suppress further clot formation. Fragment X is capable of clotting slowly and exerts an anticoagulant effect by competing with fibrinogen for thrombin. It also forms slowly polymerizing complexes with fibrin monomer. Fragment Y forms nonclottable complexes with fibrin monomer and inhibits the polymerization step. Fragment D forms abnormal complexes with fibrin monomers as it polymerizes. Fragment E is not known to have any specific anticoagulant effect. In high concentrations (>100 $\mu$g/ml), the degradation products are capable of inhibiting platelet aggregation and release. Plasmin also exerts a direct limiting effect on the coagulation process by being able to cleave proteolytically and render inactive factors V and VIII.

## Plasmin Inhibitors

Although plasmin formation characteristically takes place in the area of fibrin deposition with little free plasmin circulating, this enzyme if unchecked by the presence of specific inhibitors would result in circulating fibrinogen being digested and the blood being rendered unclottable. The primary physiologic inhibitor of plasmin in vivo is $\alpha_2$-plasmin inhibitor.[16,17] It rapidly binds to the lysine binding site on plasmin in a 1:1 molar ratio in an irreversible manner. Measurement of these plasmin:$\alpha_2$-plasmin inhibitor complexes has been suggested as an indicator for activation of the fibrinolytic system. Plasmin adsorbed onto fibrin during the fibrinolytic process appears to be protected from this inhibitor, because it binds to fibrin through the same lysine binding site. Because this binding site on plasmin is occupied, the inhibitor cannot bind and clot lysis can proceed. The overall effect is to ensure that plasmin activity is limited to the area of fibrin deposition and to prevent free plasmin from circulating. Other protease inhibitors in plasma include $\alpha_2$-macroglobulin, $C_1$-inactivator, and $\alpha_1$-antitrypsin. Of these, only $\alpha_2$-macroglobulin has a role in plasmin inhibition during normal hemostasis, and it participates only when $\alpha_2$-plasmin inhibitor binding sites for plasmin are saturated.

## CONGENITAL ABNORMALITIES

Congenital abnormalities of the fibrinolytic system are rare.[18] Only three cases of an abnormal plasminogen have been reported. In each of these reports the patient had a history of recurrent thrombotic episodes. Low levels of tissue plasminogen activator activity have been documented in two families and were associated with a similar thrombotic tendency. Deficiencies of $\alpha_2$-plasmin inhibitor have been reported in four families to date and, in contrast, are associated with a severe hemorrhagic tendency. Acquired abnormalities of the fibrinolytic system are much more common and will be discussed in the sections on disseminated intravascular coagulation and related disorders.

In summary, an integrated system of serine proteases is brought into play once the coagulation process is initiated in response to disruption of blood vessel integrity (Fig. 29–2). The response is balanced so that the same reaction that initiated thrombin formation and fibrin deposition also initiates a series of reactions to lyse the clot. Factor XII with other components of the contact phase of coagulation convert plasminogen to plasmin; protein C through its interaction with thrombin indirectly releases tissue plasminogen activator with subsequent plasmin generation. Because of the high affinity of plasmin for fibrin, most of these fibrinolytic processes take place at the site of fibrin deposition within the damaged blood vessel. The presence of plasmin inhibitors further ensures that the proteolytic process is limited to this area.

## DISSEMINATED INTRAVASCULAR COAGULATION

When there is damage to a blood vessel an ordered, integrated series of reactions involving the coagulation, fibrinolytic, kinin, and complement systems occurs (as outlined in the previous chapters) with the initial formation and subsequent lysis of fibrin deposits. The initial formation of the fibrin clot prevents further hemorrhage and promotes vascular repair. The subsequent clot lysis serves to re-establish blood flow and vascular integrity. This process is normally self-limited and localized. With certain pathologic stimuli, the coagulation response may be accentuated and the normal inhibitory mechanisms overwhelmed. Activation of the coagulation system under these circumstances causes consumption of the coagulation factors and platelets with subsequent formation fibrin thrombi not only at the site of endothelial damage, but in a random manner throughout the microcirculation.[19] This hemorrhagic syndrome has been referred to as disseminated intravascular coagulation, defibrination syndrome, or consumptive coagulopathy. Simultaneous with and secondary to the activation of the coagulation cascade, the fibrinolytic system is activated. Regardless of the nature of the inciting stimulus, the pathophysiologic effect of this process will be reflective of the balance between fibrin deposition (action of thrombin) and fibrinolysis (action of plasmin). The clinical manifestations thus can be one of diffuse hemorrhage **(see Color Figure 239)** due to depletion of platelets and coagulation factors, ischemic tissue damage due to vascular occlusion, or the occurrence of both simultaneously in different areas of the microvasculature.

## Triggering Mechanisms: Associated Clinical Disorders

The diverse stimuli that are capable of triggering the coagulation cascade in this manner all act through one or more of three mechanisms:[20] (1) activation of the extrinsic coagulation pathway by the release of tissue thromboplastin, (2) activation of the intrinsic coagulation pathway with factor XIIa formation, and (3) direct activation of factor X or II. The exact sequence of intermediary events by which certain of the stimuli initiate coagulation is well understood, but with other stimuli this process is unknown. Disseminated intravascular coagulation due to direct activation of factor VII seen after massive injury or in certain obstetric complications results from release of tissue thromboplastin from the

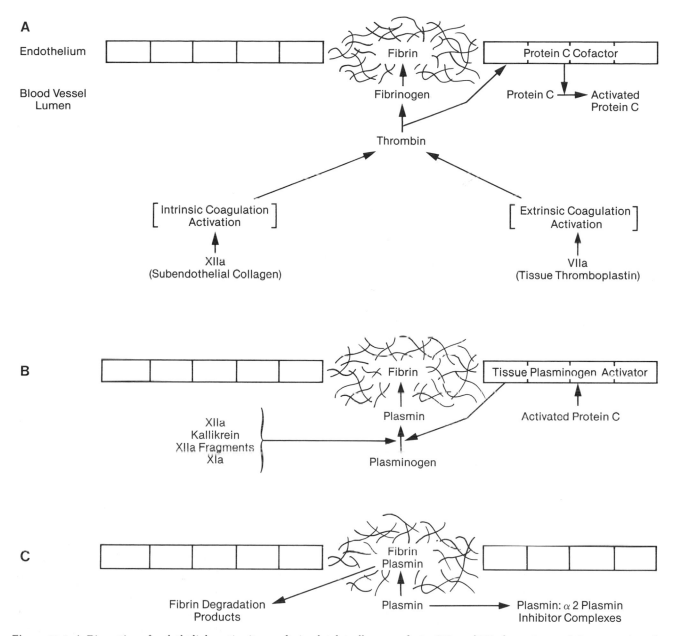

**Figure 29-2.** *A,* Disruption of endothelial continuity results in platelet adherence, factor XIIa and VIIa formation, and the generation of thrombin at the damaged site. Thrombin then converts fibrinogen to fibrin to re-establish a temporary barrier. Secondarily and simultaneously, thrombin stimulates endothelial cells to release protein C cofactor, which catalyzes activated protein C formation. *B,* Activated protein C causes release of tissue plasminogen activator from endothelial cells. An additional plasminogen activator is formed through the interaction of the contact phase components. Both of these activators then convert plasminogen in and on the surface of the fibrin clot to plasmin. *C,* Plasmin-induced proteolysis of the fibrin clot results in the formation of fibrin-degradation products. Re-endothelialization of the damaged blood vessel begins as clot dissolution is occurring. Excess plasmin is irreversibly complexed with its inhibitor, $\alpha_2$-plasmin inhibitor, preventing proteolysis of circulating fibrinogen.

injured tissue or from amniotic fluid entering the circulation. Certain tumors, particularly mucinous adenocarcinomas, are rich in thromboplastin-like material and may act through the same mechanism. The coagulopathy seen with red cell lysis may be due to the release of thromboplastin-like activity from the stroma of these cells.

All pathologic stimuli that result in activation of the intrinsic system probably do so indirectly by means of first inducing endothelial cell damage with subsequent exposure of the subendothelium. Platelet adherence and aggregation and factor XII activation can then occur. This is the proposed mechanism of disseminated intravascular coagulation associated with sepsis, anoxia, and immune complex formation. Direct activation of coagulation factors can also occur in the presence of proteolytic enzymes. The venoms of certain snakes act through this mechanism (e.g., Russell's viper venom activates factor X, whereas venom from the sand rattlesnake causes direct conversion of prothrombin to thrombin). Certain malignancies have also been reported to have direct factor X–activating capability, and this property may account for the disseminated intravascular coagulation seen in patients in these conditions. A list of clinical conditions associated with these triggering mechanisms is shown in Table 29–2.

## Clinical Presentation

The clinical presentation will to a great extent depend on which of the proteolytic processes (coagulant or fibrinolytic) is dominant. This allows for a wide spectrum ranging from an acute, severe hemorrhagic disorder to a low-grade disorder with predominantly thrombotic manifestations. A number of factors are important in determining the final clinical picture, including the magnitude and duration of the triggering stimulus; the functional ability of reticuloendothelial system, particularly the liver, to remove from circulation activated coagulation factors, fibrin monomers, fibrin/fibrinogen products, and immune complexes; the compensatory ability of the liver and bone marrow to accelerate clotting factor and platelet production, respectively; and finally, the extent to which any particular organ is involved with hemorrhage or thrombus.[19]

Table 29–2. CLINICAL CONDITIONS ASSOCIATED WITH DIC

| THROMBOPLASTIN RELEASE–FACTOR VII ACTIVATION | |
| --- | --- |
| Placental abruption | Retained dead fetus syndrome |
| Trauma | |
| Fat emboli syndrome | Acute intravascular hemolysis* |
| Mucin-secreting adenocarcinoma | Amniotic fluid embolus* |
| Sepsis* | Cardiopulmonary bypass surgery |
| Promyetocytic leukemia | |
| ENDOTHELIAL CELL DAMAGE–FACTOR XII ACTIVATION | |
| Immune complex disease | Burns |
| Intravascular hemolysis* | Vasculitis |
| Liver disease* | Anoxia |
| Heat stroke | Acidosis |
| Sepsis* | |
| FACTOR X/II ACTIVATION | |
| Snake venoms | Liver disease* |
| Acute pancreatitis | Fat emboli syndrome* |

*More than one mechanism may be involved.

## Laboratory Diagnosis

The laboratory findings in patients with disseminated intravascular coagulation reflect the direct or indirect effects of excess thrombin and plasmin generation (Table 29–3). The constellation of abnormalities in any particular patient, however, will depend on the nature, magnitude, and duration of the triggering stimulus; the compensatory capacity available; and the underlying disease state. Although the ultimate confirmatory test would be the direct demonstration of fibrin deposition in biopsy material from an involved blood vessel, this is not practical. As a result, a multitude of tests have been used by various laboratories to make this diagnosis.[15,21] It should be pointed out that no single test is diagnostic of disseminated intravascular coagulation; however, in the appropriate clinical setting (patient history and the type of bleeding) a battery of tests can ensure a diagnosis of disseminated intravascular coagulation. Indirect tests that lack specificity for thrombin action include the prothrombin, activated partial thromboplastin, and thrombin/reptilase clotting times. Use and depletion of the clotting factors in the disseminated intravascular coagulation process result in prolongation of each of these tests. Because platelets are also consumed during the coagulation process and their contents released, the findings of thrombocytopenia and elevated plasma levels of the platelet specific proteins beta thromboglobulin and platelet factor 4 would be expected. The plasma inhibitor antithrombin III will complex with thrombin and activated factor X, resulting in diminished plasma levels. If the fibrin deposition does not completely occlude the lumen of the damaged blood vessel, red cells may undergo a shearing effect as they traverse this area, with resultant fragmentation and the development of a microangiopathic hemolytic anemia **(see Color Figure 240).**

Specific tests for direct evidence of thrombin activity relate to the action of thrombin on fibrinogen. Other than certain snake venoms, thrombin is the only enzyme that releases the specific peptides fibrinopeptide A and B from the fibrinogen molecule. Radioimmunoassays are available to measure each fibrinopeptide.[22] The major drawback to measuring these peptides, paradoxically, is the extreme sensitivity of the assay such that elevated levels can be seen in clinical conditions when thrombin is only transiently generated. As a consequence of fibrinopeptide release, soluble fibrin monomers are formed that are capable of forming complexes with intact fibrinogen molecules or with fibrin/fibrinogen degradation products. The ability to precipitate these complexes from plasma is the basis for two paracoagulation assays, the ethanol gelation test and the protamine sulfate test.[23] Positive tests are indirect indications that thrombin was generated;

Table 29—3. LABORATORY TESTS TO DETECT EXCESS THROMBIN AND/OR PLASMIN ACTIVITY

| Excess Protease | Effect | Laboratory Tests |
|---|---|---|
| 1. Thrombin | Fibrinogen use | Fibrinogen concentration; thrombin/reptilase time; PT and APTT |
| | Use of other coagulation factors | PT and APTT |
| | | Coagulation factor assays |
| | Fibrin monomer generation | Ethanol gelation and protamine sulfate tests |
| | Fibrinopeptide A/B release | Radioimmunoassays for fibrinopeptides A and B |
| | Platelet aggregation/release | Platelet count, radioimmunoassays for beta thromboglobulin and platelet factor 4 |
| | Activation of protein C | Tissue plasminogen activator activity |
| | | Factor V/VIII assays |
| 2. Thrombin/Plasmin | Proteolysis of fibrinogen/fibrin | Fibrin-degradation products; D-D dimer concentration; B-beta 15-42 peptide assay; fibrinopeptide A and B assays |
| | Indirectly activate plasminogen activators | Euglobulin lysis time |
| | Soluble fibrin monomer/fibrinogen/FDP complexes | Protamine sulfate precipitation; ethanol gelation test |
| 3. Plasmin | Plasminogen use | Plasminogen concentration |
| | Proteolysis of fibrinogen/fibrin | Fibrin-degradation products thrombin and reptilase times B beta 15-42 peptide assay platelet aggregation and release tests |
| | Complexes with inhibitor | $\alpha_2$-Plasmin inhibitor concentration, $\alpha_2$-plasmin inhibitor: plasmin complexes |
| | Proteolysis of factors V/VIII | Factor assays |

therefore, the coagulation system had to have been activated.

Tests for the secondary activation of the fibrinolytic system in disseminated intravascular coagulation are primarily directed at demonstrating the action of plasmin on fibrin/fibrinogen. As already mentioned, a series of cleavage products, the fibrin/fibrinogen–degradation products are formed. The anticoagulant action of these fragments has been noted in the previous section. A number of immunologic tests are available to measure one or more of the fibrinogen fragments, and this can yield quantitative information on the degree of fibrinolysis. A recent development has been the recognition of an early cleavage product of the B beta chain of the fibrinogen dimer, peptide B beta 15-42.[14] Clinical assessment of the utility of the B beta 15-42 radioimmunoassay for this peptide in diagnosing accelerated fibrinolysis is ongoing. Direct measurement of the plasminogen concentration in plasma can also be performed, and assays for measuring plasmin levels are being used. An indication of increased plasminogen activator activity seen in early stages of disseminated intravascular coagulation can be obtained by performing a euglobulin lysis time.[24] The euglobulin fraction of plasma contains plasminogen, plasminogen activator, plasmin, and fibrinogen without the respective inhibitors. The rapidity of lysis of the fibrin clot is directly related to plasminogen activator levels. Assays for $\alpha_2$-plasmin inhibitor levels and for circulating plasmin $\alpha_2$-plasmin inhibitor complexes are under investigation for clinical use.

Table 29—4 summarizes laboratory tests available to diagnose disseminated intravascular coagulation and the constellation of results one can find in this syndrome depending on the balance between thrombin and plasmin activities and the compensatory capacity of the patient. This table describes three generalized clinical states of disseminated intravascular coagulation with the typical laboratory abnormalities associated with each. The decompensated DIC state refers to a condition in which active hemorrhage is evident and in which the consumption of the coagulation factors and platelets exceeds the capacity to increase the synthesis of these components. In the compensated state, laboratory evidence of an accelerated coagulation and fibrinolytic process exists (increased FPA, positive protamine sulfate test, increased beta thromboglobulin, increased FDPs, presence of plasmin $\alpha_2$-plasmin inhibitor complexes), but the rate synthesis of the coagulation components is balanced with the rate of destruction. Because of this balance the prothrombin time (PT); activated partial thromboplastin time (APTT), thrombin time, and platelet count are usually normal. The hypercoagulable state is the result of excess thrombin present in the plasma with a delayed or lessened plasmin response. A characteristic finding in this form of DIC is a shortened APTT, although this is by no means sensitive or specific. It should be realized that these clinical states are not static, and it is not unusual for one to evolve into one of the others depending on the nature of the underlying disease process and the response to therapy.

Table 29-4. LABORATORY TESTS TO DIAGNOSE DIC

|  | Decompensated | Compensated | Hypercoagulable |
|---|---|---|---|
| **Routine Tests** | | | |
| PT | I | N | N |
| APTT | I | N | D |
| Thrombin/Reptilase times | I | N/I | N/I |
| Fibrinogen | D | N | I |
| Platelet count | D | N/D | N |
| Fibrin-degradation products | I | I | N/I |
| Euglobulin lysis test | N/I/D | N/D | N |
| Protamine sulfate test | P | P/Ng | P/Ng |
| **Special Tests** | | | |
| Coagulation factor levels | D | N/D | I |
| Fibrinopeptide A | I | I | I |
| B-Beta 15-42 peptide | I | I | N |
| Plasminogen | D | N/D | N |
| Plasmin: $\alpha_2$-plasmin inhibitor complexes | I | I | N |
| Beta thromboglobulin/platelet factor 4 levels | I | I | I |
| Antithrombin III | D | N/D | N/D |

I = increased; D = decreased; N = normal; P = positive; Ng = negative.

## Therapy

Therapy of disseminated intravascular coagulation is essentially twofold: treatment or removal of the underlying pathologic stimulus and maintenance of blood volume and hemostatic function.[19,20] Dramatic improvement in the patient's clinical status with abrupt cessation of bleeding and normalization of the coagulation abnormalities can be seen in certain cases of DIC with removal of the underlying pathologic stimulus alone (e.g., DIC associated with retained dead fetus). In cases of DIC associated with septicemia, appropriate antibiotic therapy is imperative in order to control the pathologic process (i.e., bacterial or endotoxin-induced vascular damage). Blood component replacement therapy with transfusion of packed red blood cells, fresh frozen plasma, and platelets to maintain blood volume and to support hemostatic function is indicated in those patients with active bleeding or whose compensatory capacity is limited. In addition to fresh frozen plasma, cryoprecipitate (enriched in fibrinogen, factor VIII, and fibronectin) and prothrombin complex (enriched in vitamin K-dependent clotting factors) are often used as supplemental sources of blood component therapy. The administration of heparin in DIC has been advocated by a number of investigators, but its use is controversial. On the premise that the underlying pathologic basis for DIC is generation of excess thrombin, heparin theoretically should slow or stop the coagulation process by complexing with antithrombin III and thrombin or Xa. In control studies, however, it does not appear that heparin therapy influences the clinical outcome.[25] Its use can result in increased bleeding and because heparin itself affects a number of coagulation tests, it is often difficult to monitor the effect of

conventional therapy. Heparin should be used and is most effective in those cases of DIC that present with clinical evidence of a hypercoagulable state with evident vascular thrombosis. Heparin has also been shown to be effective in DIC associated with acute progranulocytic leukemia (M3). When major peripheral vessels are occluded as part of the hypercoagulable process, the use of fibrinolytic agents (streptokinase or urokinase) may be indicated as an initial management choice with subsequent heparinization, but clinical experience with this form of therapy is minimal. Table 29-5 summarizes the previously described profile of DIC.

## RELATED DISORDERS

Primary fibrinolysis is an unusual situation in which plasmin is formed in the absence of coagulation taking place. The clinical presentation in this disorder is similar to that in disseminated intravascular coagulation, with diffuse hemorrhage occurring as a result of increased plasma fibrinolyic activity. Several mechanisms may possibly initiate this process. The presence of proteolytic enzymes in plasma, which are capable of either directly or indirectly converting plasminogen into plasmin, can occur in certain disease states. The genitourinary system is enriched in urokinases, which can enter the systemic circulation following various urologic procedures. The fibrinolytic state seen in patients with metastatic prostatic carcinoma is another example of this mechanism. The basis for the hemorrhagic state seen following cardiopulmonary bypass surgery is complex, but activation of the plasminogen-plasmin system with increased fibrinolytic activity is well documented. The failure of the hepatic

Table 29–5. PROFILE OF DIC

| Synonyms | Conditions Associated With DIC | Suggested Triggering Mechanisms | Clinical Manifestations | Clinical Laboratory Findings | Sequential Therapy |
|---|---|---|---|---|---|
| 1. "Consumptive Coagulopathy" 2. Defibrination Syndrome | Obstetric accidents Intravascular hemolysis Septicemia Viremia (varicella) Leukemias: Acute Promyelocytic Other Solid malignancy Acidosis/alkalosis Burns Crush injury and tissue necrosis Vascular disorders | Amniotic fluid, which possesses thrombo-plastic activity Retained fetus, which possesses thrombo-plastic activity Byproduct of red cell hemolysis (phospho-lipid) Antigen/antibody complexes Endotoxin release Chronic stasis Complement activation | 1. *General signs:* significant hemorrhaging (usually from 3 unrelated sites: melena and hematemesis, epistaxis, or hemoptysis) fever, hypotension, acidosis, hypoxia, proteinuria, hematuria 2. *Specific signs:* petechiae, purpura, gangrene, wound bleeding, venipuncture bleeding, subcutaneous hematomas 3. *Microthrombi* 4. *End organ dysfunction* | Hypofibrino-genemia Abnormal PT Abnormal PTT Abnormal thrombin time Abnormal platelet count Abnormal tourniquet test Abnormal clot retraction Abnormal factors V and VIII Positive fibrin(ogen)-split products Positive protamine sulfate test Positive ethanol gelatin test Antithrombin III consumption Leukocytosis Schistocytosis Thrombo-cytopenia Reticulocytosis | 1. Remove or treat triggering process 2. Stop or slow coagulation process a. Miniheparin b. Heparin c. Antiplatelet drugs d. AT-III concentrates 3. Blood component replacement a. Platelets b. Fibrinogen c. Prothrombin complex d. AHF 4. Antifibrinolytic therapy* a. Epsilon amino caproic acid (EACA) |

*Sequential therapy used only after clotting is stopped. (3% of patients may require this therapy.)

clearance mechanism to remove plasminogen activator accounts for the increased fibrinolytic activity seen in a variety of hepatic disorders, particularly cirrhosis. Under normal circumstances, the hepatic reticuloendothelial system removes not only activated clotting proteins but also plasminogen activator from the systemic circulation. In impairment of this function, as in patients who have hepatic disease or portocaval shunting procedures, the removal of plasminogen activator is less than adequate and hyperplasminemia may occur with resultant hemorrhage. These mechanisms are by no means clear-cut, and many hematologists doubt the existence of primary fibrinolysis.

The coagulation abnormalities seen in these fibrinolytic disorders are similar to those in disseminated intravascular coagulation, with prolonged PT, APTT, and thrombin times. These defects result from the hypofibrinogenemic state induced by the proteolytic cleavage of fibrinogen by excess plasmin in addition to the catabolic effect of this enzyme on factors V and VIII. Fibrin-degradation product concentrations are increased and, as previously noted, will further interfere with coagulation by acting as antithrombins. With the excess plasmin activity, the euglobulin lysis time is typically shortened. Since thrombin is not generated during this pathologic process, several laboratory tests can serve readily to distinguish primary fibrinolysis from disseminated intravascular coagulation. The platelet count is typically normal, fibrinopeptides A and B levels are not elevated, and circulating fibrin monomer complexes are absent in primary fibrinolysis, in contrast to the results in disseminated intravascular coagulation.

Thrombotic thrombocytopenic purpura (TTP) is a syndrome of unknown etiology in which fibrin and platelet thrombi are formed diffusely throughout the microvasculature, in contrast to the localized thrombus formation seen in disseminated intravascular coagulation.[26,27] The clinical picture consists of a pentad of findings: (1) fever, (2) microangiopathic hemolytic anemia, (3) thrombocytopenia, (4) azotemia, and (5) and vacillating neurologic deficits. Despite fibrin and platelet deposition, this disorder is not typically associated with excessive activation of the coagulation system. Supportive evidence that this syndrome represents an abnormality of the fibrinolytic system is suggested by the finding of diminished or absent fibrinolytic activity, particularly of tissue plasminogen activator, in plasma and blood vessels affected with microthrombi. Therapy has not been standardized, but antiplatelet drugs (e.g., aspirin or dipyridamole), plasmapheresis, and exchange transfusion have been used either singularly or in combination, with variable success (see Chapter 27). Table 29–6 summarizes the other causes of fibrinolytic activation.

Table 29–6. OTHER CAUSES OF FIBRINOLYTIC ACTIVATION

| Clinical Condition | Mechanism | Clinical Manifestation | Other Hemostatic Alterations |
|---|---|---|---|
| 1. Chronic liver disease | Abnormal fibrinolytic inhibitor ($\alpha$-2-macroglobulin) Abnormal hepatic clearance of plasminogen activators | Often fulminant hemorrhage with massive hemoptysis, hematochezia, melena, or epistaxis. May also demonstrate petechiae, purpura, spider telangiectasia, ecchymoses | 1. Hypofibrinogenemia (due to lysis) 2. Elevated FDP (X, Y, D, and E) a. Defective fibrin monomer/polymerization b. Platelet dysfunction 3. Proteolysis of factors V, VIII, IX, XI 4. Platelet defects a. Thrombocytopenia b. Platelet dysfunction (FDP, PF3) 5. Coagulation protein defects a. Decreased synthesis of II, VII, IX, and X b. Decreased synthesis of Fletcher factor c. Decreased or dysfunctional synthesis of AT-III |
| 2. Cardiopulmonary bypass (CPB) | Unclear; possibly direct activation of fibrinolysis by the oxygenation system or pump-induced accelerated flow rates may activate plasminogen to plasmin or may alter endothelial plasminogen activator activity | Hemorrhage; hematuria, petechiae/purpura, and oozing from intravenous site in conjunction with increased chest tube loss | 1. Hyperfibrinolysis results in a. Elevated FDP b. Hypofibrinogenemia c. Low factors V and VIII 2. Functional platelet defect a. CPB-induced b. Drug-induced 3. Thrombocytopenia 4. Hyperheparinemia-heparin rebound(?) 5. DIC (?) |
| 3. Malignancy | Poorly understood, in several instances tumor extracts possess the ability to activate directly or indirectly the fibrinolytic system (e.g., gastric carcinoma, sarcomas, and prostatic carcinoma) | Thrombosis/hemorrhage | 1. Thrombocytopenia 2. Platelet function defects 3. Elevated FDP 4. Decreased AT-III 5. DIC(?) |

## CASE STUDY

A 32-year-old Caucasian female, gravida 3, para 2, in her 36th week of gestation noted the sudden onset of lower abdominal pain and profuse vaginal bleeding. She was rushed to the emergency room. On examination, she was noted to be hypotensive with a blood pressure of 70/40 and a marked tachycardia. Large ecchymoses and continuous oozing of blood from venipuncture sites were evident. A fetal heart tone was barely audible. Births of her other children were uncomplicated, and the family history was negative for a hemorrhagic diathesis.

Initial coagulation studies revealed PT 26 sec (normal 11 to 13 sec); APTT 84 sec (normal 24 to 30 sec); platelet count 20,000 (normal 140 to 440,000/$\mu$l); fibrinogen 85 mg/dl (normal 145 to 350 mg/dl); FDPs >40 $\mu$g/ml (normal <10 $\mu$g/ml); and protamine sulfate test result positive (normal negative). Blood smear showed numerous red cell fragments present.

A diagnosis of disseminated intravascular coagulation was made based on the patient's clinical presentation and the supportive laboratory data. The patient was placed on intravenous fluids to maintain her blood pressure and was given 2 units of fresh frozen plasma and 10 units of platelets. She was taken to the operating room where she underwent a cesarean section. Her bleeding abated postoperatively and all coagulation parameters returned to normal within 36 hours.

This case is illustrative of an obstetric complication, placental abruption, which resulted in an acute disseminated intravascular coagulation syndrome. Several triggering mechanisms have been postulated as an explanation for the underlying coagulopathy in this disorder, including the release of thromboplastin-like material from the amniotic fluid and tissue necrosis in the area of the retroperitoneal hemorrhage. The laboratory parameters are consistent with a consumptive coagulopathy and secondary fibrinolysis. With the delivery and removal of the placenta the source of the triggering mechanism was removed, and the pathologic process stopped. Restoration of normal hemostatic parameters results within hours postoperatively, and usually no further blood component replacement therapy is required.

# References

1. Kaplan, AP, Silverberg, M, Dunn, JI, et al: Interaction of the clotting, kinin forming, complement and fibrinolytic pathways. NY Acad Sci 389:25, 1982

2. Sundsmo, JS and Fair, DS: Relationships among the complement, kinin, coagulation and fibrinolytic systems. Springer Semin Immunopathol 6:231, 1983.

3. Castellino, FJ: Recent advances in the chemistry of the fibrinolytic systems. Chem Rev 81:431, 1981.

4. Miller, JL: Normal fibrinolysis. In Henry JB (ed): Clinical Diagnosis and Management by Laboratory Methods. Ed 17. WB Saunders, Philadelphia, 1984, p 769.

5. Mandle, RJ and Kaplan, AP: Hageman factor-dependent fibrinolysis: Generation of fibrinolytic activity by the interation of human activated factor XI and plasminogen. Blood 54:850, 1979.

6. Bachman, F and Kruithof, IEKO: Tissue plasminogen activator: Chemical and physiological aspects. Sem Thromb Hemost 10:6, 1984.

7. Owen, WG: The control of hemostasis. Arch Pathol Lab Med 106:209, 1982.

8. Owen, WG and Esmon, CT: Functional properties of an endothelial cell cofactor for thrombin-catalysed activation of protein C. J Biol Chem 256:5532, 1981.

9. Prowse, CV and Cash, JD: Physiologic and pharmacologic enhancement of fibrinolysis. Sem Thromb Hemost 10:51, 1984.

10. Rickli, EE: The activation mechanism of human plasminogen. Thromb Diath Haemorrh 34:386, 1975.

11. Brogden, RN, Speight, TM, Avery, GS, et al: Streptokinase: A review of its clinical pharmacology, mechanism of action and therapeutic uses. Drugs 5:357, 1973.

12. Gonzalez-Gronow, M, Violand, BN, Castellino, FJ, et al: Purification and some properties of the glu- and lys- human plasmin heavy chains. J Biol Chem 252:2175, 1977.

13. Marder, VJ, Shulman, NR, Carroll, WR, et al: High molecular weight derivatives of human fibrinogen produced by plasmin. I. Physicochemical and immunologic characterization. J Biol Chem 244:2111, 1969.

14. Kudryk, B, Robinson, D, Netre, C, et al: Measurement in human blood of fibrinogen/fibrin fragments containing the B beta 15-42 sequence. Thromb Res 25:277, 1982.

15. Ockelford, A and Carter, J: DIC: Application and utility of diagnostic tests. Sem Thromb Hemost 8:198, 1982.

16. Bini, A and Collen, D: Measurement of plasmin-$\alpha_2$-antiplasmin coupled in human plasma. A comparison of latex agglutination inhibition and hemagglutination inhibition tests. Thromb Res 12:389, 1978.

17. Aoki, N and Harpel, PC: Inhibitors of the fibrinolytic enzyme system. Sem Thromb Hemost 10:24, 1984.

18. Kwaan, HC: Disorders of fibrinolysis. Med Clin North Am 56:163, 1972.

19. Brozovic, M: Disseminated intravascular coagulation. In Bloom, AL and Thomas, DP (eds): Haemostasis and Thrombosis. Churchill Livingstone, New York, 1981, p 415.

20. Muller-Berghaus, G: Pathophysiology of generalized intravascular coagulation. Sem Thromb Hemost 3:209, 1977.

21. Farood, L, Walenga, JM, Blck JI, et al: Impact of automation on the quantitation of low molecular weight markers of hemostatic defects. Sem Thromb Hemost 9:355, 1983.

22. Hirsh, J: Blood tests for the diagnosis of venous and arterial thrombosis. Blood 57:1, 1981.

23. Jacobsen, CD and Southers, NJ: Ethanol gelation and protamine sulfate tests. Thromb Diath Haemorrh 29:130, 1973.

24. Buckell, M: The effect of citrate on euglobulin methods of estimating fibrinolytic activity. J Clin Pathol 11:403, 1958.

25. Mant, MJ and King, EG: Severe, acute disseminated intravascular coagulation. A reappraisal of its pathophysiology, clinical significance and therapy based on 47 patients. Am J Med 47:557, 1979.

26. Kwaan, HC, Gallo, G, Potter, E, et al: The nature of the vascular lesion in thrombotic thrombocytopenic purpura. Ann Intern Med 68:1169, 1968.

27. Bukowski, RM: Thrombotic thrombocytopenic purpura: A review. Prog Hemost Thromb 6:287, 1982.

# CHAPTER 30

BETTY E. CIESLA, B.S., M.T.(ASCP), S.H.(ASCP)

# Evaluation of Red Cell Morphology and Summary of Platelet and White Cell Morphology

It is the job of hematology atlases to guide the student through red cell morphology in a step-by-step fashion; however, this is not the intent of this chapter. Although some basic mechanics in estimating morphology will be discussed, the emphasis will be placed on interpretative morphology and its relevance to clinical conditions. By providing physiologic mechanisms, an attempt will be made to demonstrate the cause of a particular morphologic picture. This description of blood cell morphology will facilitate the overall assessment of the patient's condition.

## ANISOCYTOSIS VERSUS POIKILOCYTOSIS

By definition, anisocytosis implies a variation in size of erythrocytes seen in a well-stained, well-dispersed smear. Poikilocytosis is defined as a variation in shape of erythrocytes seen in a well-stained, well-dispersed smear. The majority of institutions use either qualitative remarks or a numerical grading (1+ to 4+) to describe anisocytosis and poikilocytosis; then they proceed to quantify the red cell changes observed. I suggest that a simple statement of the terms "aniso" and "poik" be adopted when applicable. I advise that the quantification or use of qualitative adjectives be reserved only for the more important assessment of the actual numbers and types of morphologically abnormal cells. What is paramount in the examination of the peripheral smear is the type of cells seen. Valid morphologic findings need to be reproducible from field to field. Why is a new approach to red cell morphology necessary? First, it is very difficult to explain to the new student what a 1+ variation in size of red blood cells is as opposed to a 2+ variation in size. Proponents of the quantitative methods instruct an analysis of size and shape changes in 10 oil immersion fields, by tallying up those changes (e.g., first field 6macro-5macro; second field 7macro, 8macro; and so on), dividing by 10, and then assessing anisocytosis. Likewise, the qualitative genre applies the adjective "slight," "moderate," or "marked" to the words "aniso" and "poik." It becomes apparent that time spent in either of these endeavors for purposes of recording the presence of aniso or poik in a differential might be better spent in assessing the numbers and types of cells that make these variations obvious.

## THE NORMAL RED BLOOD CELL

The mature erythrocyte (red blood cell, normocyte, erythron) is a remarkable structure. Its simplistic appearance is deceiving. It is one of the few cells that passes from a nucleated to a non-nucleated status upon maturity, with decreasing size, and a dramatic change in cytoplasmic color. On a Wright-stained blood smear, this mature red cell has a reddish-orange appearance. The red cell has an average diameter of 6.0 to 8.0 $\mu$ and an average volume of 90 $\mu^3$. The area of central pallor is approximately 2 to 3 $\mu$ in diameter and size variation of red cells from a normal patient is approximately 5 percent.

Fundamental to the red cell is the formation of hemoglobin, which functions primarily as the oxygen-carrying capacity of the cell; yet a minimum amount of hemoglobin is required for maintenance

of structural integrity. The red cell membrane is a lipid bilayer whose skeleton is composed of actin and spectrin. Spectrin, the dominant membrane protein consists of two high molecular weight polypeptides and functions prominently in the maintenance of cell shape and deformability.

## SIZE VARIATIONS

### Macrocytes

#### Physiologic Mechanism

Macrocytes may be defined as cells approximately 9 $\mu$ or larger in diameter, having an MCV of greater than 100 $\mu^3$. They may arrive in the peripheral circulation by several mechanisms. Three of the most distinct are (1) impaired DNA synthesis leading to a decreased number of cellular divisions and, consequently, a larger cell (megaloblastic erythropoiesis); (2) accelerated erythropoiesis in the face of anemic stress yielding a reticulocytosis, which in the Wright-stained smear is manifested as polychromatophilic macrocytes; and (3) increased membrane cholesterol and lecithin (however, conditions using this mechanism may not be reflective of "true" macrocytosis, e.g., obstructive liver disease).

#### Peripheral Blood Findings

A careful evaluation of the type of macrocyte seen in the peripheral blood smear can give many clues as to the underlying mechanism. Macrocytes should be evaluated for shape (oval versus round), color (red versus blue), and the presence or absence of pallor and of inclusions.

Common clinical conditions in which macrocytes, particularly oval macrocytes can be found include the megaloblastic anemias (those due to vitamin $B_{12}$ or folate deficiency) and myelodysplasia. Thin macrocytes with some targetting may be seen in patients with liver disease or hyposplenic conditions, as well as postsplenectomy. In patients undergoing chemotherapy, a macrocytosis invariably develops, as these drugs interfere with folate metabolism or DNA synthesis. Additionally, macrocytes may be seen in the following conditions: scurvy, metastatic marrow infiltration in neonatal blood, and hypothyroidism **(see Color Figure 73)**.

### Microcytes

#### Physiologic Mechanism

A microcyte is defined as a small cell having a diameter of less than 7 $\mu$ and an MCV of less than 80 $\mu^3$. Any defect that results in impaired hemoglobin synthesis will result in a microcytic hypochromic blood picture. When developing erythroid cells are deprived of any of the "essentials" in hemoglobin synthesis (see Chapter 4), the results are increased cellular division and, consequently, a smaller cell in the peripheral blood. Hemoglobin synthesis involves multiple steps, and microcytosis develops from (1) ineffective iron utilization, absorption, or release; and (2) decreased or defective globin synthesis. Effective porphyrin synthesis is of course vital for hemoglobinization; however, the porphyrias generally do not cause a microcytic erythrocyte.

### Peripheral Blood Findings

There are only three clinical conditions that produce a microcytic blood picture: iron-deficiency anemia, thalassemia syndromes, and anemia of chronic disease. A significant number of microcytes may be seen in patients with lead poisoning and iron-loading anemias. However, the number of microcytes in these conditions is not large enough to cause microcytic blood indices **(see Color Figure 66)**.

## STAIN VARIATIONS
## Hypochromia
### Physiologic Mechanism

Any red blood cell having a central area of pallor of greater than $3\,\mu$ is said to be hypochromic. There is a direct relationship between the amount of hemoglobin deposited in the red cell and the appearance of the red cell when properly stained. For this reason, any aberration of hemoglobin synthesis will lead to some degree of hypochromia. Most clinicians choose to assess hypochromia based on the MCHC, which by definition measures hemoglobin content in a given volume (100 ml) of red cells. In general, this is very reliable; however, it does not take into account the situation when a true hypochromia is observed in the presence of a normal MCHC. Suffice to say that not all hypochromic cells are microcytic. Target cells possess some degree of hypochromia, and some macrocytes and normocytes can be distinctly hypochromic.

### Peripheral Blood Findings

The most common and severe changes in hypochromia are seen in patients with iron-deficiency anemia. In patients with severe cases of iron-deficiency anemia, red cells exhibit an inordinately thin band of hemoglobin. Patients with iron deficiency will have a variety of hypochromic cells, depending on the magnitude of the deficiency.

Hypochromia in patients with thalassemia syndromes is much less pronounced. In the alpha thalassemias and beta thalassemia trait, the MCHC is normal. The sideroblastic anemias show a prominent dimorphic blood picture: macrocytic, normocytic, and microcytic cells together, only some of which show true hypochromia. Some hypochromic cells may be seen in victims of lead poisoning; however, the association of microcytosis with lead poisoning, irrespective of any other underlying process, is being questioned.

The morphologist should not be unduly influenced by the red blood cell indices in the evaluation of hypochromia. In many cases, the MCHC will not be concordant with what is observed on the peripheral smear. True hypochromia will appear as a delicate shaded area of pallor as opposed to pseudohypochromia (the water artifact), in which the area of pallor is distinctly outlined **(see Color Figure 66)**.

## Polychromasia
### Physiologic Mechanism

When red blood cells are delivered to the peripheral circulation prematurely, their appearance in the Wright-stained smear is distinctive. Red cells showing polychromatophilia are gray-blue and usually larger than normal red cells. The basophilia of the red cell is the result of the residual RNA involved in hemoglobin synthesis. Polychromatophilic macrocytes are actually reticulocytes; however, the reticulum cannot be visualized with Wright's stain. A supravital stain such as new methylene blue must be used to stain the residual aggregates of RNA **(see Color Figure 241)**.

### Peripheral Blood Findings

It is not uncommon to find a few polychromatophilic cells in a normal peripheral blood smear, since regeneration of red cells is a dynamic process. The reticulocyte count should reflect the degree of polychromasia. In the blood smear polychromatophilic red cells come in varying shades of blue. Any clinical condition in which the marrow is stimulated, particularly red blood cell regeneration, will produce a polychromatophilic blood picture. This represents effective erythropoiesis. Examples of several conditions in which polychromasia is noted include acute and chronic hemorrhage, hemolysis, and any regenerative red cell process. In the latter case, treating such conditions as iron-deficiency anemia, folate and vitamin $B_{12}$ deficiency anemias, and "responding" aplastic processes the degree of polychromasia is an excellent indication of the therapeutic effectiveness of the particular treatment **(see Color Figure 115)**.

## SHAPE VARIATIONS
## Target Cells (Codocytes)
### Physiologic Mechanism

Target cells appear on the peripheral blood as a result of increase in red blood cell surface membrane. Their true circulating form is a bell-shaped cell. In air-dried smears, however, they appear as "targets" with a large portion of hemoglobin displayed at the rim of the cell and a portion of hemoglobin either central, eccentric, or banded. Target cells are always hypochromic.

The mechanism of targetting is related to excess membrane cholesterol and phospholipid and decreased cellular hemoglobin. This is well documented in patients with liver disease, in which the cholesterol-phospholipid ratio is altered. Mature red cells are unable to synthesize cholesterol and phospholipid independently. As cholesterol accumulates in the plasma, as is the case with liver dysfunction, the red cell is expanded by increased membrane lipid, resulting in increased surface area. Consequently, the osmotic fragility is also decreased.

### Peripheral Blood Findings

The presence of target cells is a common clinical finding in any of the conditions in which hemoglobin synthesis is abnormal: thalassemia major and minor, sickle cell anemia, heterozygous and homozygous hemoglobin C disease. Targets may also be observed postsplenectomy and in patients with liver disease and iron deficiency **(see Color Figure 100)**.

## Spherocytes

### Physiologic Mechanism

Spherocytes have several distinctive properties and, in contrast to the target cell, the lowest surface area–to–volume ratio. They are smaller than the normal red cell, and their hemoglobin content seems to be relatively concentrated. Because there is no visible central pallor, they are easily distinguished in a peripheral smear. Their shape change is irreversible.

There are several mechanisms for the production of spherocytes, each sharing the mutual defect of loss of membrane. In the normal aging process of red cells, spherocytes are produced as a final stage before senescent red cells are detained in the spleen and trapped by the reticuloendothelial system. Coating of the red cells with antibodies and the detrimental effect of complement activation will produce spherocytes as the red cell membrane loses cholesterol, and consequently surface area, owing to splenic sequestration.

Perhaps the most detailed mechanism for sphering is the congenital condition known as hereditary spherocytosis. This autosomal dominant condition is an intrinsic defect in the red cell membrane that causes the spheroidal red cell to be trapped prematurely and destroyed in the spleen. Erythrocytes from patients with hereditary spherocytosis have a mean influx of sodium twice that of normal cells. It is thought that this increased permeability to sodium results from some sort of membrane "lesion." As these cells travel through plasma, they are able to handle their increased sodium content, because it has been documented that spherocytes have 35 times the ability of normal cells to metabolize glucose, producing enough energy to pump sodium out of the cell. However, once these cells reach the microenvironment of the spleen, where glucose is deficient, the active-passive transport system is invariably "hurt," and the cells swell and hemolyze (see Chapter 7).

### Peripheral Blood Findings

Spherocytes may be seen in patients with the immune hemolytic anemias, the hemoglobinopathies, hereditary spherocytosis, and severe burns. They may also be observed in any of the "splenic states," hypersplenism, or postsplenectomy, as well as in any of the microangiopathic processes **(see Color Figure 87)**.

## Ovalocytes/Elliptocytes

### Physiologic Mechanism

Many investigators consider "ovalocytes" and "elliptocytes" to be interchangeable terms; however, these two items will be dealt with distinctly and separately.

Ovalocytes have many capabilities; they may appear normochromic or hypochromic, normocytic or macrocytic. The exact physiologic mechanism is not well defined. When these erythrocytes are incubated in vitro, they reduce adenosine triphosphate (ATP) and 2,3-DPG more rapidly than do normal cells. Hemoglobin seems to have a bipolar arrangement in these cells and there seems to be a reduction in membrane cholesterol.

Ovalocytes are more egg-shaped and have a greater tendency to vary in their hemoglobin content than elliptocytes. Elliptocytes, on the other hand, are pencil-shaped and invariably not hypochromic.

### Peripheral Blood Findings

Ovalocytes may be found in patients with megaloblastic anemias, and appear as oval macrocytes in those with thalassemia major and postsplenectomy. They may be seen in patients with sickle cell anemia and myelodysplasias. Elliptocytes are seen in those with hereditary elliptocytosis, iron-deficiency anemia, and myelofibrosis **(see Color Figure 88)**.

## Stomatocytes

### Physiologic Mechanism

The stomatocyte is defined as a red cell of normal size that in wet preparation appears bowl-shaped.

This peculiar shape is manifested in air-dried smears as a "slit-like" area of central pallor. Many facts are known about stomatocytes; however, their exact physiologic mechanism in vivo has not been elucidated. Many chemical agents may induce stomatocytosis in vitro (phenothiazine and chlorpromazine); however, these changes are reversible. Stomatocytes are known to have an increased permeability to sodium; consequently, their osmotic fragility is increased.

## Peripheral Blood Findings

Stomatocytes are more often artifactual than a true manifestation of a particular pathophysiologic process. The artifactual stomatocyte will have a distinct slit-like area of central pallor, whereas the area of pallor in the true stomatocyte will appear shaded. Stomatocytes may be associated with several disease states, including hereditary spherocytosis (the stomatospherocyte viewed best in wet preparations); hereditary stomatocytosis, which is usually a benign, occasionally hemolytic, condition; acute alcoholism; and in patients with the Rh null phenotype (see Color Figure 90).

## Sickled Cells (Drepanocytes)

### Physiologic Mechanism

Sickle cells or drepanocytes are red cells that have been transformed by hemoglobin polymerization into rigid, inflexible cells with at least one pointed projection. Patients may be homozygous or heterozygous for the presence of the abnormal hemoglobin, hemoglobin S. Conditions of low oxygen tension (in vivo or in vitro) cause the abnormal hemoglobin to polymerize to form tubules, which line up in bundles to deform the cell. The surface area of the transformed cell is much greater, and the normal elasticity of the cell is severely restricted. Most sickled cells possess the ability to revert to the discocyte shape when oxygenated; however, approximately 10 percent are incapable of reverting to their normal shape. These irreversibly sickled cells (ISC) are the result of repeated sickling episodes. In the peripheral smear they appear as crescent-shaped cells with long projections. When reoxygenated, ISC may undergo fragmentation.

Classically sickled cells are best seen in wet preparations. Many of the cells observed in the Wright-Giemsa stain are the oat cell or the boat-shaped form of the sickled cell. In this form the projections are much less pronounced, and the central area of the cell is fairly broad. This shape is reversible. During a symptomatic period the percentages of irreversibly sickled cells vary tremendously and consequently do not correlate with symptomatology.

## Peripheral Blood Findings

Sickled cells are naturally seen in patients homozygous for hemoglobin S and are rarely seen in the heterozygous states (see Color Figures 96 and 98). Several other hemoglobinopathies may exhibit sickling, such as hemoglobin C Harlem and hemoglobin I. Hemoglobin O Arab does not sickle but facilitates the sickling process and therefore increases the severity of the S heterozygous state. Varying numbers of sickle cells may be seen in combination with other hemoglobinopathies and with the thalassemias.

## Acanthocytes

### Physiologic Mechanism

An acanthocyte is defined as a cell of normal or slightly reduced size possessing 3 to 12 spicules of uneven length distributed along the periphery of the cell membrane (see Color Figures 92 and 130). The uneven projections of the acanthocyte are blunt rather than pointed, and the acanthocyte can easily be distinguished from the peripheral smear background because it appears to be saturated with hemoglobin. The MCHC is, however, always in the normal range.

A specific mechanism related to the formation of acanthocytes is unknown. There are, however, some details about these peculiar cells that are of interest. Acanthocytes contain an excess of cholesterol and have an increased cholesterol to phospholipid ratio. Their surface area is increased. The lecithin content of acanthocytes is decreased. The only inherited condition in which acanthocytes are seen in numerous numbers in congenital abetalipoproteinemia. Most cases of acanthocytosis are acquired, such as the deficiency of L-CAT (lecithin–cholesterol acyltransferase), which has been well documented in patients with severe hepatic disease. This enzyme is synthesized by the liver and is directly responsible for esterifying free cholesterol; when this enzyme is deficient, cholesterol builds in the plasma.

The red cell responds to this excess cholesterol in one of two ways, depending on the balance of other lipids in the membrane. It will become a target cell or an acanthocyte. Once an acanthocyte is formed it is very liable to splenic sequestration and fragmentation, and the fluidity of the membrane is directly affected.

## Peripheral Blood Findings

As previously mentioned, acanthocytes are seen in congenital abetalipoproteinemia in high percentages (see Color Figure 92). Variable numbers of acanthocytes may be observed in patients with severe liver disease (see Color Figure 130), hypothyroidism, and vitamin E deficiency, as well as in splenectomized patients. It may be pointed out that in patients in whom acanthocytes are acquired, some type of plasma factor may be operative. Evidence for this is suggested by the fact that blood cells transfused to these patients within five days showed some acanthocyte formation.

## Fragmented Cells (Schistocytes, Burr Cells (Echinocytes), Helmet Cells)

### Physiologic Mechanism

It may seem unusual to have these three red cell forms under the same heading; however, the choice for such a grouping becomes reasonable with an expanded definition of fragmentation. Fragmentation may be defined as "loss from the cell of a piece of membrane which may or may not contain hemoglobin" **(see Color Figures 121, 122, and 240)**. These events may occur repeatedly without the loss of hemoglobin; however, each successive loss of membrane (each fragmentation that occurs) leaves the red cell more rigid and more likely to become entrapped in the splenic sinuses. It is recognized that not all membrane alterations occur pathologically. Indeed, the echinocytic transformation of normal red cells in stored plasma is known to be reversible. Likewise, discocyte to echinocyte transformation is part of normal red cell senescence. However, there are certain triggering events in disease that invariably lead to fragmentation. Two pathways are recognized. First, alteration of normal fluid circulation occurs, which may predispose to fragmentation. Examples of this include vasculitis, malignant hypertension, thrombotic thrombocytopenic purpura, and heart valve replacement.

Second, intrinsic defects of the red cell make it less deformable and therefore more likely to be fragmented as it traverses the microvasculature of the spleen. Spherocytes, antibody-altered red cells, and red cells containing inclusions have significant alterations that decrease their red cell survival, and these serve as examples of the second pathway.

### Peripheral Blood Findings

Burr cells (echinocytes) are red cells with approximately 10 to 30 spicules evenly placed over the surface of the red cells **(see Color Figure 123)**. They are normochromic and for the most part normocytic. They may be observed as an artifact but may also occur in small numbers in patients with uremia, heart disease, cancer of the stomach, or bleeding peptic ulcer, immediately following an injection of heparin, and in a number of patients with untreated hypothyroidism. In general, they may occur in situations that cause a change in tonicity of the intravascular fluid (e.g., dehydration and azotemia).

Helmet cells are recognized by their distinctive projections—usually two—surrounding an empty area of the red cell membrane that looks as if it has been bitten off **(see Color Figures 93, 125, and 126)**. In hematologic conditions in which large inclusion bodies (Heinz bodies) are formed helmet cells are visible in the peripheral smear. Fragmentation occurs by the pitting mechanism of the spleen. Helmet cells may also be seen in patients with pulmonary emboli, myeloid metaplasia, and DIC.

Schistocytes are the extreme form of red cell fragmentation **(see Color Figures 122, 125, 126, and 240)**. Whole pieces of red cell membrane appear to be missing, and very bizarre red cells are apparent. Schistocytes may be seen in patients with microangiopathic hemolytic anemia, DIC, heart valve surgery, hemolytic uremic syndrome, thrombotic thrombocytopenic purpura, as well as those with severe burns.

## Teardrop Cells

### Physiologic Mechanism

Teardrop cells appear in the peripheral circulation as "pear-shaped" red cells **(see Color Figures 132 and 185)**. The extent to which a portion of the red cell forms a tail is variable; and these cells may be normal, reduced, or increased in size. The exact physiologic mechanism is unknown, yet teardrop formation from inclusion-containing red cells is well documented. As cells containing large inclusions attempt to pass through the microcirculation, the portion of the cells containing the inclusion gets pinched, leaving a tailed end as it continues its journey. For some reason, the red cell is unable to maintain the discocyte shape once this has occurred.

### Peripheral Blood Findings

Teardrop cells are seen especially in myelofibrosis with myeloid metaplasia **(see Color Figures 132 and 185)**. This type of morphologic finding can also be seen in patients with thalassemia syndromes, iron deficiency, and conditions in which inclusion bodies are formed.

## VARIATIONS IN RED CELL DISTRIBUTION

## Agglutination

If an erythrocyte antibody is present in a patient's plasma and a corresponding erythrocyte antigen is represented, agglutination will take place. Such is the case with cold antibody syndromes such as cold hemagglutinin disease. The agglutination occurs at room temperature in EDTA sample preparation and will appear as interspersed areas of clumping throughout the peripheral smear **(see Color Figure 116)**. The use of saline will not disperse these agglutinated areas; however, warming the sample helps to break up the agglutinins.

## Rouleaux

Rouleaux formation is the result of elevated globulins or fibrinogen in the plasma. Red cells that are constantly bathed in this abnormal plasma appear as stacks of coins in the peripheral smear **(see Color Figure 193)**. These stacks are rather evenly dispersed throughout the smear. The use of a saline dilution of the serum will disperse rouleaux. Rouleaux formation correlates well with a high erythrocyte sedimentation rate and occurs as a direct result of protein deposition or adsorption on the erythrocyte membrane. This lowers the zeta potential, thus facilitating the stacking effect. Patients with multiple myeloma, Waldenström's macroglobulinemia, chronic inflammatory disorders, and some lymphomas will show rouleaux.

## RED CELL INCLUSIONS
### Howell-Jolly Bodies

Howell-Jolly bodies are nuclear remnants containing DNA. They are 1 to 2 $\mu$ in size and may appear singly or doubly in an eccentric position on the periphery of the cell membrane **(see Color Figures 74, 76, and 128)**. They are thought to develop in periods of accelerated or abnormal erythropoiesis. A fragment of the chromosome becomes detached and is left floating in the cytoplasm after the nucleus has been extruded. Under ordinary circumstances, the spleen effectively pits these nondeformable bodies from the cell. However, during periods of erythroid stress, the pitting mechanism cannot keep pace with inclusion formation. Howell-Jolly bodies may be seen following splenectomy and in patients with thalassemic syndromes, hemolytic anemias, megaloblastic anemias, and functional hyposplenia.

## Basophilic Stippling

Red cells that contain ribosomes can potentially form stippled cells; however, it is thought that the actual stippling is the result of the drying of cells in preparation for microscopic examination. Coarse, diffuse, or punctate basophilic stippling may occur, consisting of ribonucleoprotein and mitochondrial remnants.

Diffuse basophilic stippling appears as a fine blue dusting **(see Color Figure 120)**, whereas coarse stippling is much more outlined and easily distinguished **(see Color Figure 242)**. Punctate basophilic stippling is a coalescing of smaller forms and is very prominent and easily identifiable.

Stippling may accompany any condition showing defective or accelerated heme synthesis, lead intoxication, and thalassemia syndromes.

## Siderotic Granules/Pappenheimer Bodies

Siderotic granules are small, irregular magenta inclusions seen along the periphery of red cells **(see Color Figure 64)**. They usually appear in clusters, as if they have been gently placed on the red cell membrane. Their presence is presumptive evidence for the presence of iron. However, the Prussian blue stain is the confirmatory test for determining the presence of these inclusions. These granules in red blood cells are nonheme iron resulting from an excess of available iron throughout the body. They are designated "Pappenheimer bodies" when seen in a Wright-stained smear and "siderotic granules" when seen in Prussian blue stain.

Siderotic granules are found in patients with sideroblastic anemias and any condition leading to hemochromatosis or hemosiderosis. They may also be seen in those with hemoglobinopathies (e.g., sickle cell anemia and thalassemia), and following splenectomy.

## Heinz Bodies

Heinz bodies are formed as a result of denatured or precipitated hemoglobin. They can be formed experimentally by incubation with phenylhydrazine. They are large (0.3 to 2 $\mu$), rigid inclusions that severely distort the cell membrane. Upon initial exposure to phenylhydrazine, small crystalline bodies appear, coalesce, and migrate to an area beneath the cell membrane. They may not be visualized in Wright's stain but may be seen with crystal violet and brilliant cresyl blue **(see Color Figure 94)**.

Heinz bodies may be seen in patients with the thalassemia syndromes, G-6-PD deficiency under oxidant stress, and any of the unstable hemoglobin syndromes. They may also accompany red cell injury resulting from chemical insult.

## Cabot Rings

The exact physiologic mechanism in Cabot ring formation has yet to be elucidated. Cabot rings are found in heavily stippled cells, and they appear in a figure-eight conformation like the beads of a necklace **(see Color Figure 78)**. They are not composed of DNA, but they do contain arginine-rich histone and nonhemoglobin iron. Cabot rings may be found in those with megaloblastic anemias and homozygous thalassemia syndromes, and postsplenectomy.

## PLATELET MORPHOLOGY
### General Comments

The normal platelet has several morphologic characteristics. It measures approximately 2 to 4 $\mu$, with a discoid shape and even blue granules dispersed

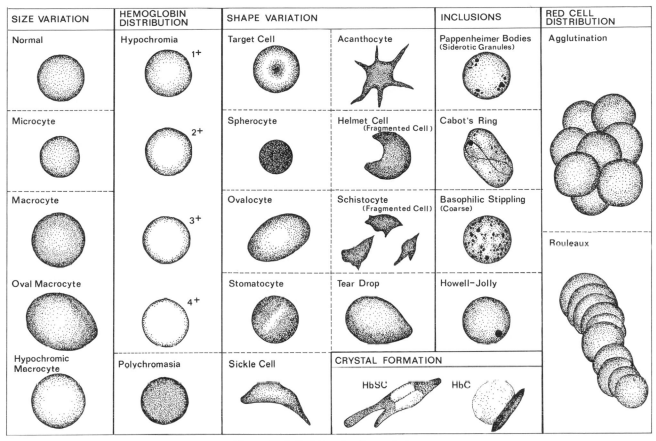

**Figure 30-1.** Red blood cell morphology.

throughout a light-blue cytoplasm. In pathologic states they may appear as blue agranular fragments and may be extremely large **(see Color Figures 142 and 233)**, with tailing or streaming of the cytoplasm. In rare instances, one may see megakaryocytic fragments in the peripheral circulation **(see Color Figure 186)**.

A close and thorough examination of platelet morphology will provide important information as to the patient's hemostatic capability. Gross variation in platelet morphology may be seen in infiltrative disease of the bone marrow (e.g., myelofibrosis or metastatic infiltrates). Large platelets may be seen in any disorder associated with increased platelet turnover as may occur with ITP or bleeding disorders. In addition to the elevated platelet count, morphologic changes may also occur postsplenectomy.

Figure 30–1 pictorially summarizes the normal and abnormal red cell morphology previously discussed in this chapter.

## WHITE BLOOD CELL (WBC) MORPHOLOGY

Morphologic changes of leukocytes—primarily of neutrophils—are associated with various pathologic processes. Severe infections, inflammatory states; and other leukemoid reactions may be accompanied by toxic granulation **(see Color Figure 136)**, toxic vacuolization **(see Color Figure 138)**, and Döhle bodies **(see Color Figure 137)** (see Chapter 16). Toxic granulation and Döhle bodies are generally considered as nonspecific toxic changes, whereas vacuolization strongly indicates a serious bacterial infection.

"Toxic granulation" is a term used to describe the prominent, dark-staining, relatively small granules diffusely scattered throughout the cytoplasm of the segmented neutrophils (PMNs). Toxic vacuolization refers to the round, usually empty vacuoles or spaces that vary in size and appear in the cytoplasm of neutrophils. Döhle bodies are usually oval, blue or blue-gray cytoplasmic inclusions (aggregates of rough endoplasmic reticulum) found in segmented neutrophils, which measure an average of 1 to 2 $\mu$m. Döhle bodies have been reported in the peripheral smear of patients with severe infections and burns, of those receiving cytotoxic drugs, and of pregnant women. In these conditions they represent toxic changes; however, Döhle bodies are also characteristically observed in inherited qualitative white cell disorders, such as the May-Hegglin anomaly and the Chédiak-Higashi disorder (see Chapter 17).

In addition to these morphologic changes, severe bacterial infections are also commonly associated with a moderate leukocytosis and a "shift to the left" in the granulocytes. A mild infection is characterized by a slight leukocytosis with or without a shift to the left. A shift to the left refers to the release of younger granulocytes from the bone marrow storage pool reflected in an increase in band forms and occasional metamyelocytes, which is frequently observed during an infection or an inflammatory process. The presence of more immature forms, such as promyelocytes or myeloblasts, in the absence of severe infection or metabolic stress strongly suggests direct marrow architectural alteration and involvement, indicative of an infiltrative, neoplastic, or myeloproliferative process.

The degree of leukocytosis or neutrophilia is also helpful in discriminating among these various conditions. Leukocytosis is most commonly defined as an increase in white blood cell (WBC) count of greater than 10,000. Acute infection, the most frequent cause of neutrophilia, generally has a WBC count below 50,000/mm$^3$ (average 25,000/mm$^3$, with a "shift to the left" of granulocytes from the *nondividing* bone marrow storage pool. The appearance of cells in the WBC count as immature as myelocytes is unusual. Fungal infections may also be associated with neutrophils and an increased WBC count but are more commonly reflected in a monocytosis **(see Color Figure 243)**. Generally, viral infections are not associated with neutrophilia but rather a lymphocytosis (see Chapter 18).

Leukemoid reactions, an elusive term, is characterized by a peripheral neutrophilia reflected in a WBC count between 50,000 and 100,000 cells/mm$^3$. A leukemoid reaction is defined as a leukocytosis with the presence of immature leukocytes or a leukemia-like peripheral blood picture in the absence of leukemia. Acute infections or chronic infections such as tuberculosis (TB) and chronic osteomyelitis, as well as severe metabolic, inflammatory, and neoplastic processes have all been associated with a leukemoid reaction. Extremely elevated WBC counts (greater than 100,000) are more suggestive of a myeloproliferative process (see Chapter 21), although exceptions have been reported.

Physiologic leukocytosis is defined as an increased WBC count *without* a shift to the left or any associated morphologic changes previously described for granulocytes. Physiologic leukocytosis may be associated with such stimuli as exercise, intense emotional stress, or the administration of epinephrine or glucocorticoids.

## Bibliography

Aarts, PA, Bolhuis, PA, Sakariassen, KS, et al: Red blood cell size is important for adherence of blood platelets to artery subendothelium. Blood 62(1):214, 1983.

Bauer, JD: Clinical Laboratory Methods. CV Mosby, St Louis, 1982.

Beck WS: Hematology. MIT Press, Cambridge, MA, 1981.

Bell, RE: The origin of burr erythrocytes. Br J Hematol 9:552, 1963.

Bessis, M, Weed, RI, and Leblond, PF: Red Cell Shape Physiology, Pathology, Ultrastructure. Springer-Verlag, New York, 1973.

Beutler, E, West, C, Tavassoli, M, et al: The Woronets trait: a new familial erythrocyte anomaly. Blood Cells 6(2):281, 1980.

Bolton, FG, Street, MS, and Pace, AJ: Changes in erythrocyte volume and shape in pregnancy. Br J Obstet Gynecol 89(12):1018, 1982.

Branton, D: Erythrocyte membrane protein associations and erythrocyte shape. Harvey Lect 77:23, 1981–82.

Bretcher, G and Bessis, M: Present studies of spiculated red cells and their relationship to the discocyte-echinocyte transformation. Blood 40:333, 1972.

Chanarin, I, England, JM, and Hoffbrand, AV: Significance of large red blood cells. Br J Hematol 25:351, 1973.

Christensen, RL and Triplett, DA: Neutrophil dysfunction: Quantitative and qualitative disorder. Lab Med 13(11):666, 1982.

Cohen, AR, Trotzky, MS, and Pincus, D: Reassessment of the microcytic anemia of lead poisoning. Pediatrics 67(6):904, 1981.

Cooper, RA: Hemalytic syndromes and red cell membrane abnormalities in liver disease. Semin Hematol 17:103, 1980.

Dacie, JF, Grimes, AJ, Meisler, A, et al: Hereditary Heinz body anemia. Br J Hematol 10:388, 1964.

Eichner, ER: The hematologic disorders of alcoholism. Am J Med 54:621, 1973.

Fairbanks, VF: Is the peripheral blood reliable for the diagnosis of iron deficiency anemia. Am J Clin Pathol 55:447, 1971.

Florane, RK: Hemolytic manifestations of an RBC defect. Diagn Med 6(3):99, 1983.

Howard, J: Myeloid series abnormalities: Neutrophilia. Lab Med 14(3):147, 1983.

Inauen, W, Stauble, M, Descoeudris, C, et al: Erythrocyte deformity in dialysed and non-dialysed uraemic patients. Eur J Clin Invest 12(2):173, 1982.

Jacob, HS: Abnormalities in the physiology of the erythrocyte Membrane in hereditary spherocytosis. Am J Med 41:734, 1966.

Jandl, JH: The pathophysiology of hemolytic anemias–a forward symposium on disorders of the red cell. Am J Med 41:657, 1966.

Jensen, WN: Fragmentation and the freakish probilocyte. Am J Med Sci 257:355, 1969.

Jensen, WN, Moreno, GD, and Bessis, MC: An electron microscopic description of basophilic stippling in red cells. Blood 25:933, 1965.

Johnson, CS, Tegos, C, and Beutler, E: Thalassemia minor: Routine erythrocyte measurements and differentiation from iron deficiency. Am J Clin Pathol 80:31, 1983.

Kapff, CT: Blood Atlas and Sourcebook of Hematology. Little, Brown, Boston, 1981.

Kass, L: Origin and composition of cabot rings in pernicious anemia. Am J Clin Pathol 64:53, 1975.

Koeffler, HP and Golde, DW: Human preleukemia. Ann Intern Med 93:347, 1980.

Lloyd, EM: How flowcharts improve RBC morphology reporting. MLO 49, 1982.

O'Conner, BH: A Color Atlas and Instruction Manual of Peripheral Blood Cell Morphology. Williams & Wilkins, Baltimore, 1984.

Ozer, FL and Mills, GL: Elliptocytosis with hemolytic anemia. Br J Hematol 10:468, 1964.

Pearson, HA: Red cell "rubbish" as a key to splenic function. Lab Man 25, 1982.

Reich, PR: Hematology: Physiopathologic Basis for Clinical Practice. Little, Brown, Boston, 1984.

Rifkind, RA and Danon, D: Heinz body anemia — an ultrastructural study. 1. Heinz body formation. Blood 25:885, 1965.

Salt, HB and Wolf, OH: On having no beta lipoprotein: A syndrome comprising a beta-lipoproteinemia acanthocytosis and steatorrhea. Lancet 2:325, 1968.

Smith, CM II, Kuettner, JF, Turkey, DP et al: Variable deformability of irreversibly sickled erythrocytes. Blood 58(1):71, 1981.

Spivak, JL: Fundamentals of Clinical Hematology. Philadelphia, Harper & Row, 1984.

Wardrop, C and Hutchinson, HE: Red cell shapes in hypothyroidism. Lancet 1:1243, 1969.

Weed, RI: The importance of erythrocyte deformability. Am J Med 49:147, 1970.

Weed, RI and Reed, C: Membrane alterations and red cell destruction. Am J Med 41:681, 1966.

Westerman, MP and Bacus, JW: Red blood cell morphology in sickle cell anemia as determined by image processing analysis: The relationship to painful crisis. Am J Clin Pathol 79:667, 1983.

Williams WJ, Beutler, E, Erslev, AJ, et al: Hematology. McGraw-Hill, New York, 1977.

# CHAPTER 31

JANIS WYRICK-GLATZEL, M.S., M.T.(ASCP) AND
SANDRA GWALTNEY-KRAUSE, M.A., M.T.(ASCP)

# Laboratory Methods in Hematology and Hemostasis

Our goal in this chapter is to present the student with basic hematologic and coagulation procedures. Emphasis has been placed on interpretation as well as on procedural methods. At the end of some of the procedures we have included a comment section, which serves as a "potpourri" highlighting general points of information concerning the procedure, its limitations, and interpretation.

The intention was never to make this section all-inclusive. We realize that with the rapid expansion of automation, some of these procedures have become antiquated. We believe, however, that the understanding of these basic procedures will serve as a sound building block for the application of more advanced technology.

# MANUAL BLOOD CELL COUNTS
## Hemacytometer

The *hemacytometer* counting chamber is used for cell counting. It is constructed so that the distance between the bottom of the *coverslip* and the surface of the counting area of the chamber is 0.1 mm (Fig. 31-1). The surface of the chamber contains two ruled areas separated by an H-shaped moat (Fig. 31-1). These are the *primary* squares. The primary square consists of a total area of 9 mm$^2$ (3 mm on each side, length $\times$ width), which is divided into nine *secondary* squares (Fig. 31-2). Each of these secondary squares measures 1 mm on each side, with the total area being 1 mm$^2$. The four corner secondary squares are further divided into 16 smaller *tertiary* squares to aid in cell counting; they are used for counting leukocytes. The four corner and center tertiary squares of the center secondary square are used when counting erythrocytes. The center secondary square differs from the four corner squares in that it is divided into 25 tertiary squares, each with an area of 0.2 mm; all 25 tertiary squares of the center secondary square are used to count platelets. Each of the 25 squares is further divided into 16 smaller *quarternary* squares.

The boundary lines of the central secondary square are either double or triple. When the boundary line is double, all the cells within the squares and those touching the innermost line are counted. When the boundary line is triple, all the cells within the squares and those touching the middle line inward are counted.

Both hemacytometers and coverslips should meet the specifications of the National Bureau of Standards and are so marked by the manufacturer. Always use the coverslip that accompanies the hemacytometer. It has been ground to fit the specifics of the hemacytometer in order to ensure a uniform depth and therefore a constant volume. A regular coverslip cannot be used.

## Manual Cell Counting Using the Hemacytometer

With the introduction of sophisticated electronic equipment such as the Coulter Counter S-Plus* and the Ortho ELT-8† into the field of hematology, there is a diminished need for manual cell counting. However, a knowledge of this method is still important in the field of hematology. Manual cell counts are often performed in patients with extreme cases of thrombocytosis, thrombocytopenia, leukocytosis, and leukocytopenia. Perhaps the most necessary reason for performing manual cell counts is that body fluids such as cerebral spinal fluid (CSF) and

---

*Coulter Electronics, Inc., P.O. Box 2145, Hialeah, FL 33012.
†Ortho Diagnostic Systems, Inc., Westwood, MA 02090.

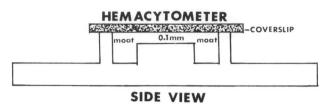

### SIDE VIEW

**Figure 31–1.** Hemacytometer side view. (Prepared by J. McMichael.)

pleural fluid can be counted only by manual methods.

## Diluting Pipettes

Dilution of the blood sample is accomplished by the use of a cell-diluting pipette. Both the RBC and WBC pipettes are made up of a stem that is divided into 10 equal parts and a mixing chamber containing a red,

white, or clear bead, which aids in mixing the diluent, and blood.

When using the *WBC pipette*, blood is drawn to either the 0.5 or the 1.0 mark and the diluent to the 11 mark, making dilutions of 1 : 20 and 1 : 10, respectively.

When using the *RBC pipette*, blood is drawn to the 0.5 and the 1.0 mark and the diluent to the 101 mark, making dilutions of 1 : 200 and 1 : 100, respectively.

In calculating the dilution, only the volume contained in the bulb is considered, as the stem will contain only diluent and its contents will be discarded before charging the chambers. The *dilution factor*, used in calculating the cell/mm³, is the reciprocal of the *dilution* and therefore can be calculated using the following formula.

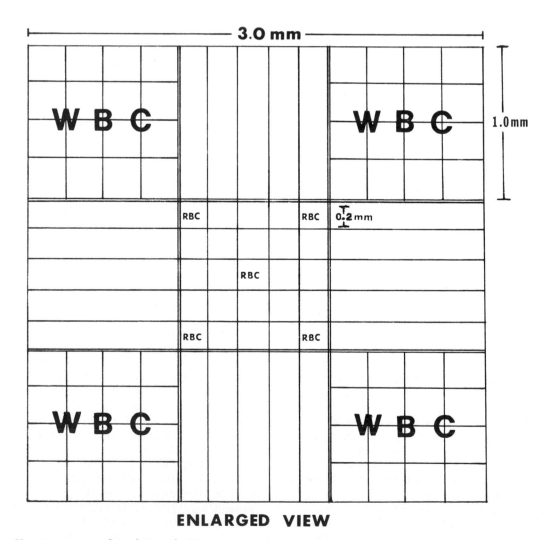

### ENLARGED VIEW

**Figure 31–2.** Hemacytometer enlarged view of primary square. This view represents one of the two primary squares of the hemacytometer. The four corner secondary squares are used for counting white cells. The five tertiary squares of the center secondary square are used for counting red cells. All tertiary squares of the center secondary square are used in counting platelets. (Prepared by J. McMichael.)

$$\text{Dilution} = \frac{\text{Amount of Blood}}{\text{Total Volume}}$$

WBC Pipette $\dfrac{0.5 \text{ (Blood)}}{10 \text{ (Volume)}} = \dfrac{1}{20}$ (Dilution)

RBC Pipette $\dfrac{1.0 \text{ (Blood)}}{100 \text{ (Volume)}} = \dfrac{1}{100}$ (Dilution)

## RBC Count Using the Hemacytometer

### Definition

The red blood cell (RBC) count is the determination of the number of erythrocytes in 1 mm³ of blood.

### Principle

Using an RBC diluting pipette, venous or capillary blood is mixed with a diluting fluid. The hemacytometer is then charged with this dilution and the cells counted with a microscope.

For RBC counts, the solution that is used is isotonic with the erythrocytes. The diluting fluids used do not lyse the leukocytes. Normally, the leukocytes are too few to interfere with the RBC count. In cases of leukocytosis, however, the leukocytes are easily identified and are not counted.

### Reagents

The following diluents can be used in counting RBCs: Gower's, Hayem's, and isotonic saline. In our laboratory we prefer using isotonic saline owing to its accessibility.

### Equipment

RBC diluting pipettes
Hemacytometer and coverslip
Aspirator tubing and mouthpiece
Alcohol pads
Lint-free wipes
Hand counter
Microscope

### Procedure

1. Clean the hemacytometer and its coverslip with an alcohol pad and then dry with a wipe. The pipettes are cleaned using pipette washers.
2. The blood specimen must be mixed just prior to use to ensure even cell suspension. Mixing is accomplished by gentle inversion of the tube 10 to 20 times. Never vigorously shake the sample, as this could cause cell lysis and give erroneous results.
3. After attaching the aspirator tubing and mouthpiece to the pipette, blood is aspirated to the 0.5 mark without letting any bubbles into the pipette.
4. The outside of the pipette is wiped clean with a wipe, being careful not to contact the bore of the pipette. If the wipe contacts the bore, fluid *and not cells* will be pulled out of the pipette, causing a false increase in cell concentration.
5. If the blood overshoots the 0.5 mark by no more than 1 to 2 mm, the excess blood can be removed by tapping the pipette tip with any nonabsorbent material (usually a fingertip) but not a wipe. Overshooting the 0.5 mark by more than 2 mm will require you to clean the pipette and start over.
6. When the specimen is at the 0.5 mark the diluting solution is then quickly and carefully aspirated to the 101 mark, with a steady suction and rotation of the pipette between your fingers, without overshooting the mark or letting any bubbles into the pipette.
7. The outside of the pipette is again carefully wiped clean, without contacting the bore of the pipette with the wipe.
8. If the 101 mark is overshot by no more than 1 to 2 mm, you may correct it by tapping the pipette tip with any nonabsorbent material.
9. The aspirator tubing is removed from the pipette by rolling it off—*not* by pulling or pinching, as this will expel fluid, changing the dilution.
10. With a finger over each end of the pipette, vigorously shake the pipette for 2 to 3 minutes, or shake the pipette on a mechanical shaker for 45 seconds. When manually shaking the pipette, do not shake it in an end-to-end fashion, but rather in a figure-8 pattern or by rotating between the fingers.
11. Discard 4 to 5 drops from the pipette before charging the hemacytometer chamber, to expel any undiluted diluent.
12. The two chambers on the hemacytometer are charged by touching the tip of the pipette to the coverslip edge where it meets the chamber floor. To aid in charging the hemacytometer, the pipette is held at a 45-degree angle. The chamber will fill by capillary action, if the hemacytometer and coverslip are clean. Overcharging the hemacytometer will result in fluid flowing into the moat, requiring you to clean and recharge the hemacytometer.
13. You can keep the remaining fluid in the pipette should you need to repeat a count. Place the pipette in a horizontal position when not in use. To reuse, shake the pipette as stated before; again discarding 4 to 5 drops prior to charging the chambers.
14. Mount the hemacytometer on the microscope and lower its condenser.
15. Let the hemacytometer sit for 1 to 2 minutes to allow the cells to settle.
16. Procedure for counting RBCs:

a. Cells are scanned under a 10× objective to ensure even distribution.
b. Use a 40× objective to count the erythrocytes in the four corner and center tertiary squares of the center secondary square. This counting procedure is repeated on the opposite side of the hemacytometer. In actuality you will be counting 80 quarternary squares; i.e., five tertiary squares of the center secondary square (see Fig. 31-4).
c. To count the cells in the quarternary squares, use the following pattern:
   (1) Count cells starting in the upper left corner square; continue counting to the right hand square; drop down to the next row; continue counting from the right hand square to the left square. Continue in this fashion until the total area in that tertiary square has been counted.
   (2) Count all cells that touch any of the upper and left lines. Do not count any cell that touches a lower or right line.
d. The difference between the highest and lowest number of cells of the 10 squares should be no greater than 25.
17. Calculate the RBCs/mm³ on the basis of the number of cells counted, area, and the dilution made, as previously outlined.

## Calculations

The following formula may still be used to calculate the RBC count:

$$\text{Count (cells/mm}^3) = \text{Cells/mm}^2 \times 10 \times \text{Dilution}$$

In the case of a normal RBC count, the factor can be determined by the following calculation:

$$\begin{aligned}\text{Factor} &= 1/\text{area} \times \text{Depth factor} \times \text{Dilution factor} \\ &= 1/0.2 \text{ mm}^2 \times 10 \times 200 \\ &= 10,000\end{aligned}$$

## Example

Blood is drawn to the 0.5 mark of the RBC pipette, and the number of cells counted in the four corner and center tertiary squares equals 300 RBCs.

$$\begin{aligned}\text{Cells/mm}^3 &= \text{Cells/mm}^2 \times \text{Depth factor} \times \\ &\quad \text{Dilution factor} \\ &= (300/0.2 \text{ mm}^2) \times 10 \times 200 \\ &= 3.0 \times 10^6/\text{mm}^3\end{aligned}$$

In this example, the area equals 0.2 mm², because the length of each of the small squares counted is equal to 0.2 mm. Thus, the area of each square is 0.04 mm². Since five of these squares were counted, the total area counted is 0.04 times 5, or 0.2 mm².

## Interpretation

Normal values:

| | |
|---|---|
| Newborn | 4.4 to 5.8 million/mm³ |
| Infant/Child | 3.8 to 5.5 million/mm³ |
| Adult Male | 4.7 to 6.1 million/mm³ |
| Female | 4.2 to 5.4 million/mm³ |

# WBC Count Using the Hemacytometer

## Definition

The white blood cell or leukocyte (WBC) count is the determination of the number of WBCs in 1 mm³ of blood.

## Principle

Using a WBC diluting pipette, venous or capillary blood is mixed with a diluting fluid. The hemacytometer is then charged (filled) with this dilution and the cells counted with a microscope.

For WBC counts, Turk's solution is used. This diluting fluid contains an acid solution that lyses the non-nucleated RBCs and a stain that stains the nuclei of the WBCs and allows for easy identification and counting.

## Reagents

The preferred diluent is Turk's solution, when counting WBCs. A useful formula for this reagent is given below.

| | |
|---|---|
| Glacial Acetic Acid | 1 ml |
| Gentian Violet (Aqueous) | 2 ml |
| Distilled Water to | 100 ml |

## Equipment

WBC diluting pipette
Hemacytometer and coverslip
Aspirator tubing and mouthpiece
Alcohol pads
Lint-free wipes
Hand counter
Microscope

## Procedure

1. Clean the hemacytometer and its coverslip with an alcohol pad and then dry with a wipe. The pipettes are cleaned using pipette washers.
2. The blood specimen must be mixed just prior to use to ensure even cell suspension. Mixing is accomplished by gentle inversion of the tube 10 to 20 times. Never vigorously shake the sample, as this could cause cell lysis and give erroneous results.
3. After attaching the aspirator tubing and mouthpiece to the pipette, blood is aspirated

to the 0.5 mark without letting any bubbles into the pipette.

4. The outside of the pipette is wiped clean with a wipe being careful not to contact the bore of the pipette. If the wipe contacts the bore, fluid and not cells will be pulled out of the pipette, causing a false increase in cell concentration.

5. If blood overshoots the 0.5 mark by no more than 1 to 2 mm the excess blood can be removed by tapping the pipette tip with any nonabsorbent material — usually a fingertip, but not a wipe. Overshooting the 0.5 mark by more than 2 mm will necessitate cleaning the pipette and starting over.

6. When the specimen is at the 0.5 mark, Turk's solution is then quickly and carefully aspirated to the 11 mark, with a steady suction and rotation of the pipette between the fingers, without overshooting the mark or letting any bubbles into the pipette.

7. The outside of the pipette is again carefully wiped clean without contacting the bore of the pipette with the wipe.

8. If the 11 mark is overshot by no more than 1 to 2 mm, you may correct it by tapping the pipette tip with any nonabsorbent material.

9. The aspirator tubing is removed from the pipette by rolling it off — not by pulling or pinching, as this will expel fluid, changing the dilution.

10. With a finger over each end of the pipette, vigorously shake the pipette for 2 to 3 minutes or shake the pipette on a mechanical shaker for 45 seconds. When manually shaking the pipette, do not shake it in an end-to-end fashion, but rather in a figure-8 pattern or by rotating it between the fingers.

11. Discard 4 to 5 drops from the pipette before charging the hemacytometer chamber to expel any undiluted diluent.

12. The two chambers on the hemacytometer are charged by touching the tip of the pipette to the coverslip edge where it meets the chamber floor. To aid in charging the hemacytometer, the pipette is held at a 45-degree angle. The chamber will fill by capillary action, if the hemacytometer and coverslip are clean. Overcharging the hemacytometer will result in fluid flowing into the moat, requiring you to clean and recharge the hemacytometer.

13. You can keep the remaining fluid in the pipette should you need to repeat a count. Place the pipette in a horizontal position when not in use. To reuse, shake the pipette as stated before, again discarding 4 to 5 drops prior to charging the chambers.

14. Mount the hemacytometer on the microscope and lower its condenser.

15. Let the hemacytometer sit for 1 to 2 minutes to allow the cells to settle.

16. Procedure for counting WBCs:
    a. Cells are scanned under a $10\times$ objective to ensure even distribution.
    b. Use the $40\times$ objective to count the white cells in each of the four corner secondary squares on both sides of the chamber.
    c. In counting the cells in the tertiary squares use the following pattern:
       (1) Count cells starting in the upper left corner square; continue counting to the right hand square; drop down to the next row; continue counting from the right-square to the left square. Continue in this fashion until the total area in that secondary square has been counted.
       (2) Count all cells that touch any of the upper and left lines. Do not count any cell that touches a lower or right line.
    d. The difference between the highest and lowest number of cells of the eight squares should be no greater than 15.

17. Calculate the WBCs/mm³ on the basis of the number of cells counted, area, and the dilution made, as previously outlined.

## Calculations

There are several ways to calculate direct cell counts. The preferred method is to convert the number of cells counted in 1 mm² to cells in 1 mm³ by correcting for the dilution made and the area counted. The following formula is used to calculate any type of cell count:

$$\text{Count (cells/mm}^3) = \text{Cells/mm}^2 \times 10 \times \text{Dilution}$$

In this equation:

$$\text{Cells/mm}^2 = \frac{\text{Cells counted}}{\text{Area counted (mm}^2)}$$

The number of cells/mm² is multiplied by 10 (the reciprocal of the depth of the chamber, 0.1) thus giving the cells in 1 mm³, and then multiplied by the dilution thus giving the number of cells/mm³. The count per cubic millimeter is then multiplied by a factor of $10^6$ to yield cells/liter ($10^9$).

The second method of calculating direct cell counts involves a factor dependent on the area counted and the dilution of the sample. The factor is then multiplied by the total number of cells counted, yielding the number of cells/mm³. The determination of a factor is not the method of choice, especially in situations involving severe leukopenia, leukocytosis, or for use with body fluids where variations in the dilution as well as the area counted are made. In the case of a normal WBC count, however, the factor can be determined by the following calculation:

Factor = 1/Area × Depth factor × Dilution factor
        = 1/4 mm² × 10 × 20
        = 50

## Example

Blood is pipetted to the 1.0 mark of the WBC pipette and the number of cells counted in the four large corner secondary squares equals 100 WBCs.

Cells/mm³ = Cells/mm² × Depth factor × Dilution factor
          = (100/4) × 10 × 10
          = 2500 WBC/mm³

## Interpretations

Normal values:

| | |
|---|---|
| Newborn | 9,000 to 30,000/mm³ |
| 1 week | 5,000 to 21,000/mm³ |
| 1 month | 5,000 to 19,500/mm³ |
| 6–12 months | 6,000 to 17,500/mm³ |
| 2 years | 6,200 to 17,000/mm³ |
| Child/adult | 4,800 to 10,800/mm³ |

## Comments

1. Discard any damaged pipettes (e.g., with chipped tips), to avoid inaccurate counts.
2. The hemacytometer, coverslip, and pipette must be clean and dry prior to use. Errors are introduced by fingerprints, lint, and dirt. Check the diluting fluid to ensure that it is free from contamination.
3. Never aspirate blood into the pipette unless using the aspirator tubing.
4. Use the coverslip that accompanies the hemacytometer.
5. When counting cells, follow the procedure as outlined before. This will prevent counting the same cell more than once or missing a cell that should be counted, therefore giving erroneous results.
6. Allow the cells to settle in the counting chamber for 1 to 2 minutes prior to counting to ensure accurate counts.
7. When using anticoagulated blood, ensure proper mixing of specimen before sampling.
8. In cases of leukopenia, with a count below 4000/mm³, the dilution factor is 10.
9. In cases of leukocytosis, with a count in excess of 11,000/mm³, a red cell pipette is used and the dilution factor is 100 or even 200 (depending on the degree of leukocytosis).
10. There are physiologic variations to consider when performing WBC counts. Higher counts are seen following exercise, emotional stress, anxiety, and food intake. Blacks generally show slightly lower WBC counts than whites.

## Manual Determination of the Platelet Count

### Principle

The reference method for determining manual platelet counts uses the phase contrast microscope. When whole blood is added to 1 percent ammonium oxalate, *mature* red cells are hemolyzed. Platelets, leukocytes, and reticulocytes, however, are preserved. By use of phase microscopy, platelets can easily be counted in a special counting chamber as described by Brecher and Conkite.[1]

### Equipment

Phase contrast microscope equipped with a 40× annulus, 40× phase objective, and 10× oculars (total of 400×).

Special thin flat-bottom counting chamber
No. 1 glass coverslip
RBC diluting pipettes
1 percent ammonium oxalate (W/V)
Petri dish and cover with moist filter paper

To prepare 1 percent ammonium oxalate, weigh 10 g ammonium oxalate (reagent grade) in a weighing boat. Transfer to a 1000 ml volumetric flask. Add about 500 ml distilled water and mix to dissolve. Fill the flask to mark and mix. Store in the refrigerator to prevent growth of microorganisms. Filter before use.

### Procedure

1. Use thoroughly mixed venous blood collected in EDTA, or peripheral blood from a freely flowing skin puncture.
2. *Duplicate* red blood cell pipettes are filled to the 1 mark with blood and diluted to the 101 mark with 1% ammonium oxalate.
3. Shake the two pipettes for 2 to 3 minutes and fill the chamber. Fill one side of the chamber with each pipette.
4. Place the counting chamber in a petri dish containing a moistened filter paper and let stand for 15 minutes, but no more than 20 minutes.
5. With the phase contrast microscope set at 400×, count the platelets in the *entire center square millimeter* (center secondary square) on both sides of the chamber. Duplicate counts or a sample (for example, both sides of the hemacytometer) should agree within *10%* for the counts to be acceptable. Platelets appear as dense, dark bodies or round, oval, or rod shape, with a diameter of about 2 to 4 μm.
6. Calculate the number of platelets per cubic millimeter using the following factor formula:

$$Cells/mm^3 = \frac{\text{No. cells counted} \times \text{Dilution} \times \text{Depth factor}}{\text{No. squares counted} \times \text{Area (0.04 mm}^2\text{)}}$$

## Interpretation

Normal Values: 150,000 to 450,000/mm³

## Comments:

1. Platelets appear round, oval, or rod-like, sometimes showing dendritic processes. Their internal *granular* structure and pearlescent sheen allows the platelets to be distinguished from debris, which is often refractile. RBCs will appear as ghost cells.
2. If platelet clumping is observed, the count should be rediluted. If clumping is still present a fresh specimen must be obtained. Because of the adhesive quality of platelets, finger-stick specimens are least desirable.
3. The phase platelet determination should be compared with a review of the blood film for correction of count and morphology.
4. EDTA is the anticoagulant of choice when performing phase platelet counts. The student should be aware of the phenomenon of "platelet satellitosis" when using this anticoagulant.[2] Platelet satellitosis appears as neutrophils ringed with adhering platelets. Correct platelet counts may be obtained by collecting a fresh specimen with sodium citrate as the anticoagulant.
5. Ordinary light microscopy may be used; however, differentiation and enumeration is made more difficult.
6. In cases of thrombocytopenia (less than 100,000/mm³) the count should be repeated with a 1:20 dilution of blood using a WBC pipette.

## Eosinophil Count

The absolute number of eosinophils per cubic millimeter of blood can be calculated by two methods. The first is an estimate using the number of eosinophils from the differential and the total leukocyte count. The second is obtained by a direct hemacytometer count. The former is the least accurate, owing to the nature of a 100 white cell differential count.

The absolute eosinophil count uses a stain in which the red cells are lysed and the eosinophils are stained. In this method eosinophils can be directly counted in a hemacytometer.

## Reagents and Equipment

WBC-diluting pipettes
Hemacytometer and coverslip

Eosinophil diluting fluid (Pilot's solution)
| | |
|---|---|
| Propylene glycol | 50 ml |
| Distilled water | 40 ml |
| Phloxine, 1% aqueous solution | 10 ml |
| Sodium carbonate, 10% aqueous solution | 1 ml |

Filter and store at refrigerator temperature. Discard after one month.

## Procedure

1. Aspirate blood to the 1.0 line in the WBC-diluting pipette. Place the tip of the pipette in diluting fluid, and aspirate until it reaches the 11 line.
2. Shake the pipette briefly and let it stand for 15 minutes.
3. Shake again for 30 seconds in a mechanical shaker.
4. Load the hemacytometer chamber and allow it to stand for two minutes to permit cells to settle.
5. Scan for an even distribution prior to counting.
6. Count the eosinophils in all nine of the large secondary squares (1 mm² each) on both sides of the hemacytometer, using the 10× objective. If the eosinophil count is extremely low, it is advisable to fill and count several chambers. It is recommended that at least 50 eosinophils be counted.
7. Calculate the absolute eosinophil count using the equation below.

## Interpretation

Normal Values: The eosinophil count of normal blood ranges from 50 to 400/ml.

## Comments

1. It is important to note that eosinophils will take a deep-red stain with Pilot's solution.
2. A good-quality control point would be to check the eosinophil count obtained from the leukocyte and differential counts. To check the accuracy of the hemacytometer count, take the percentage of eosinophils counted on the differential smear and multiply by the total white cell count. This is the relative eosinophil count.

For example:
| | |
|---|---|
| WBC count: | 7500 |
| Differential: | 4% |
| 7500 × 0.04 = 300 | |

$$\text{Cells/mm}^3 = \frac{\text{Cells counted} \times \text{Dilution} \times \text{Dilution factor}}{\text{Area}}$$

$$\text{Absolute reticulocyte count} = \frac{\text{Reticulocytes (\%)}}{100} \times \text{Red cell count (mm}^3\text{)}$$

Allow for one more or one less eosinophil on the differential (e.g., if the count had been 3 or 5, the estimated count from the differential smear would have been 225 to 375). A differential count of 3, 4, or 5 eosinophils giving a relative range of 225 to 375 would be a good verification of accuracy.

## Reticulocytes

### Principle

Reticulocytes are immature red cells that contain remnant cytoplasmic RNA and organelles such as mitochondria and ribosomes. Reticulocytes are visualized by staining with vital dyes (e.g., new methylene blue) that precipitate the RNA and organelles forming a filamentous network of reticulum. The reticulocyte count is a means of assessing erythropoietic activity of the bone marrow.

### Reagents

New Methylene Blue (CI 52030 Hartman-Leddon Company, Philadelphia)

1. Dissolve 0.5 g of new methylene blue and 1.6 g of potassium oxalate in distilled water and Q. S. to 100 ml.
2. Filter before use. Store at room temperature.

### Equipment

Whole blood anticoagulated with EDTA
6-inch capillary tubes
Microscope slides
12 × 75 test tubes

### Procedure

1. Mix equal amounts of blood and new methylene blue staining solution in a test tube.
2. The blood-dye mixture is drawn up into a capillary pipette. Allow the mixture to stand for 10 minutes at room temperature.
3. Prepare thin wedge smears of blood-dye mixture using 1 small drop. Air dry. Do not fix or counterstain slides.
4. Under oil immersion, count all red cells in each field where the cells do not overlap, inclusive of reticulocytes. The Miller eyepiece[3] will facilitate counting.
5. Count 1000 red cells in consecutive oil immersion fields. Record the number of reticulocytes seen.

6. Calculate the percent of reticulocytes as follows:

$$\frac{\text{Reticulocyte count/1000 RBCs}}{10} = \%\text{ Reticulocytes}$$

*Note:* Counting 1000 red cells is sufficient for normal or increased reticulocyte counts; however, for decreased reticulocyte counts 2000 or more red cells should be counted.

### Interpretation

Normal values are as follows:
Newborn: 2.5 to 6.0 percent (falls to normal adult values in 2 weeks)
Adult: 0.5 to 2.0 percent
The absolute reticulocyte count may be calculated by the formula above. The absolute reticulocyte count expresses the number of reticulocytes in 1 mm³ of whole blood rather than as a percentage of red cells. The normal value is 60,000/mm³.

The reticulocyte count is most often expressed as a percentage of total red cells. In states of anemia the reticulocyte percentage is not a true reflection of reticulocyte production. A correction factor must be used so as not to "overestimate" marrow production, since each reticulocyte is released into whole blood containing fewer red cells (a low hematocrit) thus relatively increasing the percentage. The "corrected reticulocyte count" may be calculated by the formula below.

For example, if a patient presents with a reticulocyte count of 12 and a hematocrit of 24, the corrected reticulocyte count would be 12(%) × (24/45), or 6.4%. In other words, the patient who presents with a reticulocyte count of 12 and a hematocrit of 24 would have the equivalent of a reticulocyte count of 6.4% in a patient with a hematocrit of 45.

An estimation of red cell production by using the corrected reticulocyte count may yield erroneously high values in patients when there is a premature release of younger reticulocytes from the marrow (owing to increased erythropoietin stimulator). These premature reticulocytes are called *stress* or *shift reticulocytes*. These result when the reticulocytes of the bone marrow pool are shifted to the circulatory pool to compensate for anemia. The younger "stress" reticulocytes present with more

$$\text{Corrected reticulocyte count} = \text{Reticulocytes (\%)} \times \frac{\text{Patient HCT}}{45 \text{ (average normal HCT)}}$$

filamentous reticulum. The mature reticulocyte may present with granular dots representing reticulum. Normally, reticulocytes lose their reticulum within 24 to 27 hours in the peripheral circulation. The premature "stress reticulocytes" have increased reticulum and require 2 to 2½ days to lose their reticulum, resulting in a longer peripheral blood maturation time. The peripheral smear should be carefully reviewed for the presence of many polychromatophilic "macrocytes," thus indicating "stress reticulocytes" and the need for a correction. When using the reticulocyte count as a means of evaluating erythropoiesis, a correction should be made for both the red cell count and the presence of "stress reticulocytes." The value obtained is called the "reticulocyte production index" (RPI). To calculate the RPI the following formula is used:

$$RPI = \frac{\text{Reticulocyte count (\%)} \times \dfrac{\text{Patient's HCT}}{45 \text{ (Normal HCT)}}}{2 \text{ ("Stress reticulocyte" maturation time)}}$$

## Comments

The reticulocyte count is elevated (1) in patients with hemolytic anemia, (2) in those with hemorrhage (acute and chronic), (3) following treatment of iron-deficiency anemia and the megaloblastic anemias, and (4) in patients with uremia (Fig. 31 – 3).

The reticulocyte count is decreased in cases of (1) aplastic anemia, (2) aplastic crises of hemolytic anemias, and (3) ineffective erythropoiesis as seen in thalassemia, pernicious anemia, and sideroblastic anemia.

Reticulocytopenia in the presence of a suggested hemolytic anemia may often make diagnosis difficult. The diagnosis of a hemolytic anemia can be made because the combination of both hemolysis and reticulocytopenia results in a rapidly falling hemoglobin and hematocrit.

By convention, "single dot" reticulocytes are not counted. A reticulocyte must contain two or more discrete blue granules. The granular reticulum of the reticulocyte may be confused with Heinz bodies. Heinz bodies will stain as light blue-green granules present at the periphery of the red cell.

According to the pattern of reticulum and the degree of maturation, reticulocytes can be divided into four categories, from the youngest to the most mature.

There is a high degree of inaccuracy in the reticulocyte count owing to error (±2 percent in low counts and ±7 percent in high counts) and lack of reproducibility. Because of the inaccuracy of the blood film, flow microfluorometry has been adapted to automatically count reticulocytes. The principle is based on staining of the RNA by an acridine orange dye, which fluoresces when exposed to UV light.

## Red Blood Cell Indices

### Principle

The values obtained for the erythrocyte count, hematocrit, and hemoglobin concentration can be fur-

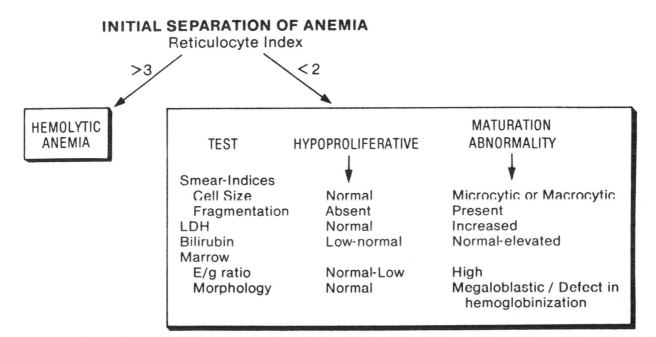

**Figure 31 – 3.** The initial separation of anemia. Anemias may be broadly classified on the basis of the reticulocyte index as hemolytic (index greater than 3) or impaired production, either a hypoproliferative or maturation abnormality (index less than 2). Further tests are required to separate the latter two functional defects as shown.

ther used to calculate *red blood indices*, which define the size and hemoglobin content of the average red blood cell in a given specimen of blood. The values for the red cell indices are useful tools in the classification of anemias.

The three most commonly used red blood cell indices are (1) mean corpuscular volume (MCV), (2) mean corpuscular hemoglobin (MCH), and (3) mean corpuscular hemoglobin concentration (MCHC).

### Definitions

**Mean Corpuscular Volume (MCV).** This is the average volume of the RBC, in cubic microns $(\mu^3)$ or femtoliters (fl). Normal erythrocytes have an MCV of 80 to 98 fl (replaces old units, $\mu^3$). Results below 80 fl indicate a smaller than normal MCV; that is, the cells are on the average *microcytic*. Similarly, an MCV of greater than 100 fl indicates the cells are *macrocytic*.

It is imperative to interpret the value for MCV along with a careful inspection of the peripheral blood smear, since the MCV is only a *mean volume* measurement. It is possible, for example, to have a wide variation in cell size—from cells that are microcytic to some that are macrocytic—and still have a MCV within the normal range. This may be true if there is a large number of reticulocytes in the peripheral blood, since reticulocytes usually have a larger volume than in adult cells.

$$ MCV = \frac{\text{Hematocrit (\%)} \times 10}{\text{RBC count (in millions/mm}^3)} $$

This value is reported in fl $(\mu^3)$ to the nearest whole number.

**Mean Corpuscular Hemoglobin (MCH).** This is the average weight of hemoglobin, in absolute units, in the RBC. The result gives the average content of hemoglobin per erythrocyte in picograms (pg) or micromicrograms $(\mu\mu g)$. The normal MCH in adults is 27 to 31 pg. This value is generally higher in newborns and infants, because their MCV is higher than in adults.

$$ MCH = \frac{\text{Hemoglobin (g/100 ml)} \times 10}{\text{RBC count (in millions/mm}^3)} $$

**Mean Corpuscular Hemoglobin Concentration (MCHC).** This is the average concentration of hemoglobin in each individual red cell. It is a ratio of the weight of hemoglobin to the volume of the red blood cell.

$$ MCHC = \frac{\text{Hemoglobin (g/100 ml)} \times 100}{\text{Hematocrit}} $$

This value is reported to the nearest 10th of a percent. The normal MCHC is 32 to 36 percent (Fig. 31-4).

### Comments

Determination of the MCV, MCH, and MCHC gives valuable information that helps to characterize red blood cells. According to the MCV, erythrocytes

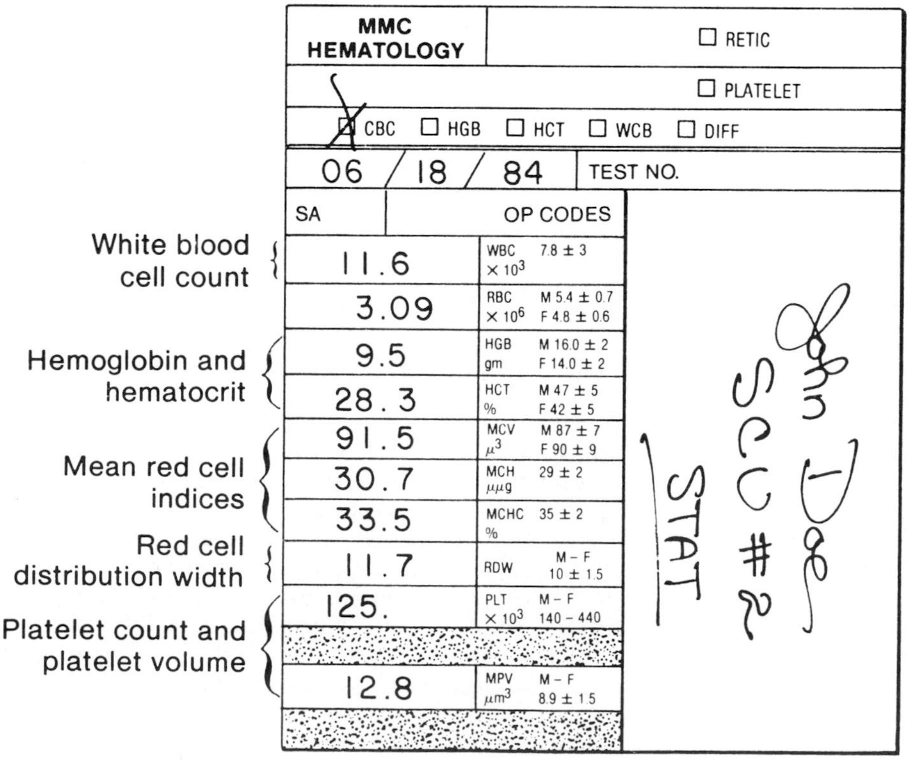

| MMC HEMATOLOGY | | | ☐ RETIC |
|---|---|---|---|
| | | | ☐ PLATELET |
| ☒ CBC ☐ HGB ☐ HCT ☐ WCB ☐ DIFF | | | |
| 06 / 18 / 84 | TEST NO. | | |

| | SA | | OP CODES | |
|---|---|---|---|---|
| White blood cell count | 11.6 | | WBC × 10³ | 7.8 ± 3 |
| | 3.09 | | RBC × 10⁶ | M 5.4 ± 0.7 F 4.8 ± 0.6 |
| Hemoglobin and hematocrit | 9.5 | | HGB gm | M 16.0 ± 2 F 14.0 ± 2 |
| | 28.3 | | HCT % | M 47 ± 5 F 42 ± 5 |
| Mean red cell indices | 91.5 | | MCV μ³ | M 87 ± 7 F 90 ± 9 |
| | 30.7 | | MCH μμg | 29 ± 2 |
| | 33.5 | | MCHC % | 35 ± 2 |
| Red cell distribution width | 11.7 | | RDW | M – F 10 ± 1.5 |
| Platelet count and platelet volume | 125. | | PLT × 10³ | M – F 140 – 440 |
| | 12.8 | | MPV μm³ | M – F 8.9 ± 1.5 |

**Figure 31-4** Results of blood cell counts and indices.

may be classified as normocytic, microcytic, or macrocytic. Based on the MCHC, erythrocytes may be classified as normochromic or hypochromic. The MCH only expresses the mean weight of hemoglobin per erythrocyte.

# Erythrocyte Sedimentation Rate (ESR)

## Principle

When anticoagulated blood is allowed to stand undisturbed, the red cells will normally settle out to the bottom of the tube. This principle is the basis for the erythrocyte sedimentation rate (ESR). By definition, the ESR is the distance in millimeters that red cells fall per unit of time, which is usually 1 hour. Various factors will affect the ESR, such as red cell size and shape, plasma fibrinogen, and globulin levels, as well as mechanical and technical factors.

The rate of sedimentation is directly proportional to the red cell mass and inversely proportional to plasma viscosity. In normal whole blood, red cells do not rouleaux; the mass of the red cell is small and therefore the ESR is decreased (cells settle out slowly). In abnormal conditions when red cells can rouleaux, the mass of the red cell is greater, therefore increasing the ESR (cells settle out faster).

Historically there have been two methods to perform an ESR—the Westergren method[4] and the Wintrobe and Landsberg method.[5]

## Stages of Sedimentation

1. *Initial period of aggregation.* Rouleaux is formed with minimal sedimentation. This phase lasts about 10 minutes.
2. *Period of fast settling.* At this stage the settling rate is constant and lasts about 40 minutes.
3. *Final stage.* The remaining amount of time is a period of packing at the bottom of the tube.

## Reagents and Equipment

Wintrobe tubes, disposable, 3 mm bore, 110 mm long flat-bottom (American Dade, Division of American Hospital Supply Corp., Miami, FL)
9-inch glass Pasteur pipettes
Sedimentation tube rack
Patient EDTA specimen

## Sedimentation Rate Determinations (Method from American Dade)

1. Blood should be collected with proper anticoagulant in proportion to volume of blood to avoid shrinkage of erythrocytes. EDTA (0.5 mg/ml of blood) is suggested.
2. Thoroughly mix blood with anticoagulant immediately before filling tube.
3. Use a filling needle, a 9-inch Pasteur pipette or other cannula that will reach the bottom of the tube. Slowly fill the tube with blood, avoiding air bubbles in the column.
4. Adjust the meniscus of the specimen to the "0" line at the top of the tube.
5. Place tube in upright position, in rack that will maintain the tube in this position.
6. At the end of 1 hour read the fall of erythrocytes by recording the level of erythrocytes in the tube. The erythrocyte sedimentation rate is read on the same side of the tube as the "0" line. Reading from the top downward, the ESR is read as the fall of cells in mm per 1 hour of time.
7. If the demarcation between plasma and red cell column is hazy, the level is taken where the full density is first apparent.

Rapid sedimentation will occur with large bore tubes and tall columns of blood. It is important to keep the position of the tube vertical at all times. Slight degrees of tilting will accelerate the ESR.

Normal Values:
| | |
|---|---|
| Adult males | 0 to 9 mm/hr |
| Adult females | 0 to 15 mm/hr |

## Comments

The erythrocyte sedimentation rate is not a very specific or diagnostic test. Despite the time constraints and the lack of specificity among disorders that can cause an abnormal ESR, this test is still used in many institutions as a screening test.

Perhaps the usefulness of this test lies in its ability to differentiate between diseases with similar symptoms or to monitor the course of an existing disease. For example, early in the course of an uncomplicated viral infection the ESR is usually normal, but it may rise later with a superimposed bacterial infection. Within the first 24 hours of acute appendicitis, the ESR is not elevated, but in the early stage of acute pelvic inflammatory disease or ruptured ectopic pregnancy it is elevated. The ESR is elevated in established myocardial infarction but normal in angina pectoris. It is elevated in rheumatic fever, rheumatoid arthritis, and pyogenic arthritis but not in osteoarthritis. The ESR can be an index to disease severity. In many cases it can be an index of the activity of pulmonary tuberculosis. In general, there is no direct correlation between fever and the ESR.

## Interpretation

**Factors that Affect Sedimentation Rate.** *Plasma Factors.* Increased plasma concentration of fibrinogen, and immunoglobulin, will result in rouleaux formation and an increased ESR. It can therefore be expected that disease states that are characterized by hyperfibrinogenemia or elevated immunoglobulin levels will result in an increased ESR.

*Extreme increases in plasma viscosity slow down the ESR, thus resulting in a decreased ESR.

***Red Cell Factors.*** When rouleaux formation cannot occur, owing to the shape or size of the RBC, a decreased or low ESR is expected. This is observed with sickle cells and spherocytes. The ESR is of little diagnostic value in severe anemia or in hematologic states noted by poikilocytosis.

***Anticoagulants.*** Sodium citrate or EDTA can be used without an effect on the sedimentation rate. Sodium or potassium oxalate can cause shrinkage of the red cells. Heparin causes only a slight amount of shrinkage but a falsely elevated ESR. EDTA is our anticoagulant of choice because of its routine use in the hematology laboratory.

***Mechanical Factors.*** Different normal values are given for various methods due to variations in the caliber of the tube and height of the column of blood.

A number of years ago Wintrobe and Landsberg[6] proposed a method of correcting the ESR for anemia, based on the patient's hematocrit level. The significance of a corrected ESR is still debatable, because the hematocrit can vary for the type and severity of anemia seen and therefore influence the corrected ESR. As a result, we do not correct the ESR for anemia in our laboratory.

## Hematocrit

### Principle (Centrifugal Microhematocrit Method)

Hematocrit is defined as the volume occupied by erythrocytes (RBCs) in a given volume of blood and is usually expressed as a percentage of the volume of the whole blood sample.

The hematocrit is usually determined by spinning a blood-filled capillary tube in a centrifuge. The Coulter Counter S* series provides an indirect measurement, whereas Ortho Instrument's ELT-8† provides a direct measurement of the hematocrit (see section on automated cell counting).

### Reagents and Equipment

Capillary tubes, heparinized or plain (75 mm)
Microhematocrit centrifuge
Microhematocrit reader (needed only if centrifuge does not have one incorporated in the tube holder)

### Procedure

1. Venous blood is drawn from an antecubital vein and into potassium EDTA. Care should be taken to avoid tourniquet stasis since this can elevate venous hematocrit results. The blood is then carefully mixed, preferably on a mechanical rotator. Venous blood may also be obtained through capillary puncture using a heparinized capillary tube to collect the specimen.

2. Once adequately mixed, the unmarked end of a plain capillary tube is placed in the blood and permitted to fill rapidly to approximately three quarters of its length. Tipping the tube horizontally will speed filling. The tube is then removed from the blood and wiped clean of excess blood.

3. The unmarked end is then plugged with modeling clay and placed in the centrifuge, clay-filled end against the rubber gasket (i.e., against the peripheral rim). For accuracy, each determination should be done in duplicate or triplicate.

4. Centrifuge for 5 minutes at a set speed (force is approximately 14,500 rpm). This separates red cells from plasma and leaves a band of *buffy coat* at the interface consisting of white cells and platelets.

5. Allow the centrifuge to stop on its own; *do not hand brake.*

6. The hematocrit is read as the percent of whole venous blood occupied by red cells. With a constant bore capillary tube this can be done by obtaining a distance ratio on a microhematocrit reader. The reader is first set with the clay-red cell interface at 0 percent. Next, shift the ruled scale or etched line to 100 percent and align it with the plasma meniscus. Read down to the percent spiral line that intersects with the red cell–white cell interface. This percent is the hematocrit value. Do not include the buffy coat layer in this value. If it exceeds 2 percent it should be recorded and noted as volume of packed white cells (VPW).

7. Results should duplicate within 1 percent.

### Interpretation

Normal Values:

| | |
|---|---|
| Newborn | 53 to 65% |
| Infant/Child | 30 to 43% |
| Adult Male | 42 to 52% |
| Female | 37 to 47% |

### Comments

1. Incomplete sealing of the capillary tubes will give falsely low results because in the process of spinning, red cells and a small amount of plasma will be forced from the tube.

2. Process of centrifugation will give falsely elevated results.

3. If the buffy coat is included in the red cells when reading the result, the hematocrit will be falsely elevated.

4. The microhematocrit centrifuge should never be forced to stop by applying pressure to the metal cover plate. This will cause the red cell layer to "sling" forward and results in a falsely elevated result.

---

*Coulter Electronics, Inc., P.O. Box 2145, Hialeah, FL 33012
†Ortho Diagnostic Systems Inc., Westwood, MA 02090

## PRINCIPLES OF AUTOMATED CELL COUNTING

### Coulter Counter Model S-Plus

Over the past two decades, the hematology laboratory has witnessed the evolution of the Coulter Counters from the Model A to the sophisticated Coulter Counter Model S-Plus series. Despite the technologic advances, the principles of these instruments remains the same: one-by-one, *nonoptical* particle counting based on volumetric impedence. The Coulter principle of volumetric impedance uses the principle that the measure of volume displacement is directly proportional to cell size (Fig. 31–5). An electric current exists between two electrodes immersed in a conductive (saline) solution and contained in an aperture tube. Blood cells are also suspended in this fluid and are directed through an orifice in the aperture tube. As a blood cell passes through the orifice, it displaces its own volume of solution. This displacement increases the resistance between the electrodes which results in an electrical pulse. The pulse, or signal, is a precise measurement of cell volume. Pulses are then electronically amplified and transmitted to a scaling circuit with adjustable threshold levels. Particles with counts (volumes) below a selected size are separated out from the cell counts. In the Coulter S-Plus series, each cell count is performed in triplicate, compared, and if in agreement, averaged for the best result. Instances in which three counts are not in agreement result in the operator being alerted to the problem.

The Coulter S-Plus series directly measures RBCs, WBCs, and platelets. Hematocrit, MCH, and MCHC are electronically computed from the other data. Hemoglobin concentration is measured photometrically after lysis for the WBC determination (see section on Hemoglobinometry). The MCV is directly measured from the amplitude of the pulse signals from the second and third RBC aperture tubes.

This instrument can also include red cell distribution width (RDW) and mean platelet volume (MPV) as parameters in its profile. The RDW is an index of anisocytosis, and the MPV can provide information on the distribution of the platelets.

The Coulter S-Plus consists of five basic interconnecting units (Fig. 31–6):

1. Diluter unit: In this unit, blood is aspirated, diluted, mixed, lysed, and sensed.
2. Analyzer unit: It is here that counting, measuring, and computing functions occur.

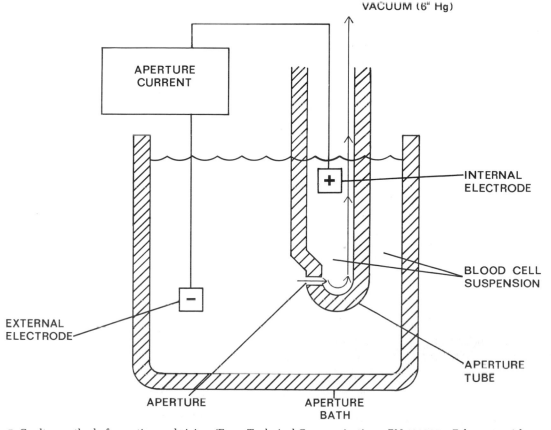

**Figure 31–5.** Coulter method of counting and sizing. (From Technical Communications, PN 4235051, Feb 1982, with permission.)

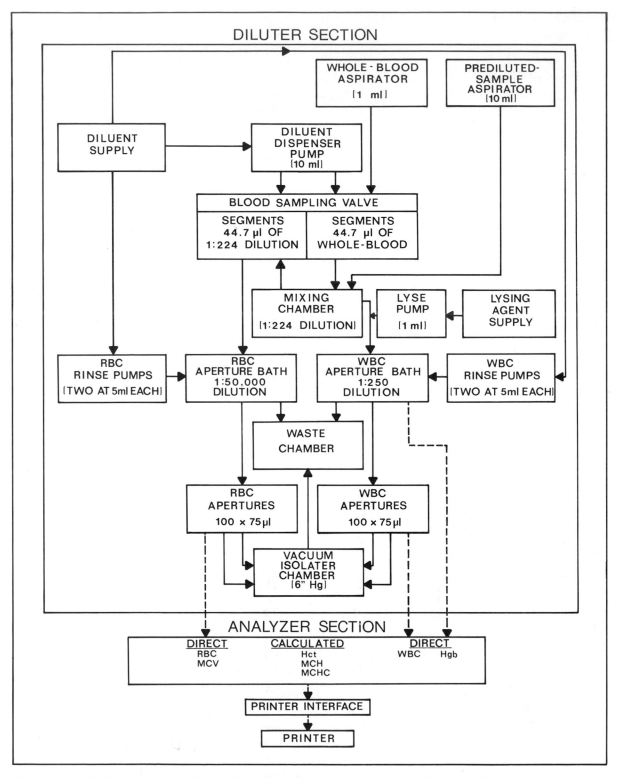

**Figure 31–6.** The five basic units of the Coulter S-Plus: diluter, analyzer, power unit, pneumatic power supply, printer.

3. Power supply: Furnishes the electrical power for all circuits.
4. Pneumatic power supply: Provides vacuum and pressure for the diluter unit.
5. Printer: Provides numerical printout as a result of signal conversion from voltage information to digital data.

In some of the more advanced Coulter S-Plus systems, automated differentials can be performed by the instrument. A size-referenced histogram is provided which includes lymphocytes, mononuclear cells, and granulocyte subpopulations for each specimen and is reported in percentages and absolute numbers.

The Coulter S-Plus uses an EDTA patient sample and aspirates 1 ml for testing. When the sample is aspirated, it is split into two segments before it reaches the sampling valve. One half of the sample is for WBC counting, the other half for RBC and PLT determinations. From the WBC segment, 10 ml of diluent enters the valve and picks up 42.9 lambda of whole blood and carries it to the WBC aperture bath (the bath on the *right* side of the diluter unit). Simultaneously, 10 ml of diluent picks up 1.6 lambda of whole blood from the second segment and enters the RBC aperture bath (the bath on the *left* side of the diluter unit). As the dilution from the WBC count enters the WBC aperture bath, 0.7734 ml of lyse reagent is also pumped into the aperture bath. Bubbles are introduced into each aperture bath to completely mix the diluted blood sample. At the same time the aperture baths are being filled, the hemoglobin cuvette is drained into the waste chamber and then filled with diluent for the hemoglobin blank reading. The counting cycle can now begin in each of the aperture baths. There are three apertures in each aperture bath so that the counts can be performed in triplicate and averaged. Each aperture contains an internal electrode, and there is one external electrode in each aperture bath. The vacuum draws the diluted blood sample through each $100 \mu$ aperture. When a cell passes through the aperture, a volume of electrolyte is displaced proportional to the cell volume. This reduces the electrical current flow and changes the resistance between the internal and external electrodes. The result is a voltage change proportional to the size of the cell. While the red cells are being counted, the MCV is determined from the amplitude of the voltage pulses. Since red cells and platelets are passing through simultaneously, those particles measuring 2 to 20 $\mu m^3$ are counted as platelets and all particles greater than 36 $\mu m^3$ are considered red blood cells. After the counting cycles have taken place the RBC bath empties to waste and the WBC bath empties into the hemoglobin cuvette, which is filled with WBC diluent. The hemoglobin lamp is set at 520 nm,

and a reading is taken for hemoglobin concentration.

If 1 ml of whole blood cannot be obtained, 44.7 lambda of whole blood can be volumetrically pipetted to 1 ml of diluent. By pressing the 1 : 224 dilution button and aspirating the entire specimen, the initial dilution is bypassed.

## Ortho ELT-8 Hematology Analyzer (ELT-8)

The ELT-8 Laser Hematology Counter is produced by Ortho Instruments for in vitro diagnostic use in clinical laboratories. This instrument *optically* detects WBCs, RBCs, and platelets using a narrow beam helium/neon laser as a light source. The MCV, MCH, and MCHC are calculated from the test data. Hematocrit determinations are obtained by using the red cell detection signals. Hemoglobin concentration is measured by the colorimetric cyanmethemoglobin method, which employs a light emitting diode and a photomultiplier tube.

Physically, the ELT-8 consists of two basic units (Figs. 31–7, 31–8). One unit, the sample processor, actually processes the blood sample and performs the testing. A second unit, the data handler, is the electronic unit that processes the test data and displays it on the cathode ray tube (CRT) screen. The data handler can also provide a hard copy of the test results. The ELT-8 can test 60 samples per hour using a volume of less than 100 $\mu l$ for a sample and provide eight parameters (WBC, RBC, platelet counts, HCT, Hb, MCV, MCH, MCHC). In addition, this instrument can provide a printed copy of histograms for RBC, WBC, or platelet distribution. Calibration is automatic, and quality control programs include moving range studies.

A routine sample collected with EDTA is used for testing. The ELT-8 uses Isolac, Lysac, and Cyanac reagents for platelet, red cell, white cell, hemoglobin, and hematocrit determinations. Isolac is a buffered saline reagent used as a diluent for RBC, platelet, and HCT determinations. It is also used as a flow channel sheath reagent. Lysac is the lysing reagent and diluent for the WBC determination. Cyanac is the reagent used for the hemoglobin determination. Samples should be processed within 8 hours and maintained at room temperature.

The sample processor begins testing by aspirating approximately 100 ml of sample. An air segment from the previous cycle prevents premature dilution by Isolac at the leading edge of the sample. The sample is then split into two aliquots. Half of the sample and its protective air bubble goes to the RBC/platelet determining channel. Isolac reagent is introduced into the sample yielding a 1 : 63 dilution. Pressure forces the diluted sample through the

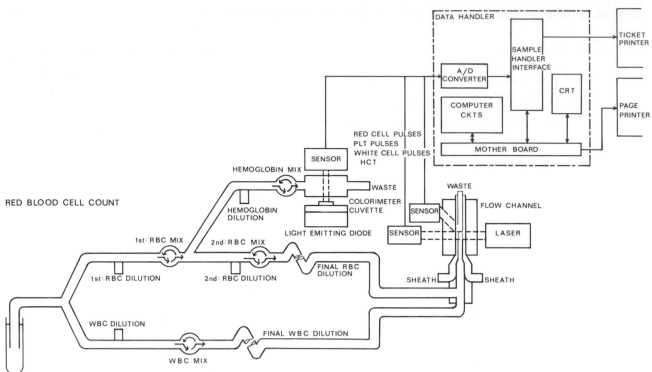

**Figure 31–7.** Overall system operation for Ortho ELT-8. This is a schematic diagram of the pathway a specimen follows from the point of aspiration to the printing of patient values. (From Ortho Diagnostic Systems: Laser Hematology Analyzer Operator Reference Manual. Westwood, MA, March 1981, pp. 3–25, with permission.)

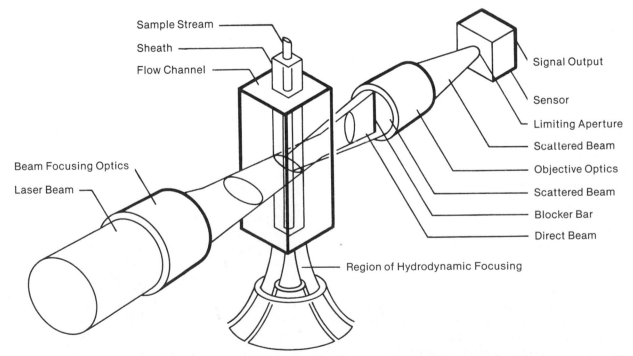

**Figure 31–8.** Schematic diagram of the ELT-8 optical subsystem. This illustrates the optical detection of cells by the scattering of light from the laser. The intensity of the scattered light is detected, processed, and converted to electrical pulses which ultimately results in a printed value. This diagram also shows the region of hydrodynamic focusing of cells into a single file line through the flow channel. (From Ortho Diagnostic Systems, Inc.: Laser Hematology Analyzer Operator Reference Manual. Westwood, MA, March 1981, pp. 3–23, with permission.)

mixing station, where on its exit the sample is split a second time. A portion goes to the colorimeter for hemoglobin testing, where an equal volume of Cyanac is metered into the sample yielding a 1 : 126 dilution. It is then sent to the cuvette in the colorimeter. The other portion continues on to the RBC/platelet determination. A second RBC/platelet dilution with Isolac results in a sample that consists of 1 part diluted sample to 6.3 parts diluent; a final sample dilution of 1 : 440. After passing through a mixing station, the sample is held for a short time before entering a flow channel, where counting and sizing of cells is performed to determine RBC, platelets, and HCT.

When the sample was originally split, half was sent for RBC, platelet count (PLT), IIb, and HCT; the other half was directed into the WBC-determining channel. As part of the WBC sample is pushed through the conveyor tube, Lysac is added to dilute and lyse the red cells so that white cells can be counted. This yields a 1 : 19 dilution. The treated sample passes through a mixer and then enters into the WBC storage lines, where it is retained for stabilization and transport to the laser/optics for cell counting.

## Counting Methods

**Cell Counting Method.** After dilution and stabilization, the RBC, platelet, and WBC dilutions are held for sequential entry into the flow channel, where the actual cell counting occurs. The laminar-flow effect begins when the sample enters the channel. The laminar sheath flow technique allows the actual orifice to be $250\,\mu$, which is still wide enough to prevent clogging. Faster-flowing Isolac carries the slower-moving sample upward until the sample stream is only wide enough for the cells to flow in "single file." Transportation of the cells in "single file" ensures a minimum of coincidence, owing to more than one cell passing in front of the laser optics at once and being counted as only one cell. As each cell passes through the laser beam, forward angle scattering of the light by the cell causes a change in the light intensity directed toward the sensor. These changes in sensor signals are forwarded to the electronic subsystem to be counted. Red cell sizing is performed at the same time that red cells and platelets are counted.

Red cells are differentiated from platelets and white cells based on the following criteria[7]:

1. A voltage threshold is present in the instrument. When counting the RBC/PLT dilution, all voltage values lower than the voltage threshold are counted as platelets, and all values higher than the threshold are classified as red blood cells.
2. The ELT-8 differentiates the refractive index of red cells from that of the platelets.
3. The time of flight through the counting zone is determined by measuring the time when the forward tip of the cell enters the counting zone and the time when the end of the cell leaves the counting zone.

Automatic correction for coincidence is incorporated into the RBC and platelet counts, but this has not been done for WBC counts.

**Hematocrit Determination.** Each of the pulses generated during the RBC count phase is integrated to determine the area under the scattered light signal. The sum of the integrals is directly proportional to the percent hematocrit. This concept can be further explained by the fact that the greater the total number of pulses counted, the higher the RBC count. The greater the sum of their integrals, the greater the percent hematocrit.

**Hemoglobin Determination.** The hemoglobin concentration of a sample is determined by comparing its optical density with that of a reference solution of Isolac and Cyanac. The light beam from the light emitting diode (LED) is passed through the cuvette and onto the photomultiplier tube (PMT). Output from the PMT is sent to the data handler for conversion and storage.

## HEMOGLOBINOMETRY

### Principle

Hemoglobin, the main component of the red cell, transports oxygen and $CO_2$ to and from the body's tissues. Hemoglobin in circulating blood is a mixture of hemoglobin, oxyhemoglobin, carboxyhemoglobin, and minor amounts of other forms of this pigment. It is necessary to prepare a stable derivative involving all forms of hemoglobin in the blood in order to measure this compound accurately. The cyanmethemoglobin derivative can be conveniently and reproducibly prepared and is widely used for hemoglobin determination. All forms of circulating hemoglobin are readily converted to cyanmethemoglobin (HiCN) except for sulfhemoglobin, which is rarely present in significant amounts. Cyanmethemoglobin can be measured accurately by its absorbance in a colorimeter.

The basic principle of the cyanmethemoglobin (HiCN, hemoglobin-cyanide method) is that blood is diluted in a solution of potassium ferricyanide and potassium cyanide. The potassium ferricyanide oxidizes hemoglobin to methemoglobin (Hi, hemoglobin) and the potassium cyanide converts methemoglobin to the stable cyanmethemoglobin, which is read on a spectrophotometer at 540 nm.

### Reagents and Equipment

Hemoglobin calibrator (American Scientific Products, McGraw Park, IL)
Cyanmethemoglobin reagent (Drabkin's reagent)
5 ml pipettes

Spectrophotometer
Cuvettes
Test tubes
20 $\mu$l pipette

### Cyanmethemoglobin Reagent (Drabkin's Reagent)

| | |
|---|---|
| Sodium bicarbonate | 1.00 g |
| Potassium cyanide | 0.05 g |
| Potassium ferricyanide | 0.02 g |
| Distilled water | 1000 ml |

### Procedure

**Standard Curve.** Prepare a standard curve by diluting S/P hemoglobin standard with cyanmethemoglobin reagent. Measure the absorbance of each dilution at 540 nm. The dilutions should be made to yield a linear curve.

The hemoglobin concentration of a blood sample is measured by diluting 0.02 ml of blood with 6.0 ml of cyanmethemoglobin reagent, measuring the absorbance of the resulting cyanmethemoglobin solution at 540 nm, and comparing its absorbance with the absorbance of the standard. For example, if the concentration of the standard is 80 mg/dl of cyanmethemoglobin, then in 5 ml there are:

$$\frac{80}{100} \times 5 = 4 \text{ mg of cyanmethemoglobin}$$

This amount of cyanmethemoglobin is formed from 4 mg of hemoglobin. If a 0.02 ml sample contains 4 mg of hemoglobin, then 100 ml contains 20 g (see below).

1. Prepare tubes containing 5 ml of the cyanmethemoglobin reagent and label them "blank," "controls" (high and low), and for each unknown sample.
2. Using a 20 $\mu$l pipette, add 20 $\mu$l (0.02 ml) of mixed whole blood (EDTA) to the reagent, rinsing the pipette at least three times.
3. Mix thoroughly by vortexing or inversion with "parafilm" and allow the tube to stand at least 10 minutes before reading.
4. Using cyanmethemoglobin reagent as a *blank*, adjust the spectrophotometer to read 100 percent T at wavelength 540 nm. Invert sample to be analyzed and aspirate into a cuvette. Read percent transmittance.
5. Determine hemoglobin values of the test sample and controls from the standard curve.

Normal Values (in g/100 ml blood):

| | |
|---|---|
| Adult male | 14 to 17 |
| Adult female | 12.5 to 15 |
| Newborn | 17 to 23 |
| At 3 months of age | 9 to 14 |
| At 10 years of age | 12 to 14.5 |

### Special Considerations and Comments

Before the test sample is read, the solution should be clear:

1. *A high white blood cell count.* The specimen should then be centrifuged and the supernatant used for reading.
2. *HbS and HbC.* The mixture should be diluted 1:1 with distilled water and then read in the colorimeter; the reading is multiplied by 2.
3. *Abnormal globulins.* 0.1 g of potassium carbonate should be added to the solution.

## Hemoglobin Electrophoresis

### Principle

Electrophoresis is defined as the movement of charged particles in an electric field. The different normal and abnormal hemoglobins show different mobilities or migration patterns in an electric field at a fixed pH. The usual support medium is cellulose acetate at an alkaline pH of 8.5. The following procedure is that of Helena Laboratories, and all reagents and apparatus are available from them.

### Reagents

1. Hemolysate reagent
2. Controls: $A_1$FSC: normal $A_1A_2$ patient
3. Buffer: SupreHeme buffer. One envelope is dissolved in distilled water and diluted to 980 ml tris–EDTA–boric acid buffer, pH 8.4.
4. Ponceau S stain
5. Destain: 5 ml glacial acetic acid (Mallinckrodt) per 100 ml distilled water. A 5 percent solution.
6. Dehydrating agent: absolute methanol (Mallinckrodt)
7. Clearing solution: 150 ml glacial acetic acid, 350 ml absolute methanol, and 20 ml Clear Aid
8. Titan III-H cellulose acetate plates

### Apparatus

All are available from Helena Laboratories.

1. Cliniscan
2. Helena Titan Power Supply
3. Incubator-oven-dryer
4. Electrophoresis chamber
5. Super Z sample well plate
6. Super Z aligning base
7. Applicator
8. Zip-zone chamber wicks

---

$$\frac{4}{0.02} \times 100 \text{ ml} = 20 \text{ g (i.e., the standard is equivalent to 20 g/dl)}$$

## Procedure

1. Preparation of hemolysate: Spin EDTA blood for 20 minutes at 3000 rpm to pack the red cells. Remove the plasma and buffy coat. Add 6 drops of hemolysate reagent to 1 drop of packed red cells. Let stand for 1 minute; then vortex for 1 minute. Hemolysate may be frozen and then thawed to ensure complete hemolysis.
2. Preparation of electrophoretic chamber: Pour 100 ml of buffer into each outer compartment. Soak a wick in each compartment, and then drape it over the bridge, making sure it contacts the buffer. Cover the chamber.
3. Preparation of cellulose acetate plates: Number the plates on the bottom right of the glossy side. Wet the plates by slowly lowering the rack into a container of buffer. Allow to soak for at least 5 minutes.
4. Preparation of sample well plates: Clean with distilled water and dry each well with a cotton swab. Prepare two rinse plates by filling the wells with distilled water. Prepare the patient samples by using a 5 lambda microdispenser to fill the wells on clean dry plates. Patients should be run in duplicate, and an $A_1A_2$ and $A_1FSC$ control should be run on each plate. Cover with a glass slide to prevent evaporation.
5. Loading of cellulose acetate plates:
   a. Prime the applicator by depressing several times into the sample well plate then depressing once on a blotter.
   b. Remove the cellulose acetate plate from the buffer; blot once firmly; place on the aligning base with the number at the bottom left.
   c. Load the applicator by depressing three times into the sample well plate; then transfer the applicator to the aligning base, and depress the bar firmly for 5 seconds.
   d. Place the plate, glossy side up, across the bridge in the electrophoresis chamber.
6. Electrophorese at 350 volts for 25 minutes.
7. Staining:
   a. Ponceau S for 5 minutes. Drain 5 to 10 seconds.
   b. Four successive washes of 5 percent glacial acetic acid to destain. Leave in each for 2 minutes, draining for 5 seconds between each wash.
   c. Two successive washes of absolute methanol to dehydrate. Leave for 2 minutes in each, draining for 5 seconds between each wash.
   d. Clearing solution for 5 minutes.
   e. Dry vertically for 1 to 2 minutes.
   f. Dry in the oven for 3 to 4 minutes, acetate side up.
8. Scan the plate with the Cliniscan using a 525 nm filter, slit size 5, and optics filter wheel V-2 O.D.
9. Label the plate and store in a plastic envelope as a permanent record.

## Results

Hemoglobinopathies are reported out in relative-percentages.

| | |
|---|---|
| $HbA_1$ | 96.0 to 98.6 percent |
| $HbA_2$ | 1.5 to 4.0 percent |
| HbF | 60.0 to 90.0 percent at birth |
| | 1.0 to 2.0 percent after 1 year of age |

## Comments

At an alkaline pH, hemoglobin S and hemoglobin D have the same mobility, as do hemoglobins $A_2$, C, E, and O Arab. These hemoglobins may be separated by electrophoresing on citrate agar at an acid pH (Fig. 31–9). Hemoglobin $A_2$ may also be quantitated by column. It should be kept in mind that $HbA_1$ and HbF cannot be separated on cellulose acetate. Separation and quantitation of HbF is performed, based on acid and or alkali resistance. (See HbF denaturation.)

## Citrate Agar Hemoglobin Electrophoresis

### Principle

Electrophoresis is the movement of charged particles in an electric field. Using citrate agar at an acid pH facilitates the separation of hemoglobins that migrate together on other media (cellulose acetate) at a different pH (alkaline). The following procedure is that of Helena Laboratories, and all reagents and apparatus are available from them.

### Reagents

1. Hemolysate reagent
2. Controls: $A_1FSC$: normal $A_1A_2$
3. Buffer: Citrate buffer. Dissolve one package in distilled water and dilute to 1 liter.
4. Stain:
   a. 10 ml of 5 percent glacial acetic acid
   b. 5 ml of tolidine in methanol
   c. 1 ml of sodium nitroferricyanide in water
   d. 1 ml of 3 percent hydrogen peroxide
   e. Prepare fresh on day of use.
5. Titan IV citrate agar plates

### Apparatus

All are available from Helena Laboratories.

1. Helena Titan Power Supply
2. Electrophoresis chamber
3. Sample well plate
4. Aligning base

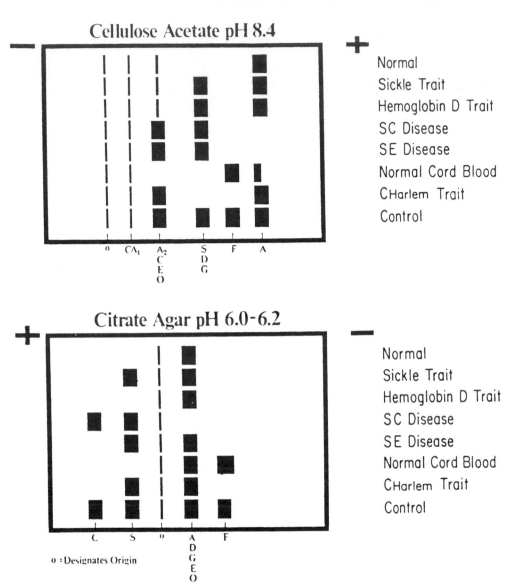

**Figure 31–9.** Comparative hemoglobin electrophoresis. Hemoglobin electrophoresis on cellulose acetate and citrate agar indicating patterns of mobility. The width of the band is not indicative of hemoglobin concentration. (From Schmidt, RM, and Brosious, E: Basic Laboratory Methods of Hemoglobinopathy Detection. Dept. of Health and Human Services, Atlanta, 1972, with permission.)

5. Applicator
6. Sponge wicks

## Procedure

1. Preparation of hemolysate: Spin EDTA blood for 20 minutes at 3000 rpm to pack the red cells. Remove the plasma and buffy coat. Add 10 drops of hemolysate reagent to 1 drop of packed red cells. Let stand for 1 minute, then vortex for 1 minute. Hemolysate may be frozen and then thawed to ensure complete hemolysis.

2. Preparation of electrophoresis chamber: Pour 100 ml of buffer into each outer compartment. Soak a sponge wick in each compartment then place it so that the top of the sponge protrudes

over the inner ridge of the compartment. Cover the chamber.

3. Preparation of sample well plates: Clean all wells with distilled water and dry with cotton swabs. Prepare the patient samples by using a 5 lambda microdispenser to fill the wells. Patient hemolysates should be run in duplicate, plus an $A_1FSC$ and an $A_1A_2$ control should be run on each plate. Cover the plate with a glass slide to prevent evaporation.

4. Loading of citrate agar plates:
   a. Prime the applicator by pressing several times into the sample well plate, and then dispensing once on a blotter.
   b. Place the Titan IV citrate agar plate on the aligning base.

c. Load the applicator by pressing three times into the sample well plate; then transfer applicator to the aligning base.
d. Depress the applicator onto the gel surface using no pressure, and allow hemolysate to absorb for 1 minute.
5. Place the plate gel side down across the inner ridges of the electrophoresis chamber with the application point near the anode.
6. Electrophorese for 40 minutes, at 40 milliamps per plate and 50 volts per plate.
7. Staining:
a. Place the plate in a staining dish and puddle the stain over the surface. Let stand for 5 to 10 minutes.
b. Rinse with distilled water for 10 minutes.
c. Cover with another gel plate and seal with tape to store.

## Results

Using this procedure, hemoglobins S and D can be separated. Hemoglobin D, instead of migrating with hemoglobin S as in an alkaline buffer, will migrate with hemoglobin A. This procedure also separates hemoglobins $A_2$ and E from hemoglobin C, as hemoglobins $A_2$ and E will migrate with hemoglobin A, leaving hemoglobin C by itself. The pattern distributes thus from cathode to anode: C, S, $A_1$, $A_2$, D, E, and F (Fig. 31–9).

# Hemoglobin $A_2$ by Column

## Principle

This is an anion exchange chromatography method. The anion exchange resin is a preparation of cellulose covalently coupled to small positively charged molecules, which will attract negatively charged molecules. Hemoglobins have positive or negative charges, owing to properties of their component amino acids. Here buffer and pH favor net negatively charged hemoglobins, which are attracted and bound to the resin. Once bound, the hemoglobins can be selectively eluted and measured on a spectrophotometer. This procedure (the Sickle-Thal Column method) is that of Helena Laboratories.

## Reagents

1. Control: Quik column control
2. Sickle-Thal Quik column
3. Hemoglobin $A_2$ developer
4. Hemoglobin S developer
5. Hemolysate Reagent-C

All are available in a kit from Helena Laboratories.

## Apparatus

1. Column rack and collection tubes
2. Digispec, a spectrophotometer

## Procedure

1. Preparation of hemolysate: Add 50 lambda EDTA blood plus 200 lambda Hemolysate Reagent-C to a small test tube. Vortex vigorously and allow to stand 5 minutes before use.
2. Preparation of columns:
a. Allow to come to room temperature.
b. Turn each column upside down twice, place it in the rack, remove top cap, and resuspend with a pipette.
c. Remove the bottom cap and allow the buffer to drain out.
d. After the resin repacks, remove any buffer remaining at the top, being careful not to disturb the resin.
3. Slowly apply 100 lambda of patient hemolysate to the column and allow to absorb into the resin.
4. Put 100 lambda of patient hemolysate in a large collection tube and Q.S. to 15 ml with distilled water. Label this tube "total fraction."
5. Elution of hemoglobin $A_2$:
a. Slowly apply 3 ml of hemoglobin $A_2$ developer and allow to pass through the column into the small collection tube (approximately 30 minutes).
b. Q.S. the tube to 3 ml with distilled water.
6. Elution of hemoglobin S (optional):
a. Slowly add 10 ml of hemoglobin S developer to the column in aliquots of 3 ml, 3 ml, and 4 ml.
b. Allow it to pass through the column into a large collection tube (approximately 1½ to 2 hours).
c. Q.S. the tube to 15 ml with distilled water.

7. Using the spectrophotometer at 415 nm, record the absorbance of the $A_2$ eluate, the S eluate, and the total fraction.

## Results

$$\% \text{ HbA}_2 = \frac{\text{O.D. HbA}_2 \text{ eluate}}{5 \times \text{O.D. total fraction}} \times 100$$

$$\% \text{ HbS} = \frac{\text{O.D. HbS eluate}}{\text{O.D. total fraction}} \times 100$$

O.D. = optical density.

The hemoglobin S eluate is optional, as it can be picked up on alkaline electrophoresis.

The normal range for hemoglobin $A_2$ is 1.7 to 3.3 percent. This can be used to separate hemoglobin $A_2$ from hemoglobin C or hemoglobin E. Elevated levels of hemoglobin $A_2$ may be useful in diagnosing a beta thalassemia.

## Differential Solubility Test for Hemoglobin S (Sicklequik by General Diagnostics)

### Principle

This particular test is a rapid, self-contained tube test manufactured by General Diagnostics as a modification of the solubility test. It is a biphasic (that is, two layer) system, with an upper organic layer of toluene and a lower aqueous layer of phosphate buffer, saponin, and reducing agents. When whole blood is added and mixed, the red cells are lysed by toluene and saponin, and the hemoglobin is reduced by sodium hydrosulfite. If any insoluble S hemoglobin is present, it rises to the top of the aqueous layer and forms a dark interface between the layers.

### Reagents

None are required. A ready-to-use tube comes from General Diagnostics.

### Procedure

1. Add 0.1 ml EDTA blood to the tube.
2. Shake vigorously for 10 seconds.
3. Let the tube stand for 5 minutes.
4. Centrifuge for 5 minutes at 3400 rpm.
5. A positive and negative control should be run.

### Results

A negative result (indicating no sickling hemoglobin) shows a gray-pink interface with a dark-red aqueous layer.

A positive result (indicating the presence of a sickling hemoglobin) will show one of two patterns. The homozygous state shows a dark-red interface with a pale straw aqueous layer. All of the hemoglobin is abnormal and is picked up at the interface. The heterozygous state shows a dark-red interface with an aqueous layer of varying shades of pink to red, depending on the amount of nonsickling hemoglobin.

## Sodium Metabisulfite Slide Test

### Principle

The addition of a reducing agent (sodium metabisulfite) to cells containing hemoglobin S causes them to sickle.

### Reagents

Sodium metabisulfite solution: Dissolve 200 mg of sodium metabisulfite in 10 ml distilled water. This solution is stable for 24 hours.

### Procedure

1. Make a very dilute suspension of EDTA blood in the sodium metabisulfite solution on a slide.

The tip of an applicator stick swirled through a drop of the solution is sufficient.
2. Coverslip the drop and seal with permount.
3. Examine the slide immediately, then every 15 minutes for 1 hour, and again at 2 hours.

### Results

In patients with sickle cell disease the sickling process will be immediate with obvious sickled, elongated, and holly-leaf shapes. In sickle cell trait or a combination, the process will be slower. This test cannot be used to differentiate the homozygous and heterozygous states and is only used to show the presence of a sickling hemoglobin.

## Acid Elution for Hemoglobin F

### Principle

Hemoglobin F in red cells is resistant to acid elution; therefore, it can be precipitated and stained. Hemoglobin A will be eluted from the red cells. This is a modification of the original Kleinhauer stain and is available in kit form from Simmler, Inc.

### Reagents

1. Fetal cell fixing solution: 80 percent reagent alcohol
2. Fetal cell buffer solution: citrate buffer 0.027M
3. Fetal cell stain: erythrosin B
4. Control: 0.1 ml of cord blood plus 0.9 ml of normal adult blood

*Note*: All reagents are available in the Simmler Fetal Cell Stain Kit.

### Procedure

1. Add 2 drops of EDTA blood to 3 drops of 0.85 percent saline.
2. Prepare a monolayer film of this suspension. Allow to air dry.
3. Immerse film in fixing solution for 5 minutes at room temperature.
4. Rinse in distilled water and allow to air dry.
5. Immerse in buffer solution for 8 to 10 minutes at room temperature.
6. Immediately immerse in staining solution for 3 minutes at room temperature.
7. Rinse in distilled water and allow to air dry.
8. Examine for the presence of cells staining for fetal hemoglobin.

### Results

Cells containing hemoglobin F will stain bright pink-red. Cells containing only hemoglobin A will be very light pink. The stain may be useful in distinguishing hereditary persistence of fetal hemoglobin (HPFH, where most red cells show an even distribution of hemoglobin F) from a high level of hemoglobin F in thalassemia minor (where the distribution of hemoglobin F is uneven). The percentage of fetal cells may be calculated if this stain is to be used to assess fetal cells in maternal circulation.

## Staining for Heinz Bodies

### Principle

Heinz bodies are denatured hemoglobin precipitated in the red cell and attached to the red cell membrane. They are not visible with Wright's stain but show up with vital staining and phase microscopy.

### Reagents

1. Crystal violet solution: 1.0 g of crystal violet dissolved in 50 ml of a 0.85 percent saline solution, which is shaken for 5 minutes and filtered before storage.
2. Methyl violet solution: 0.5 g of methyl violet dissolved in 100 ml of a 0.85 percent saline solution, which is shaken for 5 minutes and filtered before storage.

Note: A 0.75 percent saline solution may be used. This slightly hypotonic solution swells the cells slightly.

### Procedure

1. Mix equal volumes of EDTA blood and stain in a small test tube. Either stain may be used.
2. Incubate for 20 minutes at room temperature.
3. Make several smears. Let them air dry, then examine for Heinz bodies.
4. Alternately, make a wet prep. Place a drop of the blood and stain mixture on a slide, coverslip, seal with permount, and examine for Heinz bodies.

### Results

Heinz bodies appear as irregular, refractile, purple inclusions, 1 to 3 microns in diameter, located on the periphery of the cell. They may even seem to be outside the cell. Reticulocytes should not stain.

The presence of Heinz bodies indicates exposure of the red cells to various oxidizing agents or the presence of an unstable hemoglobin.

## Heinz Body Induction Test

### Principle

Heinz bodies can be induced in great numbers in susceptible individuals by incubating the blood in various reducing substances. Susceptible individuals such as those with a G-6-PD deficiency are those who would hemolyze following administration of aniline derivatives such as primaquine, phenacetin, or sulfanilamides.

### Reagents

1. Buffer solution:
   a. Dissolve 0.908 g of $KH_2PO_4$ in 100 ml of distilled water.
   b. Dissolve 0.824 g of $Na_2HPO_4$ in 87 ml of distilled water.
   c. Mix 13 ml of the $KH_2PO_4$ solution with 87 ml of the $Na_2HPO_4$ solution.
2. Acetylphenylhydrazine solution: Dissolve 0.1 g of acetylphenylhydrazine in 100 ml of the buffer solution. Make fresh on day of use and use within 1 hour.
3. Crystal violet solution: Dissolve 1.0 g of crystal violet in 50 ml of a 0.85 percent saline solution. Shake for 5 minutes and filter before use. A 0.75 percent saline solution may be used. This is slightly hypotonic and swells the cells a little.

### Procedure

1. Add 0.1 ml of EDTA blood to 2 ml of acetylphenylhydrazine solution. Whiffle mix by blowing air into the suspension (aerate).
2. Incubate at 37°C for 2 hours.
3. Whiffle mix again and incubate a further 2 hours at 37°C.
4. Mix equal volumes of cell suspension and crystal violet in a small tube. Incubate for 10 minutes.
5. Make a wet prep (a drop of stained suspension plus a coverslip) and let settle. Examine and count under oil immersion.

### Results

A normal control subject will have at least one Heinz body in each red cell. A susceptible patient (e.g., G-6-PD deficiency, defects of glutathione reductase enzyme, or unstable hemoglobins) will have five or more Heinz bodies in 40 percent or more of the red cells. The Heinz bodies appear as irregular, refractile, purple inclusions, 1 to 3 microns in diameter, and located either on the periphery or bulging out of the red cell.

## TESTS FOR HEMOLYTIC ANEMIAS
## Osmotic Fragility

### Principle

Whole blood is added to a series of saline dilutions. The presence or absence of hemolysis is an effective measure of erythrocyte susceptibility to hypotonic damage. This test is more than just an index of cell shape; it is also a measure of the surface-to-volume ratio. When a red cell's membrane surface decreases and its volume remains the same or increases, the cell becomes more turgid and less deformable. This is because the red cell membrane is flexible but not elastic. The result of this loss of surface-to-volume ratio is similar to what happens to a small plastic bag that is filled with more and more water—a rupture of the cell membrane.

Spherocytes, which have a *decreased* surface-to-volume ratio, demonstrate an *increased* osmotic fragility. This is due to their inability to swell in a hypotonic medium before leaking hemoglobin. Sickle cells, target cells, and other poikilocytes are relatively resistant to osmotic change and therefore demonstrate a *decreased* fragility.

## Reagents and Equipment

24 12 × 75 mm test tubes
Two 5 ml serologic pipettes (TD)
Parafilm squares
1 heparinized normal control sample
1 heparinized patient sample
Linear graph paper

**1 Percent NaCl Solution.** Weigh 1.0 g NaCl crystals on an analytical balance. Place crystals in a 100 ml volumetric flask and fill to the mark with distilled water. Stir to completely dissolve NaCl.

## Procedure

1. Arrange two series of 12 tubes in the rack. Label both sets of tubes 1 to 12. The first series of tubes, 1 to 12, is for the patient and the second series of 12 tubes is the control.
2. With a 5 ml pipette add 1 percent NaCl solution, and with the other 5 ml pipette add distilled water into the series of patient tubes according to the following schedule:

| Tube | 1% NaCl (ml) | Distilled Water (ml) | NaCl%, Final Concentration |
|---|---|---|---|
| 1 | 4.25 | 0.75 | 0.85 |
| 2 | 3.5 | 1.5 | 0.70 |
| 3 | 3.25 | 1.75 | 0.65 |
| 4 | 3.0 | 2.0 | 0.60 |
| 5 | 2.75 | 2.25 | 0.55 |
| 6 | 2.5 | 2.5 | 0.50 |
| 7 | 2.25 | 2.75 | 0.45 |
| 8 | 2.0 | 3.0 | 0.40 |
| 9 | 1.75 | 3.25 | 0.35 |
| 10 | 1.5 | 3.50 | 0.30 |
| 11 | 1.25 | 3.75 | 0.25 |
| 12 | 0.75 | 4.25 | 0.15 |

3. Thoroughly mix the contents of each tube by covering with parafilm and inverting several times.
4. With a 3 ml pipette transfer 2.5 ml of solution from the first set of tubes to the corresponding second set. Only one pipette is necessary if you start to transfer with the most dilute solution.

5. Blood is drawn into a tube containing heparin. Immediately add 50 $\mu$l of blood into each tube of the first set. It should drop directly into the solution. Do not allow the blood to drop onto the sides of the tube. Cover each tube with parafilm and invert gently.
6. Add 50 $\mu$l of known normal blood, collected in the same manner, to each tube in the second set.
7. Let the tubes sit at room temperature for half an hour.
8. Mix gently and centrifuge at 2000 rpm for 5 minutes.
9. When interpreting results, note which tubes show *initial* and *complete* hemolysis. *Initial* hemolysis is recognized by a faintly pink supernatant and a cell button at the bottom of the tube. *Complete* hemolysis is seen as a red supernatant with possibly a button of cell stroma at the bottom of the tube.
10. This test may be quantitated by measuring each tube on the spectrophotometer. If this is done, two additional tubes are necessary. The first is a blank containing 50 $\mu$l of blood to which 2.5 ml of 0.9 percent NaCl is added, which will result in no hemolysis. The second blank is for complete (100 percent) hemolysis and is obtained by adding 50 $\mu$l of blood to 2.5 ml of distilled water.
11. These blanks are run in parallel with the other tubes.
12. After centrifugation, the supernatant of each tube is removed, and its optical density is read in a spectrophotometer using a 540 nm filter. The percentage of hemolysis in each tube is calculated using the following equation:

$$\% \text{ Hemolysis} = \frac{\text{O.D.}_{(x)} - \text{O.D.}_{\cdot 0.85\%}}{\text{O.D.}_{\cdot(o)} - \text{O.D.}_{\cdot 0.85\%}} \times 100$$

An osmotic fragility curve may be drawn by plotting the percent hemolysis in each tube against the corresponding concentration of NaCl solution as shown (Fig. 31–10). It is helpful to plot the normal control with the patient so that any difference can be seen more clearly.

## Interpretation

1. Patient values are always reported with the value of the control. With normal samples, initial hemolysis is generally around 0.45 percent, with complete hemolysis occurring at 0.30 percent or 0.35 percent.
2. Examples of initial and complete hemolysis in various conditions follow:

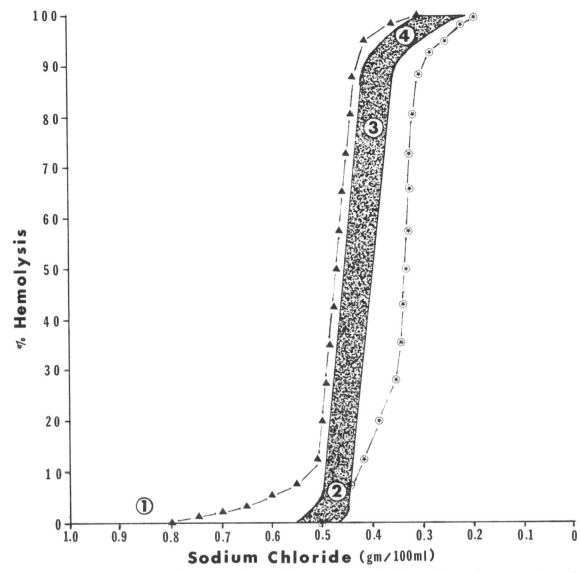

**Figure 31–10.** Comparative osmotic fragility curve. ⊛ ⊛ ⊛ sickle cell anemia; ▲ ▲ ▲ hereditary spherocytosis. Normal range is indicated by shaded area. 1 = normal biconcave disc; 2 = disc-to-sphere transformation; 3 = disc-to-sphere transformation; 4 = lysis. (Prepared by J. McMichael.)

|  | Initial Hemolysis (% NaCl) | Complete Hemolysis (% NaCl) |
|---|---|---|
| Normal | 0.45 | 0.35 |
| Hereditary spherocytosis | 0.65 | 0.45 |
| Acquired hemolytic anemia | 0.50 | 0.40 |
| HDN | 0.55 | 0.40 |
| Thalassemia | 0.35 | 0.20 |
| Sickle cell anemia | 0.35 | 0.20 |

It may be necessary in some cases to incubate the patient's heparinized blood for 24 hours at 37°C. This will enhance increased osmotic fragility, which may reveal a subtle but abnormal osmotic fragility not apparent upon initial testing.

## Comments

1. Fresh heparinized blood is recommended, but defibrinated blood may be used. EDTA, oxalate, or citrate should not be used because of the additional salts present.
2. This test should be performed immediately, because cell shape and osmotic conditions change with time.
3. Osmotic fragility can be altered by pH and temperature.
4. If the plasma is significantly jaundiced it is suggested that the plasma be replaced with isotonic saline before testing to prevent interference.
5. Hemolytic organisms in a blood specimen can

cause erroneous results owing to hemolysis, which is not attributed to test conditions.

6. If the patient has a low hemoglobin level, wash patient and control cells once with isotonic saline and resuspend with equal volumes of red cells and saline for both specimens. This will correct for the anemia.

7. In some anemias, when poikilocytosis accompanies a low hemoglobin level, decreased osmotic fragility may be seen. This may be due in part to the decreased hemoglobin concentration and not to the presence of poikilocytes.

## Acidified Serum Test (Ham Test) for Paroxysmal Nocturnal Hemoglobinuria (PNH)

### Principle

Confirmation of a diagnosis of PNH is dependent on a positive acidified serum test. The red cells of patients with PNH are complement sensitive. In this test, complement will affix to the red cells at a slightly acidic pH, become activated by the alternate pathway, and result in lysis of the red cells.

### Equipment and Reagents

Venous patient specimen
Venous normal control
Five 12 × 75 test tubes
0.2N HCl
1 ml serologic pipettes
Two Erlenmeyer flasks
Glass beads

### Procedure

1. Collect venous specimens from patient and control in a plastic syringe and defibrinate by swirling in an Erlenmeyer flask that contains glass beads.
2. Centrifuge the defibrinated blood and separate serum from cells. Save the normal control serum, the patient's serum, and red cells.
3. Wash the red cells from the patient and control three times with isotonic saline, and dilute to a 50 percent cell suspension.
4. Label test tubes 1 through 5.
5. Add the reagents to the five tubes in numerical order, as shown below.
6. Cover with parafilm and incubate all tubes for 1 hour at 37°C.

7. Centrifuge and examine supernatant for hemolysis.

### Interpretation

1. Patients with PNH will demonstrate hemolysis in tubes 1 and 3. Tube 3 was run in the event the patient had decreased complement levels.
2. Little or no hemolysis will be seen in tubes 2 and 4.
3. No hemolysis should be seen in your control, tube 5.

### Comments

1. The optimum pH for this test is 6.5 to 7.0.
2. Blood containing a large number of spherocytes, as seen in hereditary spherocytosis, may result in a false-positive result.
3. The test result may be positive also in hereditary erythroblastic multinuclearity with positive acidified serum test (HEMPAS). There are, however, two differentiating features; in HEMPAS the red blood cells are not lysed by the patient's own acidified serum, and the sugar-water test result is negative.

## Sugar-Water Test for Paroxysmal Nocturnal Hemoglobinuria (PNH)

### Principle

In patients with PNH, the sucrose solution provides a low ionic strength environment that allows complement to bind to the red cells. These abnormal cells are extremely complement sensitive, which results in complement-mediated lysis.

### Reagents and Equipment

"Sugar-Water" Solution: Dissolve 10 g table sugar in 100 ml distilled water. Prepare fresh daily.
Patient and control venous, clotted specimens, fresh
Test tubes, 12 × 75
1 ml serologic pipettes

### Procedure

1. Obtain clotted specimens, centrifuge, and separate serum from clot.
2. Prepare 50 percent red cell suspensions from the clots.
3. In separate labeled tubes, add 0.85 ml of sugar solution, 0.5 ml of autologous serum, and 0.1

| | TUBES | | | | |
|---|---|---|---|---|---|
| REAGENTS | 1 | 2 | 3 | 4 | 5 |
| 1. Patient serum | 0.5 ml | 0.5 ml | | | |
| 2. Normal serum | | | 0.5 ml | 0.5 ml | 0.5 ml |
| 3. 0.2N HCl | | 0.05 ml | 0.05 ml | | 0.05 ml |
| 4. Patient's RBCs (50%) | 1 drop | 1 drop | 1 drop | 1 drop | |
| 5. Normal RBCs (50%) | | | | | 1 drop |

ml of the corresponding red cell suspensions. Mix thoroughly but gently.

4. Incubate at 37°C for 30 minutes. Centrifuge for 1 to 2 minutes at 3400 rpm.
5. Examine the supernatant for any hemolysis.

### Interpretation

1. The presence of marked hemolysis in the patient tube is indicative of PNH. No hemolysis should be evident in the control.
2. Slight hemolysis is not usually indicative of PNH and is considered questionable.

### Comments

1. Fresh samples must be used in order to retain complement activity.
2. The sugar-water solution must be made fresh daily; otherwise false-negative results will occur.
3. This is a screening test and is considered diagnostic only when used in conjunction with the acidified (Ham's) serum test.

## Autohemolysis Test

### Principle

When defibrinated blood is incubated at 37°C for 48 hours, only minimal hemolysis will occur. In patients with hereditary spherocytosis (HS), autohemolysis is increased. The addition or glucose or ATP to the incubation state will decrease the percentage of the abnormal hemolysis seen in the spherocytes of HS patients.

### Reagents and Equipment

1. Ammonia Water: Add 0.4 ml concentrated ammonium hydroxide to 1 liter of deionized $H_2O$.
2. 0.239M ATP: Weigh out 121 mg of ATP, dilute with 1 ml saline, and carefully neutralize to pH 7.5 to 8.0 with 1M NaOH. This solution must be sterilized through a 0.45 $\mu$m pore filter unit syringe.
3. Sterile 10 percent dextrose in 0.85 percent NaCl solution
4. Sterile 125 ml Erlenmeyer flasks with approximately 25 glass beads (4 mm)
5. Sterile polypropylene tubes with caps (12 × 75 mm)
6. Sterile 5 ml pipettes
7. Sterile 3 ml syringes
8. Spectrophotometer set to read at 540 nm
9. Assorted volumetric flasks, test tubes, and Pasteur pipettes

### Procedure

**Day 1**

1. Draw 25 ml of blood from the patient, and carefully defibrinate by swirling blood in a sterile 125 ml Erlenmeyer flask with glass beads. Repeat the same procedure for a control sample.
2. Prelabel six sterile 12 × 75 polypropylene tubes for each patient, and control and dispense the appropriate reagents as follows:

   tubes 1, 2   Plain
   tubes 3, 4   0.1 ml of 10% dextrose in saline
   tubes 5, 6   0.1 ml of 0.239M ATP

3. Add 2 ml of the appropriate defibrinated blood to each tube and gently rotate to mix.
4. Incubate for 24 hours in a 37°C incubator.
5. Prepare a 1:100 dilution of defibrinated blood by pipetting 0.5 ml of whole blood into a 50 ml volumetric flask, and bring it to volume with ammonia water. This is done for both the control and the patient blood.
6. Centrifuge remaining defibrinated blood, and remove serum.
7. Prepare a reagent blank by making a 1:10 dilution of serum with 4.5 ml ammonia water. This is done for both the control and the patient serum.
8. Refrigerate serum for use on day 3.
9. Read the optical density (O.D.) of the whole blood dilutions against the serum blanks at 540 nm. Record these results.

**Day 2**

1. Rotate incubated samples gently, and reincubate for an additional 24 hours.

**Day 3**

1. Gently mix incubated samples, and pool pairs.
2. Perform a spun hematocrit on each sample (total three hematocrits per patient and control). Record results.
3. Pour each sample into a tube, and centrifuge for 5 minutes at 2500 rpm.
4. Remove the serum from each tube, and prepare a 1:10 dilution of each serum with ammonia water (0.5 ml serum with 4.5 ml ammonia water).
5. Make a 1:10 dilution of original serum saved from day 1. This will be your serum blank.
6. Read the O.D. of the serum samples made in step 4 at 540 nm using the sample prepared in step 5 as the reagent blank.

### Calculations

The percentage of hemolysis for each tube is calculated as shown below.

$$\% \text{ Hemolysis} = \frac{(100 - \text{HCT of tube}) \times \text{O.D. serum sample}}{\text{O.D. of whole blood} \times 10}$$

Normal Values: Lysis at 48 hours
Without added dextrose     0.2 – 2.0%
With added dextrose        0 – 0.9%
With added ATP             0 – 0.8%

## Comments

When normal blood is incubated for 48 hours under sterile conditions, the amount of hemolysis is relatively small. If dextrose or ATP is added, hemolysis is further slowed.

Increased autohemolysis occurs in many types of hemolytic anemia. The patterns that may be observed, according to Dacie,[7] are as follows:

1. Dacie's type I — Patients whose red cells show slight autohemolysis, corrected by dextrose as seen in those with G-6-PD deficiency, hexokinase deficiency, and acquired nonspherocytic hemolytic anemia.

2. Dacie's type II — Patients with moderate autohemolysis without dextrose and in whom correction with dextrose does not take place, as seen in those with pyruvate kinase deficiency and acquired spherocytic hemolytic anemia.

3. The third type demonstrates marked autohemolysis without dextrose correction, seen in patients with hereditary spherocytosis and in those with triose phosphate isomerase deficiency (Fig. 31–11).

The autohemolysis test is no longer used in the

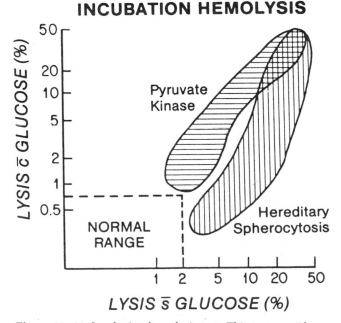

**INCUBATION HEMOLYSIS**

Figure 31–11. Incubation hemolysis test. This test provides a further measure of cell resistance to hemolysis. Pyruvate kinase–deficient blood demonstrates an abnormal rate of hemolysis that is independent of the presence or absence of glucose in the incubation media. In contrast, the blood from a patient with hereditary spherocytosis shows more marked hemolysis when glucose is absent.

differential diagnosis of nonspherocytic congenital hemolytic anemia, because specific enzymatic assays are now available that are considerably more accurate. It is, however, a useful screening test for some RBC enzyme deficiencies related to hemolysis.

## PREPARATION OF BLOOD SMEARS AND GROSS EXAMINATION

### Preparation and Examination of the Peripheral Blood Smear

The preparation and examination of a peripheral blood smear is one of the most frequently requested tests in the hematology laboratory. This procedure not only is requested for the diagnosis of hematologic disorders but also is an essential tool in providing information for a diagnosis in nonhematologic diseases, in indicating side effects in chemotherapy, and in monitoring patient therapy. Reasons such as these make it essential that a blood smear be prepared correctly and examined in such a way as to provide the physician with an accurate interpretation.[8]

There are four methods used to prepare blood smears:

1. Slide-to-slide
2. Coverslip-to-slide
3. Coverslip-to-coverslip
4. Automated spinner

Blood smears are prepared with EDTA anticoagulated blood to minimize degenerative changes in the blood cells. The collection tube must be completely filled with the appropriate amount of blood so that it can mix with the anticoagulant. If there is an excess of anticoagulant, artifacts will occur. To ensure good preservation of cellular morphology, differential smears should be made as soon as possible and no later than 3 hours after collection.[9]

### Slide-to-Slide Method

#### Principle

A small drop of blood is placed near the frosted end of a clean glass slide. A second slide is used as a spreader. The blood is streaked in a thin film over the slide. The slide is allowed to air dry and is then stained.

#### Equipment

Glass slides, 3 × 1 inch (precleaned with frosted edge)
Capillary tubes, plain

#### Procedure

1. Fill a capillary tube three quarters full with the anticoagulated specimen.

2. Place a drop of blood, about 2 mm in diameter, approximately one third inch from the frosted area of the slide.
3. Place the slide on a flat surface, and hold the narrow side of the nonfrosted edge between the left thumb and forefinger.
4. With your right hand, place the smooth clean edge of a second (spreader) slide on the specimen slide, just in front of the blood drop.
5. Hold the spreader slide at a 30 degree angle, and draw it back against the drop of blood.
6. Allow the blood to spread almost to the edges of the slide.
7. Push the spreader forward with one light, smooth, and fluid motion. A thin film of blood in the shape of a bullet with a "feathered" edge will remain on the slide.
8. Allow the blood film to air dry completely before staining (Fig. 31–12).

### Comments

1. A good blood film preparation will be thick at the "drop" end and thin at the opposite end.
2. The blood smear should occupy the central portion of the slide and should not touch the edges.
3. The thickness of the spread when pulling the smear is determined by the (1) angle of the spreader slide (the greater the angle, the thicker and shorter the smear),[10] (2) size of the blood drop, and (3) speed of spreading.
4. This is one of the easiest and most popular methods for producing a blood smear, but it does not produce quality smears. The white cells are unevenly distributed, and red cell distortion is seen at the edges. Smaller WBCs such as lymphocytes tend to reside in the middle of the feathered edge. Large cells such as monocytes, immature cells, and abnormal cells can be found on the outer limits of this area.

## Coverslip-to-Coverslip Method

### Principle

A drop of blood is placed in the middle of a clean glass coverslip. A second coverslip is placed over the first coverslip to form an octagon. The blood drop is allowed to spread between the two coverslips and quickly pulled apart horizontally.

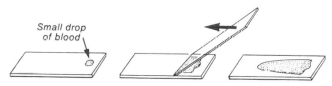

Small drop of blood

**Figure 31–12.** Preparation of a peripheral blood smear; slide-to-slide technique.

### Equipment

Coverslips, clean, 22 × 22 mm
Capillary tubes, plain

### Procedure

1. Hold a coverslip by two sides between the thumb and forefinger of the right hand. Place a drop of blood from a capillary tube in the center of the coverslip.
2. With the left hand pick up a second coverslip at one corner, holding the slide with your thumb and forefinger.
3. Quickly place the second coverslip over the first so that they are superimposed to form an octagon. Allow 2 to 4 seconds for the blood drop to spread; then quickly pull them apart in a rapid, smooth, and horizontal motion. Lifting either coverslip during this process will ruin the smear, owing to an uneven distribution of cells.
4. Allow the coverslips to air dry, smear side up.
5. Wright stain the smear, using staining jars instead of an automatic stainer.
6. Mount on a 3 × 1 inch glass slide.

### Comments

1. This method, when performed correctly, results in an even distribution of white cells. However, this method is difficult to master, and technologists find it awkward working with fragile coverslips.
2. An advantage to this method is that one can end up with two smears on the same glass slide, if they were mounted side by side.
3. A disadvantage is that an automatic slide stainer cannot be used. It is more time consuming to stain the smears by hand and therefore less efficient for a high-volume laboratory.

## Coverslip-to-Slide Method

### Principle

This method is similar to the coverslip-to-coverslip method. It differs in that two drops of blood are placed approximately one inch apart on a slide. A coverslip is placed, with three of its corners touching the slide, on top of one drop of blood and allowed to spread. The coverslip is quickly pulled off the slide in a quick horizontal motion. The coverslip is then immediately turned over, and the same sequence is repeated on the other drop of blood. As with the coverslip-to-coverslip method, two smears are obtained for evaluation.

### Equipment

Glass slides; 3 × 1 inch, precleaned and without a frosted edge
Coverslips, 22 × 22 mm
Capillary tubes, plain

## Procedure

1. Hold a $3 \times 1$ inch glass slide lengthwise between the thumb and forefinger of the left hand. A capillary tube with the blood sample is held in the right hand, and two drops of blood are placed approximately 1 inch apart on the slide.
2. Pick up a coverslip by one edge with the thumb and forefinger of the right hand, and place it on top of the blood drop. Three corners of the coverslip should cover the blood drop, and the fourth corner should extend slightly from the edge of the slide.
3. Allow the blood to spread evenly, and then grasp the extended corner of the coverslip between the thumb and forefinger and pull it from the slide in a quick, smooth, horizontal motion.
4. Turn the coverslip over and repeat the procedure on the adjacent blood drop.
5. Allow both smears on the slide to air dry and stain.

## Comments

1. This procedure yields an even distribution of WBCs and two blood smears on one slide, which can facilitate evaluation.
2. If an automatic stainer is used, care must be taken not to place one of the blood drops too close to the edge of the slide. If this slide happens to be toward the bottom of the staining plate, the stain may not cover it sufficiently. This would result in only one smear being completely stained.

## Automatic Spinner Technique

### Principle

Although there are several automatic slide spinners out on the market, the basic principle remains the same. A small quantity of patient blood is placed in the middle of a $3 \times 1$ inch glass slide. The slide is held in a horizontal position by a platen. The motor of the spinner is activated and accelerates rapidly to a predetermined speed. When the slide has spun for its predetermined time, the motor quickly stops.

A slide with a monolayer of cells is produced, which is suitable for evaluation. An even distribution of cells over the entire slide makes this preparation ideal for performing differentials on samples with low white cell counts, as well as normal and abnormal specimens. The only disadvantage is that the slides must be extremely clean to prevent the sheering and spreading of cells as they are spun.

## Examination of the Peripheral Blood Smear

There are several necessary steps in the examination of a peripheral blood smear.

### Low-Power ($\times$10) Scan

1. Determine the overall staining quality of the blood smear.
2. Determine if there is a "good distribution" of cells on the smear.
   a. Scan the edges and center of the slide to be sure there are no clumps of red cells, white cells, or platelets.
   b. Scan the edges for abnormal cells.
3. Find an optimal area for the detailed examination and enumeration of cells.
   a. The red cells should not quite touch each other.
   b. There should not be areas containing large amounts of broken cells or precipitated stain.
   c. The red cells should have a graduated central pallor.

### High-Power ($\times$40) Examination

1. Determine the white cell estimate.
2. Correlate the white cell estimate with the white cell count/mm³.
3. The morphology of the WBCs should be evaluated and any abnormalities, e.g., toxic granulation or Döhle bodies, should be recorded.

### Oil Immersion ($\times$100) Examination

1. Perform a 100 white cell differential count.
   a. *All white cells* are to be included.
2. Evaluate red cell anisocytosis, poikilocytosis, hypochromasia, polychromasia, and inclusions.
3. Perform a platelet estimate and evaluate platelet morphology.
   a. Count the number of platelets in 10 oil immersion fields.
   b. Divide by 10.
   c. Multiply by 15,000/mm³ if smear was prepared by an automatic slide spinner; multiply by 20,000/mm³ for all other blood smear preparations.
4. Correct any total white cell count/mm³ that has greater than *one* nucleated red cell (NRBC)/100 WBCs.
   a. When performing the white cell differential, do not include NRBCs in your count.
   b. Use the formula below to correct a white cell count:

$$\frac{WBC/mm^3 \times 100}{100 + \#NRBCs/100\ WBCs} = \text{Corrected WBCs/mm}^3$$

The examination of the peripheral blood smear is performed as part of the hematologic laboratory workup called the complete blood count (CBC) (Fig. 31-13).

## The LE Cell Preparation

### Principle

The LE cell is a neutrophil (or eosinophil) that has ingested a mass of nuclear material. These cells can be formed when the LE plasma factor is present in blood or body fluids. The LE factor is considered an antinuclear antibody and may be present in the plasma of patients with systemic lupus erythematosus (SLE). When leukocytes are suspended in plasma containing the LE factor, depolymerization of DNA and liberation of the nuclear material occurs. This homogeneous globular mass of altered nuclear material is termed a "hematoxylin body." When neutrophils phagocytize this hematoxylin body, LE cells are formed.

### Equipment and Reagents

Glass beads (4 mm)
Test tube rotator
Microscopic slides
Pipettes
10 ml heparinized vacutainer tube
Wintrobe sedimentation rate tubes, 10 mm disposable (American Dade, Division of American Hospital Supply Corp., Miami, FL)
Wright's stain

### Procedure

1. Collect approximately 10 ml of patient blood in a 10 ml heparinized vacutainer tube.
2. Add 10 glass beads to the patient specimen, and place on a tube rotator for 20 minutes.
3. Allow the specimen to sit at room temperature for 1 hour.
4. Transfer the mixed specimen to two or more Wintrobe tubes and spin for 5 minutes at 1500 rpm, or until three distinct layers can be seen (serum, buffy coat, and red cells).

*Note:* To spin the Wintrobe tubes place three of the tubes in a 15 × 100 mm test tube and pack tightly with gauze so tubes will not break. Spin for desired time.

5. With a pipette, discard all but 1 mm of serum above the buffy coat, so that few red cells will be present on the blood smear.
6. Transfer a drop of the buffy coat onto a slide and make smears. Use the additional Wintrobe tubes for additional smears.
7. Stain with Wright's stain.
8. Scan blood smears at low and high power, to locate possible LE cells. Examine questionable areas with the oil immersion objective to confirm suspected LE cells.

### Interpretation

1. LE cells must follow certain strict criteria to be classified as such:
   a. A neutrophil or granulocyte must be intact and contain a homogenous, velvety, hematoxylin body.
   b. Generally, the hematoxylin body will be large enough to push the nucleus of the neutrophil out to the rim of the cell membrane.
   c. The hematoxylin body may not retain any of its nuclear characteristics such as chromatin pattern, nucleoli, or nuclear membrane.
   d. The hematoxylin body must be completely engulfed.
2. Microscopic examination of the blood smear may reveal phagocytosis of whole or fragmented nuclei by monocytes and occasionally

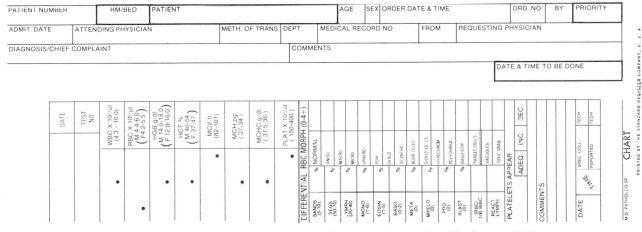

**Figure 31–13.** Hematology laboratory report form illustrating the complete blood count (CBC).

the neutrophil or the eosinophil. This is termed a "tart cell." It can be distinguished from an actual LE cell, because the phagocytized nucleus lacks homogeneity and does not have the characteristic "velvety" appearance of a hematoxylin body. The nuclear material in a "tart cell" may also retain some structures of a nucleus such as chromatin pattern or nucleoli.

3. Hematoxylin bodies surrounded by neutrophils, but not engulfed by any *one* cell, are termed "rosettes." Rosette formation is not diagnostic of the LE phenomenon or of SLE; it strictly suggests the *possibility* of the LE factor being present.

## Comments

1. LE cells are observed in some patients with SLE and also in patients with other connective tissue diseases.
2. A negative result from an LE cell preparation does not rule out the diagnosis of SLE. In many cases, these patients may demonstrate fluorescent antinuclear antibody titers and patterns diagnostic of SLE.
3. Certain drugs may give a positive LE cell test result.

## SPECIAL STAINS SECTION (see also Chapter 19)*

## Cytochemistry

### Leukocyte Alkaline Phosphatase (LAP) Stain

Alkaline phosphatase is located in the specific granules of neutrophils. It is combined with the substrate at an alkaline pH. A colored precipitate is formed at the site of hydrolysis of the substrate.

The purpose of this procedure is to distinguish the cells of a leukemoid reaction from those of chronic myelocytic leukemia (CML). One hundred mature neutrophils are counted on the blood smear and are scored on the following basis:

| | |
|---|---|
| 0 | Colorless |
| 1 | Diffuse, slight positivity; or occasional granules |
| 2 | Diffuse positivity and moderate number of granules |
| 3 | Strongly positive (granules fill cell) |
| 4 | Very deep staining, nucleus is almost obscured |

The score values for various disease states may vary, and each laboratory must establish its own limits. The chart below is a general guide.

**Purpose.** This stain is used to determine cytoplasmic LAP enzyme activity. LAP activity is decreased in patients with CML and increased in those with leukemoid reactions.

**Principle.** The LAP within the cell hydrolyzes the substrate naphthol AS-BI phosphate. The hydrolyzed substrate then couples with the dye (fast red-violet salt L.B.) and precipitates out at the site of enzyme activity.

**Specimen.** Fingerstick specimens are ideal. Heparinized blood may be used. Do not use EDTA anticoagulated blood. If staining is to be delayed, fix slides and store at $-20°C$ within 2 hours of specimen collection. Smears should be thin.

**LAP Control**

Establishing limits for LAP control:

1. Obtain fresh, heparinized blood from an individual who has an elevated LAP score (e.g., pregnant female in last trimester or person with leukemoid reaction). The control is usually stable for 12 months.
2. Make smears, dry, fix with LAP fixative, and rinse. Allow fixed smears to air dry, then store at $-22°C$.
3. Run a new control with an old control at least five times. Calculate the mean LAP score and set control limits at $±15$ percent.
4. When LAP control is outside the acceptable range ($±$ a mean of 15 percent), the following action should be taken:
   a. Have a second technologist count. If still out of limits, then:
   b. Repeat LAP stain on patient and control. If this action fails to bring control to within acceptable limits, new reagents may be necessary.

**Reagents**

Control: Heparinized blood with score close to 200. Fix and store at $-20°C$:

1. Fixative: Store at room temperature. Expires in 90 days, pH 4.2 to 4.5.

   | | |
   |---|---|
   | a. Sodium citrate F.W. 294.10 | 0.282 g |
   | b. Citric acid F.W. 210.14 | 1.058 g |
   | c. Deionized water | 200 ml |
   | d. Acetone | 300 ml |

   Allow dry reagents to dissolve in water before adding acetone.
2. Substrate solution: Aliquots of 45 ml are stored at $-20°C$. Expires in 8 months.

| | Leukemoid Reaction | CGL | AGL | PRV | Myelofibrosis | PNH | Pregnancy |
|---|---|---|---|---|---|---|---|
| LAP score | ↑ | ↓ | Varies | ↑ | Varies | ↓ | ↑ |

*Courtesy of Mary L. Perkins, M.T.(ASCP), S.H., provided in correlation with Chapter 19; Joe Marty, M.S., M.T.(ASCP), Technical Director from University of Utah Medical Center, Hematopathology Laboratory, Salt Lake City, Utah.

2-amino-2-methyl-1,3-propanediol    13.15 g
0.1N HC1    125 ml
Check the pH (9.5 to 9.7) before adding 0.2 g
naphthol AS-BI phosphate dissolved in 10 ml
N,N-dimethylformamide. Q.S. with deionized
water to 2500 ml.

3. Dye: 40 mg aliquots of fast red-violet salt L.B. are stored at −20°C.
4. Hematoxylin: See hematoxylin counterstain procedure.
5. Glycerol-Gelvatol mounting media: Good for 5 months at 4°C.
   a. Dissolve 996 mg Trizma 9.0 in 160 ml deionized water.
   b. Add 40 g of Gelvatol and stir overnight.
   c. Add 80 ml of glycerol and stir overnight.
   d. Spin at 10,000 Gs for 30 minutes and store in syringes.

### Procedure

1. Allow smears to dry for 30 minutes. (This helps to keep the cells from falling off the slides when rinsing after fixation.)
2. Fix smears in fixative for 30 seconds at room temperature.
3. Rinse with distilled H₂O.
4. Thaw substrate solution to room temperature (22° to 24°C); check with thermometer.
5. Add dye to substrate solution, agitate, filter, and use immediately.
6. Place slides, including control, in mixture for 15 minutes at room temperature.
7. Rinse slides in deionized water.
8. Counterstain with hematoxylin for 2 minutes.
9. Rinse slides in deionized water.
10. Air dry and mount with Gelvatol.

### Interpretation

Score 100 cells from 0 to 4+, and add the scores on the sample.

| | |
|---|---|
| 0 | No staining |
| +1 | Faint staining |
| +2 | Moderate staining |
| +3 | Strong staining (some cytoplasm background visible) |
| +4 | Brilliant (no cytoplasm background visible) |

Report patient score if control is within previously established limits and report normal value.

Normal values:
Males:    22–124
Females:    33–149

LAP activity is decreased in patients with CML, PNH, and hereditary hypophosphatasia. Increased activity is seen in those with polycythemia vera, myelofibrosis, and leukemoid reactions.

### Comments

1. Controls are obtained from blood smears of patients in the third trimester of pregnancy. Control slides are stable for 1 year at −40°C. Re-

peat stain if control values are not within ± 15 percent of control average.
2. Blood smears should be made thin so that WBCs do not touch erythrocytes. Thick smears may falsely elevate results.
3. The control used should score high. If it does not score as high as previous runs, the test should be repeated after new reagents are made.
4. Only segmented and band form neutrophils are scored. Do not include other cells. Monocytes and eosinophils do not stain.
5. LAP slides need to be scored as quickly as possible. The dye tends to fade, especially if Permount is used as a mounting media.

## Peroxidase Stain

**Purpose.** The peroxidase reaction is positive for myeloid cells and negative for lymphoid and erythroid cells. It is, therefore, useful in identifying granulocytic leukemias.

**Principle.** The enzyme peroxidase is present in the primary granules of myeloid cells. These primary granules first appear in the early promyelocyte and persist through subsequent stages. In the presence of hydrogen peroxide, the enzyme peroxidase oxidizes the substrate 3-amino-9-ethylcarbazole to a red-brown color. Some of the oxidized substrate remains at the site of enzyme activity.

**Specimen.** Smears or imprints may be used. Fresh capillary blood is best for smears, however, smears made from EDTA, heparinized, or oxalated blood are adequate. The fresher the specimen, the more reliable are the results.

### Reagents

1. Fixative (buffered formalin acetone pH 6.6). Store at 4° to 10°C. Good for 90 days.
   a. Na₂HPO₄ anhydrous (F.W. 141.96)    0.2 g
   KH₂PO₄ anhydrous (F.W. 136.09)    1.0 g
   Deionized water    300 ml
   b. Add 250 ml reagent grade formalin 37 percent.
   c. Add 450 ml reagent grade acetone.
   d. pH should be 6.6. If necessary, adjust the pH with appropriate buffer salt.
2. 0.02M acetate buffer pH 5.2. Store at 4° to 10°C. Good for 90 days.
   a. 900 ml distilled water.
   b. 2.72 g sodium acetate (F.W. 136.08).
   c. Adjust the pH to 5.2 with dilute acetic acid.
   d. Bring the volume to 1000 ml with distilled water.
3. Hydrogen peroxide 30 percent.
4. 3-amino-9-ethylcarbazole.
5. Dimethylsulfoxide.
6. Mayer's hematoxylin.
7. Glycerol-Gelvatol mounting media. Good for 5 months at 4°C.
   a. Dissolve 996 mg Trizma 9.0 in 160 ml deionized water.

b. Add 40 g of Gelvatol and stir overnight.

c. Add 80 ml of glycerol and stir overnight.

d. Spin at 10,000 Gs for 30 minutes and store in syringes.

**Procedure**

1. Fix smears or imprints for 15 seconds.
2. Rinse with deionized water.
3. Incubate smears for 8 minutes at room temperature in a freshly made filtered mixture containing the following:
   a. 3-amino-9-ethylcarbazole (AEC)        10 mg
   b. Dimethylsulfoxide (DMSO)              6 ml
   c. Acetate buffer                        50 ml
   d. Hydrogen peroxide 30 percent          0.005 ml
4. Rinse with deionized water.
5. Stain with Mayer's hematoxylin for 2 minutes. (Do not differentiate.)
6. Rinse in deionized water.
7. Air dry and mount with glycerol-Gelvatol.

**Interpretation**

1. Red-brown peroxidase positive granules are found in promyelocytes, myelocytes, metamyelocytes, neutrophils, eosinophils, and monocytes. Monocytes stain less intensely than neutrophils and eosinophils. Auer rods are peroxidase positive.
2. Early myeloblasts, lymphoblasts, lymphocytes, basophils, and plasma cells are peroxidase negative.
3. In acute and chronic leukemia, some mature neutrophils may be peroxidase negative.

**Notes**

1. Peroxidase enzyme is sensitive to light. Smears should be stained immediately or kept in the dark. Smears that are older than 2 weeks or that have been exposed to excessive light should not be reported as peroxidase negative. If smears are to be stained at a later date, they should be fixed, air dried, and stored in an envelope in the freezer.
2. Permount must not be used for mounting. Color usually fades before microscopic observation can be made. In addition, xylene should not be used to clean unmounted slides.
3. A 2-minute stain with 1 percent methyl green may be used instead of Mayer's hematoxylin.
4. A normal patient should be run as a positive control.
5. If some of the RBCs are peroxidase positive, the incubation period was too long.
6. Handle DMSO with care.

### Alternative Method—Peroxidase Stain

**Purpose.** The peroxidase reaction is positive for myeloid cells and negative for lymphoid and erythroid cells. It is, therefore, useful in identifying granulocytic leukemias. Use this alternative method only when the regular procedure does not stain blasts that are still suspected to be myeloid.

This procedure requires approval by a hematopathologist.

**Principle.** The enzyme peroxidase is present in the primary granules of myeloid cells. These primary granules first appear in the early promyelocyte and persist through subsequent stages. In the presence of hydrogen peroxide, the enzyme peroxidase oxidizes the substrate benzidine dihydrochloride to a black crystal. The oxidized substrate essentially remains at the site of the enzyme activity.

**Specimen.** Smears or imprints may be used. A fresh specimen is best. Capillary blood is best when staining smears; however, EDTA, heparinized, or oxalated blood are adequate.

**Reagents**

1. Fixative (store at room temperature, good for 90 days).
   Formaldehyde (37 percent)         10 ml
   Absolute ethyl alcohol            90 ml
2. Zinc sulfate solution
   Zinc sulfate ($ZnSO_4\ 7H_2O$)        0.38 g
   Deionized water                   10 ml
3. Substrate solution: Filter and store at room temperature, good for 6 months. Add reagents in order, mixing well after each addition.
   Ethyl alcohol (30 percent)            100 ml
   Benzidine dihydrochloride             0.3 g
   Zinc sulfate solution                 1.0 ml
   Sodium acetate (F.W. 136.1)           1.0 g
   Hydrogen peroxide (30 percent)        0.005 ml
   Sodium hydroxide (1.0N)               1.5 ml
   Safranin O                            0.2 g

*Note:* Benzidine is a potential carcinogen, and the following precautions should be taken when handling the reagent or its solutions.

a. Wear protective clothing. This includes gloves, lab coat, and mask when weighing out powders.

b. Use mechanical aids for all pipetting.

c. Clean up spills immediately.

d. Wash hands after completion.

e. Weigh benzidine in hood.

The 30 percent alcohol may be warmed with hot tap water to help dissolve the benzidine.

**Procedure**

1. Fix smears or imprints for 60 seconds.
2. Rinse with deionized water.
3. Incubate for 30 seconds in substrate solution at room temperature.
4. Rinse with deionized water.
5. Air dry and mount with Permount.

**Interpretation.** Peroxidase positive granules are black.

### Sudan Black B Stain

**Purpose.** Sudan black B stain is the most sensitive stain for granulocytic precursors.

**Principle.** Sudan black stains phospholipids and other lipids. This is believed to be due to physical solubility of the dye in the lipid particles. These lipid particles occur both in primary and secondary granules. They also occur to some extent in monocytic lysozomal granules. They may rarely occur in lymphocytes.

**Specimen.** Smears or imprints may be used. Fresh capillary smears are best; however, smears made from EDTA or heparinized blood are also adequate.

### Reagents

1. Plasdone: K-29-33 (polyvinyl pyrrolidone) GAF Corp., 140 West 51 St., New York, NY 10020.
2. Phosphate buffer, pH 7.2
   a. 0.15M $Na_2HPO_4$ (21 g/l)          7.0 ml
   b. 0.15M $NaH_2PO_4 \cdot H_2O$ (20.7 g/l)   3.0 ml
   c. Distilled water                     30.0 ml
3. Fixative, pH 5.5; store at room temperature in amber bottle; good for 90 days.
   a. Dissolve 10 g of Plasdone in 400 ml of absolute ethanol.
   b. Add 75 ml of 37 percent formaldehyde.
   c. Add 10 ml phosphate buffer pH 7.2.
   d. Add 15 ml liquified phenol or 13.2 g.
4. Sudan black B solution, good for 1 year.
   a. Dissolve 1.5 g of Sudan black B in 500 ml of absolute ethanol.
   b. Stir with a magnetic stirrer for 60 minutes; filter before use.
5. Phosphate: Phenol buffer; good for 6 months.
   a. Dissolve 0.48 g anhydrous $Na_2HPO_4$ (F.W. 141.96) in 400 ml of distilled water.
   b. Dissolve 64 g of crystalline phenol (or 72.8 ml of liquified phenol in 120 ml of absolute ethanol) and mix with the phosphate.
6. Nuclear counterstain, good for 1 year.
   a. 1 percent aqueous cresyl violet.
7. Background stain, good for 1 year.
   a. 0.2 percent aqueous light-green to which 2 drops of glacial acetic acid have been added.

### Procedure

1. Fix slides or coverslip smears for 60 seconds.
2. Rinse three times with tap water.
3. Incubate slides in the following mixture for 60 minutes (prepare daily):
   a. 20 ml phosphate-phenol buffer
   b. 30 ml Sudan black B solution
   c. Filtering solution is not necessary.
4. Rinse in 70 percent ethanol.
5. Air dry.
6. Counterstain for 10 seconds in 1 percent violet. Wash three times in tap water. Air dry.
7. Counterstain for 10 seconds in 0.2 percent light-green. Wash three times in tap water. Air dry, and mount in Permount.

**Interpretation.** Lymphoid cells rarely stain. Brownish-black cytoplasmic granules occur in myelocytic precursors. Monocytes have a few small brownish-black granules. Eosinophilic granules are brown and usually show central pallor.

### Comments

1. The peroxidase reaction parallels the Sudan black B stain except in that the peroxidase enzyme is only found in primary granules.
2. Mayer's hematoxylin, or Giemsa stain, may be used as counterstains.
3. Normal blood smears should always be run as a control.
4. Ideally, smears should be made and stained as soon as possible.

## Specific Esterase (Naphthol AS-D Chloroacetate)

**Purpose.** This is used to aid in differentiation of granulocytes, lymphocytes, and monocytes.

**Principle.** The esterase enzyme within the cell hydrolyzes the substrate naphthol AS-D chloroacetate. The hydrolyzed substrate then couples with the diazo salt (hexazotized pararosaniline). The diazo dye precipitates out at the site of enzymatic activity.

**Specimen.** This consists of paraffin sections, smears, and imprints. For smears, fresh capillary blood is best; however, anticoagulated blood is acceptable.

### Reagents

1. Esterase fixative, pH 6.6; store at 4°C; good for 90 days.
   a. In 120 ml of deionized water dissolve:
   | | |
   |---|---|
   | $Na_2HPO_4$ (F.W. 141.96) | 0.08 g |
   | $KH_2PO_4$ (F.W. 136.09) | 0.40 g |
   | Formaldehyde 37 percent | 100 ml |
   | Acetone | 180 ml |
   b. Adjust pH to 6.6 if necessary with appropriate buffer salt.
2. Phosphate buffer, 0.1M pH 6.5; store at 4°C; good for 90 days. Discard if mold develops.
   a. $NaH_2PO_4 H_2O$ (F.W. 137.99)   9.45 g
   b. $Na_2HPO_4$ (F.W. 141.96)       4.4 7 g
   c. Deionized water                1000 ml
   d. Check pH, and adjust to 6.5 if necessary with appropriate buffer salt solution.
3. Substrate solution. Store in glass stoppered bottle at 4°C. (Not plastic!) Good for 1 month.
   a. Dissolve 100 mg of naphthol AS-D chloroacetate in 10 ml of $N,N$-dimethylformamide (F.W. 73.1).
4. Pararosaniline solution: Store in brown bottle at 4° to 10°C. Good for 3 months.
   **Caution:** Pararosaniline is a potential carcinogen.
   a. Dissolve 1.0 g pararosaniline HCl (F.W. 323.8) in 20 ml distilled water plus 5 ml concentrated HCl. Solution may be gently heated to dissolve pararosaniline.
   b. Filter.
5. Sodium nitrite solution. Prepare daily.
   a. Dissolve 1.0 g $NaNO_2$ (F.W. 69.0) in distilled water to a volume of 25 ml.

6. Mayer's hematoxylin.
7. Acid alcohol stock
   a. Concentrated HCl                                        1 ml
   b. Deionized water                                       100 ml
8. Acid alcohol working solution.
   a. Acid alcohol stock                                      5 ml
   b. Deionized water                                       995 ml
9. Blueing agent
   a. NaHCO$_3$                                                1 g
   b. Deionized water                                       100 ml

**Procedure**

1. Deparaffinize and hydrate sections. The fixative B5 can be used if the fixation time is short and if the mercury precipitate is not removed with iodine.
2. For blood smears and imprints, fix in esterase fixative and wash well with deionized water at 4°C for 30 seconds.
3. Incubation mixture:
   a. To 40 ml of buffer add 1.0 ml of substrate solution.
   b. In a separate test tube add 0.1 ml of sodium nitrite solution to 0.1 ml of pararosaniline solution. Wait 1 minute and add buffer substrate solution.
   c. Filter.
4. After 30 minutes at room temperature, check control slide microscopically. If the reacting cells are not red enough, refilter the solution and replace slides for 15 to 30 minutes.
5. Wash slides in running tap water for 5 minutes.
6. Counterstain for 2 minutes in Mayer's hematoxylin.
7. Rinse well with deionized water.
8. Dip in blueing solution until counterstain turns from purple to blue (approximately 10 dips).
9. Wash, dry, and mount smears with Permount. Tissue sections must be dehydrated and cleared in xylene before mounting with Permount.

**Interpretation.** The cytoplasm of granulocytes and tissue mast cells appears red. Nuclei are counterstained blue.

**Comments.** Esterase is inhibited to varying degrees by mercury, acid solutions, heat, and iodine. Poor or false-negative results occur when:

1. Slides are overheated when drying.
2. "Mercury" crystals are removed from tissues with an iodine solution.
3. Tissues are fixed in an acid fixative such as Zenker's (formalin or acetic), or Bouin's fixative.
4. Tissues are decalcified in an acid solution. Use EDTA.
5. Using solutions that are too old.
6. Tissue may be dezenkerized after incubation in substrate solution.

## Nonspecific Esterase (Alpha-Naphthol Butyrate)

**Purpose.** The purpose of nonspecific esterase is to aid in differentiation of granulocytes, lymphocytes, and monocytes.

**Principle.** The esterase enzyme within the cell hydrolyzes the substrate alpha-naphthol butyrate. The hydrolyzed substrate then couples with the diazo salt (hexazotized pararosaniline). The diazo dye formed precipitates out at the site of enzymatic activity.

**Specimen.** Smears or imprints may be used. A fresh specimen is best. Capillary blood is preferred when staining smears; however, EDTA, heparinized, or oxalated blood is adequate.

**Reagents**

1. Esterase fixative, pH 6.6; store at 4°C; good for 90 days
   a. In 300 ml of deionized water dissolve:
      Na$_2$HPO$_4$ (F.W. 141.96)                           0.2 g
      KH$_2$PO$_4$ (F.W. 136.09)                             1.0 g
      Formaldehyde 37 percent                              250 ml
      Acetone                                              450 ml
   b. Adjust pH to 6.5 if necessary with appropriate buffer salt. (*Note:* pH has tendency to increase if allowed to sit. If pH is near 6.5, allow to stand overnight, and then Q.C. new fixative on known positive.)
2. Phosphate buffer 0.15M, pH 6.3; store at 4°C; good for 90 days. Discard if mold growth is observed.
   a. NaH$_2$PO$_4$ H$_2$O (F.W. 137.99)                     8.02 g
   b. Na$_2$HPO$_4$ (F.W. 141.96)                             2.4 g
   c. Deionized water                                      1000 ml
   d. Check the pH and adjust to 6.3 if necessary with appropriate buffer salt.
3. Substrate solution: Store in glass stoppered bottle at 4° to 10°C. Good for 1 month. Dissolve 250 mg alpha-naphthol butyrate in 12.5 ml ethylene glycol monomethyl ether (Eastman Kodak). If alpha-naphthol butyrate is in liquid form, then use 0.225 ml/12.5 ml of solvent.
4. Sodium nitrite solution. Prepare daily.
   a. Dissolve 1.0 g NaNO$_2$ (F.W. 69.0) in distilled water to a volume of 25 ml.
5. Pararosaniline solution (possible carcinogen; see Comments). Store in brown bottle at 4° to 10°C; good for 90 days.
   a. Dissolve 1.0 g pararosaniline HCl (F.W. 323.8) in 20 ml distilled water plus 5 ml concentrated HCl. Solution may be gently heated to dissolve pararosaniline.
6. Mayer's hematoxylin.
7. Acid alcohol working solution
   a. 70 percent ethanol                                     5 ml
   b. Deionized water                                      995 ml
   c. Concentrated HCl                                     0.05 ml
8. Blueing agent
   a. NaHCO$_3$                                                1 g

b. Deionized water      100 ml

**Procedure**

1. Fix smears for 30 seconds at 4° to 10°C in esterase fixative.
2. Wash three times with deionized water.
3. Air dry smears and place in Coplin jar.
4. a. To 40 ml of buffer (pH 6.3) add 2 ml of substrate solution.
   b. In a separate container, add 0.2 ml sodium nitrite solution to 0.2 ml pararosaniline solution. Wait 1 minute and add to buffer substrate solution.
   c. Filter into Coplin jar.
5. Incubate for 45 minutes at room temperature.
6. Wash well with deionized water.
7. Counterstain with hematoxylin for 2 minutes.
8. Wash well with deionized water.
9. Place slides in blueing reagent for 30 seconds
10. Wash well with deionized water.
11. Air dry and mount with Permount.

**Interpretation.** Megakaryocytes, histiocytes, macrophages, and monocytes stain brick-red. Lymphocytes have punctate staining. Granulocytes have little or no activity. Histiocytes are fluoride resistant, and monocytes are fluoride sensitive.

**Comments**

1. Pararosaniline is a possible carcinogen and the following precautions should be taken when handling the reagent or its solutions.
   a. Wear protective clothing. Wear gloves, lab coat, or smock. Wear mask when weighing out powders.
   b. Mechanical pipetting aids used for all pipetting.
   c. Immediate clean-up of all spills.
   d. Washing of hands after completion.
2. A control must be run to ensure reagents are working.
3. Hexazotized reagents are unstable and must be used immediately.
4. Fixation keeps the enzyme from washing out of the cell during staining and improves the morphological preservation of the cells.
5. Smears should be fixed after drying, even if staining is to be performed at a latter date.
6. Since this stain depends on an enzymatic reaction, we must take care to preserve the enzyme activity by avoiding light, heat, and aging. Store fixed smears in freezer.
7. For sodium fluoride inhibition studies add NaF 1.5 mg/ml of incubation mixture.

## Combined Esterase

**Purpose.** The purpose of combined esterase is to aid in differentiation of granulocytes, lymphocytes, and monocytes. It is especially valuable when a limited number of coverslips are available.

**Principle.** The esterase enzymes within the cell hydrolyze the substrates alpha-naphthol butyrate and naphthol AS-D chloroacetate. The hydrolyzed substrate then couples with the dye, fast blue BB or paraosaniline, and the colored complex formed precipitates out at the site of enzymatic activity.

**Specimen.** This may be a fresh smear or an imprint. For smears, fresh capillary blood is best; however, anticoagulated blood is acceptable.

**Reagents**

1. Esterase fixative pH 6.6. Store 4°C. Good for 3 months.
   a. In 120 ml of deionized water dissolve:
      $Na_2HPO_4$ (F.W. 141.96)    0.08 g
      $KH_2PO_4$ (F.W. 136.09)    0.40 g
   b. Formaldehyde 37 percent    100 ml
   c. Acetone    180 ml
   d. Adjust pH to 6.6 if necessary with appropriate buffer salt.
2. Phosphate buffer M/15, pH 7.4. Store at 4°C. Good for 90 days. Discard if any mold is observed.
   a. $NaH_2PO_4$ $H_2O$ (F.W. 137.99)    1.67 g
   b. $Na_2HPO_4$ (F.W. 141.96)    7.74 g
   c. Deionized water    1000 ml
   d. Adjust pH to 7.4 if necessary with appropriate buffer salt solution.
3. Naphthol AS-D chloroacetate. Store at −0°C.
4. Substrate solution. Store at 4°C in glass stoppered bottle. Good for 30 days.
   a. Naphthol AS-D chloroacetate    20 mg
   b. N,N-dimethylformamide (F.W. 73.1) 10 ml
5. Fast blue BB salt. Store at −0°C.
6. Mayer's hematoxylin.
7. Blueing agent:
   a. $NaHCO_3$    1 g
   b. Deionized water    100 ml
8. See nonspecific esterase procedure for reagents needed for step one of this combined esterase procedure.

**Procedure**

1. Do a nonspecific esterase, but do not counterstain.
2. Incubate slides in the following filtered mixture for 20 minutes:
   Buffer    38 ml
   Substrate solution    2 ml
   Fast blue BB    20 mg
3. Wash well with deionized water.
4. Counterstain with hematoxylin for 2 minutes.
5. Wash well with deionized water.
6. Place slides in blueing reagent for 30 seconds.
7. Wash, air dry, and mount with Permount.

**Interpretation.** Monocytes, histiocytes, macrophages, and mesothelial cells stain diffusely brick-red. T cells usually stain with a punctate red granule. Mast cells, early promyelocytes, and later granulocytes stain a granular blue.

## Acid Phosphatase Stain/TRAP (for Smears, Imprints, and Frozen Sections)

**Purpose.** This procedure is useful for making a diagnosis of leukemic reticuloendotheliosis (hairy cell leukemia). It may also be of use in T-cell identification and in multiple myeloma.

**Principle.** The acid phosphatase within the cell hydrolyzes the substrate naphthol AS-BI phosphoric acid. The hydrolyzed substrate then couples with the dye (hexazotized pararosaniline), and because the colored complex is insoluble, it precipitates out at the site of enzymatic activity. Tartaric acid, when added to the incubation mixture, will not inhibit the enzyme fraction found in hairy cell leukemia (isoenzyme 5).

**Specimen.** Smears, imprints, or frozen sections may be used. Fresh capillary smears are best; however, smears made from EDTA or heparinized blood are also adequate.

**Reagents**

1. Acid phosphatase fixative, pH 5.4; store at 4° to 10°C; good for 90 days. Discard if RBC morphology is poor.
   a. Dissolve 0.63 g citrate acid (F.W. 210.14) in 30 ml of deionized water.
   b. Add 10 ml of methanol and 60 ml of acetone.
   c. Mix and adjust the pH to 5.4 with concentrated NaOH solution.
2. 0.1N acetate buffer, pH 5.2; store at 4°C; good for 90 days.
   a. 600 ml distilled water.
   b. 13.6 g sodium acetate (F.W. 136.1)
   c. Adjust the pH to 5.2 with 1.0M acetic acid. Bring the volume to 1000 ml with distilled water.
3. "Tartrate" sodium acetate buffer, pH 5.2; store at 4° to 10°C; good for 3 months.
   a. Dissolve 3.75 g of L-(+)-tartaric acid in 490 ml of 0.1N acetate buffer.
   b. Adjust the pH to 5.2 with concentrated NaOH.
   c. Bring the volume to 500 ml with distilled water.
4. 0.1M acetic acid
   a. 200 ml distilled water
   b. 1.25 ml glacial acetic acid (F.W. 60.05, 16N).
5. L-(+)-tartric acid.
6. Substrate solution: Store in glass stoppered bottle at 4° to 10°C; good for 30 days. Discard if it turns pink.
   a. Dissolve 100 mg naphthol AS-BI phosphoric acid in 10.0 ml N,N-dimethylformamide.
   b. When used infrequently, make up fresh by adding 10 mg naphthol AS-BI phosphoric acid in 1.0 ml N,N-dimethylformamide.

7. 4 percent sodium nitrate solution: Prepare daily.
   a. Dissolve 1.0 g $NaNO_2$ (F.W. 69.0) in distilled water to a volume of 25 ml.
8. 4 percent pararosaniline solution (possible carcinogen; see Comments under Nonspecific Esterase). Store in brown bottle at 4° to 10°C; good for 90 days.
   a. Dissolve 1.0 g pararosaniline HCl (F.W. 323.8) in 20 ml distilled water plus 5 ml concentrated HCl. Solution may be gently heated to dissolve pararosaniline. Filter.
9. Mayer's hematoxylin.
10. Acid alcohol solution
    a. Concentrated HCl                    0.05 ml
    b. 100 percent ethanol                 3.5 ml
    c. Deionized water                    996.5 ml
11. Blueing reagent
    a. $NaHCO_3$                              1 g
    b. Deionized water                     100 ml

**Procedure**

1. Fix smears, imprints, or frozen section for 30 seconds with cold fixative.
2. Wash three times with deionized water. Air dry.
3. Incubate smears or imprints at 37°C in the appropriate filtered mixture:
   a. Acid phosphatase stain
      Acetate buffer                      50 ml
      Stock substrate solution            2 ml
   In a separate container add 0.2 ml of 4 percent sodium nitrate solution to 0.2 ml of 4 percent pararosaniline solution. Wait 1 minute, and then add to buffer substrate solution.
   b. Acid phosphatase with tartrate stain (TRAP)
      Acetate-tartrate buffer             50 ml
      Stock substrate solution            2 ml
   In a separate container add 0.2 ml of 4 percent sodium nitrate solution to 0.2 ml of 4 percent pararosaniline solution. Wait 1 minute, and then add to buffer substrate solution.
4. Incubate for 60 minutes at 37°C.
5. Wash three times in tap water.
6. Counterstain with hematoxylin for 2 minutes.
7. Rinse well with deionized water.
8. Place in blueing solution for 30 seconds.
9. Wash, dry, and mount with Permount. Frozen tissue sections must be dehydrated and cleared in xylene before mounting with Permount.

**Comments**

1. A control must be run to ensure reagents are working.
2. Hexazotized reagents are unstable and must be used immediately.
3. Fixation keeps the enzyme from washing out of the cell during staining and improves the morphologic preservation of the cells.

4. Because these stains depend on enzymatic reactions, we must take care to preserve the enzyme activity by avoiding light, heat, and aging.
5. Smears can be kept at room temperature for at least 2 weeks without apparent loss of enzymatic activity.
6. After a couple of weeks, reaction products may precipitate out (salting out phenomenon). This false-positive result should not be confused with the original stain.
7. Controls should be fixed, air dried, and stored at −50°C.
8. Increasing the temperature beyond 37°C causes inactivation of the enzyme and decomposition of the azo dye, resulting in nonspecific precipitation.
9. Mayer's hematoxylin as a counterstain gives a light gray tint to the cytoplasm of the leukocytes; which at times may mask some weak enzymatic activity. Methyl green gives poor nuclear detail, but it does not mask weak enzymatic activity in the cytoplasm.

**Interpretation.** Acid phosphatase activity is shown by an orange-red precipitate with pararosaniline. The test result is considered positive when two or more cells are found with 4+ activity. Seven acid phosphatase isoenzymes have been identified in various blood cells. The fraction found in leukemic reticuloendotheliosis is resistant to the addition of L-(+)-tartaric acid (isoenzyme 5). In addition, when acid phosphatase is present in a localized (dot-like) fashion, i.e., in the Golgi zone, there is evidence that this may be a marker for T lymphocytes. Increased activity is seen in myeloma cells.

## Periodic Acid–Schiff Reaction (PAS Stain)

**Purpose.** Used in identifying M-6 leukemias, negative in Burkitt's lymphoma.

**Principle.** PAS stains glycogen. Periodic acid oxidizes glycols to aldehydes. The aldehydes react with Schiff's reagent.

**Specimen.** Smears or imprints may be used. Anticoagulants do not inhibit activity. Paraffin tissue sections may also be used but sections must first be hydrated.

**Reagents**
1. Fixative: Store at room temperature. Expires in 1 year.
   a. 37 percent reagent grade formalin  50 ml
   b. Absolute ethanol  450 ml
2. 1 percent periodic acid: Store at room temperature. Expires in 3 months.
   a. Periodic acid  5 g
   b. Deionized water  500 ml

3. Schiff's reagent: Store at 4°C. Expires in 3 months.
   a. Basic fuschin CI 42500  2.5 g
   b. Deionized water  500 ml
   c. Sodium metabisulfite  5 g
   d. 1N HCl  50 ml
   Stir ingredients a through d for 2 hours, or until solution turns yellow (light amber). Add 4.0 g of activated charcoal. Filter until all charcoal is removed from solution. Do not use solution if it turns pink.
4. 0.5 percent sodium metabisulfite $(Na_2S_2O_5)$: Store at room temperature. Expires in 3 months.
   a. Sodium metabisulfite  2.5 g
   b. Deionized water  500 ml
5. Hematoxylin (see hematoxylin counterstain).
6. Acid alcohol solution: Store at room temperature. Expires in 6 months.
   a. 1 percent HCl in 70 percent ethanol 2.5 ml
   b. Deionized water  497.5 ml
7. 1 percent sodium bicarbonate solution. Store at room temperature. Expires in 6 months.
   a. Sodium bicarbonate  5 g
   b. Deionized water  500 ml

**Procedure**
1. Fix smears for 15 minutes. Paraffin tissue sections need to be hydrated but have already been fixed.
2. Rinse gently in deionized water. Take extra care to rinse gently to avoid causing the smear partially to lift off the slide.
3. Place in periodic acid for 10 minutes.
4. Rinse in deionized water and dry.
5. Place dried smears in Schiff's reagent for 30 minutes.
6. Place in three 10-minute changes of metabisulfite solution.
7. Wash in deionized water for 10 minutes.
8. Counter stain with hematoxylin for 2 minutes.
9. Rinse in deionized water.
10. Place in sodium bicarbonate (blueing) solution for 30 seconds.
11. Rinse in deionized water, dry (tissue needs to be dehydrated), and mount with Permount.

**Interpretation.** PAS-positive material appears bright-red. If PMNs are present, they serve as a good "auto" positive control. The staining pattern may be granular, diffuse, or block. Lymphocytes, granulocytes, monocytes, and megakaryocytes may be positive. Normal erythroid precursors are negative. In M-6, the normoblasts are usually positive, but normoblasts may also be positive in sideroblastic anemia, iron deficiency, thalassemia, and severe hemolytic anemias. Burkitt's lymphoma cells are PAS negative. Ewings sarcoma cells are PAS positive. Lymphocytic leukemia cells may or may not stain with a block pattern. Since PAS positivity may occur in ALL and AML, the PAS stain should not be used to distinguish AML from ALL.

### Terminal Deoxynucleotidyl Transferase (TdT) Test

**Purpose.** TdT is an enzyme marker for primitive lymphocytic cells.

**Principle.** TdT is a DNA polymerase present in lymphocytic cells. Rabbit antibody to TdT is incubated with cold methanol fixed cells. Then FITC-labeled goat antirabbit antibody is incubated with the cells. If TdT is present in the nucleus of the cells, the positive cells will fluoresce.

**Specimen.** A nonheparinized bone marrow aspirate or one in which the cells have been separated and washed three times with RPMI and 2 percent fetal calf serum may be used. Peripheral blood may also be used; however, it requires special specimen collection. Store the slides at 4°C in the dark. Slides should be stained within a few days of preparation.

#### Reagents

1. Antiserum:
   Kit #9311 SB
   Bethesda Research Laboratories
   411 North Stonestreet Avenue
   Rockville, MD 20850
   
   *or*

2. P-L Biochemicals, Inc.
   Subsidiary of Pharmacia, Inc.
   800 Centennial Avenue
   Piscataway, NJ 08854
   a. Rabbit anticalf TdT, affinity purified IgG.
   b. Goat antirabbit IgG, FITC conjugated
   c. Antisera dilutions (for P-L Biochemicals antisera)
      (1) Every time a new batch of antisera is received, the plateau end point of antibody activity should be determined. This is the highest dilution at which optimum staining occurs. If the antibody concentration is the same as the previous batch, it is usually acceptable to run one higher and one lower dilution, in addition to the regular one.
      (2) Dilute antisera at optimum dilution using diluting media. An 8- to 10-fold dilution is recommended for the rabbit anticalf TdT, and a 70- to 100-fold dilution for the goat antirabbit.
      (3) Store anti-TdT at 4°C. Aliquot antirabbit antisera (20 $\lambda$) and store at −20°C.

3. Diluting media: RPMI with 2 percent fetal calf serum and 0.1 percent sodium azide.

4. Phosphate buffered solution, pH 7.4

   | | |
   |---|---|
   | $NaH_2PO_4 \cdot H_2O$ | 0.4 g |
   | $Na_2HPO_4$ | 1.6 g |
   | NaCl | 8.0 g |
   | Deionized water | 1000 ml |

5. Mounting media (buffered glycerol)

   | | |
   |---|---|
   | Glycerol | 90 ml |
   | 0.05M Trizma 9.0 | 10 ml |

6. Control
   a. Make cytopreps from a known ALL with a positive TdT.
   b. Air dry cytopreps.
   c. Wrap with plastic wrap.
   d. Freeze and store at −70°C.
   e. Bring to room temperature before unwrapping.
   f. Follow test procedure and treat like unknown sample.

#### Procedure

1. Circle an area rich in nucleated cells on the slide with a diamond scribe. Fix slides in methanol at 4°C for 30 minutes.
2. Rinse well in PBS to remove all fixative. Do not air dry.
3. Hydrate the fixed slides in PBS for 5 minutes at room temperature.
4. Carefully wipe off all the sample on the slide outside the circle. Apply 10 $\mu$l of primary antibody (rabbit, anticalf TdT) onto this area and distribute it over the circle. Incubate for 30 minutes at room temperature in a humid chamber. *It is very important that the slide does not dry out!*
5. Wash slides with three changes of PBS over a period of 15 minutes to remove excess antibody. Wipe off all the excess PBS around the circle, being especially careful not to let the sample dry out.
6. Apply 15 $\mu$l of secondary antibody (FITC F(ab')$_2$ goat, antirabbit IgG) to the circled area of the slide and incubate for 30 minutes at room temperature in a humid chamber.
7. Repeat wash as in step 5.
8. Apply a small drop of mounting media and cover with a coverslip.
9. Examine the nuclei for fluorescence at 495 nm excitation with a Barrier filter. Record the intensity of fluorescence, 0 to 4+, and the percentage of cells that are positive. The preparation can be stored in the dark in the refrigerator for several days.

**Interpretation.** The majority of patients with T and null ALL and lymphoma will have positive TdT activity. In addition, patients with pre-B ALL, 50 percent of patients with acute undifferentiated leukemia, and 30 percent of patients in CML blast crisis will also have TdT activity. Approximately 5 percent of patients with AML will have TdT activity. In summary, TdT is a marker for primitive lymphoid cells.

#### Comments

1. Peripheral blood, bone marrow aspirate smears, or touch preps can be examined for TdT activity. The slides should be stored no

## CYTOCHEMICAL REACTIONS OF NORMAL CELLS

| | Granulocytes | Monocytes | Lymphocytes | Platelets or Megakaryocytes | Erythroid Cells |
|---|---|---|---|---|---|
| Px | 4+ | 2+ | − | − | − |
| SBB | 4+ | 2+ | − | − | − |
| PAS | 4+* | 2+* | −/+ | 2+ | − |
| "Specific" esterase (NCA) | 4+ | − | − | − | − |
| "Nonspecific" esterase (αNA or αNB) | (+/−) | 4+ | −/+("dot") | +/− | − |
| αNA with NaF | (+/−) | − | −/+("dot") | | − |

## CYTOCHEMICAL REACTIONS OF LEUKEMIC BLASTS AND IMMATURE CELLS

| | ALL | AML | AMML | AMoL | EL |
|---|---|---|---|---|---|
| Px | − | + | + | + | − |
| SBB | − | + | + | + | − |
| PAS | −/+* | +* | +* | +* | + |
| "Specific" esterase (NCA) | − | + | + | − | − |
| αNA or αNB | −/+("dot") | (+/−) | + | + | − |
| αNA or αNB with NaFl | −/+("dot") | (+/−) | +/− | − | − |

Px: peroxidase; SBB: Sudan black B; PAS: periodic acid–Schiff; NCA: naphthol AS-D chloroacetate; NA: α naphthol acetate; NB: α naphthol butyrate; NaF: sodium fluoride; ALL: acute lymphoblastic leukemia; AML: acute myelogenous leukemia; AMML: acute myelomonocytic leukemia; AMoL: acute monocytic leukemia; EL: erythroleukemia.
*Diffuse background staining of cytoplasm and fine PAS granulation.
"dot" = staining reaction confined to small circular area of cytoplasm.
Courtesy of Mary Jo Fackler, B.Sc., M.T.(ASCP), S.H.

longer than 7 days at room temperature. It is best to stain them as soon as possible.

2. A control slide should be run periodically and with each new lot number of reagents.

## Cytochemical Stains

See tables above.

## Immunologic Surface Markers

### E Rosettes for Evaluation of T Cells

**Purpose.** E rosettes are to identify T cells that have receptors for sheep red blood cells (SRBCs).

**Principle.** Washed lymphocytes are incubated with washed sheep red blood cells. The percentage and population of cells forming rosettes is determined.

**Specimen.** This includes blood, bone marrow aspirates, or fluids that have been anticoagulated with heparin or EDTA. The specimen should be less than 48 hours old.

**Reagents**
1. Culture media (RPMI 1640) is purchased from Microbiological Associates, Walkersville, MD 21793.
2. Heat-inactivated fetal calf serum (Microbiological Associates). Thaw, dispense into 1 ml aliquots, store −20°C.
3. Sheep red blood cells (must be less than 2 weeks old). Obtain from R. Kent Richards, 135 North 100 West, Pleasant Grove, UT 84062.
4. Trypan blue solution stock solutions.
   a. Trypan blue 0.2 percent
      1.0 g trypan blue
      500 ml deionized water
   b. NaCl 4.25 percent
      21.25 g NaCl
      500 ml deionized water
   c. Working solution: Make fresh.
      Add 100 $\mu$l 4.25 percent NaCl to 400 $\mu$l 0.2 percent trypan.

**Procedure**
1. Wash SRBC with RPMI 1640 three times.
2. Add 50 $\mu$l of SRBC pellet to 5 ml of RPMI. Mix suspension.
3. Add an equal volume of SRBC suspension to an equal volume of a 4000 cell/mm³ lymphocyte suspension. (When there is ample lymphocyte suspension, use 0.5 ml of SRBC and 0.5 ml of lymphocyte suspension.)
4. Incubate at 37°C for 15 minutes.
5. Centrifuge for 10 minutes at 1000 rpm.
6. Remove half of the supernatant, replace with an equal amount of heat inactivated fetal calf serum. Do not disturb the cell button.
7. Incubate for 2 hours or overnight in refrigerator at 4°C.
8. Gently resuspend the button with a Pasteur pipette. Stop resuspension while there are still small visible clumps of cells present.
9. Add 100 $\mu$l of cell suspension to 100 $\mu$l of fresh

trypan solution. Gently make a wet prep and record the percentage of viable cells that have three or more SRBCs attached.

10. Take 2 drops of the resuspended button (not trypan) and make a cytocentrifuge prep for a Wright's stain. Make extra preps if special stains are needed.

**Comments**

1. The Wright-stained cytocentrifuge prep is valuable in determining what population of cells is rosetting.
2. On a cytocentrifuge prep, true rosettes will be surrounded by SRBCs that have a "stretched" appearance.
3. Healthy individuals should be run as controls. They should have 60 to 80 percent T cells.
4. Viable cells do not stain with trypan. Dead cells cannot exclude trypan and stain blue.

### Cytoplasmic Immunoglobulin (CIg) (Immunofluorescent Method)

**Purpose.** The purpose of this procedure is to detect cytoplasmic immunoglobulin. Some lymphocytes lack surface immunoglobulins and sheep red blood cell receptors but do contain cytoplasmic immunoglobulins. These cells are believed to be pre-B cells. Plasma cells also contain cytoplasmic immunoglobulin.

**Principle.** Cells are fixed to expose cytoplasmic immunoglobulins. Fluorescein conjugated F(ab')$_2$ fragment antihuman IgM (or other immunoglobulin chain) is incubated with fixed cells, and examined for the presence of cytoplasmic fluorescence.

**Specimen.** Use a fresh smear, tissue imprint, or cytocentrifuge preparations of cells. A cytocentrifuge prep made from a washed cell suspension is best, giving less background staining. Smears must be fresh. As the specimen ages, background fluorescence becomes a problem.

**Reagents**

1. Fluorescein conjugated antisera, produced in goat, F(ab')$_2$ fragment: Antihuman IgM, IgG, IgA, IgD, IgE, kappa, lambda (purchased from Kallestad).
   a. Determine optimal dilution with each new lot (usually between 1:5 and 1:20).
   b. Make appropriate dilution using RPMI 1640, with 0.1 percent sodium azide, and 2 percent fetal calf serum.
   c. Aliquot (150 to 200 $\mu$l) and store at $-20°C$.
2. RPMI 1640 Medium, purchased from Microbiological Associates Bioproducts.
3. Heat inactivated fetal calf serum (FCS), purchased from Sterile Systems, Inc., 750 W. 2nd N., Logan, UT 84321.
4. RPMI with 2 percent FCS and 0.1 percent azide

| | |
|---|---|
| RPMI 1640 | 500 ml |
| FCS | 10 ml |
| Sodium azide | 500 mg |

5. Fixative: Make fresh

| | |
|---|---|
| a. Absolute ethanol | 47.5 ml |
| b. Acetic acid | 2.5 ml |

6. PBS, 0.14M, pH 7.4.

| | |
|---|---|
| a. NaH$_2$PO$_4$ H$_2$O (F.W. 137.99) | 4 g |
| b. Na$_2$HPO$_4$ (F.W. 141.96) | 16 g |
| c. NaCl | 80 g |
| d. Deionized water | 10 l |

7. Glycerol-Gelvatol mounting media; good for 5 months at 4°C.
   a. Dissolve 1.5 g Trizma 9.0 in 240 ml deionized water.
   b. Add 60 g of Gelvatol and stir overnight to dissolve.
   c. Add 120 ml glycerol and stir overnight.
   d. Spin at 10,000 Gs for 30 minutes, and store in syringes.

**Procedure**

1. With a diamond marker, etch a circle around the cells to be stained. Wipe off extra cells with a Kimwipe.
2. Fix smear for 10 minutes at 4°C.
3. Rinse smear in PBS.
4. Do not allow smear to air dry.
5. Wash smear for 10 minutes with PBS.
6. Distribute 100 $\mu$l of antiserum onto the inside of circle. Incubate for 30 minutes at room temperature in a humid chamber.
7. Wash smear for 15 minutes with PBS.
8. Apply a small drop of mounting media and coverslip smear.
9. Using the 63 oil objective, and epifluorescence with FITC filter, examine the cytoplasm of the cells for fluorescence. Do not mistake the autofluorescence of eosinophilic granules for cytoplasmic fluorescence.
10. Report the degree and pattern of fluorescence, and the percentage of cells positive.

**Comments.** Smears should be fresh. As the smear ages, background fluorescence becomes a problem. Immediately after fixation, it is important to rinse smears before they are allowed to dry.

### Surface Immunoglobulins

**Purpose.** This procedure is to identify B cells that have surface-bound immunoglobulins.

**Principle.** Monospecific fluorescein-conjugated F(ab')$_2$ antisera are incubated at 4°C to detect surface-bound immunoglobulins.

**Specimen.** Blood, bone marrow aspirates, or fluids that have been anticoagulated with heparin or EDTA. The specimen should be less than 48 hours old.

**Reagents**

1. The following antiserum may be purchased from:
   Kallestad
   1000 Hazeltine Drive
   Chaska, MN 55318

a. Anti-Human IgG, fluorescein-conjugated antisera, produced in goat F(ab')$_2$ fragment.

b. Anti-Human IgA, fluorescein-conjugated antisera, produced in goat F(ab')$_2$ fragment.

c. Anti-Human IgM, fluorescein-conjugated antisera, produced in goat F(ab')$_2$ fragment.

d. Anti-Human IgD, fluorescein-conjugated antisera, produced in goat F(ab')$_2$ fragment.

e. Anti-Human Albumin, fluorescein-conjugated antisera, produced in goat.

f. Anti-Human Kappa (k) light chain, fluorescein-conjugated antisera, produced in goat F(ab')$_2$ fragment.

g. Anti-Human Lambda light chain, fluorescein-conjugated antisera, produced in rabbit (may substitute goat). F(ab')$_2$ fragment.

h. Fluorescein-conjugated antiserum to total human gamma globulins. Produced in goat F(ab')$_2$ fragment.

i. Normal rabbit serum, 2.5 ml vial.

2. Ficoll-Hypaque, purchased from Pharmacia, Piscataway, NJ 08854.

3. RPMI 1640, purchased from Microbiological Associates, Walkersville, MD 21793. Store at 4°C.

4. Fetal calf serum, heat-inactivated. Keep at 20°C for long-term storage.

5. Diluting media: RPMI with 2 percent FCS, 0.1 percent azide, store at 4°C.

| | |
|---|---|
| RPMI 1640 | 500 ml |
| Fetal calf serum (heat-inactivated) | 10 ml |
| Sodium azide | 500 mg |

6. Mounting media (buffered glycerol); store at 4°C.

| | |
|---|---|
| Glycerol | 90 ml |
| Trizma 9.0, 0.05 M | 10 ml |

7. RPMI with 0.5 percent sodium azide; store at 4°C.

| | |
|---|---|
| RPMI | 500 ml |
| Sodium azide | 250 mg |

**Procedure**

1. Separate cells by using Ficoll-Hypaque density gradient procedure.

2. Incubate the cell suspension in RPMI at 37°C on rocket for 45 minutes to remove cytophilic antibodies.

3. Spin down cell suspension at 1000 rpm for 10 minutes and pour off supernatant. Adjust cell count to $4.0 \times 10^6$/ml with 37°C RPMI.

4. Place 500 μl of the cell suspension in microfuge tubes. Centrifuge for 5 seconds. Remove the supernatant. (The pellicles will contain approximately $2.0 \times 10^6$ cells.) Centrifuge antiserum for 4 minutes before using.

5. Add 100 μl of supernatant of a 1:10 dilution of fluorescein-conjugated antiserum to the cell button and gently resuspend the cells. (Antiserum is diluted with RPMI and aliquots of 200 μl are stored frozen at −20°C.)

6. Cap the tubes and incubate at 4°C for 45 minutes. (For patients known to have CLL, incubate for 60 minutes.)

7. Make cytocentrifuge preparation of the cell suspension for Wright's and special stains.

8. Following incubation, wash the cells three times with cold RPMI containing 0.05 percent sodium azide (25 mg azide/50 ml RPMI).

9. After the last wash, remove all of the supernatant and add 1 drop of buffered glycerol.

10. Resuspend the cells and make a wet mount.

11. Examine the preparation under a fluorescent microscope. (Xenon epifluorescence is recommended.) If wet prep is not to be looked at immediately, store slides on slide tray in refrigerator.

**Comments**

1. Avoid excessive exposure of antiserum to light.

2. For best results, the slides should be read immediately.

3. The Wright's stain cyto prep should be examined and a differential done.

4. By using F(ab')$_2$ fragment antiserum, the nonspecific binding of lymphocytes and monocytes for the Fc portion of the antibody can be eliminated.

5. Immunoglobulin bearing lymphocytes (B cells) have a stippled or "dusty" stained pattern (apple-green fluorescence) around the circumference of the cell. Some cells, especially lymphoma cells, may show prominent capped staining.

### Indirect Immunofluorescence Using Monoclonal Antibodies (for Evaluation of Lymphocyte Subsets)

**Purpose.** This procedure is used to recognize lymphocyte cell types by identifying specific antigens on the surface of the cells.

**Principle.** Cells are separated from blood or tissue and incubated with monoclonal antibodies produced by mouse hybridoma cell lines. Indirect immunofluorescence and phase microscopy are used to identify the cell types.

**Specimen.** Bone marrow aspirate, or peripheral blood with adequate numbers of the cells in question may be used. A cell suspension is prepared using the Ficoll-Hypaque method of cell separation to obtain a mononuclear cell population.

**Reagents**

1. Antisera

a. HTA antiserum, Boehringer Mannheim, 7941 Castleway Drive, Indianapolis, IN 46250

b. OKT antisera, Ortho Diagnostics Systems, Inc., Customer Service Department, Route 202, Raritan, NJ 08869

c. Calla antiserum (J-5), Jerome Ritz, M.D.,

Dept. of Medicine, Sidney Farber Cancer Institute, 44 Binney Street, Boston, MA 02115
   d. Coulter clone antisera, Coulter Immunology, 440 West 20th Street, Hialeah, FL 33010
   e. Becton Dickinson Antisera, B.D. Monoclonal Center, Inc., 2375 Garcia Avenue, Mountain View, CA 94043
   f. Secondary antibody, FITC-conjugated antimouse IgG
2. RPMI 1640, purchased from Microbiological Associates, Walkersville, MD 21793
3. Fetal calf serum (FCS), heat-inactivated, purchased from Sterile Systems, Inc., 750 W. 2nd No., Logan, UT
4. Sodium azide
5. Diluting media: RPMI with 2 percent FCS and 0.1 percent sodium azide. After optimal dilutions are determined, the remaining concentrated antisera may be diluted, aliquoted, and stored at $-20°C$. For dilution of all antisera, the following diluting media should be used:

| | |
|---|---|
| RPMI | 500 ml |
| FCS, heat-inactivated | 10 ml |
| Sodium azide | 500 mg |

6. Antisera dilutions
   a. Every time a new batch of antisera is received, the plateau end point of antibody activity should be determined. This is the highest dilution at which optimum staining occurs. If the antibody concentration is the same as the previous batch, it is usually acceptable to run one higher and one lower dilution, in addition to the regular one.
   b. Protocol for freezing reconstituted Coulter clone monoclonal antibody
      (1) Reconstitute the antibody with 500 $\mu l$ of distilled water.
      (2) Dilute the reconstituted antibody solution prior to freezing as follows:

| Vial Test Size | Volume of Reconstituted Antibody for Each Test | Volume of 2% FCS with 0.1% Azide to be Added |
|---|---|---|
| 10 | 50 $\mu l$ | 200 $\mu l$ |
| 25 | 20 $\mu l$ | 200 $\mu l$ |
| 50 | 10 $\mu l$ | 200 $\mu l$ |
| 100 | 5 $\mu l$ | 200 $\mu l$ |

      (3) Alliquot 110 to 120 $\mu l$ of antibody solution into micro eppendorf centrifuge tubes. Store at $-20°C$.
      (4) To use this material, allow the solution to return to room temperature. Centrifuge for 4 minutes at 4000 rpm.

**Procedure**
1. Follow the cell separation procedure and adjust cell concentration to $4 \times 10^6$ cells/ml.
2. Place 0.5 ml of the cell suspension in microfuge tubes. Centrifuge for 15 seconds and remove supernatant.
3. Add 0.100 ml of the thawed monoclonal aliquot. Resuspend cells and incubate at 4°C for 30 minutes. (*Note:* If antiserum is stored at $-20°C$, it should be centrifuged for 4 minutes after thawing.)
4. Wash cells once with 4°C RPMI.
5. Add 0.100 ml of the secondary antibody to each monoclonal that was set up. Resuspend cells and incubate at 4°C for 30 minutes.
6. Wash cells three times with 4°C RPMI.
7. After last wash, remove all of the supernatant and add 1 drop of buffered glycerol to cell button.
8. Resuspend the cells and make a wet mount.
9. Examine the preparation with a fluorescent microscope (blue light excitation). If the wet prep is not to be examined immediately, store the slides in the refrigerator.

**Interpretation.** Positive cells stain green with a granular appearance on the surface of the cell. Dead cells fluoresce diffusely and should not be included in the count. It is important to use phase microscopy in addition to fluorescent microscopy to determine what population of cells is positive. This is especially important when one is working with cell suspensions that have more than one cell type (i.e., cell suspensions of CLL patients with low white cell counts generally have a higher percentage of normal lymphocytes than do CLL patients with high white cell counts). Low counts generally make it more difficult to assess the surface marker phenotype of the malignant cells. Correlate all findings. It is unusual for cells to be E-rosette positive and HTA negative. Cells positive for SIg should be HTA negative, except for CLL.

**Comments**
1. Avoid excessive exposure of antiserum to light.
2. For best results, the slides should be read immediately.

## LASER-BASED FLOW CYTOMETRY

Flow cytometry is an automated method used to measure cells or particles as they flow single file through a sensing area. Sensing can be accomplished electronically, as done by the Coulter principle, or optically. The term "flow cytometry" (FCM) is commonly used to denote the optical type. Optical sensing is done with an intense light source, usually a laser or mercury-arc lamp. These instruments measure light scatter and fluorescent signals generated as cells pass through a light beam. This review will focus on the main components of laser-based FCM and its clinical applications.

## Flow Cytometry Components

The four main components of FCM (Fig. 31–14) include the fluidics (or cell transportation system), a laser for cell illumination, photodetectors for signal detection, and a computer-based management system. The fluidics are regulated by pressurized gas, usually nitrogen. Cells suspended in fluid are transported to a flow tip where the sample is surrounded by a liquid sheath. The sheath and sample stream both exit the flow chamber through a small orifice (usually 75 microns). This laminar flow design confines cells to the center of the sheath and can be adjusted to obtain single-file alignment of cells.

As a cell enters the laser beam, light is scattered through 360 degrees. Forward-angle light scatter (FALS, 2 to 10 degrees) provides information relevant to the cell size. Light scattered at 90 degrees (90LS) reflects cellular structure or granularity. In addition to light scatter, fluorescent signals can also be measured when cells are tagged with appropriate dyes. Fluorescence occurs when a chemical absorbs light, causing its electrons to be excited briefly to a higher, less-stable energy state. As the electrons return to their resting state, light at a longer wavelength (lower energy) than the initial exciting light is emitted. Laser-based FCM is well adapted for measurement of fluorescence, because it provides a stable source of coherent monochromatic light. Proper alignment of this intense light beam with the sample stream is required for optimal signal production. Many flow systems use argon gas, which generates a strong laser line at 488 nm. Fluorescein isothiocyanate (FITC), phycoerythrin (PE), and propidium iodide (PI) are popular dyes for these systems, because they are excited at 488 nm.

Detection and conversion of light signals into electrical signals are accomplished by a series of photodetectors and photomultiplier tubes (PMTs).

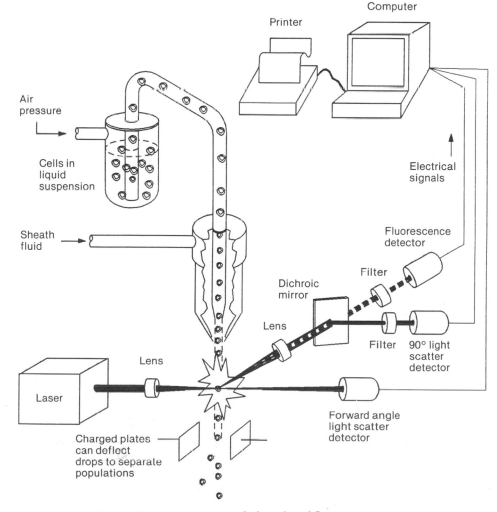

**Figure 31–14.** Components of a laser-based flow cytometer.

The PMTs also serve to amplify the light signals. An assembly of filters and mirrors directs the light to various detectors. A clinical FCM system typically has a photodetector for FALS, a PMT for 90LS, and one or two PMTs for fluorescence detection. These photodetectors can be adjusted to manipulate the intensity of single output. The filter assembly used in conjunction with the photodetection system can also be adjusted for sensitivity to different fluorescent emissions.

The heart of the FCM system is the computer, which controls the instrument's operation, data collection, storage, and analysis. The computer capabilities vary among different instruments, and computer software is in a constant state of development. The beauty of FCM lies in the user's ability, through computer control, to create different test systems or profiles for the analysis of multiple sample types. Different combinations of parameters can be measured as needed. For example, simultaneous evaluation of FALS and 90LS allows for separation of peripheral blood leukocytes on the basis of size and granularity. Lymphocytes, monocytes, and granulocytes fall into three separate populations by these criteria (Fig. 31–15). Further manipulation can be done by placing "electronic gates" around the population of interest. In this way, fluorescence of just lymphocytes, or of another population, can be measured. Other combinations of parameters and gating can be used, depending on the needs of the investigator.

Some FCM systems have the additional option of cell sorting. Cells flow through the laser beam, where they produce light scatter and fluorescent signals, and then continue with their movement downstream. Vibration of the sample stream causes droplets to form that contain single cells. Those droplets that have cells meeting the "sorting criteria" are electronically charged and deflected in an electromagnetic field. In this way, purified cell populations can be collected for further studies.

## Clinical Applications

Laser-based FCM is relatively new to the clinical laboratory. Its greatest contribution has been in the detection of lymphocyte cell surface markers and DNA analysis. Other clinical uses of flow technology include assessment of phagocytosis, reticulocyte counts, HLA crossmatching, detection of platelet autoantibodies, evaluation of spermatogenesis, cell kinetic studies, and rare event analysis such as detection of small numbers of lymphoma cells in the peripheral blood. This is only a partial list and one that is still growing.

The basis of cell surface marker studies is the existence of specific proteins on the surface of cells that distinguish one cell line from another. Evaluation of lymphocyte subsets most clearly exemplifies this. Helper and suppressor lymphocytes have glycoproteins on their surface that are unique to each. Using monoclonal antibodies against these proteins coupled with fluorescent dyes, it is possible to distinguish and quantitate these subsets. Lymphocyte subset evaluation is useful for investigating a number of immunologic conditions and disorders, including leukemias and lymphomas, acquired immune deficiency syndrome (AIDS) and other immunodeficiencies, transplant rejection, and autoimmune diseases.

Cells for evaluation of surface markers can be obtained from whole blood, Ficoll-Hypaque separation, bone marrow aspirates, body fluids, or from solid tissue such as lymph nodes that are disrupted to release cells into suspension. Samples can be evaluated rapidly (up to 10,000 cells per second) and quantitatively, eliminating some of the human subjectivity encountered with the microscope.

Flow cytometric DNA analysis is accomplished by exposing cellular DNA to dyes such as propidium iodide that stoichiometrically bind to DNA. The more DNA present, the stronger the fluorescent signal produced. Cells at different stages of the cell cycle have different but predictable amounts of DNA. Thus, a normal resting cell will produce a 2N peak (diploid); whereas a cell in mitosis, just before cell division, will have twice as much DNA (4N, or tetraploid). Malignant cells tend to have abnormal amounts of DNA (aneuploidy). Measurement of DNA ploidy and cell proliferation in tumors has been applied to cancer detection and attempts to grade some cancers. Frequency of aneuploidy varies with the type of neoplasm, and its detection depends on the resolving power of the FCM system.

In summary, laser-based FCM systems provide a versatile and powerful tool for laboratory studies.

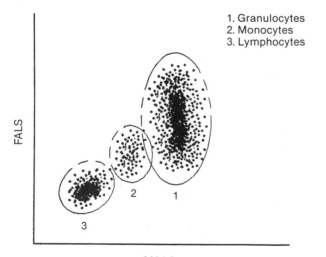

1. Granulocytes
2. Monocytes
3. Lymphocytes

FALS

90° LS

**Figure 31–15.** Peripheral blood leukocyte analysis by simultaneous evaluation of FALS and 90LS.

Any particle that can be put into suspension and tagged with a fluorescent marker is fair game for analysis by this technique. Clinical laboratories are currently using these systems for a vast array of studies. Undoubtedly, as more laboratories gain access to these new instruments, the number of clinical uses will grow.

## General Points Regarding Coagulation Procedures

1. The exact procedure will vary depending on the method used to measure fibrin formation.
2. The endpoint for most tests of coagulation is the formation of a fibrin clot.
3. Most coagulation procedures are performed on plasma, thereby requiring the addition of calcium in order to perform the tests.
4. Testing is performed at $37°C \pm 1°$.
5. Each laboratory should develop its own normal values reflective of the methodology, reagents, instrumentation, and patient population.
6. Sodium citrate (3.2 percent or 3.8 percent) is the anticoagulant used for routine coagulation procedures. Other anticoagulants (e.g., EDTA, heparin, and oxalate) are unacceptable.
7. The ratio of blood to anticoagulant should be 9:1. This may vary, as long as the final concentration of sodium citrate remains 3.2 percent or 3.8 percent of the final blood mixture. The disproportion of anticoagulant to blood is seen in patients with polycythemia and those with moderate to severe anemia.
8. Immunologic assays are currently available for several coagulation factors, inhibitors, and proteins involved in fibrinolysis. Because these assays determine the presence or absence of these proteins and not their biologic activity, the tests should be performed in conjunction with various clotting tests.
9. Chromogenic assays using synthetic substrates have been developed for measurement of proteases involved in coagulation and fibrinolysis and for the inhibitors of these systems. The development of more highly specific substrates and advances in automated technology should simplify techniques and help to make more sophisticated techniques available for routine use.

## PLATELET FUNCTION TESTS

### Bleeding Time

#### Principle

Bleeding time is defined as the time taken for a standardized skin wound to stop bleeding. Upon vessel injury, platelets adhere and form a hemostatic platelet plug. Bleeding time measures the ability of these platelets to arrest bleeding and therefore measures platelet number and function. Capillary contractility, as well as both the intrinsic and the extrinsic systems of coagulation, function in a minor capacity in the bleeding time. Bleeding time is performed as a screening procedure used to detect both congenital and acquired disorders of platelet function. The bleeding time assesses in vivo platelet function.

There are several methods of performing the bleeding time. The Duke method[11] is performed by puncturing the earlobe with a lancet, making a 3 mm–deep incision. This method is not easily standardized and is rather insensitive. Prolonged bleeding times occur in severe platelet disorders. The Ivy method[12] is slightly more sensitive and easier to standardize. This method is performed under constant venous pressure with the incisions being made on the forearm, where the skin is more uniform in thickness. Three 3 mm–deep incisions are made, and the bleeding times are averaged. The Duke and Ivy methods, although not routinely used in clinical practice, are discussed here for historic perspective. The template method, a modification of the original bleeding time procedure, standardized this technique. The Simplate device has further standardized bleeding time assessment.

#### Duke Method
##### *Reagents and Equipment*
Sterile disposable lancet
Circular filter paper (No. 11, Whatman Inc., Clifton, NJ)
Stopwatch
Alcohol wipes
##### *Procedure*
1. Cleanse the site (earlobe) with alcohol. Allow it to dry.
2. Pierce the earlobe with the lancet, making the incision 3 mm deep. Start the stopwatch.
3. Blot the blood with the filter paper at regular 30-second intervals. Move the filter paper so that each drop of blood touches a clean area. Do not touch the incision with the filter paper.
4. When the filter paper no longer shows signs of blood, stop the stopwatch and record the time.

**Interpretation.** Normal values of 0 to 6 minutes.
**Comments.** If the patient continues to bleed after 15 minutes, stop the test and apply pressure to the wound.

#### Ivy Method
##### *Reagents and Equipment*
Sphygmomanometer
Sterile, disposable lancet
Stopwatch
Circular filter paper (No. 11, Whatman Inc., Clifton, NJ)
Alcohol wipes

*Procedure*

1. Place a blood pressure cuff on the patient's arm above the elbow. Inflate the cuff and maintain pressure at 40 mmHg.
2. Cleanse the outer surface of the patient's forearm with alcohol. The area should be free of all superficial veins.
3. Holding the skin tightly, make three small punctures about 3 mm deep and 1.5 cm apart. Start the stopwatch.
4. Blot the blood at regular 30-second intervals with the filter paper. Move the filter paper so that each drop of blood touches a clean area. Do not touch any of the incisions with the filter paper.
5. When the filter paper no longer shows signs of blood, stop the stopwatch.
6. The average of the times for bleeding to stop from the three puncture sites is recorded as the bleeding time.

**Interpretation.** Normal values of 1 to 6 minutes.

*Comments*

If the patient continues to bleed after 15 minutes, terminate the test and apply pressure to the wound. If a superficial vein is punctured during the procedure, the bleeding time will be falsely prolonged. Repeat the test. Should bleeding not cease at any one of the puncture sites, average the bleeding time of the two other sites.

**Simplate Method.** [13] This is a standardized bleeding time procedure that is a modification of the template procedure employing a commercially available device, Simplate. *Caution:* Each patient should be informed that with any bleeding time procedure, the possibility of faint scarring exists. Keloid formation, although rare, may occur with certain patients.

*Materials*

1. Simplate is a sterile disposable device used to make uniform incisions. When the spring-loaded blade is triggered on the forearm, an incision 5 mm by 1 mm is made. Simplate II makes duplicate incisions.
2. Sphygmomanometer
3. Timer (stopwatch) with sweep second hand
4. Whatman No. 1 Filter Paper Disc, or equivalent
5. Alcohol sponge
6. Butterfly bandage and covering bandage

*Procedure*

1. The preferred site for the bleeding time test is the muscular area over the lateral aspect of the forearm approximately 5 cm below the antecubital crease. Take care to avoid surface veins, scars, and bruises. Place a sphygmomanometer cuff on the upper arm, cleanse the site with an alcohol sponge, and allow the area to air dry at least 30 seconds. If the patient has marked hair, lightly shave the area.
2. Remove the Simplate II from the blister pack, and twist off the white, tear-away tab on the side of the device. *Do not push the trigger or touch the blade slot.* Inflate the sphygmomanometer cuff to 40 mmHg. The time between inflation of cuff and incision should be 30 to 60 seconds. Monitor pressure frequently to ensure maintenance of pressure during test procedure.
3. Place Simplate II firmly on the forearm parallel to the fold of the elbow. Do not press.
4. Depress the trigger and simultaneously start the timer. Remove the Simplate II approximately 1 second after triggering.
5. At 30 seconds, blot the flow of blood with filter paper. Bring the filter paper close to the incisions without touching the edges of the wounds. (Do not disturb either platelet plug.) Blot in a similar manner every 30 seconds until blood no longer stains the filter paper. Stop timer.
6. Remove cuff, clean arm with water (do not use alcohol sponge; alcohol on open incisions will increase scarring tendency), and apply both a butterfly and a covering bandage across the incision. Ask the patient to keep the bandages in place for 24 hours. Record the bleeding time to the nearest 30 seconds and average test results. Return the device to the opened blister pack and discard.

*Hints on Technique*

1. The pressure placed on the Simplate will affect the bleeding time.
2. The incision(s) may be made either parallel or perpendicular to the fold of the elbow. Results will vary depending on the direction of the incision, therefore, one direction should be used consistently.
3. If two incisions are made, the results should be recorded within 1½ minutes of each other.
4. Blood should flow freely within 20 seconds after incision is made.

**Interpretation.** Normal values are 2.3 to 9.5 minutes. Owing to variations in technique and patient population, it is recommended that each laboratory establish its own "normal values."

**General Comments Regarding Bleeding Time.** Prolonged bleeding times are seen in patients with platelet counts of less than $100,000/mm^3$. With platelet counts below this level, the bleeding time increases proportionately to the decrease in platelet count. The use of aspirin, aspirin-containing drugs, and antihistamines causes a prolonged bleeding time. The patient should be instructed not to take any aspirin or drugs containing aspirin for 1 week prior to the test. The bleeding time should be performed in the diagnostic workup of a qualitative platelet disorder.

## Clot Retraction

### Principle

In a normal blood specimen the clot after the first hour should be firm and should retract from the walls of the tube. The process of retraction is influenced by platelet number and activity, fibrinogen concentration, packed red cell volume, and excessive fibrinolytic activity.

### Reagents and Equipment

37°C waterbath
Plastic syringe
21-gauge needle
13 × 100 test tube

### Procedure

1. A blood sample is allowed to clot in a test tube.
2. The clotted specimen is incubated at 37°C, and inspected at 1 and 24 hours.
3. Clot retraction should be recorded as normal or defective. Complete retraction occurs, when about half the total volume is serum, the other half clot (or clot retraction should be recorded as normal or defective, based on a normal retraction of about 50 percent).

### Interpretation

Normal clot retraction starts in 1 hour and is complete in 24 hours.

### Comments

Clot retraction is poor in patients whose platelet count is less than $100,000/mm^3$ ($0.10 \times 10^{12}/l$) and in those with Glanzmann's thrombasthenia. Erythrocytosis results in increased red cell fallout. Anemia facilitates clot retraction resulting in a small clot. In hypofibrinogenemic conditions, the clot is small with evidence of increased red cell fallout. In states of DIC, the clot appears small and ragged with evidence of red cell fallout. Rapid dissolution of the clot is evidence of increased fibrinolytic activity.

## Platelet Retention/Adhesion

### Principle

This in vitro test is designed to measure the ability of platelets to adhere to glass surfaces. When anticoagulated blood is passed through a column of glass beads at a constant rate, some platelets will be retained by the glass beads. The percentage of platelets retained by the glass beads is calculated from the difference between platelet counts prior to and after passage through the glass bead column. It is not certain what aspects of platelet function are involved; however, it is probable that both adhesion to the glass beads and the formation of platelet aggregates cause platelet retention.[14]

### Reagents and Equipment

All necessary reagents and equipment used in the Bowie and Owens[15] modification of platelet retention are available through Pacific Hemostasis Laboratories, Los Angeles.

### Procedure

1. 12 ml of blood from a clean venipuncture is drawn into a 20 ml plastic syringe. To prevent thrombin generation and the loss of platelet function and platelet count, the time taken to draw the sample should be no longer than 60 seconds.
2. Immediately aliquot 1.0 ml of whole blood into an EDTA tube.
3. Label this tube as the control.
4. Connect the syringe to the column. Insert the syringe into the perfusion pump.
5. Start the pump at a rate of 5.8 ml of blood per minute.
6. Collect the first 1 ml of blood after passage through the column into an EDTA tube. Label #1. Collect the second 1ml aliquot of blood into an EDTA tube labeled #2. Collect the third 1ml aliquot of blood into an EDTA tube labeled #3.
7. Perform platelet counts on tubes 1, 2, 3, and control.
8. Properly discard the rest of the blood, syringe, and column.
9. Calculate platelet retention as shown below.

### Interpretation

Normal range is 75 to 95 percent platelet retention.

### Comments

Decreased platelet retention is seen in patients with hereditary disorders such as Glanzmann's thrombasthenia, von Willebrand's disease, Bernard-Soulier syndrome, and Chédiak-Higashi syndrome. The acquired disorders associated with decreased platelet retention include some of the myeloproliferative disorders, plasma cell dyscrasias, and uremia; this can also be caused by ingestion of aspirin and other drugs. Increased platelet retention has been reported in those with thrombotic disorders such as venous thrombosis and pulmonary emboli, with hyperlipidemia, and with carcinomas; it also occurs in

$$\text{Platelet retention} = \frac{\text{Platelet count on control tube} - \text{Platelet count on tube 3}}{\text{Platelet count on control tube}} \times 100$$

patients taking oral contraceptives and those who are pregnant. Normal platelet retention is seen in patients with a factor deficiency and in those receiving anticoagulant therapy.

Factors that influence platelet retention are size of the glass beads, length of the column, type of plastic used in the column, degree of packing of the column, rate of blood flow, and the packed cell volume. The value of platelet retention in the diagnosis of von Willebrand's disease is still questionable, as different methodologies yield varying results.[16]

It is quite important that each laboratory determine its own range of normal values, as minor differences in technique yield varying results.

## Platelet Aggregation

### Principle

Platelets function in primary hemostasis by forming an initial platelet plug at the site of vascular injury. The phenomenon occurs in part by the ability of platelets to adhere to one another, a process known as aggregation. Substances that can induce platelet aggregation include collagen, adenosine diphosphate (ADP), epinephrine, thrombin, serotonin, arachidonic acid, the antibiotic ristocetin, snake venoms, antigen-antibody complexes, soluble fibrin monomer complexes, and fibrin(ogen)olytic degradation products. These aggregating agents induce platelet aggregation or cause platelets to release endogenous ADP, or both. Platelet aggregation is an essential part of the investigation of any patient with a suspected platelet dysfunction.

Platelet aggregation is studied by means of a platelet aggregometer, a photo-optical instrument connected to a chart recorder. Platelet-rich plasma, which is turbid in appearance, is placed in a cuvette, warmed to 37°C in the heating block of the instrument, and stirred by a small magnetic bar. Light transmittance through the platelet-rich plasma, relative to the platelet-poor plasma, is recorded. The addition of an aggregating agent causes the formation of larger platelet aggregates with a corresponding increase in light transmittance, owing to a clearing in the platelet-rich plasma. The change in light transmittance is converted to electronic signals and recorded as a tracing by the chart recorder.

*Note:* There are some basic requirements for platelet aggregation as an in vitro means of evaluating platelet function:

1. In performing platelet aggregation studies, a clean venipuncture is crucial. Hemolyzed samples should not be studied, because red cells contain ADP.
2. It is preferred to test plasma from fasting patients. Lipemic samples may obscure changes in optical density owing to platelet aggregation.

3. Sodium citrate is the anticoagulant used in aggregation studies. Keep in mind that in vitro aggregation is dependent on the presence of calcium ions. The concentration of calcium even after anticoagulation may be sufficient for aggregation to occur.
4. Fibrinogen must be present in the test sample for aggregation to occur.
5. The plasma sample should not come in contact with a glass surface unless siliconized. Platelets adhere to glass.
6. Aggregation studies should be performed at 37°C and a sample pH of 6.5 to 8.5. To help maintain pH values, all samples once collected should be capped to prevent $CO_2$ loss.
7. Test samples should be maintained at room temperature during processing. Cooling inhibits the platelet aggregating response. Just prior to performing the test, the plasma is incubated at 37°C in the heat block of the aggregometer.
8. Stirring is necessary to bring the platelets in close contact with one another to allow aggregation to occur.
9. All aggregation studies should be performed within 3 hours of sample collection.
10. It is essential that the patient refrain from taking any anti-inflammatory drugs 1 week prior to the test. These drugs inhibit the platelets' release reaction.
11. Thrombocytopenia makes evaluation of the aggregation responses difficult.
12. Aggregating agents should be prepared fresh daily and brought to room temperature prior to use. They must be of known potency and added in small volumes.
13. Control tests using platelet-rich plasma from a known donor must be performed with the test samples.

### Reagents and Equipment

Control and test platelet-rich plasma
Aggregometer and cuvettes
Aggregating agents
Magnetic stirring bar
Pipettes

1. ADP: adenosine 5'-phosphate, grade I, sodium salt (Sigma Chemicals, St. Louis, MO). Dissolve 4.93 mg of trisodium salt or 4.71 mg of the disodium salt in 10 ml of saline pH 6.8. Makes 1 mmol/l stock solution. Freeze in 0.5 ml aliquots in plastic vials at −20°C until use. For aggregation testing, prepare 100 $\mu$mol/l, 50 $\mu$mol/l, 25 $\mu$mol, and 10 $\mu$mol/l solutions in saline from the stock solution.
2. Collagen (Hormon-Chemie, Munich). This is a 1 mg/ml stock solution. Store at 4°C until use. For aggregation testing, dilute the stock solu-

tion with buffer supplied to obtain 40 $\mu$g/ml and a 20 $\mu$g/ml working concentration.

3. Ristocetin: antibiotic (H. Lunbeck and Co., Copenhagen). Each vial contains 100 mg of ristocetin. Dissolve in 5 ml of saline. Freeze in 0.5 ml aliquots at $-20°$C until use. For aggregation testing prepare 15 mg/ml, 12 mg/ml, and 10 mg/ml working solutions.

4. Arachidonic acid: sodium salt 99 percent pure (Sigma Chemicals, St. Louis, MO). Dissolve 4.10 mg in 25 ml of 0.1 mol/l $Na_2CO_3$ to prepare a 0.50 mmol/l stock solution. Freeze in 0.5 ml aliquots at $-20°$C until use. Use undiluted in aggregation testing.

5. Epinephrine: epinephrine tartrate (Sigma Chemicals, St. Louis, MO). Dissolve 3.33 mg in 10 ml of deionized water containing 0.1 percent sodium metabisulphite, pH 3.5. This will yield a 1 mmol/l stock solution. Freeze in 0.5 ml aliquots at $-20°$C until use. For aggregation testing, prepare 20 $\mu$mol/l and 200 $\mu$mol/l solutions in 0.1 percent sodium metabisulphite.

## Procedure

1. Centrifuge the citrated venous blood sample at room temperature (18 to 25°C) at 150 to 200 g for a period of 10 to 15 minutes. Dilute the platelet-rich plasma with platelet-poor plasma to obtain a platelet count of $250 \times 10^9$/l. Plasma may be left at room temperature in capped plastic tubes for up to 2 hours before testing. Repeat procedure for control sample.

2. Turn on heating block of the aggregometer 30 minutes before tests are to be run.

3. Pipette into a cuvette the appropriate volume of plasma and place into the 37°C heat block for 1 minute to warm the test plasma.

4. Place a magnetic stirring bar into the cuvette and turn on the motor. Adjust the speed of the stirring bar to between 800 and 1100 rpm (the speed that yields optimal platelet aggregation when strong concentrations of ADP are added to normal plasma). Adjust the absorbance of the plasma to 0.40, and adjust the chart recorder so that the difference in absorbance between platelet-rich and platelet-poor plasma causes the pen to cover the width of the paper.

5. Pipette 0.1 ml of aggregating agent to the plasma. Observe the aggregation curve for 3 minutes.

6. Tests are usually performed with three dilutions of ADP, collagen, ristocetin, and epinephrine for patient and normal plasma samples.

## Interpretation

Low concentrations of ADP induce biphasic aggregation (that is, both a primary and a secondary wave of aggregation); very low concentrations of ADP induce a primary wave followed by disaggregation;

and high concentrations of ADP induce a single, broad wave of aggregation.[17] A biphasic aggregation response to ADP is not seen in patients with platelet release disorders. Patients with Glanzmann's thrombasthenia show incomplete aggregation with ADP regardless of the final concentration. Platelet aggregation induced by collagen is characterized by a lag period prior to aggregation, followed by only a single wave of aggregation.[18] A biphasic aggregation response is seen with the antibiotic ristocetin; however, often only a single, broad wave of aggregation will occur. In patients with severe von Willebrand's disease, aggregation to ristocetin characteristically is absent. Decreased to normal aggregation can be seen in patients with mild von Willebrand's disease. Correction of the abnormal ristocetin aggregation curves can be seen by the addition of normal, platelet-poor plasma to the patient's platelet-rich plasma.

Abnormal ristocetin-induced platelet aggregation may occur in patients with Bernard-Soulier syndrome, platelet storage pool defects, and idiopathic thrombocytopenia purpura. Platelet aggregation induced with arachidonic acid causes a rapid secondary wave of aggregation. Biphasic aggregation is observed with epinephrine. One third to one half of normal, healthy patients will produce a primary wave of aggregation with epinephrine.[19] The aggregating agent thrombin induces a biphasic wave of aggregation. Platelet aggregation induced by serotonin will normally produce a wave of aggregation with a maximum of 10 to 30 percent transmittance followed by disaggregation (Figs. 31–16, 31–17).[20]

## Comments

When evaluating patients with suspected platelet disorders, the aggregating agents most commonly used are ADP in various concentrations, collagen, epinephrine, and ristocetin.

Aspirin, aspirin compounds, and anti-inflammatory drugs inhibit the secondary wave of aggregation by inhibiting the release reaction of the platelet. Reduced or absent aggregation as well as disaggregation curves may be observed in patients taking aspirin medication.

The intensity of platelet aggregation may be estimated by recording the change in absorbance as a percentage of the difference in absorbance between platelet-rich and platelet-poor plasma. This has limited usefulness, as absorbance is dependent on the size and density of platelet clumping and the number of platelets that aggregate. A more complex analysis of aggregation related to the rate of aggregation may also be obtained. However, visual interpretation of the aggregation curves suffices and can establish whether aggregation is abnormal or normal.

## Platelet Factor 3 (PF3) Availability

### Principle

Platelets serve as templates on which activation of coagulation proteins can occur by releasing a phospholipid (PF3) that acts as a partial thromboplastin, which is necessary for the intrinsic conversion of prothrombin to thrombin. PF3 is not available in normal intact circulating platelets. It is released when platelets are activated by a stimulus such as celite or kaolin, which are contact activators. The recalcification time of platelet-rich plasma (PRP) will be shortened when plasma is incubated with celite before the addition of calcium. Celite causes the release of PF3 from the patient's platelets and activation of intrinsic coagulation. PRP, a source of PF3, and platelet-poor plasma (PPP), which is low in PF3 activity, are compared with an activated partial thromboplastin reagent for activity.

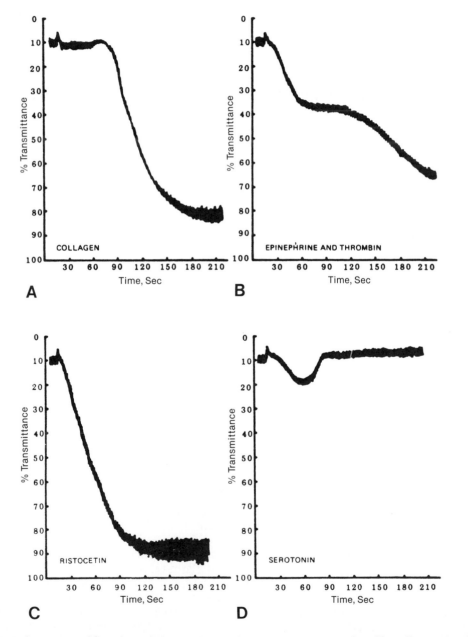

**Figure 31–16.** Aggregation curves with various aggregating agents. *A*, Aggregation curve induced by collagen. *Note:* the lag time before aggregation followed by a single wave of aggregation. *B*, Aggregation curve induced with epinephrine and thrombin. *Note:* the biphasic wave of aggregation. *C*, Aggregation curve induced by ristocetin. *Note:* a biphasic wave of aggregation as well as a single wave of aggregation may be seen. *D*, Aggregation curve induced by serotonin. *Note:* Generally a single wave of aggregation followed by disaggregation is seen. (From Triplett, DA (ed): Platelet Function: Laboratory Evaluation and Clinical Application, Chicago, The American Society of Clinical Pathologists, 1978, with permission.)

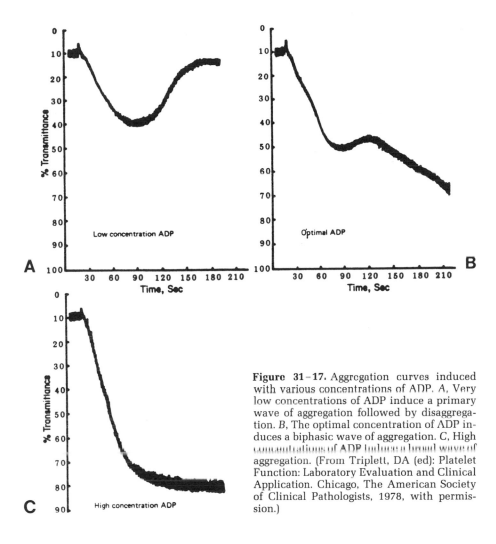

**Figure 31–17.** Aggregation curves induced with various concentrations of ADP. *A*, Very low concentrations of ADP induce a primary wave of aggregation followed by disaggregation. *B*, The optimal concentration of ADP induces a biphasic wave of aggregation. *C*, High concentrations of ADP induce a broad wave of aggregation. (From Triplett, DA (ed): Platelet Function: Laboratory Evaluation and Clinical Application. Chicago, The American Society of Clinical Pathologists, 1978, with permission.)

## Reagents and Equipment

Celite 505 (Johns-Manville), 1 percent suspension in 0.85 percent NaCl
0.025M $CaCl_2$
Platelin plus activator (General Diagnostics)
APTT assay equipment
Plastic tubes and pipettes

*Preparation of Plasma Samples:*

1. Obtain 9.0 ml of blood with a plastic syringe and place in a plastic tube containing 1.0 ml of 3.8 percent sodium citrate and mix thoroughly. Dacie states that hemolyzed samples are not satisfactory. The phospholipid of the lipid red cells may act like PF3 and yield questionable results.
2. Platelet-Rich Plasma (PRP): Spin the citrated sample at 1500 RPM for 5 minutes. Do not use the centrifuge brake and gently remove from the centrifuge. Remove as much of the plasma as possible using a plastic pipette and place in a plastic tube labeled "PRP."
3. Platelet-Poor Plasma (PPP): Re-spin the blood sample for 10 to 15 minutes at 1500 rpm. Remove as much plasma as possible with a plastic pipette and place in a plastic tube labeled "PPP."

## Procedure

Determine the clotting time for the following three assays:

1. Control: Add 0.1 ml platelin plus activator to 0.1 ml PPP and incubate for 5 minutes at 37°C. Add 0.1 ml of 0.025M $CaCl_2$. Obtain clotting time.
2. PRP: Add 0.1 ml 1 percent celite suspension to 0.1 ml PRP and incubate for 5 minutes at 37°C. Add 0.1 ml 0.025M $CaCl_2$. Obtain clotting time.
3. PPP: Add 0.1 ml 1 percent celite suspension to 0.1 ml PPP and incubate for 5 minutes at 37°C. Add 0.1 ml 0.025M $CaCl_2$. Obtain clotting time.

## Results

The PRP and celite should have a clotting time close to that of the control. Platelin acts in vitro like PF3, so by recalcifing the PRP and control, the test systems and results are similar.

The PPP will have a prolonged clotting time because of a lack of platelets and PF3. If the PRP clotting time is prolonged, close to the PPP time, there is reduced PF3 activity in the patient sample.

## TESTS TO MEASURE THE INTRINSIC SYSTEM

### Whole Blood Clotting Time

#### Principle

The whole blood clotting time is the length of time required for blood to clot in a glass test tube and measures the activity of the intrinsic system of coagulation. It is an insensitive test and not satisfactory for use as a screening procedure. It is often used as a means of monitoring heparin therapy; however, other tests such as the activated partial thromboplastin time and thrombin time are preferred for monitoring heparin. Despite the insensitivity of the test, visual inspection of the clot may reveal useful information.

#### Reagents and Equipment

    37°C waterbath
    Plastic syringes (glass or siliconized syringes)
    21-gauge needles
    Three 13 × 100 test tubes
    Stopwatch

#### Procedure

1. Label three 13 × 100 test tubes 1, 2, and 3.
2. Using a plastic syringe, draw 4 ml of blood. If blood has been withdrawn with difficulty or a poor venipuncture has been performed, the specimen of blood is unsatisfactory for this test.
3. When using a glass syringe, the stopwatch is started as blood enters the syringe. If a siliconized or plastic syringe is used, the stopwatch is started as blood is dispersed into test tube 3.
4. Remove the needle from the syringe and dispense 1 ml of blood into each tube. Fill tube 1 first, then tube 2, and then tube 3 last. Start the stopwatch as the blood is dispensed into tube 3.
5. Place the tubes in the 37°C waterbath.
6. Tilt tube 3 at 30-second intervals until the blood clots. Then tilt tube 2 in the same manner until the blood clots. Finally tilt tube 1 at 30-second intervals until the blood clots. Stop the watch when the blood in tube 1 clots.
7. The whole blood clotting time is the length of time required for the blood in tube 1 to clot. Visually inspect the clot in each tube at the end of 1 hour and again 24 hours later.

#### Interpretation

The normal value obtained by this method is between 7 and 15 minutes. A time of less than 7 minutes may be the result of poor technique. When using a siliconized syringe and test tubes, the clotting time is usually prolonged to about 30 minutes.

#### Comments

Many uncontrollable variations occur when performing the whole blood clotting time, making this a rather insensitive test. Prolongation of the whole blood clotting time occurs in patients with marked factor deficiencies, with the use of heparin, and in the presence of circulating anticoagulants.

## Activated Partial Thromboplastin Time (APTT)

### Principle

The activated partial thromboplastin time (APTT) is a screening test used to "measure" the intrinsic pathway of coagulation—more precisely, to assay all the plasma coagulation factors—with the exception of factors VII and XIII and platelet factor 3. The formation of fibrin occurs at a normal rate only if the factors involved in the intrinsic pathway (XII, XI, IX, VIII) and the common pathway (I, II, V, X) are present in normal concentrations. In the APTT, variables of plasma recalcification have been removed by modifications to the test. Optimal activation is achieved by the addition of a platelet phospholipid substitute, which eliminates the test's sensitivity to platelet number and function, as well as the addition of "activators" such as kaolin, celite, and ellagic acid, which eliminates the variability of activation by glass contact. The APTT is also used to monitor heparin therapy.

### Reagents and Equipment

    Fibrometer (Becton-Dickinson)
    Fibrometer cups and tips (Becton-Dickinson)
    Commercial activated cephaloplastin
    $CaCl_2$ 0.02M
    Citrated plasma (test plasma and control)
    Stopwatch
    Pipettes
    37°C heat block

### Procedure

1. Obtain 4.5 ml of blood by means of a clean venipuncture. Mix by gentle inversion with 0.5 ml of 0.109M sodium citrate. (B-D vacu-

tainer tubes containing sodium citrate may be used.) Oxalate is not recommended.

2. Centrifuge for 5 minutes at 1500 rpm. Collect plasma and store at 4°C until use. Testing should be performed within 4 hours.
3. Reconstitute activated cephaloplastin reagent according to directions.
4. Prewarm a small amount of activated cephaloplastin at 37°C. Prewarm a small amount of control plasma at 37°C for 3 to 5 minutes but no longer than 10 minutes. Place a tube of $CaCl_2$ into the heat block. (The major concerns are those of evaporation and contamination.)
5. With reagent, $CaCl_2$, and control plasma prewarmed at 37°C, pipette 0.1 ml of activated cephaloplastin into number of cups for tests to be performed.
6. Pipette 0.1 ml of control plasma into activated cephaloplastin. Allow the cephaloplastin-plasma mixture to warm and activate for 3 minutes.
7. Transfer cup containing cephaloplastin-plasma mixture to the reaction well. Pipette 0.1 ml $CaCl_2$ into the cup in the reaction well and simultaneously start the stopwatch. (The fibrometer system will start automatically when test plasma is added with the automatic pipette switched on, and will stop when fibrin web is formed.)
8. Record time for fibrin formation.
9. Repeat procedure with test plasma.
10. All testing, both on control and test plasma, must be performed in duplicate. (Normal duplicate results should be within ±0.5 seconds of each other; therapeutic results within ±1.0 seconds.) Calculate the mean clotting time and report results in seconds to the nearest tenth. *Note:* The exact procedure will vary depending on the methodology used to measure fibrin formation.

### Interpretation

**Normal Value.** We consider less than 35 seconds to be normal. (It is recommended that each laboratory develop its own normal range.) The test result is abnormal in patients with deficiencies of all factors involved in the intrinsic pathway. The APTT is prolonged with levels of factor IX and VIII 30 to 40 percent below normal. Hypofibrinogenemia (levels less than 100 mg/dl) will prolong the APTT. When the APTT is used to monitor heparin therapy, it is prolonged 1.5 to 2.5 times the control level.

### Comments

Both the APTT and the PT should be performed as screening procedures, since together the tests evaluate the intrinsic, extrinsic, and common pathways of coagulation.

## TESTS TO MEASURE THE EXTRINSIC SYSTEM

## One-Stage Prothrombin Time (Quick)[21]

### Principle

The prothrombin time (PT) is the time required to form a fibrin clot when plasma is added to a thromboplastin-calcium mixture. The test is a "measure" of the extrinsic pathway of coagulation involving factors II, V, VII, and X (as well as fibrinogen). Tissue thromboplastin activates factor VII, which proceeds through the cascade, ultimately generating thrombin. The thrombin thus formed converts fibrinogen to fibrin. The rate of fibrin formation therefore depends on the level of factors II, V, VII, and X, and fibrinogen, and thus measures the overall activity of these factors.

The test is a valuable screening procedure used to indicate possible factor deficiencies of the extrinsic pathway. The PT test is sensitive to the vitamin K–dependent factors of the extrinsic pathway (factors II, VII, and X) and therefore is used as a means of monitoring oral anticoagulant therapy. (The fourth vitamin K–dependent factor, factor IX, is measured by the APTT.)

### Reagents and Equipment

Fibrometer (Becton-Dickinson)
Fibrometer cups and tips (Becton-Dickinson)
Commercial thromboplastin-$CaCl_2$ reagent
Citrated plasma (test plasma and control)
Stopwatch
Pipettes
37°C heat block

### Procedure

1. Obtain 4.5 ml of blood by means of a clean venipuncture. Mix by gentle inversion with 0.5 ml of 0.109M sodium citrate. (B-D vacutainer tubes containing sodium citrate may be used.) Oxalate is not recommended.
2. Centrifuge for 5 minutes at 1500 rpm. Collect plasma and store at 4°C until use. Testing should be performed within 4 hours.
3. Reconstitute thromboplastin-$CaCl_2$ reagent according to directions.
4. Prewarm a small amount of thromboplastin-$CaCl_2$ mixture at 37°C. Prewarm a small amount of control plasma at 37°C for 3 to 5 minutes, but no longer than 10 minutes.
5. With reagent and control plasma prewarmed at 37°C, pipette 0.2 ml of thromboplastin-$CaCl_2$ mixture into the cup in the reaction well. Pipette 0.1 ml of control plasma into the cup in the reaction well and simultaneously start stopwatch. (The fibrometer system will start automatically when test plasma is added with

the automatic pipette switched on, and will stop when fibrin web is formed.)

6. Record time for fibrin formation.
7. Repeat procedure with test plasma.
8. All testing on both control and test plasma must be performed in duplicate. (Normal duplicate results should be within ±0.5 second of each other; therapeutic results within ±1.0 second.) Calculate the mean clotting time and report results in seconds to the nearest 10th.

## Interpretation

Normal prothrombin time is 12 to 14 seconds. (It is recommended that each laboratory develop its own normal range.) *Note:* There are many acceptable methods of reporting the patient's clotting time. The preferred method reports the patient's clotting time in seconds and compares with normal control time also reported in seconds. Another method is to report percent activity as compared with a prothrombin activity curve using normal pooled plasma.

The prothrombin time is prolonged in individuals with a factor deficiency involving a single factor (as in those with a congenital deficiency) or involving multiple factors (as in those with acquired deficiencies, for example, liver disease, coumarin therapy, or vitamin K deficiency), and in the presence of circulating anticoagulants such as fibrin(ogen) degradation products (FDPs) and heparin.

In patients with polycythemia, the prothrombin time is prolonged as a result of a change in the ratio of anticoagulant to plasma.

## Coagulation Factor Assays

### One-Stage Quantitative Assay Method for Factors II, V, VII, and X

**Principle.** The prothrombin time is the basis of this test system, with specific factor–deficient plasmas being used instead of a correction plasma or serum. The percentage of factor activity is determined by the amount of correction detected when specific dilutions of patient plasma are added to a factor-deficient plasma. These results are obtained from an activity curve made from dilutions of normal reference plasma and specific factor–deficient plasma.

**Reagents and Equipment**
Simplastin
Specific factor–deficient plasma (II, V, VII, X) (General Diagnostics, Warner-Lambert)
Imidazole buffered saline, pH 7.3 ± 0.1
Normal reference plasma (commercial reference plasma with known factor levels)
Equipment used for prothrombin time assay
**Procedure**
1. Preparation of activity curve:
   a. Prepare 1:10, 1:20, 1:40, 1:80, 1:160, 1:320, 1:640, and 1:1280 serial dilutions of

the normal reference plasma with imidazole buffered saline. The 1:10 dilution is considered 100 percent in factor activity.
   b. Warm Simplastin to 37°C.

## PREPARATION OF TEST DILUTIONS FOR REFERENCE PLASMA IN THE ONE-STAGE ASSAY FOR FACTORS

| Tube # | Amount of Plasma | Imidazole Buffered Saline | Dilution | % of Factor |
|---|---|---|---|---|
| (1) | 0.1 ml | 0.9 ml | 1:10 | 100.00 |
| (2) | 0.5 ml of (1) | 0.5 ml | 1:20 | 50.00 |
| (3) | 0.5 ml of (2) | 0.5 ml | 1:40 | 25.00 |
| (4) | 0.5 ml of (3) | 0.5 ml | 1:80 | 12.50 |
| (5) | 0.5 ml of (4) | 0.5 ml | 1:160 | 6.25 |
| (6) | 0.5 ml of (5) | 0.5 ml | 1:320 | 3.13 |
| (7) | 0.5 ml of (6) | 0.5 ml | 1:640 | 1.56 |
| (8) | 0.5 ml of (7) | 0.5 ml | 1:1280 | 0.78 |

   c. Perform the following test procedure on each dilution:
      (1) Add 0.1 ml of specific factor–deficient plasma to 0.1 of diluted normal reference plasma and warm to 37°C for allotted time.
      (2) Add 0.2 ml Simplastin to the sample and determine the clotting time.
      (3) Repeat procedure on duplicate sample and average results.
   d. Plot results on 2 × 3 cycle log graph paper, with percent factor activity on the X axis and seconds on the Y axis. Draw a "best fit" line. The curve will demonstrate a plateau at the least concentrated dilutions and should be plotted as such demonstrating the end of sensitivity for the assay.
2. Procedure for testing patient plasma:
   a. Prewarm Simplastin to 37°C.
   b. Prepare a 1:10 dilution of citrated patient plasma with imidazole buffered saline. It is important to keep samples and dilutions refrigerated until they are to be tested.
   c. Add 0.1 ml of specific factor–deficient plasma to 0.1 ml of diluted patient plasma. Warm for allotted time at 37°C.
   d. Add 0.2 ml Simplastin to sample and determine the clotting time.
   e. Repeat procedure on a duplicate sample and average results.
   f. Read the percent of activity directly from the activity curve (Fig. 31–18). A 35-second result on a 1:10 dilution of plasma would be interpreted as 8.3 percent activity.)

**Results.** A range of 40 to 150 percent is considered normal, but each laboratory should define its own range.
**Comments**
1. If the result is greater than 100 percent, dilute

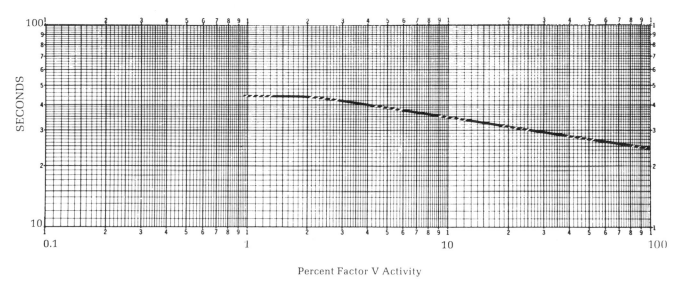

Percent Factor V Activity

**Figure 31–18.** Percent factor V activity curve. (From Lenahan and Smith,[45] with permission.)

the test sample with buffered saline until results fall within the sensitivity range of the curve.

2. Calculate the percent activity of the dilution tested, and multiply by the dilution factor for the percent activity of the patient sample.

3. These tests require the same considerations as the APTT and PT assay with regard to quality control, specimen handling, reagent preparation, and points of procedure importance. The assay should be performed on the same equipment and in the same manner as all other coagulation assays in your laboratory.

## One-Stage Quantitative Assay Method for Factors VIII, IX, XI, and XII

**Principle.** The activated partial thromboplastin time (APTT) is the basis of this test system. This method is also based on the ability of patient plasma to correct specific factor–deficient plasma. Results in percent activity are obtained from an activity curve.

**Reagents and Equipment**
APTT reagent
9.925M $CaCl_2$
Specific factor–deficient plasma (VIII, IX, XI, and XII) (General Diagnostics, Warner-Lambert)
Normal reference plasma (with known factor levels)
Imidazole buffered saline, pH 7.3 ± 0.1
Equipment for APTT assay

**Procedure**
1. Preparation of activity curve:
   a. Prepare a 1:10, 1:20, 1:40, 1:80, 1:160, 1:320, 1:640, 1:1280 serial dilution of the normal reference plasma with imidazole

buffered saline (see previous table). The 1:10 dilution is considered 100 percent in factor activity.
   b. Prewarm the $CaCl_2$ and APTT reagent to 37°C.
   c. Perform the following test procedure on each dilution:
      (1) Add 0.1 ml of specific factor–deficient plasma and 0.1 ml of diluted normal reference plasma to 0.1 ml APTT reagent. Mix well and incubate for the specified time.
      (2) Add 0.1 ml $CaCl_2$ into the mixture at the specified time, and determine the clotting time.
      (3) Repeat the procedure on a duplicate sample and average results.
   d. Plot results on 2 × 3 cycle log graph paper, with percent factor on the X axis and seconds on the Y axis. Draw a "best-fit" line. The curve will demonstrate a plateau at the least concentrated dilutions and should be plotted as such, demonstrating the end of sensitivity for the assay.

2. Procedure for testing patient plasma:
   a. Prewarm $CaCl_2$ and APTT reagent to 37°C.
   b. Prepare a 1:10 dilution of citrated patient plasma with imidazole buffered saline. It is important to keep samples and dilutions refrigerated until they are to be tested.
   c. Add 0.1 ml of specific factor–deficient plasma and 0.1 ml of diluted patient plasma to 0.1 ml APTT reagent. Mix well and incubate for the allotted time.
   d. Add 0.1 ml $CaCl_2$ into the mixture at the specified time, and determine the clotting time.

e. Repeat the procedure on a duplicate sample and average results.
f. Read the percentage of activity directly from activity curve (see Fig. 31 – 18).

**Results.** A range of 40 to 150 percent is considered normal, but each laboratory should define its own range.

## Stypven Time Test (Russell's viper venom time test)

### Principle

This test is performed to differentiate a deficiency of factor VII from a deficiency of factor X, as both of these disorders present with a prolonged prothrombin time. Russell's viper venom (Stypven) has thromboplastic activity and can be substituted for tissue thromboplastin in the one-stage prothrombin time. The thromboplastic activity of the venom is dependent on factor X, factor V, prothrombin, platelets, and phospholipid. The venom does not require factor VII for activity.[22] The Stypven time is also a useful means of measuring prothrombin plus factor V when tested on platelet-rich nonlipemic plasma.[23]

### Reagents and Equipment

Stypven (Burroughs Wellcome Co., Research Triangle Park, NC): Dilute 1 : 10,000 with distilled water according to package directions.
0.02M $CaCl_2$
Platelet-rich plasma (test plasma and control)
Equipment as needed for one-stage prothrombin time

### Procedure

1. Obtain 4.5 ml of blood by means of a clean venipuncture. Mix by gentle inversion with 0.5 ml of 0.109M sodium citrate. (B-D vacutainer tubes containing sodium citrate may be used.)
2. Centrifuge for 5 minutes at 1500 rpm. Collect the platelet-rich plasma.
3. With all reagents prewarmed at 37°C, pipette 0.1 ml of control plasma and 0.1 ml of venom into the reaction well. Pipette 0.1 ml of 0.02M $CaCl_2$ into the cup in the reaction well, and simultaneously start stopwatch.
4. Record the clotting time.
5. Repeat procedure with test plasma.

### Interpretation

The normal value is that obtained with tissue thromboplastin in the one-stage prothrombin time.

A deficiency of factor X, factor V, and prothrombin will prolong the Stypven time. In factor VII deficiency, the Stypven time will be normal.

### Comments

The use of platelet-rich plasma makes the Stypven time sensitive to both quantitative and qualitative platelet deficiencies.

## TESTS TO MEASURE FIBRIN FORMATION

### Prothrombin Consumption Test (PCT) (Serum Prothrombin Time)

### Principle

When normal whole blood coagulates, prothrombin is converted to thrombin by the interaction of *plasma thromboplastin*. Only small amounts of prothrombin will remain in the serum after clotting has occurred, and virtually all of the prothrombin will be consumed if the serum is tested 1 hour after whole blood has clotted. When there is a deficiency in any of the factors required for thromboplastinogenesis (i.e., all the intrinsic factors that activate factor X), prothrombin will have been incompletely consumed, and more than the normal amount will be present in the serum 1 hour after clotting. The prothrombin consumption test measures this residual prothrombin by a one-stage prothrombin time test. Essentially, it is a serum prothrombin time assay. In the test system, Simplastin A supplies fibrinogen, factor X, calcium, and thromboplastin, which are needed to form a fibrin clot in serum. This test is sensitive to plasma thromboplastin precursors, platelet dysfunction, and thrombocytopenia.

### Reagents and Equipment

Simplastin A
Patient and control sera
Coagulation equipment used for determining one-stage prothrombin time (PT) assay

### Procedure

1. Draw the patient's blood sample using a two-syringe technique in a nontraumatic manner.
2. Add exactly 1 ml of blood to a glass (not siliconized) tube, and allow the blood to clot undisturbed for 1 hour at 37°C.
3. After the sample has incubated for 1 hour, spin for 1 minute at 3000 rpm. Transfer serum to a clean test tube; warm to 37°C.
4. Reconstitute Simplastin A and warm 0.2 ml at 37°C for designated amount of time.
5. Add 0.1 ml of serum and simultaneously start the timer.
6. Record the time for fibrin formation.

### Results

Normal serum prothrombin time is greater than 20 seconds. A range for this assay should be determined by each laboratory based on its test system and normal population.

## Interpretation

1. The concentration of prothrombin in serum is inversely proportional to the thromboplastinogenesis activity of coagulation. Since normal serum is prothrombin depleted, a normal serum prothrombin time is prolonged.
2. A shortened or quick PCT is indicative of defects in phase I and/or phase V of coagulation. In patients with defective plasma thrombogenesis, less of the prothrombin will be converted to thrombin and is subsequently measured by supplying fibrinogen and thromboplastin (Simplastin A) to the test system.
3. The serum prothrombin time or PCT is an indicator of the entire intrinsic clotting system, platelets, and factor X.
4. The following conditions negate the need for determining the PCT:
   a. Thrombocytopenia and platelet function abnormalities will result in an abnormal PCT, as normal platelet function is necessary for thromboplastinogenesis.
   b. A patient who has a prolonged one-stage plasma PT will also have an abnormal PCT because of the inadequate amount of prothrombin complex.

## Thrombin Time

### Principle

The thrombin time is the time required for thrombin to convert fibrinogen to an insoluble fibrin clot. Fibrin formation is triggered by the addition of thrombin to the specimen and therefore bypasses prior steps in the coagulation cascade. The thrombin time does not measure defects in the intrinsic or extrinsic pathways. The test is affected by the levels of fibrinogen, dysfibrinogenemia, and the presence of circulating anticoagulants (antithrombins) (e.g., heparin, plasmin, and FDPs).

### Reagents and Equipment

Fibrometer
Fibrometer cups and tips
100 ml pipette and tips
1.0 ml disposable serologic pipette
13 × 75 mm plastic test tubes
Fibrindex thrombin-50 NIH thrombin units 1 ml (Fibrindex, Ortho Pharmaceutical Corp., Raritan, NJ)
0.85 percent NaCl
Normal control plasma
NaOH-IN (Fisher)
ACl-IN (Fisher)
TRIS base (Sigma)

TRIS base stock solution: Weigh 72.9 g TRIS base;

Q.S. to 3 l with deionized water. Stable at room temperature for 1 year.
Working TRIS buffer, 0.05 pH 7.4: Add 42.0 ml 1 N HCl to 250 ml TRIS base stock solution in a 1 liter volumetric flask.
TRIS $CaCl_2$, 0.05M: 1.38 g anhydrous $CaCl_2$; Q.S. to 500 ml with working TRIS buffer. Stable at room temperature for 1 year.
Thrombin solution, 10 NIH units thrombin/ml: To one vial of thrombin 50 NIH units, add 5 ml of physiologic saline. Mix. Aliquot 1 ml into each of 4 plastic test tubes. Store at −15°C. Stable for 2 weeks.
Working thrombin reagent: Thaw a 1 ml aliquot of thrombin solution at room temperature. Add 1 ml of TRIS buffered $CaCl_2$. Mix. Stable for 8 hours at room temperature.

### Procedure

1. Prepare platelet-poor plasma. Separate plasma and immediately refrigerate at 4°C or store on ice. Test should be performed as soon as possible; however, stoppered refrigerated plasmas are stable for 4 hours.
2. Perform all tests in duplicate. Deliver 0.1 ml of working TRIS buffer into a fibrometer cup and incubate at 37°C for a minimum of 3 minutes, but not more than 10 minutes.
3. Add 0.1 ml of test plasma to the fibrometer cup containing 0.1 ml of working TRIS buffer. Start the stopwatch.
4. Incubate at 37°C. Prior to 1 minute transfer the fibrometer cup containing the plasma–TRIS buffer mixture to the reaction well.
5. Exactly at 1 minute, add 0.1 ml of thrombin reagent.
6. Measure the clotting time.
7. If the patient's average clotting time greatly exceeds the average control time the test should be repeated using a 1 : 1 mixture of patient's plasma and normal or control plasma (see Interpretation).

### Interpretation

Normal value is approximately 15 seconds. The thrombin time is prolonged in patients with hypofibrinogenemia (usually less than 100 mg/dl), in those with dysfibrinogenemia, and in the presence of circulating anticoagulants.

If the mixing test results in a clotting time that approximates that of the control plasma, a deficiency or a molecular abnormality of fibrinogen is most likely indicated. If the mixing tests fail to "correct" the thrombin time, the presence of a circulating inhibitor is indicated.

The thrombin time does not differentiate a state of DIC from primary fibrinolysis; however, it is the most sensitive test for determining the presence of DIC.

## Reptilase Time

### Principle

The reptilase time is similar to the thrombin time, except that with the former technique clotting is initiated with the snake venom enzyme, reptilase. Reptilase, thrombin-like in nature, hydrolyzes fibrinopeptide A from the intact fibrinogen molecule in contrast to thrombin, which hydrolyzes fibrinopeptide A and B from fibrinogen. The clot that forms by the action of reptilase on fibrinogen is more fragile than that formed by thrombin's action on fibrinogen. The reptilase time is not inhibited by heparin. There is only a minimum effect on the reptilase time by fibrin(ogen) degradation products (FDPs).

### Reagents and Equipment

> Fibrometer (Becton-Dickinson)
> Fibrometer cups and tips (Becton-Dickinson)
> Reptilase-R (Abbott Laboratories, Diagnostic Division, Chicago, IL)
> Platelet-poor citrated plasma (control and test plasma)
> 37°C heat block
> Stopwatch

### Procedure

1. Obtain 4.5 ml of blood by means of a clean venipuncture. Mix by gentle inversion with 0.5 ml of 0.109M sodium citrate. (B-D vacutainer tubes containing sodium citrate may be used.) Reject any specimens that are hemolyzed.
2. Prepare platelet-poor plasma by centrifugation at 1500 rpm for 10 to 15 minutes.
3. Reconstitute a vial of reptilase-R with 1.0 ml of deionized water. Stable for 28 days at 4°C.
4. Pipette 0.3 ml of reptilase-R reagent into a fibrometer cup. Incubate at 37°C for 5 minutes.
5. Pipette 0.3 ml of control plasma into a fibrometer cup. Start the stopwatch.
6. Prior to 2 minutes, transfer the fibrometer cup to the reaction well. At exactly 2 minutes, add 0.1 ml of prewarmed reptilase-R reagent. (The fibrometer system will start automatically when reagent is added with the automatic pipette on, and will stop when fibrin web forms.)
7. Record time for clot formation.
8. Repeat procedure with test plasma.
9. All testing, both on control and test plasma must be performed in duplicate. (Duplicate results should agree within ±0.5 seconds.) Calculate the average clotting time and report results in seconds.

### Interpretation

Normal values are 18 to 22 seconds. Except for fibrinogen Oklahoma and fibrinogen Oslow, all the congenital dysfibrinogenemias have an infinite reptilase time. The reptilase time is also infinitely prolonged in cases of congenital afibrinogenemia. In states of hypofibrinogenemia the reptilase time may be variable, dependent on the levels of fibrinogen present. The reptilase time is moderately prolonged in the presence of FDPs and is unaffected by heparin.

### Comments

In the presence of heparin, thrombin is inhibited by way of antithrombin III. However, heparin does not interfere with reptilase's ability to cleave fibrinopeptide A from fibrinogen. A comparison of both thrombin time and reptilase time will aid in detecting the presence of thrombin inhibitors such as heparin.

### TEST COMPARISON

| Thrombin Time | Reptilase Time | Defect |
|---|---|---|
| Infinitely prolonged | Infinitely prolonged | Dysfibrinogenemia |
| Infinitely prolonged | Infinitely prolonged | Afibrinogenemia |
| Prolonged | Equally prolonged | Hypofibrinogenemia |
| Prolonged | Normal | Heparin |
| Prolonged | Slight to moderately prolonged | Fibrin(ogen)-degradation products |

## Fibrinogen

### Principle

Fibrinogen can be quantitatively measured by a modification of the thrombin time, because the thrombin clotting time of dilute plasma is inversely proportional to the concentration of fibrinogen. This method involves clotting dilutions of both patient's test plasma and control plasma with an excess of thrombin.[24] Results are calculated from a calibration curve.

### Reagents and Equipment

> Fibrometer (Becton-Dickinson)
> Fibro-cups and tips
> 12 × 75 test tubes
> Data-Fi Fibrinogen Determination Kit (Dade Diagnostics, Inc., Miami, FL)
> a. Thrombin, 100 NIH units/ml, bovine lyophilized: Reconstitute with 1.0 ml distilled water.
> b. Fibrinogen standard: Fibrinogen concentration is standardized by the macro-Kjeldahl method.
> Reconstitute with 1.0 ml distilled water. Mix by gentle inversion; do not shake.
> c. Owren's Veronal buffer, pH 7.35
> d. Control (with a known fibrinogen concentration)

## Procedure

1. Mix nine parts of freshly collected blood to one part 3.8 percent sodium citrate.
2. Centrifuge for 15 minutes at 1500 Gs. Collect plasma.

### Preparation of Calibration Curve

3. Make dilutions of the fibrinogen standard with Owren's Veronal buffer as follows: 1 : 5, 1 : 15, and 1 : 40. Make all transfers from the first test tube.
   a. 1 : 5 dilution (first tube): 1.6 ml buffer to 0.4 ml fibrinogen standard
   b. 1 : 15 dilution (second tube): 0.8 ml buffer to 0.4 ml mixture from the first test tube
   c. 1 : 40 dilution (third tube): 2.8 ml buffer to 0.4 ml mixture from the first test tube

### Fibrometer

4. Perform duplicate determinations on each dilution of fibrinogen standard as follows:
   a. Incubate 0.2 ml fibrinogen standard dilution at 37°C for at least 2 minutes but no more than 5 minutes.
   b. Add 0.1 ml thrombin reagent.
   c. Measure the clotting time. Average the values.

### Calibration Curve

5. Using the graph paper furnished, plot the clotting time in seconds on the vertical axis versus the concentration of fibrogen standard dilutions on the horizontal axis. Depending on the known concentration of fibrinogen in the standard, the points on the horizontal axis will approximate the three vertical lines marked 1 : 5, 1 : 15, and 1 : 40. Connecting the plotted points usually approximates a straight line. The calibration curve may be extended to a minimum of 50 mg/ml and a maximum of 800 mg/ml.

### Sample Assay

6. Make a 1 : 10 dilution of test plasmas and control using Owren's Veronal buffer as follows: 0.1 ml plasma to 0.9 ml buffer.
7. Perform duplicate determinations on each dilution of test sample.
   a. Incubate 0.2 ml sample dilution at 37°C for at least 2 minutes but no more than 5 minutes.
   b. Add 0.1 ml thrombin reagent.
   c. Measure the clotting time. Average the values.
8. Read results from calibration curve and record in mg/dl (Fig. 31–19).

## Interpretation

Normal values: 200 to 400 mg/dl

## Comments

Prolonged clotting times may indicate either a low fibrinogen concentration or the presence of inhibitors such as heparin or circulating FDPs. The effect of heparin may be excluded by performing the thrombin time using reptilase in place of thrombin, because reptilase is unaffected by heparin. A comparison of clotting times using both thrombin time and reptilase may help to delineate a fibrinogen deficiency from a dysfibrinogenemia.

If a prolonged clotting time is obtained using a 1 : 10 dilution of patient plasma, this may indicate low fibrinogen levels of 50 mg/dl or less. Retest sample using a 1 : 5 or a 1 : 2 dilution.

If a short clotting time is obtained using a 1 : 10 dilution of patient plasma, this may indicate high fibrinogen levels of 800 mg/dl or more. Retest sample using a 1 : 20 dilution.

Low fibrinogen levels are seen in infants and children and in cases of congenital afibrinogenemia or hypofibrinogenemia. Acquired deficiencies are seen in states of liver disease, disseminated intravascular coagulation, and fibrinolysis.

High fibrinogen levels are seen in pregnancy and in women taking oral contraceptives. Fibrinogen is considered an acute phase reactant, and therefore high levels may be seen in states of acute infection, neoplasms, collagen disorders, nephrosis, and hepatitis.

Other tests are available to assay fibrinogen. The classic assay measures fibrinogen concentrations by adding thrombin or calcium chloride to plasma, washing the clot, and determining the protein content by the biuret or Folin-Ciocaltea method.[25] This assay is both tedious and time consuming; however, it yields reliable fibrinogen determinations. Semiautomated instruments such as the Bio/Data Coagulation Profiler may yield fibrinogen determinations based on maximum change in optical density. The automated Dupont ACA also determines fibrinogen concentrations. The assay is based on changes in optical density after the addition of thrombin. Simple observation of the clot retraction also may yield information regarding the fibrinogen concentration of the blood. The higher the concentration of fibrinogen, the larger the fibrin web resulting in less red cell fallout.

## Factor XIII Screening Test

### Principle

Stabilization of the fibrin clot depends on plasma factor XIII, which converts hydrogen bonds to covalent bonds by transamidation. In the absence of factor XIII, the hydrogen-bonded fibrin polymers are soluble in 5M urea or 1 percent monochloroacetic acid.

### Reagents and Equipment

5M urea or 1 percent monochloroacetic acid
Bovine thrombin (200 NIH units/ml)

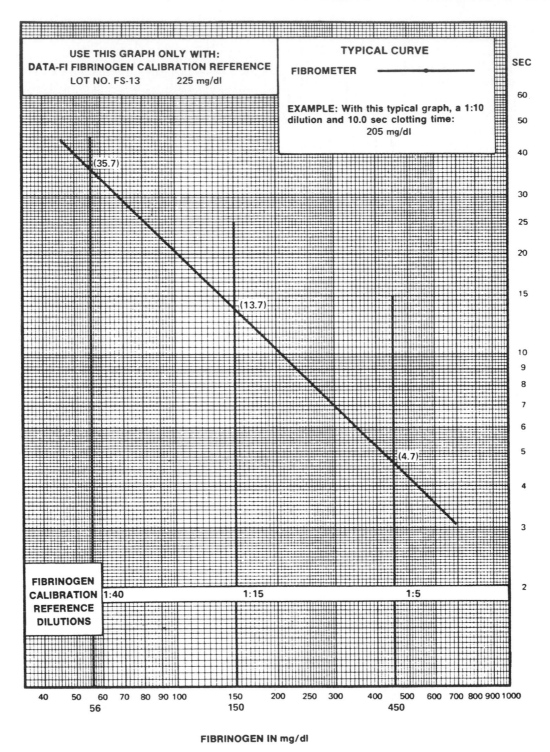

**Figure 31–19.** Fibrinogen calibration curve. (From American Dade, Hospital Supply Corp., Product #LI 0306-A, Miami, with permission.)

0.15M NaCl
Patient plasma
37°C waterbath

## Procedure

1. Add 0.5 ml of patient plasma and 0.1 ml thrombin solution to a 12 × 75 mm test tube.
2. Incubate at 37°C for 30 minutes.
3. Remove the clot from the test tube with a glass rod.
4. Wash the clot with cold saline.
5. Place the clot in a clean 12 × 75 mm test tube containing 1 ml of 5M urea or 1 ml of 1 percent monochloroacetic acid.
6. The tube is incubated at room temperature for 24 hours.

## Interpretation

After 24 hours the presence of a formed clot indicates a plasma factor XIII concentration of greater than 1 percent of normal.

## Comments

A deficiency of factor XIII is not detected by other coagulation tests; therefore, hemostatic evaluation is not complete without a factor XIII assay. Because the minimum level of XIII is about 5 percent, this assay will reliably detect those individuals with a rare factor XIII deficiency.[26]

Those patients who present with a homozygous deficiency of factor XIII show dissolution of a fibrin clot, usually within 1 hour.

# TESTS FOR VON WILLEBRAND'S DISEASE

## Measurement of Factor VIII–Related Antigen

### Principle

Factor VIII antigen, the high molecular weight component of the factor VIII molecule, is measured by Laurell rocket electrophoresis. Factor VIII antigen is electrophoresed through agar containing antisera to factor VIII. The rocket-like immunoprecipitate that forms is measured, the length of which is directly proportional to the amount of antigen present.

### Reagents and Equipment

Electrophoresis chamber and power supply
3¼ × 4 inch Kodak glass slides precoated with 0.1 percent agarose
5 μl pipette
Wicks — telfa strips
Well cutter
Template: Single row of 14 holes, 3 mm in diameter; 3 mm apart; 2 cm from edge of plate

## Reagents

1. TRIS barbital buffer, pH 8.8
   TRIS barbital buffer — 17 g
   Deionized $H_2O$ — 2000 ml
   Dissolve buffer in deionized $H_2O$. Q.S. to 2000 ml
2. Destaining Solution
   Glacial acetic acid — 200 ml
   Methyl alcohol — 1000 ml
   Distilled $H_2O$ — 1000 ml
   Mix together well.
3. Coomassie brilliant blue R 250 (Gelman Instrument Co., Ann Arbor, MI)
   Stain — 0.25 g
   Destaining solution — 1000 ml
   Dissolve stain in destaining solution. Q.S. to 1000 ml.
4. Antisera to human factor VIII–associated protein (Calbiochem-Behring Corp., San Diego, CA)
5. Patient's platelet-poor plasma
6. Pooled normal serum
7. Physiologic saline

## Procedure

1. Agarose gel slides
   a. Wash and dry the number of glass slides needed. Precoat with a thin layer of 0.1 percent agarose. Allow to air dry.
   b. Dissolve 0.15 g agarose in 15 ml of TRIS barbital buffer for agar. Heat to boiling, constantly stirring with a magnet stirring bar.
   c. When the solution is clear and the agarose dissolved, place in a 55°C waterbath.
   d. When the solution is at 50 to 55°C, add 0.5 ml of factor VIII antiserum to the solution.
   e. Mix thoroughly by swirling the solution.
   f. Place a warm precoated slide on a level work area and pour the agarose-antiserum mixture onto the slide. Allow to cool for 10 to 15 minutes at 22 to 25°C.
   g. Store overnight at 4°C in a moist chamber. Do not make slides more than 3 days prior to use.
   h. By following the pattern of the template, cut wells in the agar. Remove the agar from the wells with a pipette attached to a suction. Wells should not be cut in the agar until just prior to use.
2. Electrophoresis
   a. Pour 500 ml of TRIS barbital buffer for electrophoresis into each side of the electrophoresis chamber. Cool in refrigerator.
   b. Wet two wicks by soaking in buffer in the chamber for several minutes.
   c. Prepare dilutions of frozen normal plasma pool with TRIS buffer as follows: undiluted

(100 percent), 1:2 (50 percent), 1:4 (25 percent), and 1:8 (12.5 percent).

d. Prepare dilutions of patient plasma with TRIS buffer as follows: undiluted (100 percent) and 1:2 (50 percent).

e. 5 $\mu$l of each dilution is placed in each of the wells. Do not perform this step until the electrophoretic apparatus is ready. All samples must be applied and electrophoresis begun within 5 minutes to minimize radial diffusion.

f. Place the slide in the chamber with the sample wells toward the cathode.

g. Place the wet wicks on both the cathode and anode ends of the slide. Be sure the wicks lie flat against the agar with the other end immersed in buffer.

h. Run at 4°C for 18 hours at 8 to 10 mA.

i. When run is complete, wash slide with physiologic saline overnight.

3. Staining

a. Remove slides from saline and place on Whatman No. 1 filter paper. Cover slide with 8 to 10 layers of filter paper. Place a glass slide over filter paper and place a 1-pound weight over glass slide for 15 minutes. This sandwich effect will remove excess water from the slide.

b. At the end of 15 minutes, remove weight and filter paper and allow the slide to air dry.

c. Stain the slide for 10 minutes.

d. Destain slide in several changes of destaining solution until background is almost clear.

## Interpretation

1. Measure in millimeters the length of the rockets from the center of the wells to the apex.

2. Make a reference curve using the pooled normal plasma control. Plot the lengths of the rocket for the control dilutions against their concentrations expressed in percent of normal on log-log paper.

3. Draw a best-fit line.

4. Determine the percent of factor VIII–related antigen in the patient's sample from the reference curve. Values for sample dilutions are multiplied by the corresponding dilution factor.

Normal values are 70 to 150 percent. Patients with hemophilia A show normal levels of factor VIII–related antigen. Female carriers of hemophilia A show normal or slightly elevated levels of Factor VIII–related antigen. All patients with von Willebrand's disease were originally thought to show decreases in factor VIII–related antigen. It is now recognized that about two thirds of the patients with von Willebrand's show a decrease in the VIII antigen.[27] The remaining patients may show slightly reduced to normal VIII antigen levels.

## Comments

Some patients may show variable levels of activity. To accommodate this, undiluted plasma samples should be assayed. This test measures antigenic activity — not biologic activity.

## von Willebrand's Factor Assay

Patients with von Willebrand's disease (vWd) show abnormal platelet aggregation with ristocetin. The aggregation defect in vWd is due to a humoral factor known as von Willebrand's factor (vWf). Supporting evidence is obtained by demonstrating that the abnormal ristocetin aggregation is corrected upon the addition of normal platelet-poor plasma or factor VIII–rich plasma to the platelet-rich plasma prior to testing. Von Willebrand's factor is thought to be a required plasma cofactor for the normal adhesion of platelets to the subendothelium at sites of vascular injury. Absence of the vWf results in abnormal platelet adhesion and prolonged bleeding time. The test is based on the concept of a receptor, possibly a glycoprotein, for the vWf on the platelet membrane surface. Washed human platelets will aggregate with ristocetin when normal vWf is present and binds to its receptor.

## Principle

In this test, normal washed formalin-fixed platelets are mixed with dilutions of plasma. Ristocetin is added and the rate of aggregation is quantitated. The rate of aggregation is proportional to von Willebrand's factor activity.[28] The activity of unknown test samples are extrapolated from a reference graph obtained by testing dilutions of normal pooled plasma.

## Reagents and Equipment

Aggregometer
37°C waterbath
Refrigerated centrifuge
16 × 150 mm plastic screw-cap test tubes
Plastic centrifuge tubes
Micropipettes
Formalin fixed platelets (Bio/Data Corp., Hatboro, PA)

a. TRIS buffered saline pH 7.3 to 7.4
Mix two parts 0.85 percent NaCl to one part TRIS buffer

b. NaCl 0.15M

c. Ristocetin (Sigma Chemicals, St. Louis, MO)
Dissolve ristocetin in tris buffer to a final concentration of 10 mg/ml. Freeze at −30°C in 0.5 ml aliquots.

**467**

## Procedure

1. Obtain EDTA anticoagulated blood from both patient and normal donors. At least 10 normal donors should be drawn for reference pooled plasma. (Women should not be pregnant or taking oral contraceptives.)
2. Centrifuge at 3000 Gs for 10 minutes. Remove plasma. Do not disturb the buffy coat.
3. Prepare dilutions of reference pooled plasma in TRIS buffer as follows: 1:2, 1:4, 1:8, and 1:16. The dilution of 1:2 represents 100 percent.
4. Prepare dilutions of patient's test plasma in TRIS buffer as follows: 1:2 and 1:4.
5. Prepare the reference blank as follows: 0.25 ml fixed-platelet suspension is added to 0.25 ml of TRIS buffer in an aggregometer cuvette and mixed.
6. To a second aggregometer cuvette, pipette 0.4 ml fixed-platelet suspension. Add 0.05 ml of 1:2 reference-pool dilution to the cuvette. Incubate at 37°C for 2 minutes.
7. Add a magnetic stirring bar to the cuvette.
8. Set the baselines for 0 percent and 100 percent for the aggregometer.
9. When the 0 percent baseline has stabilized, add 0.05 ml of ristocetin. Note the point of ristocetin addition on the chart paper.
10. Observe aggregation until point of completion.
11. Repeat steps 4 through 10 on each serial dilution of reference plasma.
12. Repeat steps 4 through 10 on each serial dilution of patient's test plasma.

## Interpretation

1. The slope of the aggregation curve for each serial dilution is measured. The slope is defined as the change in optical density expressed in millimeters. The slope is determined on the steepest part of the aggregation curve measured down the middle of the curve.
2. Using log-log paper, the slope in millimeters is plotted on the vertical axis for each of the four reference dilutions, while the percent activity is plotted on the horizontal axis.
3. Draw a best-fit line through the points.
4. To determine the percent activity for both dilutions of the patient's test plasma, locate the points where the slope values intersect the reference curve. Average the results.

Normal values: 50 to 150 percent activity (compared with normal pooled plasma as reference). Patients with von Willebrand's disease range from 0 to 50 percent activity.

## Comments

There is a high degree of correlation between the activity of von Willebrand's factor in vitro and the activity in vivo, as assayed by means of the bleeding time.[29] The results also correlate well with factor VIIIR:Ag. Von Willebrand's factor activity may become normal in those with von Willebrand's disease, during inflammation, pregnancy, or following transfusion with components rich in factor VIII despite the prolonged bleeding times.[30,31] Patients who present with a variant form of von Willebrand's disease may show prolonged bleeding times in the face of decreased to normal vWf levels but increased activity to ristocetin.[32,33]

Normal or increased levels of von Willebrand's factor are found in patients with hemophilia A and in those with Bernard-Soulier syndrome.

Certain disease states such as diabetes mellitus, hyperthyroidism, liver disease, chronic renal failure, pregnancy, endothelial cell damage, and disorders of the myeloproliferative syndrome may cause an increase in the level of vWf activity. Because of these variations, it is suggested that "two or three" separate assays be performed prior to making a diagnosis.

When von Willebrand's factor is assayed by immunologic methods the protein detected is measured as VIIIR:Ag. When it is assayed through its interaction with ristocetin and platelets it is measured as VIIIR:Rcof or VIIIR:vWf.

## TESTS FOR NATURAL AND PATHOLOGIC CIRCULATING ANTICOAGULANTS
### Antithrombin III Assay

Antithrombin III (AT III) is a naturally occurring inhibitor of blood coagulation and serves an important role in maintaining blood in the fluid state. It is an $\alpha_2$-globulin synthesized in the liver, circulating in the plasma, and is the major plasma inhibitor responsible for neutralizing the activity of thrombin, factors IXa, Xa, IXa, and plasmin. AT III slowly, progressively, and irreversibly inhibits the action of thrombin by forming a 1:1 stoichiometric complex with thrombin. This complex forms when the active serine site of thrombin binds with the arginine site of antithrombin. The inhibition of thrombin by AT III is greatly accelerated by heparin.

Antithrombin III can be measured by a variety of techniques. The most frequently employed assays are (1) a clotting time based on thrombin neutralization, (2) Laurell rocket electroimmunoassay, (3) Mancini radial immunodiffusion, and (4) chromogenic substrate assays.

Assays for antithrombin III based on thrombin neutralization are not entirely specific for antithrombin III, as it comprises only 75 percent of the blood's antithrombotic activity.[34]

The use of serum instead of plasma may make the clotting tests somewhat more specific for AT III, because its activity is considered progressive. However, some AT III is thought to be consumed during the clotting process, so that AT III assays using plasma rather than serum yield higher levels. As a result of these variables a carefully standardized technique is critical with normal values established in each laboratory.

Assays for AT III based on immunologic techniques appear to be more sensitive as long as the antiserum employed is specific for AT III.

## Thrombin Neutralization

**Principle.** By measurement of the neutralization of the clotting activity of a standard solution of thrombin, antithrombin III is assayed.

### Reagents and Equipment
Thrombin (Fibrinodex, Ortho Pharmaceutical Corp., Raritan, NJ)
Lyophilized normal human serum (General Diagnostics, Division of Warner-Lambert Co., Morris Plains, NJ)
Physiologic saline
Fibrometer
Fibrometer cups and tips
Pipettes

### Procedure
1. Draw at least 5 ml of blood in a plastic syringe by means of a clean venipuncture.
2. Aliquot 5 ml of blood into a plain glass tube and allow to clot.
3. Keep the clotted sample at room temperature for exactly 2 hours.
4. Collect the serum by centrifugation. Keep at constant room temperature.
5. Prepare a solution of thrombin in saline that will yield a thrombin time of 15 to 16 seconds with normal plasma (0.2 ml normal plasma added to 0.1 ml thrombin).
6. Warm at 37°C.
7. Deliver 0.2 ml normal plasma into a fibrometer cup and incubate at 37°C.
8. Add 0.1 ml of test serum to 0.9 ml of standard thrombin solution. Mix well. Incubate at 37°C for exactly 3 minutes.
9. Move the fibrometer cup containing 0.2 ml normal plasma to the reaction well of the fibrometer.
10. Immediately at the end of the 3-minute incubation, deliver 0.1 ml of thrombin test serum solution to the 0.2 ml normal plasma and activate the fibrometer.
11. Record the clotting time.

**Interpretation.** In those individuals with normal antithrombin levels, the thrombin time is 33 ± 3 seconds. In patients with decreased antithrombin levels, the thrombin time is less than 26 seconds.

## Laurell Rocket Electroimmunoassay

**Principle.** Plasma or serum containing antithrombin III is electrophoresed through an agarose gel containing antiserum to antithrombin III. Precipitation of the antigen with the antibody in the gel results in a rocket-like immunoprecipitate, the length of which is directly proportional to the concentration of antigen in the well.

### Equipment
Electrophoresis chamber and power supply 3¼ × 4 inch Kodak glass slides precoated with 0.1 percent agarose
5 µl micropipette
Wicks—telfa strips
Well cutter, 3 mm deep
Template; single row of 14 holes; 3 mm in diameter; 3 mm apart; 2 cm from side of slide

### Reagents
a. Barbital buffer for agar, pH 8.6
   Diethylbarbituric acid          1.04 g
   Sodium diethylbarbiturate       6.57 g
   Na₂ EDTA                        1.0 g
   In 100 ml of warm distilled $H_2O$ dissolve barbituric acid. Add remaining salts and 850 ml of distilled $H_2O$. With 1N NaOH adjust pH to 8.6. Q.S. with distilled $H_2O$ to 1 liter.
b. Barbital buffer for electrophoresis, pH 8.6
   Diethylbarbituric acid          2.07 g
   Sodium diethylbarbiturate       13.14 g
   Na₂ EDTA                        1.0 g
   In 100 ml of warm distilled $H_2O$ dissolve barbituric acid. Add remaining salts and 850 ml of distilled $H_2O$. With 1N NaOH adjust the pH to 8.6. Q.S. with distilled $H_2O$ to 1 liter.
c. Agarose (Fisher Scientific Co., Pittsburgh, PA)
d. Destaining solution
   Glacial acetic acid             200 ml
   Methyl alcohol                  1000 ml
   Distilled $H_2O$                1000 ml
   Mix together well.
e. Amido black
   Amido black stain               2 g
   Destaining solution             1000 ml
   Dissolve amido black in destaining solution. Mix well.
f. Antithrombin III antiserum (Calbiochem-Behring Corp., LaJolla, CA)
g. Pooled normal serum frozen in aliquots at −20°C. This control is run on each slide undiluted (100 percent), diluted 1:2 (50 percent), and diluted 1:4 (25 percent). All dilutions are made using barbital buffer.
h. Reference plasma (Helena Laboratories, Beaumont, TX)
i. Frozen or fresh patient EDTA plasma or serum. Patient samples are run undiluted (100 percent) and diluted 1:2 (50 percent) as with pooled normal plasma.
j. Physiologic saline

### Procedure
1. Agarose gel slides
   a. Wash and dry the number of glass slides

needed. Precoat with a thin layer of 1 percent agar. Allow to air dry.

 b. Dissolve 0.15 g agarose in 15 ml of barbital buffer for agar. Heat to boiling, constantly stirring with a magnetic stirring bar.

 c. When the solution is clear and the agarose dissolved, place in a 55°C water bath.

 d. When the solution is at 50°C to 55°C, add 0.6 ml of antithrombin III antiserum to the solution.

 e. Mix thoroughly by swirling the solution.

 f. Place a warm precoated slide on a level work area and pour the agarose-antiserum mixture onto the slide. Allow to cool for 10 to 15 minutes at 25°C.

 g. Store overnight at 4°C in a moist chamber. Do not make slides more than 3 days prior to use.

 h. By following the pattern of the template, cut wells in the agar. Remove the agar from the wells with a pipette attached to a suction. Wells should not be cut in the agar until just prior to use.

2. Electrophoresis

 a. Pour 500 ml of barbital buffer for electrophoresis into each side of the electrophoretic chamber. Cool in refrigerator.

 b. Wet two wicks by soaking in buffer in the chamber for several minutes.

 c. Prepare a dilution of frozen normal serum pool as a control: undiluted (100 percent), 1:2 (50 percent), and 1:4 (25 percent).

 d. Prepare dilutions of patient's serum: undiluted (100 percent), 1:2 (50 percent).

 e. 5 μl of each dilution is placed in each of the wells. *Do not* perform this step until the electrophoretic apparatus is ready. All samples must be applied and electrophoresis begun within 5 minutes to minimize radial diffusion.

 f. Place the slide in the chamber with the sample wells toward the cathode.

 g. Place the wet wicks on both the cathode and anode ends of the slide. Be sure the wicks lie flat against the agar with the other end immersed in buffer.

 h. Run at 4°C for 6 hours at 7 to 10 mA.

 i. When run is complete, wash slide with physiologic saline for several hours or overnight.

3. Staining

 a. Remove slides from saline and place on Whatman No. 1 filter paper. Cover slide with 8 to 10 layers of filter paper. Place a glass slide over filter paper and place a 1-pound weight over glass slide for 15 minutes. This sandwich effect will remove excess water from the slide.

 b. At the end of 15 minutes, remove weight and filter paper and allow the slide to air dry.

 c. Stain slide for 5 minutes.

 d. Destain slide in several changes of destaining solution until the background is almost clear.

**Interpretation**

1. Measure in millimeters the length of the rockets from the center of the well to the apex.

2. Make a reference curve using the pooled normal serum control. Plot the lengths of the rocket for the control dilutions against their concentrations expressed in percent of normal on log-log paper.

3. Draw a best-fit line.

4. Determine the percent antithrombin III in patient sample from reference curve. Values for sample dilutions are multiplied by the corresponding dilution factor.

Normal values: 88 to 140 percent.

## Radial Immunodiffusion

### Reagents and Equipment

3¼ × 4 inch Kodak glass slides precoated with 0.1 percent agarose

5 μl pipette

Well cutter

Template

Agarose, stain, destaining solution, antithrombin III (AT III) antiserum, control serum, and patient serum (all the same as AT III) immunoelectrophoretic assay)

### Reagents

| Phosphate buffer | pH 6.5 |
|---|---|
| $K_2HPO_4$ | 0.56 g |
| $KH_2PO_4$ | 0.93 g |
| $Na_2$ EDTA | 1.0 g |

Mix salts with 1000 ml of distilled $H_2O$.

### Procedure

1. Using the procedure as described in AT III rocket assay, prepare the precoated slides with 1 percent agarose in phosphate buffer pH 6.5. Add 0.25 ml of antithrombin III antiserum to agar.

2. Make a template with 20 wells 3 mm in diameter.

3. By following the pattern of the template, cut 20 wells 3 mm in diameter in the agar. Lift the agar from the wells with suction.

4. Prepare dilutions of control serum: undiluted (100 percent), 1:2 (50 percent). Dilutions are made with phosphate buffer.

5. 5 μl of each dilution is placed in each well. The 200 percent reference well receives 10 μl of serum.

6. The slide is placed in a moist chamber and incubated at 37°C for 18 hours.

7. Dry and stain as described in AT III rocket assay.

**Interpretation**
1. Measure the diameter of the circles in two directions that are perpendicular to one another.
2. Use the mean diameter of each control sera to make a standard curve. Plot on log-log paper.
3. Determine the percent AT III in each patient sample from the standard curve.

## Chromogenic Substrates

Activated AT III develops proteolytic activity by becoming a serine protease. Methods that employ synthetic substrates exist to assay serine proteases or serine protease inhibitors. The principle depends on the cleavage of the synthetic substrate by the active serine protease to yield either a chromogenic or a fluorogenic compound. Assays that use this principle are primarily a research tool, owing to expense, specificity, and lack of standardization of the procedures.

**Comments.** Antithrombin III is the main physiologic inhibitor of thrombin in the plasma. Inherited deficiencies (autosomal recessive) are associated with an increased incidence of thromboembolic disease with levels of AT III below 50 to 60 percent.[35] Acquired deficiencies associated with significantly lowered levels have been documented in patients with DIC, liver disease, gram-negative septicemia, carcinomas, acute leukemias, hypercoagulable states, and renal disease; and in oral contraceptives. It is postulated that diminished levels of AT III contribute to a "hypercoagulable" state. Antithrombin III is an acute-phase reactant. Long-term heparin therapy has also been associated with decreases in AT III levels.[36] This phenomenon is thought to be responsible for the occurrence of thrombotic episodes during heparin therapy. A proportion of patients with an inherited deficiency of AT III have been documented as having normal immunoreactive AT III in the face of decreased biologic activity.

## Screening Test for the Detection of Circulating Anticoagulants

Circulating anticoagulants are acquired pathologic plasma proteins that inhibit normal coagulation. Circulating anticoagulants differ from naturally occurring inhibitors such as antithrombin III, $\alpha_2$-macroglobulin, $\alpha_2$-antitrypsin, and $C_1$ esterase and must be differentiated from anticoagulants such as heparin and coumarin analogues. The majority of these pathologic anticoagulants are inhibitors or autoantibodies of the IgG class whose inhibitory effects are directed against certain coagulation factors or demonstrate specific activity against phospholipids (e.g., factor VIII and the prothrombin complex).

Some of the circulating anticoagulants that have been detected thus far have been encountered in patients with hemophilia A, Christmas disease, disseminated intravascular coagulation, pregnancy, lupus erythematosus, the plasma cell dyscrasias, Waldenström's macroglobulinemia, elderly patients, and a variety of other disorders.

The circulating anticoagulant directed against the factor VIII molecule is the most common specific factor inhibitor. It is seen in patients with hemophilia A and may be related to repeated therapeutic transfusions of AHF but is also seen in nonhemophiliac patients (e.g., postpartum women, after abortions, the elderly, and immunologic disorders such as rheumatoid arthritis). Antibodies to factor VIII may also be seen in those patients known to have the severe form of von Willebrand's disease.

Other specific inhibitors have been reported against factor IX, factor XI, factor XII, factor V, factor XIII, and inhibitors of fibrin formation.

Some patients with lupus erythematosus develop an acquired circulating anticoagulant. This inhibitor demonstrates specific activity against phospholipids and thus interferes with phospholipid-dependent complexes that involve factors V and VIII.[37]

### Principle

The activated partial thromboplastin time (APTT) is useful as a screening test for all types of circulating anticoagulants. The test is based on the ability of normal plasma to correct an abnormal clotting time with a factor deficiency. The addition of normal plasma will not correct the clotting time in the presence of a circulating anticoagulant.

### Reagents and Equipment

APTT reagent
$CaCl_2$ (0.025M)
Test plasma
Normal plasma

### Procedure

1. Collect citrated plasma from patient and from a normal control.
2. Mix patient's plasma with normal control plasma in a series of six $12 \times 75$ test tubes, as follows:

|        | Patient's Plasma | Normal Control Plasma |
|--------|------------------|-----------------------|
| Tube 1 | 0.20 ml          | —                     |
| 2      | 0.15 ml          | 0.05 ml               |
| 3      | 0.10 ml          | 0.10 ml               |
| 4      | 0.05 ml          | 0.15 ml               |
| 5      | 0.02 ml          | 0.18 ml               |
| 6      | —                | 0.20 ml               |

Tube 6 is the control; tube 1 is 100 percent patient's plasma; tube 2 is 75 percent patient's plasma; tube 3 is 50 percent patient's plasma;

tube 4 is 25 percent patient's plasma; and tube 5 is 10 percent patient's plasma.

3. Incubate each tube for 1 hour at 37°C.
4. Perform APTT on each tube.

## Interpretation

If the APTT is corrected by normal plasma, a factor deficiency is indicated. The addition of normal plasma supplies the coagulation factor or factors that are deficient and thus corrects the APTT. When a factor deficiency is present, there should be correction of the abnormal APTT by only 10 to 25 percent normal plasma[38] (tubes 5 and 4).

If the APTT is not corrected by the addition of normal plasma in most of the mixtures a strong circulating anticoagulant is indicated.

A weak circulating anticoagulant is indicated by a prolonged APTT following incubation at 37°C for 1 hour. Upon incubation, a weak inhibitor progressively inactivates the coagulation factor, thus prolonging the APTT. This pattern is most typical of a factor VIII inhibitor.

## Comments

The circulating anticoagulant that inhibits factor VIII is a specific IgG antibody.[39] These antibodies are often present as weak circulating anticoagulants but are temperature and time dependent, thus causing only a slightly prolonged clotting time on fresh patient plasmas. Mixing tests may yield APTT results intermediate between the clotting times of patient and normal control. Upon incubation at 37°C, both the patient plasma and mixing plasmas will show prolonged times, but the normal control plasma will show no change. Owing to the nature of the factor VIII inhibitor, the mixture of test plasma and normal control plasma must be incubated for a period of 30 to 120 minutes to allow for the inhibitor's progressive activity.

If a factor VIII inhibitor is present, it is important to determine the level of activity periodically since the development of an inhibitor complicates the management of a hemophiliac when therapy involves AHF concentrates.

The thrombin time is also of value in the detection of circulating anticoagulants.

## TESTS FOR THE FIBRINOLYTIC SYSTEM

### Tests for Fibrin(ogen)-Degradation Products

Plasmin proteolytically cleaves fibrin(ogen) into fragments X and Y, known as early degradation products, and fragments D and E, known as late degradation products. These fibrin(ogen)-degradation products (FDPs) share antigenic determinants with both fibrin and fibrinogen, thus allowing for detection by immunologic methods by the use of antisera to highly purified preparations of human fibrinogen fragments D and E. Measurement of fibrin(ogen) degradation products provides an indirect assay of fibrinolysis.

### Thrombo-Wellcotest: Latex Agglutination Test

**Principle.** This test is a direct latex agglutination slide test for the detection and semiquantitation of FDPs. Latex particles in glycine buffer are coated with specific antibodies to human fibrinogen fragments D and E. The presence of FDPs, either in the serum or in the urine, causes the latex particles to clump yielding macroscopic agglutination. An approximate concentration of FDP in the sample can be determined by testing the sample at different dilutions. Thrombin is added to the test sample to ensure complete clotting and complete removal of fibrinogen. The addition of a proteolytic inhibitor —soybean trypsin— prevents in vitro activation of the fibrinolytic system.

**Reagents and Equipment.** Thrombo-Wellcotest kit (Burroughs-Wellcome and Co., Triangle Park, NC)

**Procedure[40] (Serum Sample)**

1. Collect 2 ml of venous blood in a special FDP sample vacutainer tube (provided with test kit). Mix immediately by gentle inversion several times.
2. Ring the clot to allow retraction to occur. Keep the sample tube at 37°C for 30 minutes, or centrifuge to separate serum.
3. If the sample is obtained from a heparinized patient, reptilase (Abbott Laboratories, North Chicago, IL) should be added to the blood. Reptilase R, an enzyme isolated from snake venom, will clot fibrinogen in the presence of heparin and other such antithrombins. 0.1 ml of reptilase R will clot 1.0 ml of blood.
4. Label two 12 × 75 test tubes. Prepare dilutions of the serum as follows:

|  | Tube 1 | Tube 2 |
|---|---|---|
| Glycine buffer | 0.75 ml | 0.75 ml |
| Serum | 5 drops | 1 drop |
| Final dilution | 1:5 | 1:20 |

To aliquot the buffer use the graduated dropper provided. To deliver the sample use the disposable pipette and bulb provided in the kit. Mix well.

5. Label two rings on the glass slide provided as #1 and #2.
6. Transfer 1 drop of the dilution from test tube 2 to position 2 on the glass slide and 1 drop from test tube 1 to position 1. Deliver the dilutions in this order.

7. Thoroughly mix the latex suspension. Add 1 drop to each position on the slide.
8. Stir the latex-serum mixture. Start with position 2 on the slide, then mix position 1. When stirring the mixture, spread to fill the circles.
9. Gently rotate the slide for 2 minutes and no longer. Observe the slide for macroscopic agglutination by viewing against a dark background.

**Interpretation.** The test is sensitive to values of 2 $\mu$g of FDP/ml. The presence of agglutination in position 1 indicates the presence of FDPs in a final concentration greater than 10 $\mu$g/ml. The presence of agglutination in position 2 indicates the presence of FDPs in a final concentration of greater than 40 $\mu$g/ml. For the test to be valid, if agglutination is present in position 2 it must also be present in position 1 on the slide.

Lack of agglutination indicates a FDP concentration of less than 2 $\mu$g/ml. The mean normal level of serum is 4.9 $\pm$ 2.8 $\mu$g FDP/ml. The normal value may be elevated during exercise and stress. The latex agglutination assay has been documented to give false-positive results with sera from patients with rheumatoid arthritis. FDPs occur in trace amounts in the blood of normal healthy adults and children as a result of physiologic fibrinolysis.

**Procedure[41] (Urine Sample)**
1. Obtain a fresh urine sample.
2. Add 2 ml of urine to a special FDP sample vacutainer tube. Mix immediately by gentle inversion several times. If the urine sample has been contaminated with blood do not accept for testing.
3. Filter the urine through a membrane filter with a pore size of $\leq$ 8 $\mu$m and freeze at $-20°$C overnight. Centrifuge the sample upon thawing. If the assay must be run immediately use the urine sample after filtering.
4. Label a 12 $\times$ 75 test tube. Prepare a dilution of the urine as follows: add 0.75 ml of glycine buffer to the test tube; add 4 drops of urine to the buffer in the test tube. Mix thoroughly. This yields a 1:5 dilution.
5. On the glass slide provided, label two rings as #1 and #2.
6. Transfer 1 drop of diluted urine to position 2 on the glass slide and 1 drop of undiluted urine to position 1.
7. Thoroughly mix the latex suspension. Add 1 drop to each position on the slide.
8. Stir the latex-urine mixture. Start with position 2 on the slide, then mix position 1. When stirring the mixture spread to fill the circles.
9. Gently rotate the slide for 2 minutes and no longer. Observe the slide for macroscopic agglutination by viewing against a dark background.

**Interpretation.** The test is sensitive to values of 2 $\mu$g of FDP/ml. The presence of agglutination in position 1 indicates the presence of FDPs in a final concentration greater than 2 $\mu$g/ml. The presence of agglutination in position 2 indicates the presence of FDPs in a final concentration greater than 10 $\mu$g/ml. For the test to be valid if agglutination is present in position 2, it must also be present in position 1 on the slide. Lack of agglutination indicates an FDP concentration of less than 2 $\mu$g/ml. Urine normally contains less than 0.25 $\mu$g FDP/ml.

**Comments.** Generally, elevated levels of FDP are associated with thrombotic episodes such as myocardial infarcts, pulmonary emboli, and deep vein thrombosis, as well as with certain complications of pregnancy.

The assay is of value in the differential diagnosis of patients with certain kidney diseases. Quantitation of urine FDP levels provides a useful clinical means of monitoring glomerulonephritis and kidney rejection following transplantation.

The detection of fibrin(ogen)-degradation products is of great clinical value in assessing patients with disseminated intravascular coagulation (DIC). A positive test result, accompanied by an elevated PT and APTT and a decrease in platelet count and fibrinogen concentration is suggestive of DIC.

There are other tests that can be used to detect the presence of fibrin(ogen)-degradation products. A test that is used to screen for FDPs is the thrombin time. The thrombin time is prolonged in the presence of a low fibrinogen concentration as well as antithrombins such as FDPs or heparin, or both. To differentiate a prolonged thrombin time due to the presence of heparin or FDPs, the reptilase time is used. The reptilase time is prolonged in the presence of FDPs but normal in the presence of heparin.

The test generally thought of as the reference method of assaying fibrinogen degradation products is the tanned red cell hemagglutination inhibition immunoassay (TRCHII).

The test performed as a microtiter procedure is sensitive to fragments X, Y, D, and E. Patient's serum is mixed with antiserum to fibrinogen and then with fibrinogen-coated tanned red cells. If the patient's serum contains FDPs, the FDPs will complex with the antisera and will not agglutinate. If the patient's serum does not contain FDPs, the antisera will complex with the fibrinogen-coated red cells and will agglutinate. Results with the latex method closely correlate with TRCHII. The TRCHII is suitable if a precise quantitation for FDP is required.

The staphylococcal clumping test uses a strain of staphylococcus that clumps in the presence of fragments X and Y, fibrinogen, and fibrin monomers. The test is insensitive to the late degradation products, fragments D and E.

Other immunologic means of assaying FDPs include immunodiffusion, immunoelectrophoresis, counterelectrophoresis, and radioimmunoassay.

## Paracoagulation Tests

### Principle

The formation of soluble fibrin monomer complexes occur through the action of thrombin on fibrinogen. Thrombin cleaves fibrinopeptides A and B from fibrinogen, resulting in the formation of fibrin monomer. Fibrin monomers are capable of polymerizing to form insoluble fibrin. During intravascular coagulation the fibrin monomers generated remain in solution by complexing with fibrinogen, or fibrin(ogen)-degradation products, or cold insoluble globulins. When plasma is cooled to 40°F, soluble fibrin monomer-fibrinogen complexes will precipitate as cryofibrinogen. Paracoagulants, such as protamine sulfate, ethanol, and products from staphylococci, will convert soluble fibrin monomer complexes into insoluble fibrin. Ethanol as well as protamine sulfate will dissociate the soluble fibrin monomer complexes, allowing the fibrin monomers to polymerize, becoming insoluble and resulting in the formation of visible fibrin strands.

Soluble fibrin monomer complexes may be detected by gelation or paracoagulation as with ethanol or protamine sulfate by cooling as in formation of cryofibrinogens or by the formation of a precipitate as in the staphylococcal clumping test.

### Ethanol Gelation Test

**Principle.** When ethanol is added to plasma containing soluble fibrin monomers, a visible gel is formed.

**Reagents and Equipment**
Ethyl alcohol 50 percent (v/v)
Platelet-poor citrated plasma from patient and normal donor as "control" (perform test within 1 hour of blood collection)
Test tube, 12 × 75 mm
Pipettes

**Procedure**
1. Add 0.5 ml of plasma to a 12 × 75 mm test tube. To this add 0.15 ml of 50 percent ethyl alcohol.
2. Mix gently. Leave at room temperature undisturbed for exactly 10 minutes. Tilt tube to check for gel formation.
3. Run a normal donor as control.

**Interpretation.** A positive test results in visible gel formation. A granular precipitate is read as negative.

**Comments.** The presence of soluble fibrin monomers is seen in patients with DIC, in some cases of acute myocardial infarct, and in patients with pulmonary emboli or those with extensive deep vein thrombophlebitis. Five to 10 percent of patients who present with acute DIC have negative paracoagulation test results.[42] The test result is negative in patients with primary fibrinolysis.

False-negative results may occur in patients with severe cases of hypofibrinogenemia. False-positive results may be seen in those with dysproteinemias or with hyperfibrinogemia. The diagnosis of DIC should be supported by other clinical and laboratory findings.

### Protamine Sulfate Test

**Principle.** When protamine sulfate is added to plasma containing soluble fibrin monomer complexes and fibrin(ogen)-degradation products, visible fibrin formation occurs.

**Reagents and Equipment**
Protamine sulfate, 1 percent solution (Eli Lilly and Co., Indianapolis, IN)
Platelet-poor plasma, patient and control
37°C incubator
Test tubes 12 × 75 mm
Pipettes

**Procedure**
1. Pipette 1.0 ml of plasma to a test tube. Place in 37°C incubator. To this add 0.1 ml of protamine sulfate solution.
2. Mix gently. Incubate at 37°C for 15 minutes.
3. Remove tube and inspect for clot formation.
4. Run normal control.

**Interpretation.** A positive test result shows definite fibrin strands. A negative result is indicated by no precipitated material in the test tube.

**Comments.** A positive test result is suggestive of DIC. The result is negative in those with primary fibrinolysis. The diagnosis of DIC should be supported by other clinical and laboratory findings.

## Euglobulin Lysis Time

### Principle

Most tests that evaluate fibrinolytic activity are based on fibrin formation in the presence of plasminogen and its activators. Under normal circumstances the dissolution of a clot occurs slowly, for the plasminogen activators must diffuse into or adsorb onto the clot and mediate lysis. The euglobulin test evaluates fibrinolytic activity and therefore is a measure of plasminogen activator concentration. The euglobulin fraction of plasma contains fibrinogen, plasminogen, and plasminogen activators, with only trace amounts of antiplasmins. In the presence of increased plasminogen activators, the lysis time is shortened.

### Reagents and Equipment

Equipment for the collection of blood
37°C waterbath
Centrifuge
Centrifuge tubes, 12-ml graduated and 10-ml tubes
Serologic pipettes
Sodium citrate, 0.11M

Buffered physiologic saline (1 part sodium barbital acetate buffer pH 7.42 and 4 parts 0.85 percent NaCl)

Thrombin (1000 NIH units in 5 ml 50 percent glycerol)

$CO_2$ — a tank fitted with a valve to control flow rate

## Procedure

1. 0.5 ml of 0.11M sodium citrate is added to a 12-ml graduated centrifuge tube. To this, 4.5M of venous blood is added.
2. Blood and anticoagulant are mixed by gentle inversion. Centrifuge immediately for 4 minutes at 1000 Gs.
3. Plasma is transferred to a clean test tube.
4. To a 50-ml Erlenmeyer flask containing 15 ml of distilled water, add 1 ml of plasma. Mix thoroughly.
5. A stream of $CO_2$ is bubbled over the surface of the plasma water mixture for 4 minutes. Slowly swirl the flask for the entire 4-minute period. This may be done by hand or with a magnetic stirrer. Avoid excessive foaming.
6. The mixture is transferred to a 40-ml centrifuge tube and spun for 3 minutes at 1000 Gs.
7. The supernatant is discarded. The tube is inverted and allowed to drain for 2 to 4 minutes.
8. Without disturbing the euglobulin fraction, wipe the inside walls of the tube clean.
9. 1 ml of buffered saline solution is added to the euglobulin fraction. Stir the mixture with a siliconized glass rod. Within 1 minute the euglobulin fraction dissolves. The remaining procedure must be performed quickly to avoid spontaneous clotting of the euglobulin fraction.
10. Transfer 0.3 ml of the mixture into two 10 × 75 mm test tubes.
11. Blow 0.01 ml of thrombin into each tube. Invert the tubes once. Clotting will occur in a few seconds.
12. Stopper the test tubes and incubate in a 37°C waterbath. Observe at 15-minute intervals for lysis. The endpoint is complete dissolution of the clot with no remaining residue.

## Interpretation

Normal euglobulin lysis time is greater than 2 hours. Complete lysis in less than 2 hours is evidence of increased fibrinolytic activity.

## Comments

States of hypofibrinogenemia or afibrinogenemia will yield results that are difficult to interpret, because dissolution of the clot may occur faster than normal. The test is most useful as a means of monitoring urokinase and streptokinase therapy.[43] A loss of fibrinolytic activity is seen in stored and frozen plasma; therefore, the test should be performed as soon as the blood is drawn.[44]

## References

1. Brecher, G and Cronkite, EP: Morphology and enumeration of human blood platelets. J Appl Physiol 3:365, 1958.
2. Dale, NL and Schumacher HR: Platelet Satellitism — New Spurious Results with Automated Instruments. Lab Med 13:5, 1982.
3. Brecher, G and Schneiderman, BS: A time saving device for the counting of reticulocytes. Am J Clin Pathol 20:1079, 1950.
4. Westergren, A: Die Senkungsreaction. Ergeb Inn Med Kinderheilkd 5:531, 1924.
5. Wintrobe, MM and Landsberg, JW: A standardized technique for blood sedimentation test. Am J Med Sci 189:102, 1935.
6. Wintrobe, MM and Landsberg, JW: A standardized technique for blood sedimentation test. Am J Med Sci 189:102, 1935.
7. Dacie, JV and Lewis, SM: Practical Hematology, ed 4. Grune & Stratton, New York, 1968.
8. O'Connor, BH: A Color Atlas and Instruction Manual of Peripheral Blood Cell Morphology. Williams & Wilkins, Baltimore, 1984.
9. Dacie, JV and Lewis, SM: Practical Hematology, ed 4. Grune & Stratton, New York, 1968.
10. O'Connor, BH: A Color Atlas and Instruction Manual of Peripheral Blood Cell Morphology. Williams & Wilkins, Baltimore, 1984.
11. Davidson, I and Henry, JB: Clinical Diagnosis by Laboratory Methods, ed 15. WB Saunders, Philadelphia, 1974.
12. Ivy, AC, Shapiro, PR, and Melnick, P: The bleeding tendency in jaundice. Surg Gynecol Obstet 60:781, 1935.
13. Lenahan, JG and Smith, K: Hemostasis, ed 16. General Diagnostics, Division of Warner-Lambert Co, NJ, 1982
14. Dacie, JV and Lewis, SM: Practical Hematology, ed 4. Grune & Stratton, New York, 1968.
15. Bowie, EJW and Owens, CA Jr: The value of measuring platelet "adhesiveness" in the diagnosis of bleeding diseases. Am J Clin Pathol 60:302, 1973.
16. Dacie, JV and Lewis, SM: Practical Hematology, ed 4. Grune & Stratton, New York, 1968.
17. Born, GVR: Aggregation of blood platelets by adenosine diphosphate and its reversal. Nature 194:927, 1962.
18. Wilner, AD, Nossel, HL, and LeRoy, EC: Aggregation of platelets by collagen. J Clin Invest 47:2616, 1968.
19. Triplett, DA, Harms, CS, Newhouse, P, et al: Platelet Function: Laboratory Evaluation and Clinical Application. American Society of Clinical Pathologists, Chicago, 1978.
20. Triplett, DA, Harms, CS, Newhouse, P, et al: Platelet Function: Laboratory Evaluation and Clinical Application. American Society of Clinical Pathologists, Chicago, 1978.
21. Quick, AJ, Stanley-Brown, M, and Bancroft, FW: A study of the coagulation defect in hemophilia and jaundice. Am J Med Sci 190:501, 1935.
22. Prentice, CMR and Ratnoff, OD: The action of Russell's viper venom on factor V and the prothrombin-converting principle. Br J Haematol 16:29, 1969.
23. Bauer, JD: Clinical Laboratory Methods, ed 9. CV Mosby, St Louis, 1982.
24. Clauss, A: Gerinnungsphysiologische Schneliomethode zur Bestimmung des Fibrinogens. Acta Haematol 17:237, 1957.
25. Quick, AJ: Hemorrhagic Diseases and Thrombosis, ed 2. Lea & Febiger, Philadelphia, 1966.
26. Kitchens, CS and Newcomb, TF: Factor XIII. Medicine 58:413, 1979.
27. Gralnick, HR, Sultan, Y, and Coller, BS: von Willebrand's disease. Combined qualitative and quantitative abnormalities. N Engl J Med 296:1024, 1977.
28. Weiss, HJ, Hoyer, LW, Rickles, FR, et al: Quantitative assay of a plasma factor, deficient in von Willebrand's disease, that is necessary for platelet aggregation. Relationship to factor VIII

procoagulant activity and antigen content. J Clin Invest 52:2708, 1973.

29. Weiss, HJ, Hoyer, LW, Rickles, FR, et al: Quantitative assay of a plasma factor, deficient in von Willebrand's disease, that is necessary for platelet aggregation. Relationship to factor VIII procoagulant activity and antigen content. J Clin Invest 52:2708, 1973.

30. Ratnoff, OD and Saito, H: Bleeding in von Willebrand's disease. N Engl J Med 290:420, 1974.

31. Weiss, HJ: Relation of von Willebrand's factor to bleeding time. N Engl J Med 291:420, 1974.

32. Ruggeri, ZM, Pareti, FI, Mannucci, PM, et al: Heightened interaction between platelets and factor VIII/von Willebrand's factor in a new subtype of von Willebrand's disease. N Engl J Med 302:1047, 1980.

33. Ruggeri, ZM and Zimmerman, TS: Variant von Willebrand's disease. Characterization of two subtypes by analysis of multimeric composition of factor VIII/von Willebrand's factor in plasma and platelets. J Clin Invest 65:1318, 1980.

34. Miale, JB: Laboratory Medicine: Hematology, ed 6. CV Mosby, St Louis, 1982.

35. Seegers, WH: Antithrombin III Function and Assay. Lab Man 9:23, 1981.

36. Seegers, WH: Antithrombin III Function and Assay. Lab Man 9:23, 1981.

37. Schleider, MA, Nachman, RL, Jaffe, EA, et al: A Clinical Study of the lupus anticoagulant. Blood 48:499, 1976.

38. Sirridge, MS and Shannon, R: Laboratory Evaluation of Hemostasis and Thrombosis, ed 3. Lea & Febiger, Philadelphia, 1983.

39. Sirridge, MS and Shannon, R: Laboratory Evaluation of Hemostasis and Thrombosis, ed 3. Lea & Febiger, Philadelphia, 1983.

40. Detection of fibrinogen degradation products and fibrinogen. Research Triangle Park, NC, Wellcome Reagents Division, Burroughs-Wellcome Co. 1977.

41. Detection of fibrinogen degradation products and fibrinogen. Research Triangle Park, NC, Wellcome Reagents Division, Burroughs-Wellcome Co, 1977.

42. Murano, G and Bick, RL: Basic Concepts of Hemostasis and Thrombosis, CRC Press, Boca Ratan, 1980.

43. Williams, JW, Beutler, E, Erslev, AJ, et al: Hematology, ed 2. McGraw-Hill, New York, 1977.

44. von Kaulla, KN and Schultz, RL: Methods for the evaluation of human fibrinolysins. Am J Clin Pathol, 29:104, 1952.

## Bibliography

Abildgard, CF, Suzuki, Z, Harrison, J, et al: Serial studies in von Willebrand's disease: Variability versus "variants." Blood 56:4, 1980.

Alami, SY, Hampton, JW, Race, GJ, et al: Fibrin stabilizing factor (Factor XIII). Am J Med 44:1, 1968.

Ambruso, DR, Leonard, BD, Bies, RD, et al: Antithrombin III deficiency: Decreased synthesis of a biochemically normal molecule. Blood 60:1, 1982.

Automated APTT, package insert. General Diagnostics, Morris Plains, NJ, 1977.

Bauer, JD: Clinical Laboratory Methods, ed 9. CV Mosby, St Louis, 1982.

Beck, WS: Hematology, ed 3. MIT Press, Cambridge, MA, 1981.

Benavides, I and Catovsky, D: Myeloperoxidase cytochemistry using 2,7-fluorenediamine. J Clin Pathol 31:1114, 1978.

Bessis, M: Blood Smears Reinterpreted. Springer International, New York, 1977.

Bessman, J: New parameters on automated hematology instruments. Lab Med 14:8, 1983.

Beutler, E: Red Cell Metabolism: A Manual of Biochemical Methods, ed 2. Grune & Stratton, New York, 1975.

Biggs, R and Rizza, CR: Human Blood Coagulation: Hemostasis and Thrombosis, ed 3. Blackwell Scientific, Boston, 1984.

Bloom, AL: The von Willebrand syndrome. Semin Hematol 27:4, 1980.

Bollum, FJ: Terminal deoxynucleotidyl transferase: Biological studies. In Meister, A (ed): Advances in Enzymology. Vol 47, John Wiley & Sons, New York, 1979, p 347.

Bowie, EJW, Owen, CA, Jr, Thompson, JH, Jr, et al: Platelet adhesiveness in von Willebrand's disease. Am J Clin Pathol 52:69, 1969.

Boyum, A: Isolation of lymphocytes, granulocytes, and macrophages. Scand J Immunol 5:9, 1976.

Brecher, G: New methylene blue as a reticulocyte stain. Am J Clin Pathol 19:895, 1949.

Brown, BA: Hematology: Principles and Procedures, ed 4. Lea & Febiger, Philadelphia, 1984.

Coleman, MS, Hutton, JJ, DeSimone, P, et al: Terminal deoxynucleotidyl transferase in human leukemia. Proc Natl Acad Sci (USA) 71:4404, 1974.

Coleman, MS, Greenwood, MF, Hutton, JJ, et al: Serial observations on terminal deoxynucleotidyl transferase activity and lymphoblastic surface markers in acute lymphoblastic leukemia. Cancer Res 36:120, 1976.

Cotter, DA: The safe use of dimethyl sulfoxide in the laboratory. Am J Med Tech 41:63, 1975.

Coulter Electronics, Inc: Coulter Counter Model S-Plus Operators Manual. Hialeah, FL, 1977.

Dacie, JV and Lewis, SM: Practical Hematology, ed 4. Grune & Stratton, New York, 1975.

Dacie, JV and Lewis, SM: Practical Hematology, ed 6. Grune & Stratton, New York, 1984.

Data-Fi Fibrinogen Determination Kit, package insert. American Dade, Division of American Hospital Supply Corporation, Miami, 1978.

Elias, JM: A rapid, sensitive myeloperoxidase stain using 4-chloro-1-naphthol. Brief scientific reports. Am J Clin Pathol 73:797, 1980.

Ellman, L, Carvalho, A, Colman, RW, et al: The Thrombo-Wellcotest as a screening test for disseminated intravascular coagulation. N Engl J Med 288:633, 1973.

Ewing, NP and Kasper CK: In vitro detection of mild inhibitors to factor VIII in hemophilia. Am J Clin Pathol 77:6, 1982.

Fannon, M, Thomas, R, and Sawyer, L: Effects of staining and storage times on reticulocytes. Lab Med 13:7, 1982.

Fischbach, DP and Fogdall RP: Coagulation: The Essentials. Williams & Wilkins, Baltimore, 1981.

Funk, A, Gmür, J, Herold, R, et al: Reptilase-R, a new reagent in blood coagulation. Br J Haematol 21:43, 1971.

Gilmer, PR, Jr and Koepke, JA: The reticulocyte: An approach to definition. Am J Clin Pathol 66:262, 1976.

Godal, HC and Abildgaard, U: Gelation of soluble fibrin in plasma by ethanol. Scand J Haematol 3:432, 1966.

Gomori, G: Microchemical demonstration of phosphatase in tissue sections. Proc Soc Exp Biol Med 42:23, 1939.

Graham, RCJ, Lundholm, U, and Karovsky, MJ: Cytochemical demonstration of peroxidase activity with 3-amino-9-ethylcarbazole. J Histochem Cytochem 13:150, 1965.

Gupta, S and Good, RA: Markers of human lymphocyte sub-populations in primary immunodeficiency and lymphoproliferative disorders. Sem Hematol 17(1):1, 1980.

Harker, L and Thompson, AR: Manual of Hemostasis and Thrombosis, ed 3. FA Davis, Philadelphia, 1983.

Hayhoe, FGJ: The cytochemical demonstration of lipids in blood and bone marrow cells. J Pathol Bacteriol 65:413, 1953.

Hellem, AJ: Platelet adhesiveness. Ser Haematol 1:2, 1968.

Henry, JB: Clinical Diagnosis and Management by Laboratory Methods, ed 17. WB Saunders, Philadelphia, 1984.

Higgy, KE, Burns, GF, and Hayhoe, FGJ: Discrimination of B, T and null lymphocytes by esterase cytochemistry. Scand J Hematol 18:437, 1977.

Hoyer, LW: The factor VIII complex: Structure and function. Blood 58:1, 1981.

Hutton, JJ, Coleman, MS, Keneklis TP, et al: Terminal deoxynucleotidyl transferase as a tumor cell marker in leukemia and lymphoma: Results from 1000 patients. In Mihich, E and Baserga, R (eds): Tumor Markers. Pergamon Press, Oxford (1979).

Hyun, BH, Ashton, JK, and Dolan, K: Practical Hematology: A Laboratory Guide with Accompanying Filmstrip. WB Saunders, Philadelphia, 1975.

Janckila, A, Chin-Yang, L, Kwok-Wai, L, et al: The cytochemistry of tartrate-resistant acid phosphatase. Am J Clin Pathol 70:45, 1978.

Kaplow, LS: Cytochemistry of leukocyte alkaline phosphatase. Use of complex naphthol HS phosphates in azo dye — coupling technics. AJCP 39:439, 1963.

Kaplow, LS: Simplified myeloperoxidase stain using benzidine dihydrochloride. Blood 26:215, 1965.

Kaplow, LS: Substitute for benzidene in myeloperoxidase stains. Am J Clin Pathol 63:451, 1974.

Kaplow, LS: Special stains for blood cells. MEDCOM, Inc, NY, 1975.

Kelly, PA and Penner, JA: Anticoagulants: Heparin and Coumadin. Dade, Division of American Hospital Supply Corporation, Miami, 1974.

Kennedy, J: Fibrinogen, Fibrin and Fibrinolysis. Dade, Division of American Hospital Supply Corporation, Miami, 1974.

Koepke, JA, Gilmer, PR, Triplett, DA, et al: The prediction of prothromin time system using secondary standards. Am J Clin Pathol 68:191, 1977.

Kowalski, E: Fibrinogen derivatives and their biologic activity. Sem Hematol 5:45, 1968.

Kung, PC and Goldstein, G: Functional and developmental compartments of human T lymphocytes. Vox Sang 39:121, 1980.

Kung, PC, Long, JC, McCaffrey, RPP, et al: Terminal deoxynucleotidyl transferase in the diagnosis of leukemia and malignant lymphoma. Am J Med 64:788, 1978.

Latallo, ZS and Teisseyre, E: Evaluation of Reptilase-R and thrombin clotting time in the presence of fibrinogen degradation products and heparin. Scand J Haematol (Suppl 13)4:261, 1971.

Laurell, CB: Quantitative estimation of proteins by electrophoresis in agarose gel containing antibodies. Ann Biochem 15:45, 1966.

Laurrell, CB: Electroimmunoassay. Scand J Clin Lab Invest 29(Suppl 124):21, 1972.

Leder, LD: The selective enzymocytochemical demonstration of neutrophil myeloid cells and tissue mast cells in paraffin sections. Klinische Wochenschrift 42(11):553, 1964.

Lee, RL and White, PD: A clinical study of the coagulation time of blood. Am J Med Sci 145:495, 1913.

Lehmann, H and Huntsman, RG: Man's Hemoglobins, ed 2. JB Lippincott, Philadelphia, 1974.

Lenahan, JG and Smith, K: Hemostasis, ed 16. General Diagnostics, Division of Warner-Lambert Company, NJ, 1982.

Li, CY, Lam KW, and Yam LT: Esterases in human leukocytes. J Histochem Cytochem 21(1):1, 1973.

Li, CY, Yam LT, and Crosby, WH: Histochemical characterization of cellular and structural elements of the human spleen. J Histochem Cytochem 20(12):1049, 1972.

Losowsky, MA, Hall, R, and Goldie, W: Congenital deficiency of fibrin stabilizing factor. Lancet 2:156, 1965.

Macfarlane, RG: A simple method for measuring clot retraction. Lancet 1:1199, 1939.

Mammen, EF: Congenital abnormalities of the fibrinogen molecule. Semin Thromb Hemost 1:184, 1974.

Mancini, G, Carbonara, AO, and Heremans, JF: Immunochemical quantitation of antigens by single radial immunodiffusion. Immunochemistry 2:235, 1965.

McGann, MA and Triplett, DA: Interpretation of antithrombin III Activity. Lab Med 13:12, 1982.

Miale, JB: Laboratory Medicine: Hematology, ed 6. CV Mosby, St Louis, 1982.

Mielke, CH, Kaneshiro, MM, Maher, IA, et al: The standardized normal Ivy bleeding time and its prolongation by aspirin. Blood 34:204, 1969.

Murano, G and Bick, RL: Basic Concepts of Hemostasis and Thrombosis. CRC Press, Boca Raton, FL, 1980.

National Committee for Clinical Laboratory Standards: Tentative guidelines for the standardized collection, transport, and preparation of blood specimens for coagulation testing and performance of coagulation assays. Vol 2, 1982, p 4.

Melvin, L: Comparison of techniques for detecting T-cell acute lymphocytic leukemia. Blood 54(1):210, 1979.

Moloney, WC, McPherson, K, and Fliegelman, L: Esterase activity in leukocytes demonstrated by the use of napthol AS-D chloroacetate substrate. J Histol Chem Cytochem 8:200, 1960.

O'Connor, BH: A Color Atlas and Instruction Manual of Peripheral Blood Cell Morphology. Williams & Wilkins, Baltimore, 1984.

Olson, JD, Brockway, WJ, Fass, DN, et al: Evaluation of ristocetin-Willebrands factor assay and ristocetin-induced platelet aggregation. Am J Clin Pathol 63:210, 1975.

Ortho Diagnostics Systems, Inc: Ortho ELT-8 Training Manual, Westwood, MA, 1984.

Ortho Diagnostics Systems, Inc: Ortho ELT-8 Hematology Analyzer Operator Manual, Westwood, MA, 1984.

Parpart, AK, Lorenz, PB, Parpart, ER, et al: The osmotic resistance (fragility) of human red cells. J Clin Invest 26:636, 1947.

Patterson, BB: Clot observation — A review of an important but neglected coagulation test. Lab Med 7:12, 1976.

Quagliano, D, and Hayhoe, FGJ: Periodic-acid – Schiff positivity in erythroblasts with special reference to di Guglielmo's disease. Br J Haematol 6:26, 1960.

Ramsey, R and Evatt, BL: Rapid assay for von Willebrand's factor activity using formalin-fixed platelets and microtitration technique. Am J Clin Pathol 72:996, 1979.

Ray, M and Noteboom, G: A modification of the erythrocyte osmotic fragility test. Am J Clin Pathol 54:711, 1970.

Reich, PR: Hematology: Physiopathologic Basis for Clinical Practice, ed 3. Little, Brown, Boston, 1984.

Reptilase-R, package insert. Abbott Laboratories, Diagnostics Division, IL, 93-4260, 1974.

Royston, I: Monoclonal antibodies for human T lymphocytes: Identification of normal and malignant T cells. Blood 54(Suppl 1):106, 1979.

Rozenszajin, L, Leibovich, M, Shoham, D, et al: The esterase activity in megaloblasts, leukaemic and normal haemopoietic cells. Br J Haematol 14:605, 1968.

Russell's Viper Venom Reagent for Factor X Assays, package insert. General Diagnostics, Morris Plains, NJ, 1976.

Salzman, ER: Measurement of platelet adhesiveness: A simple in vitro technique demonstrating an abnormality in von Willebrands disease. J Lab Med 62:724, 1963.

Schaefer, HE and Fischer, R: Peroxidase detection in smear preparations and tissue sections after decalcification and paraffin embedding. Klin Wochenschr 46:1228, 1968.

Schmidt, RM and Brocious, EM: Basic Laboratory Methods of Hemoglobinopathy Detection. HEW Pub (CDC) 75-8296, Atlanta, 1975. US Department of Health and Center for Disease Control.

Seaman, AJ: The recognition of intravascular clotting: The plasma protamine paracoagulation tests. Arch Intern Med 125:1016, 1970.

Shafer, JA and Stein, BL: Blood smear observation workshop manual. University of Rochester, Rochester, NY, 1975.

Shafer, JA: Hematology morphology workshop manual. University of Rochester, Rochester, NY, 1981.

Shapiro, SS and Hultin, M: Acquired inhibitors to the blood coagulation factors. Semin Thromb Hemost 1:366, 1975.

Shapiro, SS and Hultin, M: Acquired inhibitors to the blood coagulation factors. Clin Haematol 8:207, 1979.

Sheehan, HL and Storey, GW: An improved method of staining leukocyte granules with Sudan black B. J Pathol Bacteriol 19:336, 1947.

Shitamoto, BS, Leslie, KO, and Galloway, WB: Postpartum hemophilia. Am J Clin Pathol 78:5, 1982.

Sicklequik, package insert. General Diagnostics, Morris Plains, NJ, 1977.

Sickle-Thal Quick Column Method, package insert. Helena Laboratories, Beaumont, TX, 1981.

Simmler Fetal Cell Stain Kit, package insert. Simmler Inc, St Louis, 1979.

Simmons, A: Technical Hematology, ed 2. JB Lippincott, Philadelphia, 1976.

Sirridge, MS and Shannon, R: Laboratory Evaluation of Hemostasis and Thrombosis, ed 3. Lea & Febiger, Philadelphia, 1983.

Spero, JA, Lewis, JH, and Hasiba, V: Disseminated intravascular coagulation: Findings in 346 patients. Thromb Haemost 43:28, 1980.

Super Z and Zip Zone Hemoglobin Electrophoresis Procedure, package insert. Helena Laboratories, Beaumont, TX, 1978.

Super Z and Zip Zone Titan IV Hemoglobin Electrophoresis Procedure. Helena Laboratories, Beaumont, TX, 1978.

Sussman, LN: The clotting time — An enigma. Am J Clin Pathol 60:5, 1973.

The Fibrometer Precision Coagulation Timer, Instructions and Technical Information, BBl Division of Becton, Dickinson and Company, Cockeysville, MD, 1977.

Thomson JM: Blood Coagulation and Hemostasis: A Practical Guide, ed 2. Churchill Livingstone, New York, 1980.

Thrombo-Wellcotest, package insert. Wellcome Research Laboratories, Breckenham, England, 1974.

Triplett, DA, Harms, CS, Newhouse, P, et al: Platelet Function: Laboratory Evaluation and Clinical Application, American Society of Clinical Pathologists, Chicago, 1978.

Triplett, DA and Harms, CS: Procedures for the Coagulation Laboratory, American Society of Clinical Pathologists, Chicago, 1981.

von Kaulla, E and von Kaulla N: Deficiency of antithrombin III activity associated with hereditary thrombosis tendency. J Med 3:349, 1972.

WHO Report, 1974: Identification, enumeration and isolation of B and T lymphocytes from human peripheral blood. Scand J Immunol 3:521, 1974.

Williams, J, et al: Hematology, ed 2. McGraw-Hill, New York, 1977.

Winchester, RJ and Ross, G: Methods for enumerating lymphocyte populations. In Rose, NR, and Friedman, H (eds): Manual of Clinical Immunology. American Society for Microbiology, Washington, DC, 1976, p 64.

Wintrobe, MM, Beutler, E, Erslev, AJ, et al: Clinical Hematology, ed 8. Lea & Febiger, Philadelphia, 1982.

Wintrobe Sedimentation Tubes, package insert. American Dade, Division of American Hospital Supply Corporation, Miami.

Wislocki, GB, Rheingold, JM, and Dempsey, EW: The occurrence of the periodic acid Schiff reaction in various normal cells of blood and connective tissue. Blood 4:562, 1949.

Wolf, PL: Practical Clinical Hematology Interpretations and Techniques. John Wiley & Sons, New York, 1973.

Yam, LT, Li, CY, and Crosby, WH: Cytochemical identification of monocytes and granulocytes. Am J Clin Pathol 55(3):283, 1971.

Yam, LT, Tavassoli, M, and Jacobs, P: Differential characterization of the "reticulum cell" in lymphoreticular neoplasms. Am J Clin Pathol 64:171, 1974.

# Glossary

**Abruptio placenta:** Premature detachment of normally situated placenta.

**Acanthocyte:** An abnormal red cell that is slightly reduced in size and that possesses 3 to 12 spicules of uneven length distributed along the periphery of the cell membrane.

**Achlorhydria:** Absence of free hydrochloric acid in the stomach.

**Acholuria:** Absence of bile pigments in urine occurring when unconjugated bilirubin does not pass through the glomerular filter.

**Acrocyanosis:** Bluish tinge to the extremities.

**Activated partial thromboplastin time (APTT):** A test to evaluate the overall integrity of the clotting system that involves factors XII, XI, IX, VIII, X, V, II, and I. Commonly a means of evaluating the intrinsic system of coagulation.

**Acute phase reactant:** Plasma proteins whose concentration increases in response to a variety of stimuli.

**Adenopathy:** Swelling and morbid change in lymph nodes; glandular disease.

**Adhesion:** The molelcular attraction exerted between the surfaces of bodies in contact (e.g., platelets to connective tissue structures).

**ADP (adenosine diphosphate):** A substance used to induce platelet aggregation that may be derived from injured tissues, erythrocytes, or platelets.

**Afibrinogenemia:** A rare blood disease characterized by the absence of fibrinogen in the plasma; may be congenital or acquired.

**Agammaglobulinemia:** A rare disorder in which there is a virtual absence of gamma globulins.

**Agglutination:** The clumping together of red blood cells or any particulate matter resulting from interaction of antibody and its corresponding antigen.

**Aggregation:** A clustering or clumping together (e.g., platelet aggregation plays a critical role in hemostasis).

**Agranulocytosis:** An acute disease in which the white cell count is markedly reduced and neutropenia becomes pronounced.

**AHF:** Antihemophiliac factor; a commercially prepared source of factor VIII.

**Alkaline phosphatase:** An enzyme that is found in a number of tissues but is chiefly used in connection with diagnosis of bone and liver disease. The granules of normal granulocytic cells contain alkaline phosphatase; patients with CML have decreased phosphatase activity.

**Alkalosis:** Excessive alkalinity of body fluids, owing to accumulation of alkalies or to the reduction of acids.

**Alloantibody:** An antibody produced by an immune response that was stimulated by a foreign antigen.

**Alloimmunization:** The process in which a patient develops an antibody(ies) to foreign and/or white blood cell antigen(s) through transfusion or pregnancy.

**Allograft:** A tissue transplant between individuals of the same species.

**Alpha chain:** A type of globin chain found in hemoglobin and coded for by the alpha gene.

**Alpha methyldopa (Aldomet):** A common drug used to treat hypertension; frequently the cause of a positive direct Coomb's test result.

**Amaurotic:** Caused by the atrophying of optic nerve or vision centers.

**Ameliorate:** Moderate, improve.

**Amniocentesis:** Transabdominal puncture of the amniotic sac, using a needle and syringe, in order to remove amniotic fluid. The material may then be studied to detect genetic disorders or maternal-fetal blood incompatibility.

**Amphophilic:** Having affinity for acid and/or basic dyes.

**Amyloidosis:** A metabolic disorder marked by extracellular deposition of amyloid (an abnormal protein) in the tissues; this usually leads to loss of function and organ enlargement.

**Anamnestic (response):** An accentuated antibody response following a secondary exposure to an antigen. Antibody levels from the initial exposure are not detectable in the patient's serum until the secondary exposure, when a rapid rise in antibody titer is observed.

**Anaphylaxis:** An allergic hypersensitivity reaction of the body to a foreign protein or drug.

**Ancillary:** Auxiliary, supplementary.

**Androgenic:** Causing masculinization.

**Anemia:** A condition in which there is reduced $O_2$ delivery to the tissues. It may result from increased destruction of red cells, excessive blood loss, or decreased production of red cells.

  **Aplastic a.:** Anemia caused by aplasia of bone marrow or its destruction by chemical agents or physical factors.

  **Autoimmune hemolytic a.:** Acquired disorder characterized by premature erythrocyte destruction owing to abnormalities in the individual's own immune system.

  **Hemolytic a.:** Anemia caused by hemolysis of red blood cells resulting in reduction of normal red cell lifespan.

  **Iron-deficiency a.:** Anemia resulting from a demand on stored iron greater than can be met.

**Megaloblastic a.:** Anemia in which megaloblasts are found in the blood, usually due to a deficiency of folic acid or vitamin $B_{12}$.

**Microangiopathic hemolytic a.:** A hemolytic process associated with such conditions as TTP, prosthesis, and burns. It is visualized in the peripheral smear by fragmentation of the red cells and other bizarre morphology.

**Pernicious a.:** A type of megaloblastic anemia due to a deficiency of vitamin $B_{12}$ that is directly linked to absence of intrinsic factor (IF).

**Sickle cell a.:** See Sickle cell anemia.

**Aneuploidy:** Having an abnormal number of chromosomes.

**Angina pectoris:** Severe pain and constriction about the heart caused by insufficient supply of blood to the heart.

**Anisochromia:** Not of uniform color.

**Anisocytosis:** Variation in the size of erythrocytes when observed on a peripheral blood smear.

**Anoxia:** Without oxygen.

**Antenatal:** Occurring before birth.

**Antibody:** A protein substance developed in response to, and interacting specifically with, an antigen. In blood banking, it is found in serum, from either a commercial manufacturer or a patient. It is secreted by plasma cells.

**Cross-reacting a.:** An antibody that reacts with antigens functionally similar to its specific antigen.

**Maternal a.:** An antibody produced in the mother and transferred to the fetus in utero.

**Naturally occurring a.:** An antibody present in a patient without known prior exposure to the corresponding red cell antigen.

**Antibody screen:** Testing the patient's serum with group O reagent red cells in an effort to detect atypical antibodies.

**Anticoagulant:** An agent that delays or prevents blood coagulation.

**Antigen:** A substance that is recognized by the body as being foreign and that therefore can elicit an immune response.

**Antiglobulin test (AGT) or Anti–human globulin (AHG) test:** Test to ascertain the presence or absence of red cell coating by immunoglobulin (IgG) and/or complement. Direct AGT (DAT)—used to detect in vivo cell sensitization. Indirect AGT—used to detect antigen-antibody reactions that occur in vitro.

**Antihemophilic factor:** See Hemophilia A.

**Antihuman serum:** An antibody prepared in rabbits or other suitable animals that is directed against human immunoglobulin and/or complement. It is used to perform the antiglobulin or Coombs' test. The serum may be either polyspecific (anti-IgG plus anticomplement) or monospecific (anti-IgG or anticomplement).

**Antiplasmin:** Plasma proteins that are known to neutralize free plasmin: $\alpha_2$ antiplasmin, $\alpha_2$ macroglobulin. $\alpha_2$ **a.:** The major inhibitor of plasmin.

**Antipyretic:** An agent that reduces fever.

**Antiseptic:** Preventing decay, putrefaction, or sepsis.

**Antithrombin:** A substance that opposes the action of thrombin and thus prevents or inhibits coagulation of blood.

**Antithrombin III (AT III):** A naturally occurring inhibitor of coagulation responsible for neutralizing the activity of thrombin, factors IXa, Xa, and XIa, and plasmin. Also known as the "heparin cofactor."

**Anuria:** Absence of urine formation.

**Apheresis:** A method of blood collection in which whole blood is withdrawn, a desired component separated and retained, and the remainder of the blood returned to the donor. See also Plateletpheresis; Plasmapheresis.

**Aplasia:** Failure of an organ or tissue to develop normally.

**Ascites:** The accumulation of serous fluid in the peritoneal cavity.

**Asphyxia:** Condition caused by insufficient intake of oxygen.

**Asynchrony:** The failure of events to occur in time with each other as they usually do. In hematology, nuclear and cytoplasmic development are mismatched.

**Atypical lymphocyte:** A benign reactive change in the morphologic appearance of the lymphocyte, which is frequently secondary to a viral disease (e.g., infectious mononucleosis).

**Auer rod:** Rod-shaped alignment of primary granules that are present only in the cytoplasm of myeloblasts and monoblasts in leukemic states.

**Autohemolysis:** Hemolysis of an individual's blood corpuscles by his or her own serum.

**Autoimmune:** The production of antibodies directed against one's own tissues, usually in association with a disease state.

**Autoimmune hemolytic anemia (AIHA):** An abnormality of the immune system resulting in the production of antibodies against "self," which occurs due to a failure of the mechanism regulating the immune response.

**Autologous:** Of the self.

**Autosomal:** Relating to any of the chromosomes other than the sex (X and Y) chromosomes.

**Azotemia:** Presence of increased amounts of urea in the blood.

**Babesiosis:** A rare, often severe and sometimes fatal disease of humans, caused by the protozoal parasite of the red blood cells, Babesia microti, and perhaps other Babesia species.

**Band:** An immature neutrophilic granulocyte with a horseshoe- or sausage-shaped nucleus (also called a stab). Comprises 2 to 6 percent of the normal differential count.

**Basophil:** A mature white blood cell whose cytoplasmic granules stain deep blue-purple with basic dyes like methylene blue. Comprises 0 to 2 percent of the normal differential count.

**Basophilia:** An absolute increase in basophils.

**Basophilic normoblast:** An immature red cell precursor found only in the bone marrow that is characterized by a vivid blue cytoplasm and a high nuclear-to-cytoplasmic ratio. Synonym: Prorubricyte.

**Basophilic stippling:** Red blood cell inclusion that consists of precipitated ribonucleoprotein and mitochondrial remnants. Stippling may be fine, coarse, or punctate in form and is seen in toxic states such as metal poisoning, severe bacterial infection, drug exposure, and so forth.

**Bernard-Soulier syndrome:** A congenital bleeding disorder characterized by the presence of large platelets, thrombocytopenia of varying degrees, and a prolonged bleeding time.

**Beta chain:** A type of globin chain found in hemoglobin that is coded for by the beta gene.

**BFU-U (burst-forming unit committed to erythropoiesis):** A primitive stem cell committed to erythropoiesis and thought to be a precursor to the CFU-E.

**Bilirubin:** The orange-colored or yellowish pigment in bile, which is carried to the liver by the blood. It is produced from hemoglobin of red blood cells by reticuloendothelial cells in the bone marrow, spleen, and elsewhere.

    **Direct b.:** The conjugated water-soluble form of bilirubin.

    **Indirect b.:** The unconjugated water-insoluble form of bilirubin.

**Bilirubinemia:** Pathologic condition in which excessive destruction of red blood cells occurs, increasing the amount of bilirubin found in the blood.

**Blackwater fever:** Hemoglobinuria following chronic falciparum malaria infection.

**Bleeding time:** A test used to evaluate the hemostatic role of platelets in vivo.

**Bradykinin:** A plasma kinin.

**Buffy coat:** The layer of leukocyte and platelets lying directly on top of the red cell layer seen after sedimentation or centrifugation.

**Burr cells (echinocytes):** Red cells with approximately 10 to 30 spicules evenly distributed over the surface of the cell.

**C$_1$ esterase inhibitor:** A protein in the blood that inhibits the activity of plasmin as well as the activity of C$_1$ esterase in the complement pathway.

**C3a:** A biologically active fragment of the C3 molecule, which demonstrates anaphylactic capabilities upon liberation.

**C3b:** A biologically active fragment of the complement C3 molecule, which is an opsonin and promotes immune adherence.

**C3d:** A biologically inactive fragment of the C3b complement component formed by inactivation by the C3b inactivator substance present in serum.

**C4:** A component of complement present in serum, which participates in the classic pathway of complement activation.

**C5a:** A biologically active fragment of the C5 molecule, which demonstrates anaphylactic capabilities as well as chemotactic properties upon liberation. This fragment has also been reported to be a potent aggregator of platelets.

**Cabot rings:** A red blood cell inclusion resembling a figure eight. It is usually found in heavily stippled cells.

**Cachexia:** A condition that may result from chronic disease or certain malignancies whereby a state of malnutrition, weakness, and muscle wasting exists.

**Calmodulin:** A cytoplasmic calcium-binding protein.

**Carcinoma:** A new growth or malignant tumor that occurs in epithelial tissue. A neoplasm can infiltrate or metastasize to any tissue or organ of the body.

**Cardiac output:** The amount of blood discharged from the left or right ventricle per minute.

**Catecholamines:** Biologically active amines, epinephrine and norepinephrine, derived from the amino acid tyrosine. They have a marked effect on nervous and cardio-

vascular systems, metabolic rate, temperature, and smooth muscle.

**Celiac:** Related to the abdominal regions.

**Celite:** A substance that acts as a contact activator causing the release of PF3 and the activation of the intrinsic system.

**Central venous pressure:** The pressure within the superior vena cava reflecting the pressure under which the blood is returned to the right atrium.

**Centripetal:** Moving toward the center.

**Cerebriform:** A word that is used to describe the "brainy convolutions" of some nuclear chromatin material.

**CFU-C (colony-forming unit–culture):** Generation of stem cells using tissue culture methods. Current synonym is CFU-Gm, which is a colony-forming unit committed to the production of myeloid cells (granulocytes and monocytes).

**CFU-E (colony-forming unit committed to erythropoiesis):** A stem cell that is committed to forming cells of the red blood cell series.

**Chelation:** Combining of metallic ions with certain heterocyclic ring structures so that the ion is held by chemical bonds from each of the participating rings.

**Chemotactic:** Referring to the ability of white cells to move nondirectionally toward an attractant.

**Chemotaxis:** Describes movement toward a stimulus, particularly that displayed by phagocytic cells toward bacteria and sites of cell injury.

**Chédiak-Higashi inclusions:** Gigantic, fused lysosomal deposits seen in the cytoplasm of leukocytes.

**Cholecystectomy:** Excision of a gallbladder.

**Cholecystitis:** Acute or chronic inflammation of the gallbladder.

**Christmas factor:** Plasma thromboplastin component (PTC); factor IX. Functions in the intrinsic system of coagulation.

**Chromatin:** Located in the nucleus of the cell, this darkly staining substance contains the genetic material composed of DNA attached to a protein structure.

**Chromogenic:** Pigment-producing.

**Circulating anticoagulants:** Acquired pathologic plasma proteins that inhibit normal coagulation. The majority of these pathologic anticoagulants are inhibitors or autoantibodies of the IgG class whose inhibitory effects are directed against a specific factor or a complex of coagulation factors.

**Coagulation:** The process of stopping blood flow from a wound. This process involves the harmonious relationship of the blood clotting factors, the blood vessels and the fibrin forming and fibrin lysing system.

**Coagulopathy:** A disease affecting the blood clotting process.

**Collagen:** A fibrous insoluble protein found in the connective tissue, including skin, bone, ligaments, and cartilage. Collagen represents about 30 percent of the total body protein.

**Complement:** A series of proteins in the circulation that, when sequentially activated, causes disruption of bacterial and other cell membranes. Activation occurs via one of two pathways, and once activated, the components are involved in a great number of immune defense mechanisms including anaphylaxis, chemotaxis, and phagocytosis. Red cell antibodies that activate complement may be capable of causing hemolysis.

**Complement fixation (CF):** An immunologic test.

**Congenital:** Present at birth.

**Consanguinous:** Relationship by blood (i.e., being descended from the common ancestor).

**Contiguous:** In contact or closely associated with.

**Convulsion:** Involuntary muscle contraction and relaxation.

**Cord cells:** Fetal cells obtained from the umbilical cord at birth. They may be contaminated with Wharton's jelly.

**Corticosteroid:** Any of a number of hormonal steroid substances obtained from the cortex of the adrenal gland.

**Coumarin drugs (Warfarin, Coumadin, Dicumarol):** Oral anticoagulants that act as vitamin K antagonists and result in depression of the concentration of prothrombin and factors VII, IX, and X.

**Counterelectrophoresis (CEP):** An immunologic procedure.

**Cryoglobulin:** An abnormal protein in the blood that forms gels at low temperatures.

**Cryoglobulinemia:** An increase in the concentration of cryoglobulins in the blood.

**Cryoprecipitate:** A concentrated source of coagulation factor VIII that has been prepared from a single unit of donor blood. The product also contains fibrinogen, factor XIII, and von Willebrand's factor.

**Cryoprotein:** A protein circulating in the plasma or demonstrable in serum testing that precipitates on exposure to cold temperature.

**Cyanosis:** Slightly bluish or grayish discoloration of the skin caused by accumulation of reduced hemoglobin or deoxyhemoglobin in the blood caused by oxygen deficiency or carbon dioxide buildup.

**Cytochemistry:** The microscopic study of the chemical constituents in cells. The purpose of these studies includes differentiation of cell types and assistance in the diagnosis of hematologic diseases.

**Cytogenetics:** The study of cytology in relation to genetics, especially the chromosomal behavior in mitosis and meiosis.

**Cytomegalovirus (CMV):** One of a group of species-specific herpes viruses.

**Cytopheresis:** A procedure using a machine by which one can selectively remove a particular cell type normally found in peripheral blood of a patient or donor.

**Cytotoxicity:** Ability to destroy.

**Dacrocyte:** See Teardrop cell.

**Defibrinated:** Deprived of fibrin. The conversion of fibrinogen into fibrin is the basis for the clotting of blood.

**Delayed hemolytic transfusion reaction (DHTR):** A hemolytic reaction that occurs when previously sensitized individuals have antibody levels that are undetectable and are once again exposed to the offending antigen(s). In most cases of DHTR the antibodies implicated are IgG.

**Delta:** A type of globin chain found in hemoglobin coded for by the delta gene.

**Desferrioxamine:** Substance obtained from certain bacteria that is used to chelate iron. This substance is used orally or parenterally in treating iron poisoning.

**Diagnosis:** The use of scientific and skillful methods to establish the cause and nature of a disease process.

**Diapedesis:** The journey of the blood cells (i.e., leukocytes) through the unruptured walls of a capillary.

**Diaphoresis:** Profuse sweating.

**Dimorphism:** Existence of a two-cell population in the peripheral smear (e.g., few microcytes, few macrocytes; few hypochromic, few normochromic).

**2,3-Diphosphoglycerate (2,3-DPG):** An organic phosphate in red blood cells that alters the affinity of hemoglobin for oxygen. Blood cells stored in a blood bank lose 2,3-DPG, but once infused the substance is resynthesized or reactivated.

**Disseminated intravascular coagulation:** A pathologic form of coagulation that is diffuse rather than localized, which is characterized by generalized bleeding and shock.

**Diuresis:** Secretion and passage of large amounts of urine.

**Diuretic:** An agent that increases the secretion of urine. Action is in one of two ways: by increasing glomerular filtration or by decreasing reabsorption from the tubules.

**Diurnal:** Occurring during the daytime.

**Diverticulosis:** Outpouching of the colon without inflammation or symptoms. There are many locations of diverticula but all are saccular dilatations protruding from the wall of a tubular organ.

**Döhle bodies:** Single or multiple, round or oval, blue cytoplasmic inclusions (with Romanowsky stain) seen in neutrophils, usually associated with toxicity.

**Donath-Landsteiner antibody test:** A test usually performed in the blood bank to detect the presence of the Donath-Landsteiner antibody, which is a biphasic IgG antibody with anti-P specificity found in patient's suffering from paroxysmal cold hemoglobinuria.

**Dyscrasia:** An old term now used as a synonym for disease.

**Dyserythropoiesis:** Changes in erythroid cell nuclear chromatin pattern; some of these changes are bizarre.

**Dysfibrinogenemia:** A congenital disorder characterized by the synthesis of abnormal fibrinogen molecules with different functional characteristics.

**Dyshematopoiesis:** Abnormalities in the maturation, division, or production of blood cells.

**Dyskeratosis:** Any alteration in the keratinization of the epithelial cells of the epidermis.

**Dysostosis:** Defective ossification.

**Dyspnea:** Labored or difficult breathing.

**Dyspoiesis:** Nuclear-cytoplasmic dissociation especially in red cells.

**EACA:** Epsilon aminocaproic acid; a synthetic inhibitor of plasminogen activation.

**Early degradation products:** The large fragments X and Y that result from the proteolytic action of plasmin on fibrin or fibrinogen. Fragments X and Y have antithrombin activity.

**Ecchymosis:** A form of macula appearing in large, irregularly formed hemorrhagic areas of the skin, originally a blue-black color and changing to greenish brown or yellow.

**Eclampsia:** An acute disorder of pregnant and puerperal women, associated with convulsions and coma.

**Edema:** A local or generalized condition in which the body tissues contain an excessive amount of tissue fluid.

**Edematous:** Pertaining to swelling of body tissues.

**Electrophoresis:** The movement of charged particles

through a medium (paper, agar, gel) in the presence of an electrical field. Useful in the separation and analysis of proteins.

**Elliptocyte:** See Ovalocyte.

**Elution:** A process whereby cells that are coated with antibody are treated in such a manner as to disrupt the bonds between the antigen and antibody. The freed antibody is collected in an inert diluent such as saline or 6 percent albumin. This serum can then be tested to identify its specificity using routine methods. The mechanism to free the antibody may be physical (heat, shaking) or chemical (ether, acid), and the harvested antibody-containing fluid is called an eluate.

**Embolism:** Obstruction of a blood vessel by foreign substances or by a blood clot.

**Embolus:** A mass of undissolved matter present in a blood or lymphatic vessel brought there by the blood or lymph circulation.

**Endemic:** A disease that occurs continuously in a particular population but has a low mortality rate, such as measles. Used in contrast to epidemic.

**Endocarditis:** Inflammation of the lining membrane of the heart. May be due to invasion of microorganisms or an abnormal immunologic reaction.

**Endogenous:** Produced or arising from within a cell or organism.

**Endoplasmic reticulum:** A connecting network of microcanals or tubules running through the cytoplasm of a cell that serves in intracellular transport.

**Endothelium:** A form of squamous epithelium consisting of flat cells that line the blood and lymphatic vessels, the heart, and various other body cavities. It is derived from the mesoderm.

**Endotoxemia:** The presence of endotoxin in the blood; endotoxin is present in the cell of certain bacteria, e.g., gram-negative organisms.

**Eosinophil:** A mature type of granulocyte in which cytoplasmic granules are large, round, and refractile and stain orange or red with Wright's stain. Comprises 0 to 4 percent of the normal differential count.

**Epistaxis:** Hemorrhage from the nose; nosebleed.

**Epsilon:** A type of globin chain found in embryonic hemoglobins.

**Erythroblastosis fetalis:** See Hemolytic disease of the newborn.

**Erythrocyte:** A mature red blood cell or corpuscle.

**Erythrocyte sedimentation rate (ESR):** The rate at which red blood settles per hour. The ESR is affected by three factors: erythrocytes, plasma, and mechanical factors.

**Erythrocytosis:** Abnormal increase in the number of red blood cells in circulation, secondary to many disorders.

**Erythroid hyperplasia:** As seen in the bone marrow, an increase in the number of immature red cell forms; usually a response to anemic stress.

**Erythropoiesis:** The production and maturation of erythrocytes.

**Erythropoietin:** A hormone that regulates red blood cell production.

**Etiology:** The study of the causes of disease.

**Euglobulin:** The fraction of plasma containing fibrinogen, plasminogen, and plasminogen activators with only trace amounts of antiplasmins.

**Euglobulin lysis time:** Coagulation procedure testing for fibrinolysins.

**Exocytosis:** Secretion of the contents of cytoplasmic granules.

**Exogenous:** Originating outside an organ or part.

**Extracorporeal:** Outside of the body.

**Extramedullary hematopoiesis:** Formation of blood cells in sites other than the bone marrow (i.e., liver, spleen).

**Extravascular:** Outside of the blood vessel.

**Extravascular hemolysis:** Hemolysis occurring within the cells of the reticuloendothelial system.

**Factor VIII antigen:** The high molecular weight component of the factor VIII molecule.

**Factor assay:** Coagulation procedure to assay the concentration of specific plasma coagulation factors.

**Factor VIII concentrate:** A commerically prepared source of coagulation factor VIII.

**Favism:** An inherited condition resulting from sensitivity to the fava bean, usually seen in people of Mediterranean origin who have a deficiency in the enzyme glucose-6-phosphate dehydrogenase, which may result in a severe hemolytic episode.

**FDP (fibrinogen-degradation products):** The polypeptide fragments X, Y, D, and E that result from the proteolytic action of plasmin on fibrinogen or fibrin.

**Femto-:** A prefix used in the metric system to signify $10^{-15}$ of any unit. Femtoliter is used in reporting mean corpuscular volume (MCV) of erythrocytes.

**Ferritin:** The storage form of iron in the tissues, which is found principally in the reticuloendothelial cells of the liver, spleen, and bone marrow.

**Fibrin:** A whitish filamentous protein or clot formed by the action of thrombin or fibrinogen, converting it to fibrin.

**Fibrin monomer:** The altered molecule that results from thrombin splitting fibrinopeptides A and B from two of the three paired chains of the fibrinogen molecule.

**Fibrinogen:** A protein produced in the liver that circulates in plasma. In the presence of thrombin, an enzyme produced by the activation of the clotting mechanism, fibrinogen is cleaved into fibrin, which is insoluble protein that is responsible for clot formation.

**Fibrinolysin:** The substance, also called plasmin, that has the ability to dissolve fibrin.

**Fibrinolysis:** Dissolution of fibrin by fibrinolysin caused by the action of proteolytic enzyme system that is continually active in the body but that is increased greatly by various stress stimuli.

**Fibrinopeptides:** Peptides released when fibrinogen is converted to fibrin by thrombin. The fibrinopeptides released by thrombin are designated A and B.

**Fibrin-split products:** Those products that result from fibrin digestion.

**Fibrin-stabilizing factor (FSF):** Factor XIII.

**Fibrosis:** Excessive formation of fibrous tissue.

**Fitzgerald factor:** High molecular weight kininogen (HMWK).

**Fletcher factor:** Prekallikrein.

**Fractures:** The sudden breaking of bones.

**Fragility:** Liability to break, burst, or disintegrate as erythrocytes are prone to do when exposed to varying concentrations of hypotonic salt solutions.

**Fresh frozen plasma (FFP):** A frozen plasma product (from a single donor) that contains all clotting factors, especially the labile factors V and VIII. Useful for clotting factor deficiencies other than hemophilia A, von Willebrand's disease, and hypofibrinogenemia.

**Friable:** Easily broken or pulverized.

**Gallops:** Relating to cardiac rhythms, an abnormal third or fourth heart sound in a patient experiencing tachycardia. Gallops are indicative of a serious heart condition.

**Gamma:** A type of globin chain found in fetal hemoglobin. Two types exist: G gamma contains glycine at position 13 of the amino acid sequence, and A gamma contains alanine at the same position.

**Gamma globulin:** A protein found in plasma and known to be involved in immunity.

**Gammapathy:** Abnormalities of the immune or gamma system arising in a single disordered clone of cells that is able to synthesize immunoglobulin.

**Gastrectomy:** Surgical removal of a part or the whole of the stomach.

**Gastritis:** Inflammation of the stomach, characterized by epigastric pain or tenderness, nausea, vomiting, and systemic electrolyte changes if vomiting persists. The mucosa may be atrophic or hypertrophic.

**Gestation:** In mammals, the length of time from conception to birth.

**Gigantism:** Excessive development of the body or of a part.

**Glanzmann's thrombasthenia:** A congenital bleeding disorder characterized by impaired or absent clot retraction and a failure of the platelets to aggregate with most aggregating agents, particularly with ADP.

**Globin:** A protein constituent of hemoglobin. There are four globin chains in the hemoglobin molecule.

**Glossitis:** Inflammation of the tongue.

**Glycolysis:** Hydrolysis of sugar by an enzyme in the body.

**Glycophorin:** The principal integral blood cell protein, containing 60 percent carbohydrate and giving the red cell its negative charge. It appears on the external surface of the red cell.

**Golgi apparatus:** A lamellar membranous structure near the nucleus of almost all cells. The structure is best seen by electron microscopy. It contains enzymes that add terminal sugar sequences to protein moieties.

**Gout:** Hereditary metabolic disease that is a form of acute arthritis and is marked by inflammation of the joints. The affected joint may be at any location, but gout usually begins in the knee or foot.

**G-6-PD (glucose-6-phosphate dehydrogenase):** An intracellular red cell enzyme important in the hexose monophosphate pathway.

**Granulocyte:** A mature granular leukocyte; refers to band or polymorphonuclear neutrophil, eosinophil, or basophil.

**Granulocytopenia:** Abnormal reduction of granulocytes in the blood.

**Granulomas:** A granular tumor or growth usually of lymphoid and epithelial cells. It occurs in various infectious diseases such as leprosy, cutaneous leishmaniosis, yaws, and syphilis.

**Granulopoiesis:** The production and maturation of granulocytes.

**GVH disease (graft-versus-host disease):** A disorder in which the grafted tissue attacks the host tissue.

**Hageman factor:** Synonym for coagulation factor XII.

**Haplotypes:** A term used in HLA testing to denote the five genes (HLA-A, B, C, D, and DR) on the same chromosome.

**Hapten:** The portion of an antigen containing the grouping on which the specificity is dependent.

**Haptoglobin:** An alpha-2-glycoprotein produced in the liver, having three phenotypes with differing abilities to bind hemoglobin.

**Heinz bodies:** Large red blood cell inclusions that are formed as a result of denatured or precipitated hemoglobin. They may be seen in the thalassemia syndromes, G-6-PD deficiency, or any of the unstable hemoglobin conditions.

**Hemangioma:** A benign tumor of dilated blood vessels.

**Hemarthrosis:** Bloody effusion into the cavity of a joint.

**Hematemesis:** Vomiting of blood.

**Hematocrit:** The proportion of red blood cells in whole blood expressed as a percentage.

**Hematoma:** A swelling or mass of blood confined to an organ, tissue, or space and caused by a break in a blood vessel.

**Hematopoiesis:** Formation and development of blood cells, normally in the bone marrow. Synonym: Hemopoiesis.

**Hematuria:** Blood in the urine.

**Heme:** The iron-containing protoporphyrin portion of the hemoglobin wherein the iron is in the ferrous ($Fe^{++}$) state.

**Hemochromatosis:** A disease of iron metabolism in which iron accumulates in body tissues, causing complications and tissue damage.

**Hemoconcentration:** An increase in the number of red cells, resulting from a decrease in the volume of plasma.

**Hemodialysis:** Removal of chemical substances from the blood by passing it through tubes made of semipermeable membranes. This procedure is used to cleanse the blood of patients in whom one or both kidneys are defective or absent; and remove excess accumulation of drugs or toxic chemicals in the blood.

**Hemoglobin:** The iron-containing pigment of the red blood cells that functions to carry oxygen from the lungs to the tissues. Consists of approximately 6 percent heme and 94 percent globin.

  **H. A:** The major adult hemoglobin (95 percent), composed of two alpha and two beta chains.

  **H. A$_2$:** A small portion of adult hemoglobin (2 to 4 percent), composed of two alpha and two delta chains.

  **H. Bart's:** An abnormal hemoglobin composed of four gamma chains. This is formed in alpha thalassemia major, the most severe form of thalassemia occurring in anemic, edematous stillborn infants whose hemoglobin composition is almost all hemoglobin Bart's.

  **H. F:** The major fetal hemoglobin, composed of two alpha and two gamma chains.

  **H. Gower 1:** A type of hemoglobin found in the embryo, composed of two zeta and two epsilon chains.

  **H. Gower 2:** A type of hemoglobin found in the embryo, composed of two alpha and two epsilon chains.

  **H. H inclusions:** Red cell inclusions that are formed in the alpha thalassemias in which HbH (four beta chains) is in high concentration.

  **H. Lepore:** A type of abnormal hemoglobin that is the product of a fused delta and beta gene formed by an unequal crossing over resulting in a hemoglobin with fused delta/beta chains; a form of thalassemia.

**H. Portland:** A type of hemoglobin found in the embryo, composed of two zeta and two gamma chains.

**Hemoglobinemia:** Presence of hemoglobin in the blood plasma.

**Hemoglobinopathies:** The group of diseases caused by or associated with the presence of one of several forms of abnormal hemoglobin in the blood.

**Hemoglobin-oxygen dissociation curve:** The relationship between the percent saturation of the hemoglobin molecule with oxygen and the environmental oxygen tension.

**Hemoglobinuria:** The presence of hemoglobin (in the urine) freed from lysed red blood cells. Occurs when hemoglobin from disintegrating red blood cells, rapid hemolysis, or red cells exceed the ability of the blood proteins to combine the hemoglobin.

**Hemolysin:** An antibody that activates complement, leading to cell lysis.

**Hemolysis:** The destruction of red blood cells.

**Intravascular h.:** Refers to the disruption of the red cell membrane and release of hemoglobin into the surrounding fluid within the vasculature.

**Extravascular h.:** Refers to the phagocytosis of erythrocytes by the reticuloendothelial system (RES), primarily in the spleen and liver.

**Hemolytic:** Pertaining to, characterized by, or producing hemolysis.

**H. anemia:** Anemia caused by increased destruction of erythrocytes.

**H. disease of the newborn (HDN):** A disease characterized by anemia, jaundice, enlargement of the liver and spleen, and generalized edema (hydrops fetalis), owing to the maternal IgG antibodies that cross the placenta and attack fetal red cells when there is a fetomaternal blood group incompatibility. Usually caused by ABO or Rh antibodies. Synonym: Erythroblastosis fetalis.

**H. uremic syndrome (HUS):** A disorder that usually affects young children and is characterized by the combination of severe hemolytic anemia and renal failure. Reticulocytosis and schistocytes are the morphologic findings of this microangiopathic hemolytic anemia.

**Hemopexin:** A beta-1-globulin that has the capacity to bind hemoglobin when haptoglobin has been depleted.

**Hemophilia:** A hereditary blood disease characterized by impaired coagulability of the blood and a strong tendency to bleed.

**H. A:** A sex-linked hereditary bleeding disorder characterized by greatly prolonged coagulation time owing to a deficiency of factor VIII.

**H. B:** "Christmas disease," a hereditary bleeding disorder caused by a deficiency of factor IX.

**H. C:** A hereditary bleeding disorder caused by a deficiency of factor XI.

**Hemopoiesis:** Formation of blood cells. Synonym: Hematopoiesis.

**Hemoptysis:** Coughing and spitting of blood as a result of bleeding from any part of respiratory tract.

**Hemorrhage:** Abnormal internal or external bleeding. May be venous, arterial, or capillary from blood vessels into the tissues, into or from the body.

**Hemorrhagic diathesis:** Predisposition to spontaneous bleeding from a trivial trauma caused by a defect in clotting or in the structure or function of blood vessels.

**Hemosiderin:** An iron-containing pigment derived from hemoglobin upon disintegration of red cells. It is one method whereby iron is stored until it is needed for making hemoglobin.

**Hemosiderinuria:** The excretion of hemosiderin from disintegrated red blood cells into the urine.

**Hemosiderosis:** A condition in which the iron content of blood is increased.

**Hemostasis:** The process in which blood clots and bleeding is arrested.

**Hemotherapy:** Blood transfusion as a therapeutic measure.

**HEMPAS:** Hereditary erythrocytic multinuclearity with a positive acid serum (Ham's test). A type II congenital dyserythropoietic anemia (CDA).

**Heparin:** A sulfonated mucopolysaccharide that acts as a powerful anticoagulant at several sites in the coagulation sequence: (1) inhibition of thrombin, (2) inhibition of factor Xa, (3) inhibition of factor IXa, and (4) inhibition of factor XIIa. Used therapeutically in the treatment of thromboembolic disease.

**Hepatitis:** Inflammation of the liver.

**Hepatosplenomegaly:** Enlargement of the liver and the spleen.

**Hereditary:** Transmitted from parent to offspring.

**Hereditary angioneurotic edema:** A disease state in which there is no inhibition of C1 enzyme activity. There are increased levels of plasmin and complement activator.

**Hereditary elliptocytosis (HE):** An inherited (autosomal dominant) intracorpuscular defect of the red cell membrane that is characterized by the presence of greater than 40 percent elliptical red cells on the peripheral smear. The condition is generally asymptomatic. There is a biochemical and genetic relationship to hereditary pyropoikilocytosis (HPP).

**Hereditary hemorrhagic telangiectasia:** A congenital hemorrhagic abnormality of the vascular system characterized by localized dilation and convolution of capillaries and venules giving rise to the characteristic telangiectases.

**Hereditary persistence of fetal hemoglobin (HPFH):** A group of conditions characterized by the persistence of fetal hemoglobin synthesis into adult life.

**Hereditary pyropoikilocytosis (HPP):** A relatively rare and severe autosomal recessive hemolytic anemia characterized by striking bizarre micropoikilocytosis in which the red cells bud, fragment, and form microspherocytes. In addition, the red cells are thermally unstable when heated to 45°C and strikingly fragmented in comparison to normal red cells which fragment only at 49°C.

**Hereditary spherocytosis (HS):** An inherited (autosomal dominant) intracorpuscular defect of the red cell membrane (altered spectrin) that results in the most common hereditary hemolytic anemia found in Caucasians. The morphologic hallmark of hereditary spherocytosis is the presence of spherocytes on the peripheral blood smear.

**Hereditary stomatocytosis (hereditary hydrocytosis):** A heterogenous group of rare red cell membrane disorders inherited in an autosomal dominant fashion that are characterized by the presence of stomatocytes on the peripheral smear and alterations in the permeability of the red cell membrane to cations.

**Hereditary thrombophilia:** Antithrombin III deficiency; an autosomal dominant disorder in which there is an increased tendency toward thrombosis.

**Heterozygous:** Possessing different alleles in regard to a given characteristic.

**Histamine:** A substance normally present in the body that is released by the mast cells and basophils. It exerts a pharmacologic action when released from injured cells.

**Histiocyte:** A large fixed macrophage. See also Macrophage.

**Hodgkin's disease:** A disease of unknown etiology producing enlargement of lymphoid tissue, spleen, and liver, with invasion of other tissues.

**Homozygous:** Possessing identical alleles in regard to a given characteristic.

**Howell-Jolly bodies:** Red cell inclusions that develop in periods of accelerated or abnormal erythropoiesis. They represent nuclear remnants containing DNA.

**Humoral:** Pertaining to body fluids or substances contained in them.

**Hybridization:** The production of hybrids by crossbreeding.

**Hybridoma:** A neoplastic cell.

**Hydrops fetalis:** Erythroblastosis fetalis. A hemolytic disease of the newborn characterized by anemia, jaundice, enlargement of liver and spleen, and generalized edema.

**Hypercoagulability:** A condition in which activated coagulation factors are found intravascularly; may or may not be associated with increased incidence of thromboembolus.

**Hyperkalemia:** Excessive amounts of potassium in the blood.

**Hyperplasia:** Excessive proliferation of normal cells in the normal tissue arrangement of an organ.

**Hypersegmentation:** An increase in the number of nuclear lobes or segments (>6) in segmented neutrophils; especially characteristic in vitamin $B_{12}$ or folate deficiencies.

**Hypersplenism:** A condition arising as a result of an enlarged spleen. Red cell survival is significantly shortened.

**Hypertension:** Increase in blood pressure to above normal.

**Hyperviscosity:** Excessive viscosity or exaggeration of adhesive properties seen in anemias and inflammatory disease.

**Hypochromia:** Increased area of central pallor in red cells.

**Hypofibrinogenemia:** A congenital disorder characterized by low levels of fibrinogen, usually without any bleeding tendencies.

**Hypogammaglobulinemia:** Decreased blood levels of gamma globulins seen in some disease states.

**Hypogonadism:** Defective internal secretion of the gonads.

**Hyposplenism:** Decreased or improper splenic function. There are a variety of conditions and splenic sizes associated with hyposplenism; however, all have in common hematologic manifestations that suggest loss of many or all of the vital splenic functions (e.g., Howell-Jolly bodies, Pappenheimer's bodies, poikilocytes, increased platelet count).

**Hypotension:** Decrease in blood pressure to below normal.

**Hypothermia:** Having a body temperature below normal.

**Hypothyroidism:** A condition due to deficiency of the thyroid secretion, resulting in a lowered basal metabolism.

**Hypovolemia:** Diminished blood volume.

**Hypoxia:** Deficiency of oxygen.

**Icterus:** A condition characterized by yellowish skin, eyes, mucous membranes, and body fluids owing to deposition of excess bilirubin.

**Idiopathic:** Pertaining to conditions without clear pathogenesis or to disease without recognizable cause, as of spontaneous origin.

**Idiopathic thrombocytopenic purpura (ITP):** Bleeding due to a decreased number of platelets; the etiology is unknown, with most evidence pointing to platelet autoantibodies.

**Idiothrombocythemia:** An increase in blood platelets with unknown etiology.

**Immune response:** The reaction of the body to substances that are foreign or are interpreted as being foreign. Cell-mediated or cellular immunity pertains to tissue destruction mediated by T cells, such as graft rejection and hypersensitivity reactions. Humoral immunity pertains to cell destruction response during the early period of the reaction.

**Immune serum globulin:** Gamma globulin protein fraction of serum containing antibodies.

**Immunoblast:** A mitotically active T or B cell.

**Immunodeficiency:** A decrease in the normal concentration of immunoglobulins in serum.

**Immunogenicity:** The ability of an antigen to stimulate an antibody response.

**Immunoglobulin:** One of a family of closely related yet not identical proteins that are capable of acting as antibodies; they are IgA, IgD, IgE, IgG, and IgM. IgA is the principal immunoglobin in exocrine secretions such as saliva and tears. IgD may play a role in antigen recognition and the initiation of antibody synthesis. IgE is produced by the cells lining the intestinal and respiratory tracts and is important in forming reagin. IgG is the main immunoglobulin in human serum. IgM is a globulin formed in almost every immune response during the early period of the reaction.

**Immunologic memory:** The development of T and B memory cells that have been sensitized by exposure to an antigen and respond rapidly under subsequent encounters with the antigen.

**Immunologic unresponsiveness:** Development of a "tolerance" to certain antigens that would otherwise evoke an immune response.

**Immunoprecipitin:** An antigen-antibody reaction that results in precipitation.

**Inflammation:** Tissue reaction to injury. The succession of changes that occurs in living tissue when it is injured.

**Inhibitor:** A chemical substance that stops enzyme activity.

**Insidious:** Without warning.

**Insomnia:** Inability to sleep, or sleep prematurely ended or interrupted by periods of wakefulness.

**Interferon:** A protein or proteins formed when cells are exposed to viruses. Noninfected cells exposed to interferon are protected against viral infection.

**Intravascular hemolysis:** Hemolysis occurring within the blood vessels. See Hemolysis.

**Intrinsic factor (IF):** A protein secreted by the parietal cells of the stomach that is necessary for vitamin $B_{12}$ absorption.

**Intrinsic system:** Initiation of blood clotting that occurs through a surface-mediated pathway.

**In utero:** Within the uterus.

**In vitro:** In glass, as in a test tube.

**In vivo:** In the living body or organism.

**Ischemia:** Local and temporary deficiency of blood supply caused by obstruction of the circulation to a part.

**Isoagglutinins:** A term used to denote the ABO antibodies anti-A, anti-B, and anti-A,B.

**Isoimmune:** An antibody produced against a foreign antigen in the same species.

**Jaundice:** A condition characterized by yellowing of the skin and the whites of the eyes. One cause is excess hemolysis, which results in increased circulating bilirubin. Another cause is liver damage caused by hepatitis.

**Juvenile:** A "common usage" term that is a synonym for neutrophilic metamyelocyte.

**Kaolin:** A surface-activating substance.

**Karyorrhexis:** A necrotic stage with fragmentation of the nucleus whereby chromatin is distributed irregularly throughout the cytoplasm.

**Karyotype:** A photomicrograph of a single cell in the metaphase stage of mitosis that is arranged to show the chromosomes in descending order of size.

**Keratocyte:** A term synonymous with burr cell.

**Kernicterus:** A form of icterus neonatorum occurring in infants. Develops at 2 to 8 days of age. Prognosis is poor if untreated.

**Ketosis:** The accumulation in the body of the ketone bodies: acetone, beta hydroxybutyric acid, and acetoacetic acid.

**Kinin:** A general term for a group of polypeptides that have considerable biologic activity (for example, vasoactivity).

**Kleihauer-Betke technique:** An acid elution test used to quantitate the amount of fetal hemoglobin present. Fetal hemoglobin is more resistant than adult hemoglobin to elution at acid pH during this procedure, and stains red.

**Koilonychia:** A disorder of the nails, which are abnormally thin and concave from side to side, with the edges turned up.

**Late degradation products:** The terminal fragments D and E that result from the proteolytic action of plasmin on fibrin or fibrinogen. Fragments D and E are known to inhibit fibrin polymerization.

**Lepore:** See Hemoglobin Lepore.

**Leptocyte:** Synonymous with target cells.

**Lethargic:** Sluggish; having a lack of energy.

**Leukemia:** A chronic or acute disease of unknown etiologic factors characterized by unrestrained growth of leukocytes and their precursors in the tissues.

**Leukemoid reaction:** A moderate or advanced degree of leukocytosis in the blood that is not a result of a leukemic disease. These reactions are frequently observed as a feature of infectious disease, drug and chemical intoxication, or secondary to nonhematopoietic carcinoma.

**Leukoagglutinins:** Antibodies to white blood cells.

**Leukocytosis:** Increase in number of leukocytes (more than 10,000/mm³) in the blood.

**Leukoerythroblastosis:** Refers to the presence of immature white cells and nucleated red cells on the blood smear. This frequently denotes a malignant or myeloproliferative process.

**Leukopheresis:** Withdrawal of leukocytes from the circulation. Procedure may be used to obtain leukocytes for administration to patients with severe granulocytopenia.

**Lymphadenitis:** Inflammation of the lymph nodes.

**Lymphadenopathy:** Disease of the lymph nodes.

**Lymphocyte:** A white blood cell formed in lymphoid tissue throughout the body, generally described as nongranular and including small and large varieties. Comprises approximately 20 to 45 percent of the total leukocyte count.

**Lymphocytosis:** An increase in lymphocytes within the blood.

**Lymphoma:** Asymmetrical enlargement of a group of lymph nodes, which destroys the normal histologic lymph node architecture.

**Lysosomes:** Part of an intracellular digestive system that exists as separate particles in the cell. Even though their importance in health and disease is certain, all the precise ways lysosomes affect changes are not understood.

**Lysozyme (muramidase):** A hydrolytic enzyme destructive to cell walls of certain bacteria. It is present in body fluids and found in high concentration within granulocytes.

**Macrocyte:** A red cell 9 $\mu$ in diameter or larger.

**Macrocephaly:** Enlargement of the head.

**$\alpha_2$ Macroglobulin:** A protease inhibitor present in the blood that inhibits the activity of plasmin.

**Macroglobulinemia:** Abnormal presence of high molecular weight immunoglobulins (IgM) in the blood.

**Macrophage:** Cells of the reticuloendothelial system having the ability to phagocytose particulate substances and to store vital dyes and other colloidal substances. They are found in loose connective tissues and various organs of the body.

**Major histocompatibility complex (MHC):** Present in all mammalian and ovarian species. Analogous to human HLA complex. HLA antigens are within the MHC at a locus on chromosome 6.

**Malabsorption syndrome:** Disordered or inadequate absorption of nutrients from the intestinal tract. May be due to a disease that affects the intestinal mucosa such as infections, tropical sprue, gluten enteropathy, or pancreatic insufficiency or due to antibiotic therapy.

**Malaria:** An acute and sometimes chronic infectious disease due to the presence of protozoan parasites within red blood cells.

**Mast cell:** A tissue basophil. See Basophil.

**Mastoiditis:** Inflammation of the air cells of the mastoid process.

**Mean corpuscular hemoglobin (MCH):** A measure of hemoglobin content of red corpuscles. It is reported in picograms.

$$MCH = \frac{\text{Hemoglobin in g/100 ml} \times 10}{\text{Red blood cell count, millions}/\mu l}$$

**Mean corpuscular hemoglobin concentration (MCHC):** A measure of concentration of hemoglobin in the average red cell.

$$MCHC = \frac{\text{Hemoglobin in g/100 ml} \times 100}{\text{Hematocrit, percent}}$$

**Mean corpuscular volume (MCV):** A measure of the volume of red corpuscles expressed in cubic micrometers or femtoliters.

$$MCV = \frac{\text{Hematocrit, percent} \times 10}{\text{Red blood cell count, millions}/\mu l}$$

**Mediastinal:** Related to the mediastinum.

**Mediastinum:** A septum or cavity between two principal portions of an organ.

**Medullary:** Concerning marrow or medulla.

**Megakaryocyte:** The intermediate platelet precursor cell in the bone marrow, not normally present in peripheral blood. It is a large cell, usually having a multilobed nucleus, that gives rise to blood platelets due to a pinching off of the cytoplasm.

**Megaloblast:** A large-sized, nucleated, abnormal red cell precursor, 11 to 20 microns in diameter, oval and slightly irregular, resulting from a nuclear/cytoplasmic maturation asynchrony characteristic of vitamin $B_{12}$ or folate deficiency.

**Megaloblastoid:** Term used to describe changes in the bone marrow that are morphologically similar to, yet etiologically different from, megaloblastic change.

**Meiosis:** Type of cell division of germ cells in which two successive divisions of the nucleus produce cells that contain half the number of chromosomes present in somatic cells.

**Melena:** Black tarry feces due to the action of intestinal juices on free blood.

**Menorrhagia:** Menstrual bleeding that is excessive in number of days or amount of blood, or both.

**Menstruation:** The periodic discharge of a bloody fluid from the uterus, occurring at more or less regular intervals during the life of a woman from age of puberty to menopause.

**Metamyelocyte:** An immature neutrophilic granulocyte with a nucleus that is "kidney bean" shaped or just starts to indent, and the presence of specific granules (either neutrophilic, eosinophilic, or basophilic) in the cytoplasm (e.g., neutrophilic metamyelocyte, eosinophilic metamyelocyte, basophilic metamyelocyte).

**Metaphyseal dysostosis:** Defective bone formation in the metaphysis—the portion of a developing long bone between diaphysis or shaft and epiphysis.

**Metaplasia:** Conversion of one kind of tissue into a form that is not normal for that tissue.

**Metarubricyte:** Synonym for orthochromic normoblast. (See Orthochromic normoblast.)

**Metastasis:** Movement of bacteria or body cell, especially cancer cells, from one part of the body to another. Change in location of a disease or of its manifestations or transfer from one organ or part to another not directly connected. Spread is by the lymphatics or bloodstream.

**Metastatic:** Pertaining to metastasis which is a manifestation of a malignancy as a secondary growth in a new location. Spread is by the lymphatics or bloodstream.

**Methemoglobin:** A form of hemoglobin wherein the ferrous ion ($Fe^{++}$) has been oxidized to ferric ion ($Fe^{+++}$). This may be due to toxic substances such as aniline dyes, potassium chlorate, or nitrate-contaminated water.

**Microaggregates:** Aggregates of platelets and leukocytes that accumulate in stored blood.

**Microcephaly:** Abnormal smallness of the head, often seen in mental retardation; it is congenital.

**Microspherocytes:** Small, sphere-shaped red blood cells seen in certain kinds of anemia.

**Mitochondria:** Slender microscopic filaments or rods 0.5 $\mu m$ in diameter that can be seen in cells by using phase-contrast microscopy or electron microscopy. They are a source of energy in the cell and are involved in protein synthesis and lipid metabolism.

**Mitosis:** Type of cell division in which each daughter cell contains the same number of chromosomes as the parent cell. All cells except sex cells undergo mitosis.

**Mixed field:** A type of agglutination pattern in which there are numerous small clumps of cells amid a sea of free cells.

**MLC:** Mixed lymphocyte culture.

**MLR:** Mixed lymphocyte reaction.

**Monoclonal:** Antibody derived from a single ancestral antibody-producing parent cell.

**Monocyte:** A white blood cell that normally constitutes 2 to 10 percent of the total leukocyte staining count. This cell is 9 to 12 $\mu$ in diameter and has an indented nucleus and an abundant pale blue-gray cytoplasm containing many fine red-staining granules.

**Morbidity:** The number of sick persons or cases of disease in relationship to a specific population.

**Mortality:** The death rate; ratio of number of deaths to a given population.

**Multiparous:** Having borne more than one child.

**Multiple myeloma:** A neoplastic proliferation of plasma cells, characterized by very high immunoglobulin levels of monoclonal origin.

**Mutant:** A variation of genetic structure that breeds true.

**Mutation:** A change in a gene potentially capable of being transmitted to offspring.

  **Point m.:** A change in a base in DNA that can lead to a change in the amino acid incorporated into the polypeptide. The change is identifiable by analyzing the amino acid sequences of the original protein and its mutant offspring.

  **Frameshift m.:** A change in which a message is read incorrectly because either a base is missing or an extra base is added. This results in an entirely new polypeptide since the triplet sequence has been shifted one base.

**Myeloblast:** The first recognizable "mother cell" (precursor) of the granulocytic cell line.

**Myelocyte:** An immature neutrophilic granulocyte characterized by an eccentrically located round nucleus and specific granules, either neutrophilic, eosinophilic, or basophilic (e.g., neutrophilic myelocyte, eosinophilic myelocyte, basophilic myelocyte).

**Myelodysplasia:** Abnormal division; maturation and production of erythrocytes, granulocytes, monocytes, and platelets.

**Myelodysplastic syndrome (MDS):** A group of primary hematologic disorders associated with abnormal division, maturation, and production of erythrocytes, granulocytes, monocytes, and platelets; also referred to as preleukemic syndrome.

**Myelofibrosis:** Replacement of the bone marrow by fibrous tissue.

**Myeloperoxidase:** An enzyme that is present in the primary (azurophilic) granules of PMN, eosinophils, and monocytes-macrophages.

**Myelophthisic:** The process that occurs primarily in the bone marrow as a result of the crowding out of normal elements by a neoplasm, histiocytic type cells, and so on. A consequent reduction in normal marrow cells and release of immature hematopoietic cells (especially nucleated red cells) into the blood occurs.

**Myeloproliferative:** A group of disorders characterized by autonomous proliferation of one or more hemopoietic elements in the bone marrow. In many cases, the liver and spleen are enlarged.

**Necrosis:** The pathologic death of one or more cells of a portion of tissue or organ.

**Neonatal:** Pertaining to the first six weeks after birth.

**Neoplasm:** A new and abnormal formation of tissue, as a tumor or growth.

**Neuraminidase:** An enzyme that cleaves sialic acid from the red cell membrane.

**Neutralization:** Inactivating an antibody by reacting it with an antigen against which it is directed.

**Neutropenia:** The presence of abnormally small numbers of neutrophils in the circulating blood.

**Neutrophil:** A medium-sized mature leukocyte, with a three-to-five-lobed nucleus, and cytoplasm containing small lilac-staining granules. Normally constitutes 50 to 70 percent of leukocytes in the blood.

**Nondisjunction:** Failure of a pair of chromosomes to separate during meiosis.

**Nonresponder:** An individual whose immune system does not respond well in antibody formation to antigenic stimulation.

**Obstetric:** Referring to the branch of medicine that concerns itself with the management of women during pregnancy, childbirth, and puerperium.

**Oculocutaneous:** Relating to the eyes and the skin.

**Oliguria:** Diminished amount of urine formation.

**Oncogenic:** Tumor-forming.

**Opisthotonus:** Extreme aching in the spine.

**Opsonin:** Substance in the blood serum that acts upon microorganisms and other cells, facilitating phagocytosis.

**Organomegaly:** Enlargement of any of the specific organs of the body.

**Orthochromic (orthochromatophilic) normoblast:** An immature red cell precursor characterized by pink cytoplasm and a small round pyknotic nucleus. This stage of maturation is normally found only in the bone marrow.

**Orthodontic:** Referring to the branch of dentistry that deals with the prevention and correction of irregularities of the teeth.

**Orthostatic hypotension:** Decreased blood pressure in an erect position.

**Osmolality:** The osmotic concentration of a solution determined by the ionic concentration of dissolved substances per unit of solvent.

**Osmotic fragility:** The ability of the red cells to withstand different salt concentration; this is dependent on the volume, surface area, and functional state of the red blood cell membrane.

**Osteoclast:** Giant multinuclear cell formed in the bone marrow of growing bones.

**Osteomyelitis:** Inflammation of the bone—especially the marrow—caused by a pathogenic organism.

**Osteoporosis:** Increased porosity of the bone, seen most often in the elderly.

**Ovalocyte:** An abnormal red cell that is egg shaped or elliptical. Synonym: Elliptocyte.

**Oxyhemoglobin:** The combined form of hemoglobin and oxygen.

**P50:** The partial pressure of oxygen or oxygen tension at which the hemoglobin molecule is 50 percent saturated with oxygen.

**Pagophagia:** The craving to eat ice.

**Pallor:** Paleness; lack of color.

**Panagglutinin:** An antibody capable of agglutinating all red blood cells tested, including the patient's own cells.

**Pancytopenia:** A depression of each of the normal bone marrow elements: white cells, red cells, and platelets in the peripheral blood.

**Panel:** A large number of group O reagent red cells that are of known antigenic characterization and are used for antibody identification.

**Panmyelosis:** Increase in all the elements of the bone marrow.

**Papilledema:** Edema and inflammation of the optic nerve at its point of entrance into the eyeball.

**Pappenheimer's bodies:** Basophilic inclusions in the red blood cell that are cluster-like. They are believed to be iron particles; confirmation is made by Prussian blue stain.

**Parachromatin:** The portions of the nuclear chromatin that are nonstained or lightly stained.

**Paracoagulants:** A variety of substances capable of converting soluble fibrin monomer complexes into insoluble fibrin. These include protamine sulfate, ethanol, and material from staphylococci.

**Paracoagulation tests:** Coagulation procedures used to indicate the presence of soluble fibrin monomer complexes, which is indirect evidence of the action of thrombin on fibrinogen.

**Paraproteinemia:** A general term for abnormalities of the immunoglobulins, associated with one of several disease states.

**Parenchymal:** Relating to parenchyma, the essential parts of an organ that are concerned with its function in contradistinction to its framework.

**Parenteral:** Entry into the body through the IV or the IM route rather than the alimentary route.

**Paresis:** Partial or incomplete paralysis.

**Paresthesia:** Numbness.

**Paroxysm:** A sudden, periodic attack or recurrence of symptoms of a disease.

**Paroxysmal cold hemoglobinuria (PCH):** A type of cold autoimmune hemolytic anemia usually found in children suffering from viral infections in which a biphasic IgG antibody can be demonstrated with anti-P specificity. See also Donath-Landsteiner test.

**Paroxysmal nocturnal hemoglobinuria (PNH):** An uncommon acquired form of hemolysis caused by an intrinsic defect in the red blood cell membrane, rendering it more susceptible to hemolysins in an acid environment, and characterized by hemoglobin in the urine following periods of sleep.

**Pathogenesis:** Origination and development of a disease.

**Pathognomonic:** Specifically distinctive or characteristic of a disease or pathologic condition.

**PCT:** Prothrombin consumption test, a test that measures prothrombin activity in serum after coagulation has taken place.

**Perfusion:** Supplying an organ or tissue with nutrients and oxygen by passing blood or a suitable fluid through it.

**Perioral paresthesia:** Tingling around the mouth occasionally experienced by apheresis donors, resulting from the rapid return of citrated plasma, which contains citrate-bound calcium and free citrate.

**Peroxidase:** An enzyme that hastens the transfer of oxygen from peroxide to a tissue that requires oxygen; this process is essential to intracellular respiration.

**Petechiae:** Pinpoint hemorrhages from arterioles, venules.

**Phagocytosis:** Ingestion and digestion of bacteria and particles by phagocytes.

**Pharmacologic:** Relating to the study of drugs and their origin, natural properties, and effects on living organisms.

**Phlebotomy:** Surgical opening of a vein to withdraw blood.

**Phosphoglyceromutase (PGM):** A red cell enzyme.

**Photodermatitis:** Lesion development upon exposure to sunlight.

**Phototherapy:** Exposure to sunlight or artificial light for therapeutic purposes.

**Pica:** A perversion of appetite with ingestion of material not fit for food, such as starch, clay, ashes, or plaster.

**Pico-:** A prefix used in the metric system to signify $10^{-12}$. Picogram is used in reporting the mean corpuscular hemoglobin (MCH).

**Pinocytosis:** Process by which cells absorb or ingest nutrients and fluid.

**Pinguecula:** A yellowish discoloration near the corneal-scleral junction of the eye.

**Plaques:** Small flat growths.

**Plasma:** The liquid portion of whole blood containing water, electrolytes, glucose, fats, proteins, and gases. Contains all the clotting factors necessary for coagulation but in an inactive form. Once coagulation occurs, the fluid is converted to serum.

**Plasma cell:** A B lymphocyte–derived cell that secretes immunoglobulins or antibodies.

**Plasma protein fraction (PPF):** Also known as Plasman-

ate. Sterile pooled plasma stored as a fluid or freeze-dried. Used for volume replacement.

**Plasma thromboplastin antecedent (PTA):** See Christmas factor.

**Plasmacytomas:** Localized or generalized tumor masses of plasma cells.

**Plasmapheresis:** Removal of blood, separation of plasma by centrifugation, and reinjection of the cells into the body. Used as a means of obtaining plasma and in the treatment of certain pathologic conditions.

**Plasmin:** Fibrinolytic enzyme derived from its precursor plasminogen.

**Plasminogen:** A protein found in many tissues and body fluids. It is important in preventing fibrin clot formation.

**Plasmodium:** See Malaria.

**Platelet:** A round or oval disc, 2 to 4 microns in diameter, that is derived from the cytoplasma of the megakaryocyte, a large cell in the bone marrow. Plays an important role in blood coagulation, hemostasis, and blood thrombus formation.

**Platelet adhesion:** The interaction of platelet surface glycoproteins with connective tissue elements of the subendothelium, requiring von Willebrand's factor as a plasma cofactor.

**Platelet aggregation:** Platelet-to-platelet interaction dependent on calcium.

**Platelet concentrate:** Platelets prepared from a single unit of whole blood or plasma and suspended in a specific volume of the original plasma. Also known as random donor platelets.

**Platelet factor 3 (PF3):** A phospholipid found within the platelet membrane required for coagulation. PF3 assays are used to evaluate platelet disorders.

**Platelet plug:** Platelets that function in arresting bleeding by "plugging" any damage in the vessel wall and providing phospholipids essential for blood coagulation. The development of a hemostatic platelet plug depends on adhesion, aggregation, and consolidation.

**Plateletpheresis:** A procedure using a machine by which one can selectively remove platelets from a donor or patient.

**Platelin:** A substance that acts in vitro like PF3.

**Plethoric:** Congestion causing distention of the blood vessels.

**Pleural effusion:** Fluid in the pleural space.

**PMN (polymorphonuclear neutrophil):** A mature granulocyte with neutrophilic granules and a segmented nucleus (also called segmented neutrophil). See Neutrophil.

**Pneumonitis:** Inflammation of the lung.

**Poikilocytosis:** Variation in shape of red cells.

**Polyacrylamide gel:** A type of matrix used in electrophoresis upon which substances are separated.

**Polyagglutination:** A state in which an individual's red cells are agglutinated by all sera regardless of blood type.

**Polyclonal:** Antibodies derived from more than one antibody-producing parent cell.

**Polychromasia:** In evaluating red blood cell morphology, this term refers to the blue-gray color of some younger red cells. Increased polychromasia is a sign of a very active bone marrow.

**Polychromatophilic normoblast:** An immature red cell precursor characterized by blue-gray cytoplasm and round, eccentrically located nucleus with a distinct chromatin/parachromatin pattern of staining, and normally only found in the bone marrow. Synonym: Rubricyte.

**Polycythemia:** An excess of red blood cells in the peripheral blood.

 **P. vera:** A chronic life-shortening myeloproliferative disorder involving all bone marrow elements, characterized by an increase in red blood cell mass and hemoglobin concentration.

**Polymorphism:** A genetic system that possesses numerous allelic forms, such as a blood group system.

**Polyspecific Coombs' sera:** A reagent that contains antihuman globulin sera against IgG immunoglobulin and C3d.

**Porphyria:** A group of inherited disorders caused by excessive production of porphyrins in the bone marrow or the liver. Two types are recognized: erythropoietic and hepatic.

**Portal hypertension:** Increased pressure in the portal vein as a result of obstruction of the flow of blood through the liver.

**Postpartum:** Occurring after childbirth.

**Precipitation:** The formation of a visible complex (precipitate) in a medium containing soluble antigen (precipitinogen) and the corresponding antibody (precipitin).

**Precipitin:** An antibody formed in the blood serum of an animal by the presence of a soluble antigen, usually a protein. When added to a solution of the antigen, it brings about precipitation. The injected protein is called the antigen and the antibody produced is the precipitin.

**Preleukemia (myelodysplastic syndrome):** A clinical syndrome in which the bone marrow shows marked hypocellularity with clusters of immature cells that in many cases evolve into true nonlymphocytic leukemia.

**Priapism:** Abnormal, painful, and continued erection of the penis owing to disease, accompanied by loss of sexual desire.

**Primary fibrinolysis:** Activation of the fibrinolytic system that is not secondary to coagulation.

**Primary hemostasis:** The interaction of platelets and the vascular endothelium to stop bleeding following vascular injury.

**Proaccelerin:** Factor V; functions in the common pathway of coagulation as a cofactor.

**Proband:** The initial subject presenting a mental or physical disorder; the hereditary of this individual is studied in order to determine if other members of the family have had the same disease or carry it. Synonym: Propositus.

**Proconvertin:** Factor VII, functions in the extrinsic system of coagulation.

**Prodrome:** A symptom indicative of an approaching disease.

**Progranulocyte:** An immature white blood cell precursor found only in the bone marrow that is the characteristic stage of maturation where azurophilic nonspecific granules first appear in the cytoplasm of the granulocytic cell line.

**Pronormoblast:** The first recognizable "mother cell" (precursor) of the erythrocytic cell line. Synonym: Rubriblast.

**Prophylaxis:** Any agent or regimen that contributes to the prevention of infection and disease.

**Propositus:** The initial individual whose condition led to investigation of a hereditary disorder or to a serologic evaluation of family members. Feminine form is proposita. Synonym: Proband.

**Proprioception:** The awareness of posture, movement, and changes in equilibrium and the knowledge of position, weight, and resistance of objects in relation to the body.

**Prorubricyte:** See Basophilic normoblast.

**Prostaglandins:** A group of fatty acid derivatives present in many tissues, including prostate gland, menstrual fluid, brain, lung, kidney, thymus, seminal fluid, and pancreas.

**Prosthesis:** Replacement of a missing part by an artificial substitute, such as an artificial extremity.

**Prostration:** Absolute exhaustion.

**Protamine sulfate:** A substance used to detect the presence of soluble fibrin monomer complexes. It is also used to neutralize the effects of heparin. See also Paracoagulants.

**Prothrombin:** Factor II. Functions in the common pathway of coagulation.

**Prothrombin complex:** A commercially prepared concentrate of the vitamin K–dependent factors, prothrombin and factors VII, IX, and X in lypholized form. Preparations of prothrombin complex are used therapeutically to treat acquired and congenital hemorrhagic disorders.

**Prothrombin time (PT):** A test to evaluate the overall integrity of the clotting system that involves factors VII, X, V, II, and I. Commonly referred to as a means of evaluating the extrinsic system of coagulation.

**Protoporphyrin:** A porphyrin whose iron complex forms the heme of hemoglobin and the prosthetic groups of myoglobin and certain respiratory pigments.

**PRP:** Platelet-rich plasma.

**Pulmonary artery wedge pressure:** Pressure measured in the pulmonary artery at its capillary end.

**Pulse pressure:** The difference between the systolic and the diastolic blood pressures.

**Punctate:** Having pinpoint punctures or depressions on the surface; marked with dots.

**Purpura:** A condition with various manifestations and diverse causes, characterized by hemorrhages into the skin, mucous membranes, internal organs, and other tissues.

**Pyelogram:** A roentgen picture of the ureter and renal pelvis.

**Pyknosis (pyknotic):** Condensation and shrinkage of cells through degeneration.

**Pyoderma:** Any acute inflammatory skin disease of unknown origin. Bacteria may be cultured from the lesions, but there are normal resident flora.

**Pyogenic:** Producing pus (e.g., pyogenic infection).

**Pyroprotein:** A serum protein that precipitates upon exposure to hot temperatures.

**Raynaud's disease:** A peripheral vascular disorder characterized by abnormal vasoconstriction of the extremities upon exposure to cold or during emotional stress. A history of symptoms for at least two years is necessary for diagnosis.

**Recessive:** In genetics, incapable of expression unless carried by both members of a set of homologous chromosomes; not dominant.

**Recipient:** A patient who is receiving a transfusion of blood or a blood product.

**Red cell distribution width (RDW):** This measurement is included on some instrumentation as part of the complete blood count. It measures the distribution of red blood cell volume and is equivalent to anisocytosis on the peripheral smear. It is calculated as the coefficient of variation of the red cell volume and is expressed as a percentage (normal = $13.4 \pm 1.2$ percent).

**Refractory:** Not responsive to therapy.

**Reptilase:** An enzyme, thrombin-like in nature, derived from the venom of Bothrops atrox. Predominantly hydrolyzes fibrinopeptide A from the fibrinogen molecule, in contrast to thrombin, which hydrolyzes fibrinopeptides A and B.

    **R. time:** A coagulation procedure similar to the thrombin time except that clotting is initiated with the snake venom enzyme reptilase.

**Respiratory distress syndrome (RDS):** A condition, formerly known as hyaline membrane disease, accounting for more than 25,000 infant deaths per year in the United States. Clinical signs, including delayed onset of respiration and low Apgar score, are usually present at birth.

**Reticulocyte:** A red blood cell containing a network of granules or filaments representing an immature stage in development. Normally comprise about 1 percent of circulating red blood cells.

**Reticuloendothelial system:** Term applied to those cells scattered throughout the body that have the power to ingest particulate matter. Includes histiocytes of loose connective tissue; reticular cells of lymphatic organs; Kupffer's cells of the liver; cells lining blood sinuses of spleen, bone marrow, adrenal cortex, and hypophysis; and other cells.

**Retinopathy:** Any disorder of the retina.

**Rh immune globulin (RhIg):** A passive form of anti-D given within 72 hours of delivery to all Rh-negative mothers delivering an Rh-positive fetus.

**Ribonucleic acid (RNA):** A nucleic acid that controls protein synthesis in all living cells. There are three different types, and all are derived from the information encoded in the DNA of the cell. Messenger RNA (mRNA) carries the code for specific amino acid sequences from the DNA to the cytoplasm for protein synthesis. Transfer RNA (tRNA) carries the amino acid groups to the ribosome for protein synthesis. Ribosomal RNA (rRNA) exists within the ribosomes and is thought to assist in protein synthesis.

**Ribosome:** A cellular organelle that contains ribonucleoprotein and functions to synthesize protein. Ribosomes may be single units or clusters called polyribosomes or polysomes.

**Rickettsia:** Any of the microorganisms belonging to the genus Rickettsia.

**Ristocetin:** Drug used in platelet aggregation studies.

**Rouleau:** A group of red blood corpuscles arranged like a roll of coins, owing to an abnormal protein coating on the cell's surface; seen in multiple myeloma and Waldenström's macroglobulinemia.

**Rubriblast:** See Pronormoblast.

**Rubricyte:** See Polychromatophilic normoblast.

**Russell's viper venom (Stypven):** Snake venom with thromboplastic activity.

**Sarcoidosis:** A disease of unknown etiology characterized by widespread granulomatous lesions that may affect any organ or tissue of the body.

**Sarcoma:** Cancer arising from connective tissue such as muscle or bone. It may affect the bones, bladder, kidneys, liver, lungs, parotids, and spleen.

**Schistocyte:** An abnormal red cell that is formed when pieces of the red cell membrane become fragmented. Whole pieces of the red cell membrane appear to be missing, causing bizarre-looking red cells.

**Sclera:** A tough, white fibrous tissue that covers the so-called white of the eye. It extends from the optic nerve to the cornea.

**Scleroderma:** A chronic disease of unknown etiology that causes sclerosis of the skin and certain organs, including the gastrointestinal tract, lungs, heart, and kidneys. The skin feels tough and leathery, may itch, and later becomes hyperpigmented.

**Screening cells:** Group O reagent red cells that are used in antibody detection or screening tests.

**Scurvy:** A deficiency disease characterized by hemorrhagic manifestations and abnormal formation of bones and teeth.

**Senescence:** The aging process of the red cells.

**Sensitization:** A condition of being made sensitive to a specific substance (e.g., an antigen) after the initial exposure to that substance. This results in the development of immunologic memory that evokes an accentuated immune reponse with subsequent exposure to the substance.

**Sepsis:** Pathologic state, usually febrile, resulting from the presence of microorganisms or their poisonous products in the bloodstream.

**Septicemia:** Presence of bacteria in the blood. The microorganisms may multiply and cause overwhelming infection and death.

**Sequestration:** An increase in the quantity of blood within the blood vessels, occurring physiologically or produced artificially.

**Serine protease inhibitors:** The activity of the various enzymes (serine proteases) involved in the coagulation sequence is controlled to a variable extent primarily by plasma proteins generally known as inhibitors (e.g., antithrombin III).

**Serine proteases:** A family of proteolytic enzymes with the amino acid serine at the active site.

**Serositis:** Inflamed condition of a serous membrane.

**Serotonin:** A chemical present in platelets that is a potent vasoconstrictor.

**Serum:** The fluid that remains after plasma has clotted.

**Sex linkage:** A genetic characteristic located on the X or Y chromosome.

**Sézary syndrome:** Skin disease characterized by infiltration with atypical Sézary cells. The exfoliative dermatitis is considered a variant form of mycosis fungoides.

**Shock:** A clinical syndrome in which the peripheral blood flow is inadequate to return sufficient blood to the heart for normal function, particularly transport of oxygen to all organs and tissues.

**Sickle cell:** An abnormal red cell seen in patients who possess high quantities of hemoglobin S, an abnormal hemoglobin. The red cell is crescent- or sickle-shaped.

    **S. c. anemia:** Hereditary, chronic anemia in which abnormal sickle- or crescent-shaped erythrocytes are present. It is due to the presence of hemoglobin S in the red blood cells. The frequency of the gene that causes this disease is high in the African and Mediterranean populations.

**Sickle trait:** Blood that is heterozygous for the gene coding for the abnormal hemoglobin of sickle cell anemia.

**Sideroblast:** A ferritin-containing normoblast in the bone marrow. Comprises from 20 to 90 percent of normoblast in the marrow.

**Siderocyte:** A non-nucleated red blood cell containing iron in a form other than hematin, and confirmed by a specific iron stain such as the Prussian blue reaction.

**Siderosis:** A form of pneumoconiosis resulting from inhalation of dust or fumes containing iron particles.

**Sodium dodecyl sulfate (SDS):** An anionic detergent that renders a net negative charge to substances it solubilizes.

**Somatic:** Pertaining to nonreproductive cells or tissues.

**Specificity:** The affinity of an antibody and the antigen against which it is directed.

**Spectrin:** A large molecule found on the inner surface of red blood cell membrane, that is responsible for the bioconcave shape of the red cell as well as for its deformability.

**Spectrophotometer:** Device for measuring amount of color in a solution by comparison with the spectrum.

**Spherocyte:** An abnormal red blood cell shape. These are smaller than the normal red cell, have a concentrated hemoglobin content and have a decreased surface to volume ratio.

**Splenomegaly:** Enlargement of the spleen seen in several blood disorders.

**Sprue:** A disease endemic in many tropical regions and occurring sporadically in temperate countries, characterized by weakness, loss of weight, steatorrhea, and various digestive disorders.

**Spurious:** Not true or genuine; adulterated; false.

**Stab:** See Band.

**Staphylococcal clumping test:** A coagulation procedure used to detect the presence of fibrin-fibrinogen degradation products. The test uses a strain of staphylococcus that clumps in the presence of fibrinogen, fibrin monomers, or X and Y fragments.

**Steatorrhea:** Increased secretion of sebaceous glands; fatty stools.

**Stenosis:** Constriction or narrowing of a passage or orifice.

**Steroid hormones:** Hormones of the adrenal cortex and the sex hormones.

**Stertorous:** Pertaining to laborious breathing.

**Stomatocyte:** An abnormal red cell shape; this shape appears as having a slit-like area of central pallor.

**Strabismus:** Disorder of eye in which optic axes cannot be directed to same object. Strabismus can result from reduced visual activity, unequal ocular muscle tone, or an oculomotor nerve lesion.

**Streptokinase:** A product of beta hemolytic streptococci capable of liquefying fibrin.

**Stroma:** The red cell membrane that is left after hemolysis.

**Stuart-Prower factor:** Factor X; functions in the common pathway of coagulation.

**Stypven time test:** A coagulation procedure used to diagnose differentially a deficiency of factor VII from factor X.

**Supernatant:** Floating on surface, as oil on water.

**Supervention:** The development of an additional condition as a complication to an existing disease.

**Syncytial:** Of the nature of a syncytium, which is a group of cells in which the protoplasm of one cell is continuous with that of adjoining cells, such as the mesenchyme cells of the embryo.

**Systemic:** Pertaining to a whole body rather than to one of its parts.

**Systemic lupus erythematosus (SLE):** A disseminated autoimmune disease characterized by anemia, thrombocytopenia, increased IgG levels, and the presence of four IgG antibodies: antinuclear antibody, antinucleoprotein antibody, anti-DNA antibody, and antihistone antibody. Believed to be caused by "suppressor" T-cell dysfunction.

**Systolic pressure:** Maximum blood pressure that occurs at ventricular concentration. The upper value of a blood pressure reading.

**Tachycardia:** Abnormal rapidity of heart action, usually defined as a heart rate greater than 100 per minute.

**Tachypnea:** Abnormal rapidity of respiration.

**Target cell:** This abnormal red cell looks like a "bull's-eye," with hemoglobin concentrated in the center and on rim of the cell.

**Teardrop cell:** This abnormal red cell is seen with frequency in the myeloproliferative disorders, it is shaped like a tear. Synonym: Dacrocyte.

**Telangiectasia:** The presence of small, red focal lesions, usually in the skin or mucous membrane, caused by dilation of capillaries, arterioles, or venules.

**Template bleeding time:** The elapsed time a uniform incision made by a template and blade stops bleeding; a test of platelet function in vivo assuming a normal platelet count.

**Tertian malaria:** Malaria in which sporulation occurs every 48 hours. Symptoms are more common during the day; paroxysms divided into chill, fever, and sweating stages. Benign tertian malaria is caused by Plasmodium vivax, malignant tertian malaria by Plasmodium falciparum.

**Tetany:** A nervous affection characterized by intermittent spasms of the muscles of the extremities.

**Thalassemia:** A group of hereditary anemias produced by either a defective production rate of alpha or the beta hemoglobin polypeptide. This disorder is inherited in homozygous or heterozygous state.

> **T. major:** The homozygous form of deficient beta chain synthesis, which is very severe and presents itself during childhood. Prognosis varies; however, the younger the child when the disease appears, the more unfavorable the outcome.

**Thermal amplitude:** The range of temperature over which an antibody demonstrates serologic or in vitro activity or both.

**Thrombin:** An enzyme that converts fibrinogen to fibrin so that a soluble clot can be formed.

**Thrombin time:** A coagulation procedure that measures the time required for thrombin to convert fibrinogen to an insoluble fibrin clot.

**Thrombocytopathies:** Inherited disorders of platelets.

**Thrombocytopenia:** Decreased numbers of platelets.

**Thrombocytosis:** Increased numbers of platelets.

**Thromboembolism:** An embolism; the blocking of a blood vessel by a thrombus (blood clot) which has become detached from the site of formation.

**Thrombopoiesis:** The formation of platelets.

**Thrombosis:** The formation or development of a blood clot or thrombus.

**Thrombotic thrombocytopenic purpura (TTP):** A severe condition characterized by thrombocytopenia, microangiopathic hemolytic anemia, renal dysfunction, neurologic abnormalities, and fever.

**Thymidine:** An essential ingredient used in DNA synthesis and incorporated by T lymphocytes undergoing blast transformation in response to foreign HLA-D antigens in the mixed lymphocyte culture test.

**Thyromegaly:** Enlargement of the thyroid gland.

**Tinnitus:** Buzzing in the ears.

**Tissue plasminogen activator (TPA):** A clotting factor produced by vascular endothelial cells which selectively binds to fibrin as it activates fibrin-bound plasminogen.

**Tissue thromboplastin:** Factor III; functions in the extrinsic system of coagulation.

**Titer score:** A method used to evaluate more precisely than simple dilution by comparing the titers of an antibody. Agglutination at each higher dilution is graded on a continuous scale; the total is the titer score.

**Total iron-binding capacity (TIBC):** Transferrin is usually measured indirectly by the amount of iron that it can bind: this is referred to as the total iron-binding capacity (TIBC). TIBC = unsaturated iron-binding capacity (UIBC or amount of additional iron that transferrin can bind above that which is already complexed) + serum Fe. Normal = 250 to 360 $\mu$g/dl.

**Toxic granulation:** Medium- to large-sized metachromatic granules that are evenly distributed throughout the cytoplasm. May be seen in severe bacterial infections, severe burns, and other conditions.

**Trait:** A characteristic that is inherited.

**Transcription:** The process of RNA production from DNA, which requires the enzyme RNA polymerase.

**Transferase:** An enzyme that catalyzes the transfer of atoms or groups of atoms from one chemical compound to another.

**Transferrin:** A glycoprotein synthesized in the liver, with the primary function of iron transport.

**Transfuse:** The act of performing a transfusion.

**Transfusion:** The injection of blood, a blood component, saline, or other fluids into the bloodstream.

**T. reaction:** An adverse response to a transfusion.

**Translation:** The production of protein from the interactions of the RNAs.

**Translocation:** Transfer of a portion of one chromosome to its allele.

**Transplacental:** Through the placenta.

**Transposition:** The location of two genes on opposite chromosomes of a homologous pair.

**TRCHII:** Tanned red cell hemagglutination inhibition immunoassay; this test is the reference method for the assay of fibrinogen/degradation products.

**Ubiquitous:** Existing or being everywhere at the same time.

**Urokinase:** A trypsin-like protease, found in the urine and synthesized by the kidney, that activates plasminogen by proteolytic cleavage. Differs from tissue plasminogen activators in that urokinase reacts with plasminogen in the fluid phase of blood.

**Urticaria:** A vascular reaction of the skin similar to hives.

**Vaccine:** A suspension of infectious organisms or components of them that is given as a form of passive immunization to establish resistance to the infectious disease caused by that organism.

**Valvular:** Relating to or having a valve.

**Variable region:** That portion of the immunoglobulin light and heavy chains where amino acid sequences vary tremendously. These amino acid variations permit the different immunoglobulin molecules to recognize different antigenic determinants. In other words, the variable region determines the antigen against which the antibody will react, thus providing each antibody molecule with its unique specificity. The variable region is located at the amino terminal region of the molecule.

**Vascular:** Pertaining to or composed of blood vessels.

**Vasculitis:** Inflammation of a blood or lymph vessel.

**Vasoconstriction:** Constriction of blood vessels.

**Vasodilatation:** Dilatation of blood vessels, especially small arteries and arterioles.

**Vaso-occlusive:** Obstruction of the vasculature by some pathologic process that seriously impedes blood flow.

**Vasovagal syncope:** Syncope resulting from hypotension caused by emotional stress, pain, acute blood loss, fear, or rapidly rising from a recumbent position.

**Venipuncture:** Puncture of a vein for any purpose.

**Venom:** A poison excreted by some animals such as insects or snakes and transmitted by bites or stings.

**Venule:** A tiny vein continuous with a capillary.

**Verrucous:** Wart-like, with raised portions.

**Vertigo:** Dizziness.

**Vitamin K:** A fat-soluble vitamin required for maintenance of normal blood levels of the vitamin K–dependent factors: prothrombin, factors VII, IX, and X. Vitamin K is necessary for carboxylation of specific glutamic acid residues in the postprotein synthesis of the vitamin K–dependent factors.

**von Willebrand's disease (VWD):** A congenital bleeding disorder inherited as an autosomal dominant trait and characterized by a decreased level of factor VIII:C and a prolonged bleeding time.

**VWF (von Willebrand factor):** A component of the factor VIII molecule that mediates platelet interaction with subendothelium.

**WAIHA:** Warm autoimmune hemolytic anemia.

**Whole blood clotting time:** A test that evaluates the overall activity of the intrinsic system of coagulation.

**Xerocyte:** A dehydrated red blood cell having a peculiar morphologic appearance (i.e., hemoglobin concentration at one pole of the red cell).

**Zeta:** A type of globin chain found in embryonic hemoglobin.

# Index

A "T" following a page number indicates a table; an "F" following a page number indicates a figure.

**495**